CDC

HEALTH INFORMATION FOR INTERNATIONAL TRAVEL

THE YELLOW BOOK

2012

CDC

HEALTH INFORMATION FOR INTERNATIONAL TRAVEL

THE YELLOW BOOK
2012

Editor in Chief
Gary W. Brunette, MD, MS

Medical Editors
Phyllis E. Kozarsky, MD
Alan J. Magill, MD
David R. Shlim, MD

Managing Editor
Amanda D. Whatley, MPH

US DEPARTMENT OF HEALTH AND HUMAN SERVICES
Public Health Service
Centers for Disease Control and Prevention
National Center for Emerging and Zoonotic Infectious Diseases
Division of Global Migration and Quarantine
Atlanta, Georgia

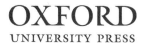

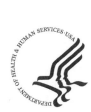

OXFORD
UNIVERSITY PRESS

Oxford University Press, Inc., publishes works that further
Oxford University's objective of excellence
in research, scholarship, and education.
Oxford   New York

Auckland Cape Town Dar es Salaam Hong Kong Karachi
Kuala Lumpur Madrid Melbourne Mexico City Nairobi
New Delhi Shanghai Taipei Toronto

With offices in
Argentina Austria Brazil Chile Czech Republic France Greece
Guatemala Hungary Italy Japan Poland Portugal Singapore
South Korea Switzerland Thailand Turkey Ukraine Vietnam

Published by Oxford University Press, Inc.
198 Madison Avenue, New York, New York 10016
www.oup.com

Oxford is a registered trademark of Oxford University Press

ISSN 0095-3539
ISBN 978-0-19-976901-8

1 2 3 4 5 6 7 8 9
Printed in the United States of America
on acid-free paper

Oxford University Press is proud to pay a portion of its sales for this book to the CDC Foundation. Chartered
by Congress, the CDC Foundation began operations in 1995 as an independent, nonprofit organization fos-
tering support for CDC through public-private partnerships. Further information about the CDC Foundation
can be found at www.cdcfoundation.org. The CDC Foundation did not prepare any portion of this book and
is not responsible for its contents.

All CDC material in this publication is in the public domain and may be used and reprinted without special permission; however, citation of the source is appreciated.

Suggested Citation

Centers for Disease Control and Prevention. CDC Health Information for International Travel 2012. New York: Oxford University Press; 2012.

Readers are invited to send comments and suggestions regarding this publication to Gary W. Brunette, Editor in Chief, Centers for Disease Control and Prevention, Division of Global Migration and Quarantine (E-03), Travelers' Health Branch (proposed), 1600 Clifton Road NE, Atlanta, GA 30333, USA.

Disclaimers

Both generic and trade names (without trademark symbols) are used in this text. In all cases, the decision to use one or the other was made based on recognition factors and was done for the convenience of the intended audience. Therefore, the use of trade names and commercial sources in this publication is for identification only and does not imply endorsement by the US Department of Health and Human Services, the Public Health Service, or CDC.

References to non-CDC Internet sites are provided as a service to readers and do not constitute or imply endorsement of these organizations or their programs by the US Department of Health and Human Services, the Public Health Service, or CDC. CDC is not responsible for the content of these sites. URL addresses were current as of the date of publication.

Notice

This material is not intended to be, and should not be considered, a substitute for medical or other professional advice. Treatment for the conditions described in this material is highly dependent on the individual circumstances. While this material is designed to offer accurate information with respect to the subject matter covered and to be current as of the time it was written, research and knowledge about medical and health issues are constantly evolving, and dose schedules for medications are being revised continually, with new side effects recognized and accounted for regularly. Readers must therefore always check the product information and clinical procedures with the most up-to-date published product information and data sheets provided by the manufacturers and the most recent codes of conduct and safety regulation. Oxford University Press and the authors make no representations or warranties to readers, express or implied, as to the accuracy or completeness of this material, including without limitation that they make no representations or warranties as to the accuracy or efficacy of the drug dosages mentioned in the material. The authors and the publishers do not accept, and expressly disclaim, any responsibility for any liability, loss, or risk that may be claimed or incurred as a consequence of the use and/or application of any of the contents of this material.

The Publisher is responsible for author selection and the Publisher and the Author(s) make all editorial decisions, including decisions regarding content. The Publisher and the Author(s) are not responsible for any product information added to this publication by companies purchasing copies of it for distribution to clinicians.

For additional copies, please contact Oxford University Press. Order online at www.oup.com/us.

Contents

1 INTRODUCTION 2

2 THE PRE-TRAVEL CONSULTATION 28

3 INFECTIOUS DISEASES RELATED TO TRAVEL 134

SELECT DESTINATIONS 398

9 HEALTH CONSIDERATIONS FOR NEWLY ARRIVED IMMIGRANTS & REFUGEES 574

APPENDICES 584

INDEX 601

List of Boxes, Figures, Maps, & Tables, by Topic

DISEASES AND CONDITIONS

Immune Compromised

Infants and Children

Medical Tourists

Military

Pregnant Travelers

Returning Travelers

Students

Travelers with Chronic Illnesses

Travelers Visiting Friends and Relatives

RESOURCES

VACCINES

General Vaccine Information

Hepatitis

Human Papillomavirus

Rabies

Tickborne Encephalitis

Typhoid

Yellow Fever

WATER TREATMENT

LIST OF MAPS

Disease Maps

Destination and Reference Maps

International Adoption

Editorial Staff

Editor in Chief: Gary W. Brunette
Medical Editors: Phyllis E. Kozarsky, Alan J. Magill, and David R. Shlim
Managing Editor: Amanda D. Whatley
Design and Production Editor: Kelly Holton
Editorial Advisor: C. Virginia Lee
Technical Writer-Editors: Ronnie Henry and Ava W. Navin
Editorial Assistant: Tricia A. Schwartz
Cartographer: Kevin Liske

CDC Contributors

Alexander, James P.
Allen, Jessica
Anderson, Alicia
Ansari, Armin
Arguin, Paul M.
Atkinson, William
Bair-Brake, Heather
Balaban, Victor
Ballesteros, Michael F.
Barskey IV, Albert E.
Barzilay, Ezra J.
Batts, Dahna
Bern, Caryn
Bhattarai, Achuyt
Blaney, David D.
Boore, Amy L.
Bowen, Anna
Brogdon, William G.
Brooks, John T.
Brown, Clive M.
Brunette, Gary W.
Buff, Ann M.
Cantor, Amanda
Chang, Loretta S.
Chiller, Tom M.
Cohn, Amanda
Czarkowski, Alan G.
Dasch, Gregory A.
Date, Kashmira
De, Barun K.
Dhara, V. Ramana
Dubray, Christine

Dunne, Eileen F.
Dykewicz, Clare A.
Eremeeva, Marina E.
Fagan, Ryan P.
Fiebelkorn, Amy Parker
Fischer, Marc
Fox, LeAnne M.
Gallagher, Kathleen M.
Gallagher, Nancy M.
Galland, G. Gale
Garrison, Laurel E.
Gee, Jay E.
Gershman, Mark
Gibney, Katherine B.
Gould, L. Hannah
Green, Michael D.
Griffith, Kevin S.
Griffin, Patricia M.
Guerra, Marta A.
Hall, Aron J.
Herwaldt, Barbara L.
Hicks, Lauri A.
Hills, Susan L.
Hlavsa, Michele C.
Holmberg, Scott
Illig, Petra A.
Jackson, Michael L.
Jentes, Emily S.
Johnson, Katherine J.
Jones, Jeffrey L.
Koumans, Emilia H.
Kozarsky, Phyllis E.

Kroger, Andrew
Kutty, Preeta K.
Lee, C. Virginia
LoBue, Philip
Lopman, Ben
Lynch, Michael
MacNeil, Adam
Mali, Sonja
Malilay, Josephine
Maloney, Susan A.
Marano, Nina
Marienau, Karen J.
Markowitz, Lauri E.
Marshall, Candace M.
Mathieu, Els
McCarron, Margaret
McLean, Huong Q.
McQuiston, Jennifer
Mead, Paul S.
Miller, Charles W.
Miller, Jeffrey R.
Mintz, Eric
Mitruka, Kiren
Montgomery, Susan
Moore, Anne
Moro, Pedro L.
Mullan, Robert J.
Nasci, Roger S.
Naughton, Mary P.
Navin, Ava W.
Nett, Randall J.
Novak, Ryan T.

Nuorti, J. Pekka
Ong, Kanyin L.
Ortega, Luis S.
Powers, Ann M.
Reef, Susan E.
Reynolds, Mary G.
Rollin, Pierre E.
Roy, Monika
Roy, Sharon L.
Rupprecht, Charles E.
Schilling, Katharine A.
Schwartz, Tricia A.
Shadomy, Sean V.
Sharapov, Umid M.
Shay, David K.
Shealy, Katherine

Skoff, Tami H.
Slaten, Douglas D.
Sleet, David A.
Smith, Jean Clare
Smith, Theresa L.
Sommers, Theresa E.
Staples, J. Erin
Steele, Stefanie F.
Stoddard, Robyn
Sutton, Madeline Y.
Tan, Kathrine R.
Teo, Chong-Gee
Teshale, Eyasu H.
Thomas, Cynthia G.
Tiwari, Tejpratap S. P.
Tomashek, Kay M.

Uzicanin, Amra
Viray, Melissa
Wallace, Gregory S.
Warnock III, Eli W.
Wassilak, Steven G. F.
Waterman, Stephen H.
Watson, John C.
Weinberg, Michelle
Weinberg, Nicholas
Whatley, Amanda D.
Wilson, Todd W.
Wirtz, Robert A.
Workowski, Kimberly
Yanni, Emad A.
Zielinski-Gutierrez, Emily

External Contributors

Acosta, Rebecca W. — Traveler's Medical Service of New York, New York, NY

Ahmed, Qanta — State University of New York, Stony Brook, NY; Glasgow Caledonian University School of Public Health, Scotland, UK; and Templeton-Cambridge Journalism Fellow, England, UK

Ansdell, Vernon E. — University of Hawaii, Honolulu, HI

Backer, Howard D. — California Health and Human Services Agency, Sacramento, CA

Barbeau, Deborah Nicolls — Tulane University, New Orleans, LA

Barnett, Elizabeth D. — Boston University School of Medicine and Boston Medical Center, Boston, MA

Borwein, Sarah T. — TravelSafe Medical Centre, Hong Kong, China

Brownstein, John S. — Children's Hospital Boston and Harvard Medical School, Boston, MA

Carroll, I. Dale — The Pregnant Traveler, Spring Lake, MI

Cersovsky, Steven B. — US Army Public Health Command, Aberdeen Proving Ground, MD

Chavez, Gilberto F. — Center for Infectious Disease, California Department of Public Health, Sacramento, CA

Connor, Bradley A. — Weill Medical College of Cornell University, New York, NY

DeFraites, Robert F. — Armed Forces Health Surveillance Center, Silver Spring, MD

Ebner, Jodi — Center for Global Education, University of California, Los Angeles, CA

Franco-Paredes, Carlos — Emory University, Atlanta, GA, and Hospital Infantil de México, Federico Gómez, México DF, México

Freedman, David O. — University of Alabama at Birmingham, Birmingham, AL

Freifeld, Clark C. — Children's Hospital Informatics Program at the Harvard–MIT Division of Health Sciences and Technology, Boston, MA

Gushulak, Brian D. — Migration Health Consultants, Cheltenham, Canada

Hackett, Peter H. — Institute for Altitude Medicine, Telluride, CO, and Altitude Research Center, University of Colorado, Denver, CO

Harriman, Kathleen H. — California Department of Public Health, Richmond, CA

Hidron, Alicia I. — Emory University and Atlanta Veteran's Affairs Medical Center, Atlanta, GA

Hochberg, Natasha — Boston University School of Public Health, Boston, MA

Howard, Cynthia R. — University of Minnesota, Minneapolis, MN

John, Chandy C.	University of Minnesota, Minneapolis, MN
Jong, Elaine C.	University of Washington School of Medicine, Seattle, WA
Kain, Kevin C.	University of Toronto, Toronto, Canada
Keystone, Jay S.	University of Toronto, Toronto, Canada
LaRocque, Regina C.	Massachusetts General Hospital and Harvard University, Boston, MA
Mackell, Sheila M.	Mountain View Pediatrics, Flagstaff, AZ
Magill, Alan J.	Walter Reed Army Institute of Research, Silver Spring, MD
McCarthy, Anne E.	Ottawa Hospital and University of Ottawa, Ottawa Canada
Neumann, Karl	Weill Medical College of Cornell University and New York Presbyterian Hospital/Cornell Medical Center, New York, NY
Nord, Daniel A.	Divers Alert Network, Durham, NC
Offit, Paul	The Children's Hospital of Philadelphia, Philadelphia, PA
Ostroff, Stephen M.	Pennsylvania Department of Health, Harrisburg, PA
Rhodes, Gary	Center for Global Education, University of California, Los Angeles, CA
Ryan, Edward T.	Massachusetts General Hospital and Harvard University, Boston, MA
Schantz, Peter M.	Rollins School of Public Health, Emory University, Atlanta, GA
Shlim, David R.	Jackson Hole Travel and Tropical Medicine, Jackson Hole, WY
Sonricker, Amy L.	Children's Hospital Informatics Program at the Harvard–MIT Division of Health Sciences and Technology, Boston, MA
Stauffer, William M.	University of Minnesota, Minneapolis, MN, and CDC, Atlanta, GA
Walker, Patricia F.	University of Minnesota, Minneapolis, MN, and HealthPartners, Center for International Health and Travel Medicine Clinics, St. Paul, MN
Wilson, Mary Elizabeth	Harvard School of Public Health, Boston, MA

All contributors have signed a statement indicating that they have no conflicts of interest with the subject matter or materials discussed in the document(s) that they have written or reviewed for this book and that the information that they have written or reviewed for this book is objective and free from bias.

Acknowledgments

The *CDC Health Information for International Travel 2012* editorial team gratefully acknowledges all the authors and reviewers for their commitment to this new edition. We extend sincere thanks to the following people for their contributions to the production of this book:

- Elise Beltrami, Clive Brown, Mark Gershman, Emily Jentes, Katherine Johnson, and Theresa Sommers for their extensive review of the text.
- Erin Carner, Samantha Dolan, Stefanie Erskine, Candace Marshall, Crystal Polite, Rhett Stoney, and Cathy Young for their assistance in preparing the text for publication.

Preface

To stay on the cutting edge of travel health information, this latest edition of *CDC Health Information for International Travel* has been extensively revised. The book serves as a guide to the practice of travel medicine, as well as the authoritative source of US government recommendations for immunizations and prophylaxis for foreign travel. As international travel continues to become more common in the lives of US residents, having at least a basic understanding of the medical problems that travelers face has become a necessary aspect of practicing medicine. The goal of this book is to be a comprehensive resource for clinicians to find the answers to their travel health–related questions.

CENTERS FOR DISEASE CONTROL AND PREVENTION
Thomas R. Frieden, MD, MPH, Director

NATIONAL CENTER FOR EMERGING AND ZOONOTIC INFECTIOUS DISEASES
Beth P. Bell, MD, MPH, Director

DIVISION OF GLOBAL MIGRATION AND QUARANTINE
Martin S. Cetron, MD, Director
Gary W. Brunette, MD, MS, Chief, Travelers' Health Branch *(proposed)*
Phyllis E. Kozarsky, MD, Expert Consultant, Travelers' Health Branch *(proposed)*
Amanda D. Whatley, MPH, CHES, Health Communications Specialist, Travelers' Health Branch *(proposed)*

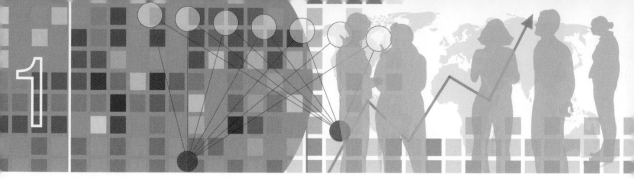

Introduction

INTRODUCTION TO TRAVEL HEALTH & THE YELLOW BOOK

Amanda D. Whatley, Phyllis E. Kozarsky

TRAVEL HEALTH

Rates of international travel have continued to grow substantially in the past decade. According to the World Tourism Organization, there were an estimated 880 million international tourist arrivals in 2009 throughout the world. In 2009, US residents made more than 61 million trips with at least one night outside the United States, an approximate 5% increase since 1999. Not only are more people traveling, but also they are seeking out areas that have rarely been visited in the past. The reasons for travel are also varied, including tourism, business, study abroad, research, visiting friends and relatives, ecotourism, adventure, medical tourism, mission work, or responding to an international disaster. Travelers range in age from very young infants to centenarians. Their health conditions are also diverse, including those who have preexisting medical conditions, are immunosuppressed, or are pregnant. The infectious disease risks that travelers face are dynamic—some travel destinations have become safer, while in other areas, new diseases have emerged and other diseases have reemerged.

The risk of becoming ill or injured during international travel depends on many factors, such as the region of the world visited, a traveler's age and health status, the length of the trip, and the diversity of planned activities. The Centers for Disease Control and Prevention (CDC) provides international travel health information to address the range of health risks a traveler may face, with the aim of assisting travelers and clinicians to better understand the measures necessary to prevent illness and injury during international travel. This publication and the CDC Travelers' Health website (www.cdc.gov/travel) are the two primary avenues of communicating CDC's travel health recommendations.

HISTORY AND ROLES OF THE YELLOW BOOK AND THE INTERNATIONAL HEALTH REGULATIONS

CDC Health Information for International Travel ("The Yellow Book") has been a trusted resource since 1967. Originally, it was a small pamphlet published to satisfy the International Sanitary Regulations' requirements and the International Health Regulations (IHR), adopted by the World Health Organization (WHO) in 1951 and 1969, respectively. The purpose of the IHR is to ensure maximum security against the international spread of diseases, with minimum interference with world travel and commerce. A copy of the current IHR and supporting information can be found on the WHO website (www.who.int/csr/ihr/en).

The IHR (1969) were originally intended to help monitor and control 6 serious infectious diseases: cholera, plague, relapsing fever, smallpox, typhus, and yellow fever. Since then, the IHR have been amended several times, and were completely revised in 2005. Under the IHR (2005), states are required to notify WHO immediately in the event of identifying smallpox, severe acute respiratory syndrome (SARS), wild poliovirus, or novel influenza within their borders. Additionally, states are required to report to WHO any other event that signifies a public health emergency of international concern (PHEIC). A PHEIC is an event that constitutes a public health risk to other member states, with international consequences such as the spread of disease, and that potentially requires a coordinated international response, as in the case of 2009 pandemic influenza A (H1N1). This definition broadens the scope of the IHR to cover existing, new, and reemerging diseases, including emergencies caused by chemical, biological, or radiologic agents and the context surrounding these events. As a member state of WHO and signatory to the IHR (2005), the United States is responsible for following these reporting requirements.

In addition to reporting health events, the United States must also inform the public about health requirements for entering other countries, such as the necessity of being vaccinated against yellow fever. Some countries require all travelers to have an International Certificate of Vaccination or Prophylaxis (ICVP) documenting yellow fever vaccine administration as a condition for entry, while other countries require vaccination against yellow fever only if travelers arrive from a country where the yellow fever virus is known to circulate. The Yellow Book and the CDC Travelers' Health website aim to communicate these requirements under the IHR (2005). Although this publication includes the most current available information, requirements can change. Current information must be accessed to ensure that these requirements are met; the CDC Travelers' Health website (www.cdc.gov/travel) may be checked for regularly updated information.

The Yellow Book is written primarily for clinicians, including physicians, nurses, and pharmacists. Others, such as the travel industry, multinational corporations, missionary and volunteer organizations, and travelers themselves, can also find a wealth of information here.

This text is authored by subject-matter experts from within CDC and outside the agency. The guidelines presented in this book are evidence-based and supported by best practices. Internal text citations have not been included; however, a bibliography is included at the end of each section for those who would like to obtain more detailed information. In addition to the hardcopy text, a searchable online version of the Yellow Book can be found on the CDC Travelers' Health website (www.cdc.gov/yellowbook).

NEW IN THE 2012 EDITION

The Yellow Book reflects the ever-changing nature of travel medicine. Each new edition notes the changes in global disease distribution, vaccine and medication guidelines, and new developments in preventing travel health risks. The CDC Travelers' Health program and the CDC Foundation are pleased to partner with Oxford University Press, Inc., for the first time to publish the 2012 edition. Finally, the editorial team is always looking for ways to adapt the publication to meet the needs of its readers.

Chapter Notes

A few chapters contain important changes in the 2012 edition and are highlighted below. Some new sections in this edition include Special Considerations for US Military Deployments, Study Abroad, and Travel to Mass Gatherings.

Topics most commonly discussed in a pre-travel consultation, with the exception of infectious diseases, are found in Chapter 2. Just as in most pre-travel consultations, general issues concerning vaccine recommendations are discussed first, then self-treatable disease topics, and finally topics generally discussed when counseling travelers about healthy behaviors that may decrease risk of illness and injury. Chapter 3 now contains all infectious diseases, including vaccine-preventable diseases, in alphabetical order.

Country-specific yellow fever requirements and recommendations, and malaria transmission information and prophylaxis recommendations, have been combined into one section and are located at the end of Chapter 3.

Chapter 4, Select Destinations, highlights some popular tourist destinations and routes discussed by authors who have lived in or visited these areas. Some of these destinations have been updated from the 2010 edition, and some are new. The purpose of this chapter is to better orient travel health providers who may not have had the opportunity to travel to these destinations, frequented by many travelers, and from which many questions are generated. Similar to a guidebook, authors discuss the destination, along with the reality of various health risks, to aid clinicians in preparing travelers. These sections are editorial in nature, containing the author's expressed opinions, and aim to present topics for consideration; they should not necessarily be taken as a prescription for pre-travel care.

Perspectives Editorial Sections

A continuing feature from the previous edition is the incorporation of editorial sections entitled Perspectives. These sections are noted by their distinctive icon and a box around the text. Although there is an increasing body of evidence-based knowledge in this new and growing field of travel medicine, there is also recognition that the practice of this specialty is not only science, but art as well. Thus, readers will notice a few sections that contain editorial discussions aiming to add depth and clinical perspective, as well as to discuss some controversies or differences in opinions and practice.

CONTACT INFORMATION FOR CDC

Questions, comments, and suggestions for CDC Travelers' Health, including comments about this publication, may be made through the CDC-INFO contact center (toll-free at 800-CDC-INFO or cdcinfo@cdc.gov). Since CDC is not a medical facility, clinicians needing assistance with patients who are preparing for travel should consider referral to a travel clinic or a clinic listed on the International Society of Travel Medicine website (www.istm.org).

Clinicians with patient questions about post-travel health issues may consider referral to a clinic listed on the American Society of Tropical Medicine and Hygiene website (www.astmh.org) or to a medical university with infectious diseases capacity. Because of the clinical complexity of malaria, the CDC Malaria Branch offers clinicians assistance with the diagnosis or management of suspected cases of malaria. Clinicians can contact CDC's Malaria Branch telephone hotline at 770-488-7788 during business hours. After hours and on weekends and holidays, a Malaria Branch clinician may be reached by calling 770-488-7100.

BIBLIOGRAPHY

1. United Nations World Tourism Organization. UNWTO World Tourism Barometer. Madrid: United Nations World Tourism Organization; 2010 [cited 2010 Aug 2]. Available from: http://www.world-tourism.org/facts/wtb.html.
2. US Department of Commerce. 2009 United States Resident Travel Abroad. Washington, DC: US Department of Commerce; 2010 [cited 2010 Nov 8]. Available from: http://tinet.ita.doc.gov/outreachpages/download_data_table/2009_US_Travel_Abroad.pdf.
3. World Health Organization. International Health Regulations (2005). 2nd ed. Geneva: World Health Organization; 2008 [cited 2010 Nov 8]. Available from: http://www.who.int/ihr/9789241596664/en/index.html.

PLANNING FOR HEALTHY TRAVEL: RESPONSIBILITIES & RESOURCES

Amanda D. Whatley, Phyllis E. Kozarsky, Gary W. Brunette

International travel encompasses a wide array of activities, including business travel, sightseeing, adventure travel, international adoption, and visiting friends and relatives. The process of planning these trips involves a relationship between the traveler, the clinicians, and the travel and tourism industry. This section outlines how these groups can work together so that travel may be safer, healthier, and more enjoyable.

RESPONSIBILITIES OF THE TRAVELER

Although studies have shown that most travelers from the United States and other countries do not seek pre-travel health advice, travelers need to understand the health risks that traveling internationally may pose and be actively involved in preparing for healthy travel.

Gathering Destination Information

Travelers should find out as many details as possible about their travel destinations, modes of travel, lodging, food, and activities during their trip. These details help the travel health provider tailor his or her advice in regard to immunizations, prophylaxis, and other health advice. Travelers can visit the CDC Travelers' Health website (www.cdc.gov/travel) for the latest health information for international destinations, which includes disease outbreaks, natural disasters, and other events with health-related concerns.

Seeking and Following Pre-Travel Health Advice

Obtaining pre-travel health care and advice from a clinician familiar with travel is an important step in preparing to travel internationally. Ideally, this visit should take place 4–6 weeks before travel, but even getting a consultation in the week before travel can be of value. The pre-travel visit includes a discussion of immunizations, prophylactic medications (such as antimalaria drugs), and specific health advice for preventing and treating travelers' diarrhea and other illnesses the traveler may encounter. Travelers who have chronic health issues or who take medications may also need to coordinate their pre-travel care with their regular doctors. CDC recommends that travelers prepare and carry a travel health kit (see Chapter 2, Travel Health Kits).

Avoiding Travel When Sick

Recently, more emphasis has been placed on advising people to avoid traveling while they are sick, if they may have a communicable disease that can be transmitted to other people. Postponing or canceling a trip can be inconvenient and may incur additional expenses, but these costs may be small compared with the public health costs of a disease outbreak, which may include a search for airline travelers who might have been exposed to the traveler's disease.

RESPONSIBILITIES OF THE CLINICIAN

Regardless of their specialty, most clinicians will encounter a traveling patient at some point in their practice. Clinicians, especially those in primary care, should know basic travel health information to determine the extent of health advice their patients should access before traveling, and be able to recognize common post-travel health symptoms and syndromes.

Incorporating Pre-Travel Care into One's Practice

At a minimum, clinicians can easily incorporate the topic of travel medicine into their practice by routinely asking patients if they are planning to travel internationally, particularly to a developing country. By doing so, clinicians can begin to raise awareness and emphasize the importance of a pre-travel consultation, and the fact that international travel can pose special health risks. Inquiring in advance also allows time for the patient to receive comprehensive pre-travel care, either at the current visit or by scheduling a pre-travel consult before the planned trip. Additionally, patients who have more complex medical histories, or who need to see a specialist in travel medicine, would have time to adequately address any special needs. Clinicians should be particularly aware of people who were born in or may be visiting friends or relatives in developing countries. For more information on this population, refer to Chapter 8, Immigrants Returning Home to Visit Friends and Relatives (VFRs).

Before evaluating a traveler for a pre-travel consultation, the clinician should determine what level of information he or she is comfortable giving to the patient. Some clinicians may base their comfort level on aspects of trips, such as location, length, and type, on the complexity of the patient's medical history, or both. Common categories of service include the following:

- Referring all travelers to a travel clinic or a travel medicine specialist.
- Offering only basic pre-travel advice and common vaccinations for less complex situations, such as advising travelers who are going on a short vacation to a popular tourist destination such as Mexico or the Caribbean.
- Providing complex pre-travel consultations and making a commitment to the practice of travel medicine.

Even if clinicians have decided to offer only pre-travel care for less complex situations and itineraries, they should take the time to give a comprehensive pre-travel consultation, incorporating vaccines, medications, and behavioral preventive recommendations. For more information, see Chapter 2, The Pre-Travel Consultation.

Clinicians who wish to provide pre-travel care in more complex consultations can extend their knowledge and expertise in several ways:

- Refer to Appendix A for additional information about the practice of travel medicine, professional resources, and certifications offered through professional organizations.
- As travel medicine is dynamic, clinicians who regularly advise travelers in pre-travel consultations need to maintain a current base of knowledge. Many different Internet resources and databases, although sometimes incomplete or in conflict with one another, are available for clinicians to use to keep abreast of the health issues in international travel (see Appendix B).
- In addition to general pre-travel consultations, some clinicians may also wish to become registered yellow fever vaccine providers. This process is initiated with one's state health department.

Incorporating Post-Travel Care into One's Practice

Recognizing common travel-related disease symptoms and syndromes is important in the primary care and emergency care settings, as these settings are usually where an ill returned traveler will initially seek medical care. When assessing a patient for a possible infectious disease, it is of paramount importance to remember to obtain a travel history. Patients with influenzalike symptoms may not remember to volunteer the fact that they have recently traveled to Africa, for example, and could have malaria, which is potentially life-threatening. Further information about post-travel medical care can be found in Chapter 5.

Additionally, clinicians should have a plan as to when they will refer a patient to a specialist and who that specialist would be, before the patient comes into the office seeking medical care. Patients needing more extensive post-travel care can be referred to a clinician in infectious diseases or clinical tropical medicine. The American Society of Tropical Medicine and Hygiene provides a listing of such clinicians on its website (www. astmh.org).

RESPONSIBILITIES OF THE TRAVEL AND TOURISM INDUSTRY

Customers often look to their travel agents to advise them on all aspects of their trip, including health risks and preventive actions they should take. Although the role of travel and tourism industry professionals is not to provide personal medical consultations, mentioning that health risks exist and referring travelers to a clinic or to the International Society of Travel Medicine website are appropriate actions. In many cases, this may be the best opportunity to help someone who was not aware that pre-travel medical advice was important. The CDC Travelers' Health website can be consulted to give a general idea of the health risks the client may encounter on a given trip (www.cdc.gov/travel).

CDC RESOURCES FOR TRAVEL HEALTH ADVICE
Travelers' Health Website
Destination Pages

CDC's Travelers' Health website features destination-specific pages with information on current CDC assessments of disease risk and recommendations for healthy travel (wwwnc.cdc.gov/travel/destinations/list.aspx).

Travel Notices

The travel notice section of the website (wwwnc.cdc.gov/travel/notices.aspx) contains the latest information about international outbreaks or other health-related issues, including recommendations for travelers.

CDC's Travel Notices are presented in 4 levels: In the News, Outbreak, Travel Health Precaution, and Travel Health Warning (Table 1–1). Most notices posted on the website are in the first 2 categories. CDC rarely issues a travel health precaution or a travel health warning.

Occasionally, travel notices may feature changes to existing recommendations, such as adding antimalarial prophylaxis for an area previously thought to be malaria free. If the outbreak resolves, the recommendation may be withdrawn. If the new recommendation becomes permanent, it is incorporated at that time into the text of the online version of *CDC Health Information for International Travel,* and added to a running list of updates to the hardcopy edition at www.cdc.gov/yellowbook. Any related recommendation changes for specific destinations are also incorporated into the relevant destination pages.

Considerations for Instituting Travel Notices

The purpose of CDC Travel Notices is to inform travel health providers and travelers about situations occurring internationally that may present a health risk to US residents traveling internationally, and to provide recommendations for protecting the health of these travelers. These notices are not meant to catalog all disease outbreaks or health-related disasters. When deciding whether to post a travel notice and at what notice level, CDC considers several factors outlined below, in consultation with relevant subject-matter experts. These factors are used to guide the decision-making process, but do not limit the process from incorporating other factors necessary in making the best possible public health decision during an event.

Disease transmission: For specific disease outbreaks, the modes of transmission and patterns of spread, as well as the magnitude and scope of the outbreak in the area, affect the decision for the appropriate level of notice. Criteria include the presence or absence of transmission outside defined settings, as well as evidence that cases have spread to other areas.

Containment measures: The presence or absence of acceptable disease outbreak control measures in the affected area can influence decisions about travel notices, including the level of the notice. Outbreak-affected areas with poor or no containment measures in place may have the potential for a higher risk of transmission to exposed people and spread to other areas.

Quality of surveillance: Considerations include whether health authorities in the outbreak-affected area have the ability to accurately detect and report cases, and conduct contact tracing of exposed people. Areas where a disease is occurring that have poor surveillance systems may have higher risk of transmission than is apparent from local reporting.

Quality and accessibility of medical care: Affected areas with inadequate medical services and infection control procedures in place, as well as remote locations without access to medical evacuation, present a higher level of risk for the US traveler or resident living abroad.

Aftermath of a natural or nonnatural disaster: In the aftermath of a disaster, an assessment of the potential for illness and injury would be used to determine if a travel notice is warranted and at what level. Certain diseases may result due to circumstances such as flooding, congregation of displaced people into small areas, and the destruction of or limitation of food, water, and medical supplies. Resulting disease situations would

Table 1-1. CDC travel notice definitions[1]

TYPE OF NOTICE	SCOPE[2]	RISK FOR TRAVELERS[3]	PREVENTIVE MEASURES	EXAMPLE OF NOTICE	EXAMPLE OF RECOMMENDED MEASURES
In the News	Reports of an isolated event, sporadic cases, or the occurrence of a disease of public health significance affecting a traveler or travel destination	No increased risk over baseline for travelers observing standard recommendations	Keeping travelers informed and reinforcing standard prevention recommendations	Report of increased cases of meningococcal meningitis in several sub-Saharan African countries in 2009	Reinforced standard recommendations for vaccination to the meningitis belt during the dry season (December–June)
Outbreak	Event in a limited geographic area or setting	Increased risk but definable and limited to specific settings	Reminders about standard and enhanced recommendations for the area, such as vaccination	Outbreak of yellow fever in 2 states in Brazil outside the reported yellow fever risk areas in 2008–2009	Reinforced yellow fever vaccine recommendations for known yellow fever risk areas in Brazil and extended recommendations for areas of the outbreak
Travel Health Precaution	Event of greater scope, affecting a larger geographic area	Increased risk in some settings or among travelers with specific risk factors, along with risk for spread to other areas	Specific precautions to reduce travelers' risk during the stay and what to do before, during, and after travel,[4] including what to do if ill; CDC may recommend that	Outbreak of avian influenza among poultry and humans in several countries in Southeast Asia in early 2004	Recommended specific precautions, including avoiding areas with live poultry, such as live animal markets and poultry farms; ensuring poultry and eggs are thoroughly cooked; monitoring health

Travel Health Warning[5]	Event with extremely serious health implications or evidence that a disease outbreak is expanding outside the area or populations initially affected	Increased risk because of evidence of transmission outside defined settings or inadequate containment measures	travelers in groups with high risks for complications consider delaying or canceling travel to certain areas	In addition to the specific precautions cited above, CDC recommends travelers postpone nonessential travel[4]	Haiti earthquake in 2010, H1N1 influenza A in 2009, and severe acute respiratory syndrome (SARS) outbreak in Asia in 2003	Recommended travelers avoid nonessential travel to affected areas because of level of risk

[1] The term "event" in the table is used for disease outbreaks and natural and nonnatural disasters with resulting health risks.

[2] The term "scope" incorporates the size, magnitude, and rapidity of spread of an event.

[3] Risk for travelers is dependent on several factors, including patterns of disease transmission, as well as severity of illness.

[4] Preventive measures other than the standard advice for the region may be recommended, depending on the circumstances (for example, travelers may be advised to monitor their health for a certain period after their return, or arriving passengers may be screened at ports of entry).

[5] The purpose of a travel health warning is to describe the situation and to reduce the volume of traffic to affected areas. For disease outbreaks, reducing the volume of travel aids in limiting the risk of spreading the disease to unaffected areas. For those who cannot avoid traveling to the affected area, the travel warning gives information about preventive measures to reduce travelers' risk for illness or injury, and what they should do if they become ill or injured. Additional preventive measures may be recommended, depending on the circumstances (for example, travelers may be requested to monitor their health for a certain period after their return; arriving and returning passengers may be screened at airports of entry).

be assessed by using the categories above, as any disease outbreak would be assessed. Additionally, environmental risks, or risks related to injuries and safety, would be considered in disaster situations.

Considerations for Downgrading or Removing Notices

Factors used in considering the institution of a travel notice are also used in considering its removal or revision. As situations resolve, international health authorities may officially declare a formal end to a disease outbreak. However, in most instances, there is no formal end or resolution. In these cases, CDC must consider whether the disease outbreak has ceased or waned to levels that existed before the notice was posted. In disaster situations, a similar assessment would take place regarding the environmental risks to travelers' health. "In the News Notices" and "Outbreak Notices" are reassessed at regular intervals, and are removed when they are no longer relevant or when the outbreak has resolved.

Since each disease is unique in characteristics such as incubation periods and transmission methods, the decision-making process for removing or downgrading notices is not an exact algorithm. For example, to downgrade a travel health warning to a travel health precaution, CDC would consider information such as the severity of the disease or event, surveillance data from the area, the extent of ongoing transmission, the public health response, and exported cases. In some situations, cases of the disease may cease, as happened during the SARS outbreak. However, in other situations, a travel health warning may no longer be needed because the disease has become endemic in affected areas, such as in the situation of 2009 pandemic influenza A (H1N1).

Malaria Website

CDC's Malaria website contains informational tools, educational materials, and cautionary tales of people who acquired malaria during or after travel without adequate prophylactic measures (www.cdc.gov/malaria/travelers/index.html). The CDC Malaria Map Application is an interactive map that provides location-specific information on current CDC assessments of malaria transmission, and recommendations for preventive malaria treatment (www.cdc.gov/malaria/map). Assessments are based largely on national surveillance reports; thus, the presence of malaria in most countries is displayed only at the national and provincial level.

BIBLIOGRAPHY

1. Hamer DH, Connor BA. Travel health knowledge, attitudes and practices among United States travelers. J Travel Med. 2004 Jan–Feb;11(1):23–6.
2. Keystone JS, Kozarsky PE, Freedman DO. Internet and computer-based resources for travel medicine practitioners. Clin Infect Dis. 2001 Mar 1;32(5):757–65.
3. Kozarsky PE, Keystone JS. Body of knowledge for the practice of travel medicine. J Travel Med. 2002 Mar–Apr;9(2):112–115.
4. MacDougall LA, Gyorkos TW, Leffondre K, Abrahamowicz M, Tessier D, Ward BJ, et al. Increasing referral of at-risk travelers to travel health clinics: evaluation of a health promotion intervention targeted to travel agents. J Travel Med. 2001 Sep–Oct;8(5):232–42.
5. Wolfe M, Wolfe Acosta R. Structure and organization of the pre-travel consultation and general advice for travelers. In: Keystone JS, Kozarsky PE, Freedman DO, Nothdurft HD, Connor BA, editors. Travel Medicine. 2nd ed. Philadelphia: Mosby; 2008. p. 35–45.

TRAVEL EPIDEMIOLOGY

David O. Freedman

To prescribe optimal pre-travel advice, preventive measures, and education, travel health providers must be aware of the absolute and relative magnitude of the many travel-related health risks. Such knowledge allows travel health care providers to perform an epidemiologic and traveler-specific risk assessment so that these measures can be appropriately prioritized for each traveler. Travel-related health problems are self-reported by 22%–64% of travelers to the developing world; most of these problems are mild, self-limited illnesses such as diarrhea, respiratory infections, and skin disorders. Approximately 8% of the more than 50 million travelers to developing regions, or 4 million people, are ill enough to seek health care, either while abroad or upon returning home.

LIMITATIONS OF CURRENT EPIDEMIOLOGIC KNOWLEDGE

Knowledge of the precise risk for a specific disease in a specific location has proved elusive, despite several decades of interest and investigation. (For additional discussion, see the Perspectives: Risks Travelers Face section later in this chapter.) A reasonably exact estimate of the number of cases of a disease or infection in all travelers over a time period at a location is difficult to determine, as many will have returned to their home countries by the time the disease manifests symptoms. Similarly difficult to obtain is an exact denominator reflecting the total number of travelers to that location. An accurate numerator must be divided by an accurate denominator to calculate a true incidence rate or risk. Even this standard population-based approach assumes that past experience predicts future risk. In addition, disease risks are not stable over time, and current or real-time data are rarely available. Much of the frequently quoted numerical data regarding the incidence of infection in travelers are based on extrapolations of limited data, collected in limited samples of travelers anywhere from a few to more than 20 years ago. This knowledge base includes morbidity studies of various methodologic designs, each with its own set of strengths and weaknesses. These studies have mostly examined a few key individual diseases in all travelers regardless of destination, profiles of disease occurrence at a few specific high-risk destinations, and disease occurrence in certain types of travelers with certain behaviors. Many have been single-clinic or single-destination studies that can lead to conclusions that are not generalizable to groups of travelers with different local, national, or cultural backgrounds.

INCIDENCE RATES AND ESTIMATES OF RISK

A compilation of best available incidence rate estimates, given the above limitations, is available and is frequently updated (Figure 1-1). With the notable exception of malaria, the major preventable travel-related diseases are associated with relatively low risks, ranging from 1 in 100 for influenza to less than 1 in 100,000 for several diseases that often concern travelers. Hepatitis A may be taken as an example of a prototypical vaccine-preventable disease, with an estimated overall uncorrected incidence of approximately 1 in 5,000 travelers to the developing world. Thus, the odds against acquiring hepatitis A on a single short trip are greatly in the traveler's favor, as many travelers realize. Any considered vaccination should be presented in context as insurance against a relatively uncommon event, but one that may result in significant illness or consequences.

For diseases with poor or fatal outcomes, such as meningococcal meningitis, rabies, or Japanese encephalitis, the context of less tolerance of even small risks needs to be communicated to travelers to help them make informed decisions about all available interventions. The incidence rates in Figure 1-1 reflect aggregate data and studies, and do not consider variations in risk behaviors, destination, season, duration of travel, or general style of travel. For many diseases, research

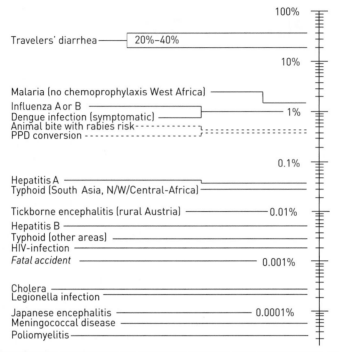

FIGURE 1-1. ESTIMATED INCIDENCE RATE PER MONTH OF INFECTIONS AND FATAL ACCIDENTS AMONG TRAVELERS IN DEVELOPING COUNTRIES, 2010[1]

[1] Unpublished; used with permission of Robert Steffen, Zurich, Switzerland.

into increased or decreased risk according to these variables is still in its infancy because of difficulties in tracking outcomes at remote destinations.

SURVEILLANCE NETWORKS AND TRACKING OF DISEASE PROFILES

A more recent and novel approach to defining disease epidemiology in travelers has involved the use of collaborative networks of specialized travel medicine clinics to collect and aggregate data on large samples of ill travelers who have been exposed in many countries, and who are seen during and after their return home. One such network, GeoSentinel, a collaborative effort of the International Society of Travel Medicine and CDC, has developed a profile of the relative likelihood of travel-related disease stratified by region of travel in the developing world (Figure 1-2).

Based on 17,353 ill returned travelers seen at 31 clinical sites on 6 continents, the destination-specific differences in relative frequencies (proportionate morbidity) are apparent for most diseases. Figure 1-2 shows destination-specific proportions of ill returned travelers with each diagnosis, rather than incidence rates, which can be used to assist with risk-profiling of prospective travelers during the pre-travel medical consultation. When individual diagnoses were collected into syndrome groups and examined for all regions together, 226 of every 1,000 ill returned travelers seen by participating clinicians had a systemic febrile illness, 222 had acute diarrhea, 170 had a dermatologic disorder, 113 had chronic diarrhea, and 77 had a respiratory disorder. Region-specific disease occurrence data indicated the following:

- Febrile illness was most likely from Africa and Southeast Asia.
- Malaria was among the top 3 diagnoses from every region.
- Over the past decade, dengue became the most common febrile illness from every region outside sub-Saharan Africa.
- In sub-Saharan Africa, rickettsial disease was second only to malaria as a cause of fever.
- Respiratory disease was most likely in Southeast Asia.
- Acute diarrhea was disproportionately seen in travelers from south-central Asia.

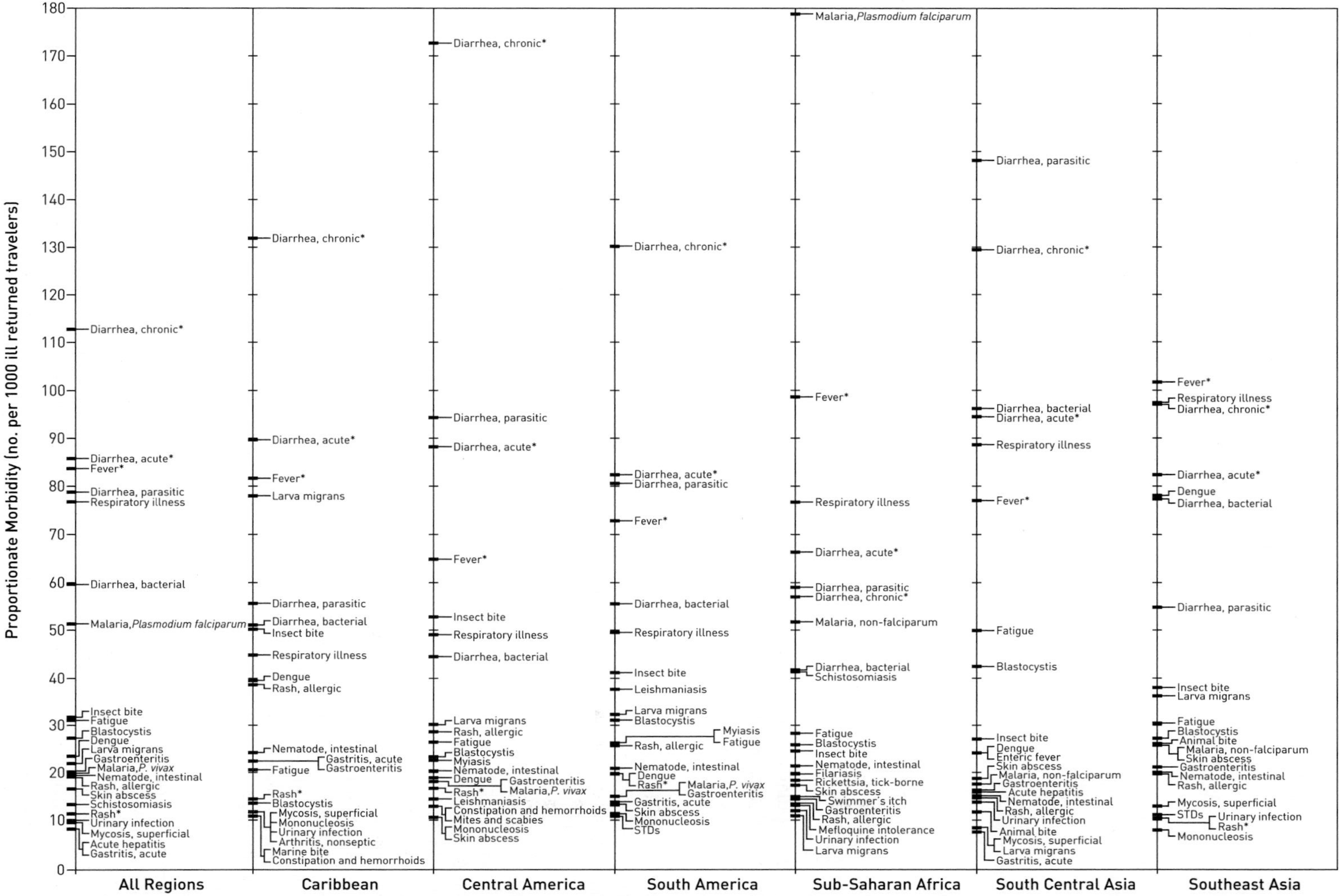

FIGURE 1-2. PROPORTIONATE MORBIDITY AMONG ILL TRAVELERS RETURNING FROM THE DEVELOPING WORLD, ACCORDING TO REGION OF TRAVEL[1,2]

[1] From Freedman DO, Weld LH, Kozarsky PE, Fisk T, Robins R, von Sonnenburg F, et al. Spectrum of disease and relation to place of exposure among ill returned travelers. N Engl J Med. 2006 Jan 12;354(2):119–130. Copyright © 2006 Massachusetts Medical Society. All rights reserved.

[2] Proportionate morbidity, not incidence rate, is shown for each of the top 22 specific diagnoses for all ill returned travelers within each region. STD denotes sexually transmitted disease. Asterisks indicate syndromic diagnoses for which specific etiologic diagnoses could not be assigned.

A recent GeoSentinel study indicated that disease profiles in European travelers, when compared with travelers from North America and other continents, did not differ, further showing that disease risk is dependent on destination and place of exposure rather than on origin country of the traveler.

FUTURE CHALLENGES AND PRIORITIES FOR TRAVEL EPIDEMIOLOGY

Issues surrounding the relative merits of different methodologic approaches to defining travel-associated disease risk have recently been reviewed at length. In order to better characterize health risks and provide guidance to travelers, some epidemiologic priorities include the following:

- Obtaining travel-related data for many existing and potentially vaccine-preventable diseases. Current data are sparse, and incidence in local populations is often not reflective of travelers' risk because of different risk behaviors, previous infection, or preexisting vaccination campaigns.
- Developing better surrogate markers for malaria exposure during travel, to facilitate interventional studies for novel malaria chemoprophylaxis drugs. Such information is difficult to obtain because of the inability to perform placebo drug studies, given the life-threatening nature of the infection.
- Studying the effect of high-risk medical conditions or immunocompromising medications on travel outcomes.
- Improving understanding of the impact of host behavior related to different types of travel, such as tourism, business travel, travel to visit friends and relatives, missionary travel, and volunteer travel.
- Conducting research to gain more insight on exposure-related factors, such as urban vs. rural travel, luxury vs. rough travel, season of travel, and organized package travel vs. self-directed travel. Recent information on long-stay vs. short-stay travel has been published.

BIBLIOGRAPHY

1. Caumes E, Ehya N, Nguyen J, Bricaire F. Typhoid and paratyphoid fever: a 10-year retrospective study of 41 cases in a Parisian hospital. J Travel Med. 2001 Nov–Dec;8(6):293–7.
2. Chen LH, Wilson ME, Davis X, Loutan L, Schwartz E, Keystone J, et al. Illness in long-term travelers visiting GeoSentinel clinics. Emerg Infect Dis. 2009 Nov;15(11):1773–82.
3. Freedman DO, Weld LH, Kozarsky PE, Fisk T, Robins R, von Sonnenburg F, et al. Spectrum of disease and relation to place of exposure among ill returned travelers. N Engl J Med. 2006 Jan 12;354(2):119–30.
4. Gautret P, Schlagenhauf P, Gaudart J, Castelli F, Brouqui P, von Sonnenburg F, et al. Multicenter EuroTravNet/GeoSentinel study of travel-related infectious diseases in Europe. Emerg Infect Dis. 2009 Nov;15(11):1783–90.
5. Greenwood Z, Black J, Weld L, O'Brien D, Leder K, Von Sonnenburg F, et al. Gastrointestinal infection among international travelers globally. J Travel Med. 2008 Jul–Aug;15(4):221–8.
6. Hill DR. Health problems in a large cohort of Americans traveling to developing countries. J Travel Med. 2000 Sep–Oct;7(5):259–66.
7. Jensenius M, Davis X, von Sonnenburg F, Schwartz E, Keystone JS, Leder K, et al. Multicenter GeoSentinel analysis of rickettsial diseases in international travelers, 1996–2008. Emerg Infect Dis. 2009 Nov;15(11):1791–8.
8. Leder K, Wilson ME, Freedman DO, Torresi J. A comparative analysis of methodological approaches used for estimating risk in travel medicine. J Travel Med. 2008 Jul–Aug;15(4):263–72.
9. Lederman ER, Weld LH, Elyazar IR, von Sonnenburg F, Loutan L, Schwartz E, et al. Dermatologic conditions of the ill returned traveler: an analysis from the GeoSentinel Surveillance Network. Int J Infect Dis. 2008 Nov;12(6):593–602.
10. Liese B, Mundt KA, Dell LD, Nagy L, Demure B. Medical insurance claims associated with international business travel. Occup Environ Med. 1997 Jul;54(7):499–503.
11. Mutsch M, Spicher VM, Gut C, Steffen R. Hepatitis A virus infections in travelers, 1988–2004. Clin Infect Dis. 2006 Feb 15;42(4):490–7.
12. Nicolls DJ, Weld LH, Schwartz E, Reed C, von Sonnenburg F, Freedman DO, et al. Characteristics of schistosomiasis in travelers reported to the GeoSentinel Surveillance Network 1997–2008. Am J Trop Med Hyg. 2008 Nov;79(5):729–34.
13. Schwartz E, Weld LH, Wilder-Smith A, von Sonnenburg F, Keystone JS, Kain KC, et al. Seasonality, annual

trends, and characteristics of dengue among ill returned travelers, 1997–2006. Emerg Infect Dis. 2008 Jul;14(7):1081–8.

14. Steffen R, Amitirigala I, Mutsch M. Health risks among travelers—need for regular updates. J Travel Med. 2008 May–Jun;15(3):145–6.

15. Steffen R, deBernardis C, Banos A. Travel epidemiology—a global perspective. Int J Antimicrob Agents. 2003 Feb;21(2):89–95.

16. Steffen R, Rickenbach M, Wilhelm U, Helminger A, Schar M. Health problems after travel to developing countries. J Infect Dis. 1987 Jul;156(1):84–91.

17. Torresi J, Leder K. Defining infections in international travellers through the GeoSentinel Surveillance Network. Nat Rev Microbiol. 2009 Dec;7(12):895–901.

18. Whitty CJ, Mabey DC, Armstrong M, Wright SG, Chiodini PL. Presentation and outcome of 1107 cases of schistosomiasis from Africa diagnosed in a non-endemic country. Trans R Soc Trop Med Hyg. 2000 Sep–Oct;94(5):531–4.

Perspectives

THE ROLE OF THE TRAVELER IN TRANSLOCATION OF DISEASE
Stephen M. Ostroff

Since humans began moving from one place to another, they have offered free passage to pathogens, on themselves or in their belongings, and the consequences of such microbial hitchhiking have, at times, altered the course of history. Among the more notable examples are the great plagues that swept into Europe from Asia during the Middle Ages, the importation of smallpox to the Americas by European explorers, and the reverse movement of syphilis into Europe in those same returning explorers.

Although the movement of pathogens through travel is not a new phenomenon, today's increasing pace and scale of global human movement have enhanced the opportunities for disease spread. HIV infection, with symptoms that may be delayed for years, spread around the world less than a decade after it was recognized. In the twenty-first century, no place on the globe is more than a day from any other location, which gives even diseases with short incubation periods unprecedented opportunities for rapid spread. The following examples from the last decade illustrate the role travel plays in the translocation of infectious diseases. They also remind us that all travelers should take steps to prevent bringing more than luggage to their destination.

INFLUENZA
Two new forms of influenza have recently emerged. One is avian influenza A (H5N1), which was first observed during a limited-scale outbreak in Hong Kong in 1997. It reappeared in Vietnam in 2003 and has been in

continuous circulation ever since. Even though H5N1 has primarily affected poultry, from 2003 through 2009, 458 human illnesses in 15 countries were reported, with an alarming case-fatality ratio of 62%. The countries with the most human disease (Indonesia, Vietnam, and Egypt) are tourist destinations, but no international travelers have become ill, largely because close contact with infected poultry is the primary risk factor for infection, and no sustained human-to-human transmission has been observed. However, movement of the virus between countries in goods carried by conveyances and animals has been documented.

In contrast, the rapid spread of 2009 pandemic influenza A (H1N1) was aided by infected travelers, both those who were symptomatic and those who were in the incubation stage. Although the virus was first identified in southern California in April 2009, human illnesses appeared weeks earlier in Mexico. Infected travelers who had visited Mexico were quickly detected in other parts of the world. An analysis of air traffic patterns found a very strong correlation between the volume of air travel from Mexico to a country and the likelihood H1N1 was identified in that location during the early stages of the pandemic. Aided by travel, this new virus found its way to dozens of countries in less than 2 months after it was identified, resulting in a June 2009 pandemic designation by the World Health Organization. The H1N1 pandemic vividly demonstrates the potential for global dissemination of pathogens in a highly interconnected world.

SARS

The severe acute respiratory syndrome (SARS) epidemic of 2003 is another major example of the role of travel in the spread of infectious diseases in the twenty-first century. In February 2003, a professor from southern China, who was caring for patients with an unrecognized respiratory illness, traveled to a family wedding in Hong Kong while he was ill. His infection spread to 10 other travelers in his hotel, who then boarded airplanes to other parts of Asia, North America, and Europe, setting off a global epidemic of SARS that resulted in 8,098 cases and 774 deaths in 29 countries. Fortunately, characteristics of the virus, transmission dynamics of the disease, and aggressive public health measures contained the virus within months, but not before SARS produced widespread fear, and economic and political turmoil. SARS had a major influence on the revisions to the International Health Regulations in 2005.

CHILDHOOD VACCINE-PREVENTABLE DISEASES

Vaccination programs have substantially reduced the global prevalence of childhood infectious diseases. In the Western Hemisphere, measles transmission has been effectively eliminated, and diseases like mumps and rubella are at historical lows. Globally, poliomyelitis has been targeted for eradication, and by the early 2000s, transmission of indigenous poliovirus was confined to only 4 countries. However, these diseases are all highly transmissible and can easily spread in infected travelers; endemic transmission has been reestablished in some previously polio-free areas.

Measles

In the United States, all recent clusters of measles have been associated with travel. These episodes have been precipitated by visitors from areas of the world where measles continues to circulate due to low vaccination coverage, susceptible US travelers going abroad, and overseas adoptees. These importations then ignite outbreaks because of waning population immunity, which is fueled largely by parents who elect not to vaccinate their children. During the first half of 2008, 13% of measles cases with an identified source were imported, and 76% of the remaining cases were the result of subsequent local transmission. In the previous decade, 20%–60% of cases were imported, and subsequent spread was much more limited.

Mumps

Several recent large outbreaks of mumps in the United States are directly traceable to travel-related importation from Great Britain. A 2006 outbreak centered in Iowa, likely fueled by spring break travel, resulted in more than 2,500 cases across 11 states. A more recent outbreak that began in mid-2009, resulting in more than 2,000 cases in New York City and surrounding states, largely centered around an Orthodox Jewish community. This outbreak was started by a single traveler to Great Britain who returned to a summer camp in New York State. Mumps then spread to campers and staff, who carried it home to New York City and ignited sustained transmission for many months.

Polio

In 2002, only 6 countries had circulating indigenous wild-type poliovirus, but from 2002 through 2007, wild-type poliovirus spread to 27 previously disease-free countries in Africa and Asia through the movement of infected travelers. Northern Nigeria was the source of most of these illnesses, which reached all the way to Indonesia. Vaccination campaigns, guided by laboratory-based surveillance, largely disrupted transmission in these places, but travel continues to result in the spread of polio. In 2008–2009, there were 47 introductions or reintroductions of the virus into 17 African countries, all originating from Nigeria or India, resulting in 255 subsequent cases. In 2010, even as polio incidence decreased in Nigeria and India, 2 large outbreaks demonstrated the risk of introduction from poliovirus reservoirs. Spread of poliovirus into Tajikistan from India caused an outbreak of 458 cases and, subsequently, 18 cases in 2 other Central Asian republics and Russia. In the Republic of the Congo, a large outbreak (more than 300 suspected cases as of late November 2010) resulted after introduction from Angola, posing further risk of spread elsewhere. Although these cases do not threaten most travelers, polio remains a serious concern for migrants, pilgrims, and people displaced by conflict; outbreaks heavily tax the public health resources of affected countries.

VECTORBORNE INFECTIONS

Several mosquito-transmitted diseases have expanded their range in the last decade. West Nile virus was introduced into New York City in 1999 and, in the next several years, spread throughout the Western Hemisphere, resulting in millions of human infections. The source and mode of introduction are unknown; an infected traveler is a distinct possibility, although importation of infected birds or mosquitoes is considered more likely.

For 2 other major vectorborne infections (dengue and chikungunya), the role of travelers is much clearer. Neither of these viruses has an avian intermediary, and humans are amplifying hosts for both viruses, effectively moving these viruses from place to place. Dengue outbreaks are expanding in scale and scope, especially in Asia and South America. Twice since 2000, the virus has made incursions into the United States via infected travelers. In 2001, local transmission was detected on Maui in Hawaii for the first time since the 1940s, resulting in 122 cases. The source was travelers from French Polynesia, which was experiencing an outbreak at the time. In 2009–2010, local dengue transmission was seen in the Florida Keys, also for the first time in decades. More than 70 cases were identified, including in tourists to the Florida Keys from other areas of the United States. The source of introduction is unknown, although many people from areas where dengue is endemic transit through the area.

Chikungunya virus was largely restricted to Africa and Asia until it began to appear in islands of the Indian Ocean in 2005, after an outbreak in Kenya in 2004. From there, it crossed to the Indian subcontinent in 2006, touching off major disease outbreaks, especially in southern India. Sizeable numbers of travelers to Indian Ocean tourist destinations and India have returned to Europe, North America, and Australia infected with chikungunya virus, and infected Indian nationals have also been seen in these locations. Chikungunya virus can be introduced into these areas in the same way that West Nile virus was introduced into the United States in 1999. Such events have taken place in several areas, including northern Italy in 2007, and southeast France and south-central China in 2010. The source for translocation in Italy was a viremic traveler from India. A total of 205 locally acquired cases were acquired through infected *Aedes albopictus* mosquitoes, an invasive species which appeared in the area in the early 1990s. In contrast to West Nile in North America, chikungunya virus does not appear to have persisted in northern Italy. Many countries that have a viable vector for chikungunya virus remain at risk for importation and local transmission. Map 1-1 shows the general pattern of how the chikungunya virus spread globally during these years.

DISEASE ASSOCIATED WITH GLOBAL GATHERINGS

The pilgrimage to Mecca is the world's largest annual event, drawing approximately 2 million Muslims from across the globe to Saudi Arabia. The history of the Hajj pilgrimage serves as an example of how diseases can spread during a global mass gathering, and can spread to home countries of returning travelers. The intermingling and close contact offer ample opportunities for transmission of infectious diseases and rapid dissemination as pilgrims return home. In 2000, this occurred with *Neisseria meningitidis* serogroup W-135, despite requirements for pilgrims to be vaccinated against meningococcal disease. Some vaccines used at that time did not cover this serogroup. After the event, 90 infections in returnees and their contacts were seen across Europe. In contrast, the number of infections in North America, where quadrivalent vaccine that covered W-135 was in use, was small. The outbreak strain of W-135 also quickly surfaced across areas of Africa, Asia, the Middle East, and the Indian Ocean, altering the epidemiologic patterns of meningococcal disease. As a result of this outbreak and similar cases in 2001, pilgrims to the Hajj are now required to be vaccinated with the quadrivalent vaccine.

These examples highlight the diversity of opportunities for microbial movement afforded by travel. No amount of vigilance is likely to eliminate such opportunities, especially since microbes can be silent travelers. However, all travelers should take precautions to prevent the spread of disease.

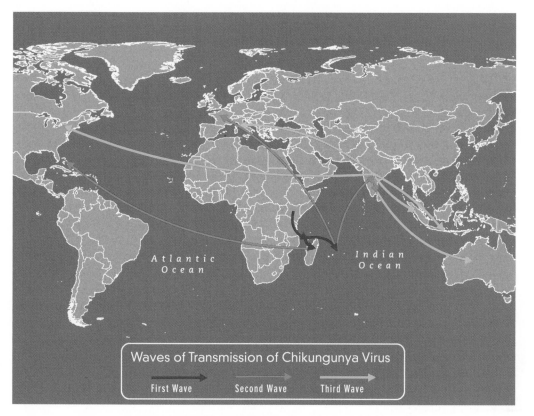

MAP 1-1. GLOBAL SPREAD OF CHIKUNGUNYA VIRUS DURING 2005–2009

BIBLIOGRAPHY

1. CDC. Resurgence of wild poliovirus type 1 transmission and consequences of importation—21 countries, 2002–2005. MMWR Morb Mortal Wkly Rep. 2006 Feb 17;55(6):145–50.

2. CDC. Update: measles—United States, January–July 2008. MMWR Morb Mortal Wkly Rep. 2008 Aug 22;57(33):893–6.

3. CDC. Update: mumps outbreak—New York and New Jersey, June 2009–January 2010. MMWR Morb Mortal Wkly Rep. 2010 Feb 12;59(5):125–9.

4. Chen LH, Wilson ME. The role of the traveler in emerging infections and magnitude of travel. Med Clin North Am. 2008 Nov;92(6):1409–32, xi.

5. Cleri DJ, Ricketti AJ, Vernaleo JR. Severe acute respiratory syndrome (SARS). Infect Dis Clin North Am. 2010 Mar;24(1):175–202.

6. Gushulak BD, MacPherson DW. Globalization of infectious diseases: the impact of migration. Clin Infect Dis. 2004 Jun 15;38(12):1742–8.

7. Khan K, Arino J, Hu W, Raposo P, Sears J, Calderon F, et al. Spread of a novel influenza A (H1N1) virus via global airline transportation. N Engl J Med. 2009 Jul 9;361(2):212–4.

8. Polgreen PM, Bohnett LC, Yang M, Pentella MA, Cavanaugh JE. A spatial analysis of the spread of mumps: the importance of college students and their spring-break-associated travel. Epidemiol Infect. 2010 Mar;138(3):434–41.

9. Rezza G, Nicoletti L, Angelini R, Romi R, Finarelli AC, Panning M, et al. Infection with chikungunya virus in Italy: an outbreak in a temperate region. Lancet. 2007 Dec 1;370(9602):1840–6.

10. Scott P, Deye G, Srinivasan A, Murray C, Moran K, Hulten E, et al. An outbreak of multidrug-resistant *Acinetobacter baumannii-calcoaceticus* complex infection in the US military health care system associated with military operations in Iraq. Clin Infect Dis. 2007 Jun 15;44(12):1577–84.

11. Stoddard ST, Morrison AC, Vazquez-Prokopec GM, Paz Soldan V, Kochel TJ, Kitron U, et al. The role of human movement in the transmission of vector-borne pathogens. PLoS Negl Trop Dis. 2009;3(7):e481.

12. Taylor WR, Burhan E, Wertheim H, Soepandi PZ, Horby P, Fox A, et al. Avian influenza—a review for doctors in travel medicine. Travel Med Infect Dis. 2010 Jan;8(1):1–12.

13. Wilder-Smith A. Meningococcal disease: risk for international travellers and vaccine strategies. Travel Med Infect Dis. 2008 Jul;6(4):182–6.

14. Wilder-Smith A, Gubler DJ. Geographic expansion of dengue: the impact of international travel. Med Clin North Am. 2008 Nov;92(6):1377–90.

Perspectives

RISKS TRAVELERS FACE

David R. Shlim

Travel medicine is based on the concept of the reduction of risk. In the context of travel medicine, "risk" refers to the possibility of harm during the course of a planned trip. Some risks may be avoidable, and others may not. Vaccine-preventable diseases may be mostly avoidable, depending on the risk of the disease and the protective efficacy of the vaccine. Non-disease risks, such as motor vehicle accidents or drowning, account for a much higher percentage of deaths among travelers than infectious diseases.

For most travelers, the perception of risk colors their choice of destinations, activities, and health concerns. Travel health providers may know statistics for a given risk, but whether the risk is considered high or low depends on the perception of the traveler. For example, the risk of dying while trekking in Nepal is 15 deaths per 100,000 trekkers, but there is no objective way to determine whether this risk is high or low. When the manuscript that reported this risk of dying while trekking was peer reviewed, one reviewer wrote, "You need to emphasize that these data show how dangerous trekking actually is." The other reviewer wrote, "You should make a point of stating that these data show how safe trekking is."

The subjective sense of risk is based on one's perception of risk ("15 per 100,000 means it's dangerous") and one's tolerance for risk ("it may be 15 per 100,000, but it's worth it"). This subjective sense of risk suffuses the field of travel medicine, from the travel health provider to the traveler, but it is rarely discussed. Some travelers canceled travel plans to Asia because of their fear of H5N1 avian influenza, even though the actual risk to travelers was extremely low. Other travelers plan to ascend Mount Everest, even though the risk of dying during an Everest climb is 1 in 40.

Regardless of the perception and tolerance of risk, the hazards associated with travel cannot be eliminated, just as the risks of staying home are not zero. Even the act of trying to prevent a risk—such as yellow fever—can lead to a fatal reaction to the vaccine in rare cases. Therefore, the goal in travel and in travel medicine should be skillfully managing risk, rather than trying to eliminate risk. The pre-travel visit is an opportunity to discuss risks and develop plans that minimize these risks. Each traveler may have individual concepts about the risks and benefits of vaccines, prophylaxis, and behavior modification.

Travelers should consider the psychological and emotional aspects of foreign travel. Culture shock can occur on either end of a journey: on arrival when one encounters an entirely strange new world, and on return when one's own world may temporarily appear unfamiliar. Travelers with underlying psychiatric conditions should be cautious when heading out to a stressful new environment, particularly if they are traveling alone.

All travelers should contemplate the concept of commitment, which describes the fact that certain parts of a journey cannot easily be reversed. A person trekking into a remote area may have to realize that rescue, if available at all, may be delayed for days. A person who has a myocardial infarction in a country with no advanced cardiac services may have a difficult time getting to definitive medical care. If the traveler has already contemplated these concerns and accepted them, it will be easier to deal with them if they come to pass.

Travel helps break down the barriers between human beings around the world and enriches the lives of travelers. Despite the risks of travel, we should never lose sight of the benefits.

Perspectives

WHY GUIDELINES DIFFER

Alan J. Magill, David R. Shlim

INTRODUCTION
Numerous international, national, and professional organizations publish guidelines and recommendations that assist travel health providers in providing the best possible advice to prospective travelers. The CDC Yellow Book is

one example of published recommendations. However, it is quickly apparent to both clinicians and patients that guidelines and recommendations differ, sometimes dramatically. Conflicting messages from authoritative sources may confuse patients and clinicians, and undermine the credibility of the source. It can be unsettling for patients to receive travel medicine advice, vaccines, and a malaria prescription from a provider, only to find that the recommendations conflict with what they have obtained from other sources, or even heard from other advisors. The skillful travel health provider will be able to help the traveler run this gauntlet of conflicting advice by knowing more about why guidelines differ.

HOW ARE GUIDELINES CREATED?

Most guidelines of interest to travel health providers and travelers focus on recommendations for immunizations, prophylactic medications, and self-treatment regimens (such as those for travelers' diarrhea). Guidelines come from many sources. A regulatory agency in each country must review and approve an application from the sponsor of a product in order for the product to be commercially distributed. Regulatory authorities review data from preli-censure clinical trials and also assess the manufacturing process. International organizations such as the World Health Organization (WHO) promote their own sets of guidelines. At national levels, agencies such as CDC make recommendations for the use of approved vaccines and medications for travelers. In addition, professional organizations may create consensus clinical practice guidelines based on published medical literature and expert opinion. Travel medicine–specific subscription services use experts to organize and present travel medicine recommendations for clinicians. However, these services can use information and sources that may not be fully validated by national and international authorities. Finally, vast quantities of unregulated opinions are published on the Internet. People new to travel medicine may not be aware of the decision-making process or the source information that results in formal recommendations from these organizations.

Regulatory Authorities

A national regulatory authority is the government body that approves vaccines and drugs. In the United States, this is the Food and Drug Administration (FDA). For the vaccines and medications commonly prescribed in a pre-travel consultation, providers are expected to use the products in accordance with the product label as approved by the FDA. The product label is a valuable source of information that is accurate at the time it is published. Manufacturers submit a detailed application that undergoes rigorous, multidisciplinary review. The approved product label reflects the information provided by the manufacturer in response to the requirements specified by a large body of regulatory law developed over many years. Since each country has different laws and requirements, approved products and their product labels may differ from country to country. This difference is then reflected in the national guidelines that relate to that product.

International Organizations

Travelers' health information is provided by WHO's publication, *International Travel and Health* (the "Green Book") and also in the WHO International Health Regulations 2005. Countries with less developed or nonexistent regulatory agencies often default to the WHO guidelines, while more developed countries with resources devoted to travelers' health may be aware of the WHO recommendations, but may not be able to reconcile WHO recommendations with their own country's recommendations in every situation.

US National Organizations

CDC provides recommendations for travelers' health and publishes those recommendations in this book. Subject-matter experts at CDC review information in their area of expertise and formulate recommendations. For vaccines, the Advisory Committee on Immunization Practices (ACIP) develops written recommendations for the administration of vaccines, including travelers' vaccines, to children and adults in the civilian population. Recommendations include age for vaccine administration, number of doses and dosing interval, and precautions and contraindications. ACIP, which is the only entity appointed by the federal government to make such recommendations, consists of 15 experts in fields associated with immunization who have been selected to provide advice and guidance to the US Department of Health and Human Services and CDC on the control of vaccine-preventable diseases (see Chapter 2, Perspectives: Vaccine Recommendations of the ACIP).

Professional Organizations

Professional organizations often develop, write, and publish practice guidelines using committees of experts from their membership. These practice guidelines typically follow an evidence-based medicine approach that links recommendations to the strength and quality of the evidence as assessed by the committee members. The Infectious Disease Society of America has published a travel medicine practice guideline that many find useful. Practice guidelines, by their nature, are consensus documents.

Peer-Reviewed Medical Literature and Open Sources

As experience with a vaccine or a drug is acquired over the years, these results are often published in the peer-reviewed medical literature. In addition, people who use these products gain experience over time and develop their own opinions ("experience-based medicine"). The data that would be most useful in deciding how to use a vaccine or medication may not be available in published reports, so expert opinion attempts to interpret available information or provide background perspective.

WHY DO GUIDELINES DIFFER?

Guidelines in different countries and organizations may differ in significant ways. Some of the reasons why guidelines differ include availability of products in different countries, a different cultural perception of risk, lack of evidence (or differing interpretations of the same evidence), and sometimes just honest differences in opinion among experts. Occasionally, public opinion may influence recommendations (for example, the widespread adverse publicity about mefloquine that was reported in the media).

Availability of Products

Travel health providers can only use the products that are available to them. Availability is determined by the regulatory approval status of the product and, to a lesser extent, the marketing and distribution plan of the manufacturer.

Among the various vaccines and antimalarial drugs commercially available worldwide, the process for regulatory approvals varies greatly. For example, registering a new vaccine or antimalarial drug in the United States is a costly and rigorous process. If the market is insufficient to justify the expense of registration, then a commercial company may not seek registration in a particular country. The standards for licensure vary, and what may be sufficient for one regulatory authority may not suffice for another. For example, primaquine, an option for antimalarial prophylaxis in the United States, is not registered or commercially available in Switzerland. Atovaquone-proguanil was available for malaria chemoprophylaxis in the United States before many other countries. On the other hand, an oral vaccine against cholera is approved for use and widely available in many countries, but is not approved by the FDA. Therefore, CDC and ACIP guidelines do not include any recommendations for the use of this vaccine.

Even when the same products are available, the recommendations for their use may differ. The capsular polysaccharide typhoid vaccine and the oral typhoid vaccine are examples. In the United States, a booster of the polysaccharide vaccine is recommended after 2 years, but in most European countries a booster is recommended after 3 years. In the United States, a packet of 4 oral typhoid capsules is dispensed, whereas in Europe, 3 doses are considered adequate. The regulatory agencies may have reviewed the same data and drawn different conclusions, or they may have reviewed different data at separate times and reached different conclusions. It is unusual for regulatory submissions to various agencies to be ready and occur at the same time; therefore, the data available for review by each agency may not be the same, for legitimate reasons.

Perception of Risk

People from varying backgrounds can view the same risk data and come to different conclusions as to the cost and benefit of preventing that risk. For example, national-level recommendations to prevent malaria while traveling to India vary widely. German recommendations are to not use standard prophylaxis for any travel to an Indian destination; standby emergency treatment (SBET or self-treatment) is the recommendation for identified risk destinations. The guidelines in the United Kingdom recommend only awareness and mosquito bite prevention for more than half the Indian subcontinent, including large cities and popular tourist destinations in the north and south, while recommending an individual risk assessment that is based on activities and types of travelers. Standard prophylaxis recommended in the UK guidelines is the combination of chloroquine plus proguanil (an option not available in the United States) for much of the middle of the subcontinent. However, CDC recommends malaria prophylaxis for any Indian destination except for some mountainous areas of northern states above 2,000 m (6,561 ft). Is one of these guidelines better than the others? Not necessarily, as the recommendations may be based on the national experience with different types of travelers, and the risk assessment approach of the organization formulating the national guidelines. For example, in 2008, CDC reported 114 malaria cases acquired in India by returning US travelers, the second highest absolute number of cases from any destination, and 194 cases of malaria acquired in Nigeria. However, when viewed as estimated relative case rates (the number of cases among US travelers attributable to each country divided by the estimated travel volume for US travelers to that country), Nigeria remains well above the median estimated risk, but India falls just below the median estimated risk due the much higher volume of travel to India. India reports active transmission in all provinces in the country. Based on the extremely large population of India, some of these provinces have high absolute numbers of cases but low case rates. Some countries base their recommendations on these relatively low case rates, but other countries believe that the high absolute numbers of cases results in large numbers of infective mosquitoes that can, in turn, infect travelers. In any case, travelers to India are likely to encounter diverse recommendations for malaria prevention on the Internet or from other travelers.

The best available data should always balance the risk of the intervention—and the costs—against the risk of the disease, so that the decision to recommend a vaccine or prophylactic medicine may be understood by the clinician and the traveler.

Lack of Evidence

In many cases, limited or no data are available to inform an evidence-based assessment. In this setting, travel health providers defer to expert opinion or an extrapolation from limited data in conjunction with expert opinion. In travel medicine, it is rare to have actual prospective numerator and denominator data on the risk of any vaccine-preventable diseases in travelers. For example, any data on the risk of hepatitis A in travelers would have to account for the immunization rate with hepatitis A vaccine. These data are rarely available, and therefore we often rely on historical data that captured few actual cases.

CAN WE HARMONIZE GUIDELINES?

The complex nature of how we obtain, evaluate, and verify data, combined with the fundamental differences in risk perception, makes it likely that multiple, overlapping, and at times conflicting guidelines will continue to exist. However, given the international nature of travel medicine and the existence of the International Society of Travel Medicine, conflicting guidelines have decreased in the past decade. In one example of an effort to harmonize guidelines, from 2008 through 2010, WHO convened an international group of yellow fever and travel medicine experts to review available data on yellow fever virus transmission. The product of this collaboration was a country-specific list of yellow fever vaccine recommendations based on the geographic distribution of risk (see Chapter 3, Yellow Fever and Malaria Information, by Country).

In summary, the role of the travel health provider is to become more sophisticated in his or her understanding of the various differences in guidelines, in interpreting this information, and in conveying it in an assured and comforting manner to travelers.

BIBLIOGRAPHY

1. CDC. Advisory Committee on Immunization Practices (ACIP). Atlanta: CDC; 2010 [updated Nov 1; cited 2010 Sep 16]. Available from: http://www.cdc.gov/vaccines/recs/ACIP/default.htm.
2. Chiodini P, Hill D, Lea G, Walker E, Whitty C, Bannister B. Guidelines for malaria prevention in travellers from the United Kingdom 2007. London: Health Protection Agency; 2007 [cited 2010 Nov 8]. Available from: http://www.hpa.org.uk/Publications/InfectiousDiseases/Travel Health/0701Malariapreventionfortravellers fromtheUK/.

3. Committee to Advise on Tropical Medicine and Travel. Canadian recommendations for the prevention and treatment of malaria among international travellers—2009. Can Commun Dis Rep. 2009 Jul;35 Suppl 1:1–82.

4. German Society for Tropical Medicine and International Health Association (DTG). Deutsche Gesellschaft für Tropenmedizin und Internationale Gesundheit e.V. 2010 [updated Nov 8; cited 2010 Sep 16]. Available from: http://www.dtg.org.

5. Hill DR, Ericsson CD, Pearson RD, Keystone JS, Freedman DO, Kozarsky PE, et al. The practice of travel medicine: guidelines by the Infectious Diseases Society of America. Clin Infect Dis. 2006 Dec 15;43(12):1499–1539.

6. World Health Organization. International Health Regulations (2005). Geneva: World Health Organization; 2008 [cited 2010 Nov 8]. Available from: http://www.who.int/ihr/9789241596664/en/index.html.

7. World Health Organization. International travel and health. Geneva: World Health Organization; 2010 [cited 2010 Sep 16]. Available from: http://www.who.int/ith/en/.

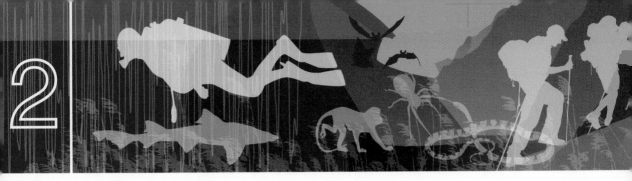

The Pre-Travel Consultation

THE PRE-TRAVEL CONSULTATION

Rebecca W. Acosta

The risk assessment is the foundation of the pre-travel consultation and allows the health care provider to customize care for each traveler based on the itinerary, health and medical history, and the traveler's concerns and needs. The goal of the pre-travel consultation is to prepare the traveler through counseling, education, vaccinations, and medications to help reduce and manage their risk of illness and injury during travel.

The well-organized and well-executed pre-travel consultation supports consistent, appropriate, and efficient pre-travel health preparation with the following 3 essential elements: risk assessment, risk communication, and risk management.

RISK ASSESSMENT

The pre-travel health risk assessment involves gathering pertinent information about the itinerary ("where, when, and what") and the traveler ("who, why, and how") to highlight the potential hazards of the trip, and alert the travel health provider to any contraindications and precautions to vaccinations or medications that may be indicated. A questionnaire designed to collect and organize the itinerary and traveler data is an essential tool to help support the risk assessment process and facilitate consistent practice.

The most important information to gather is the following:

- Itinerary data
  - > Countries and regions to be visited, in the order of travel
  - > Visits to urban versus rural areas
  - > Dates and length of travel in each area
  - > Purpose of travel (such as business, vacation, visiting friends and relatives)
  - > Modes of transportation
  - > Planned and possible activities (such as hiking, scuba diving, camping)
  - > Types of accommodations in each area (such as air-conditioned, screened, tents)

- Traveler demographics and health/medical history
  - > Age, sex
  - > Vaccination history, including dates, how many doses received in a scheduled series, and prior adverse events
  - > Medical and psychiatric history (past and current), including any conditions or medications that suppress the immune system
  - > Medications (current or taken in the past 3 months)
  - > Allergies (in particular to eggs, latex, yeast, mercury, or thimerosal)

> Pregnancy and breastfeeding (current status and plans)
> Any planned surgeries or other medical care during travel (medical tourism)

An example of using the itinerary and traveler data includes determining if there will be a risk of yellow fever disease or a country requirement for proof of yellow fever vaccination based on the planned destinations, and if there is a contraindication (such as egg allergy) or a precaution (such as age >60 years) to the traveler's receiving the vaccine. Malaria risk is another example. It is important to assess whether the traveler will be going to a region endemic for malaria, and what the appropriate measures are to help prevent malaria based on the details of the traveler's itinerary, activities, and medical history. See the respective disease sections in Chapter 3 for detailed information on yellow fever and malaria prevention.

During the risk assessment, the provider must remain alert to other factors about "who" will be traveling. Such factors include the traveler's previous travel experience, perception of risk, cultural background, peer groups, and possible barriers to care, such as economic issues, attitudes regarding vaccine safety, and language limitations. These factors may affect the traveler's ability and willingness to accept and adhere to recommendations.

Certain travelers are considered high risk, as their preexisting health and medical conditions may be uniquely impacted by travel and related activities. In some cases, risk-reduction measures may be more complicated because of increased precautions and contraindications. It is important to anticipate the special needs of the following high-risk travelers:

- People with weakened immune systems
- Women who are pregnant or breastfeeding
- People with certain preexisting medical issues such as diabetes, and certain pulmonary and cardiac conditions
- People visiting friends and relatives (VFRs). These travelers have typically migrated from a less-developed area to a developed area, and are now returning to the region of their birth. The traveler returning to his or her country of origin may not appreciate the dynamics of risk and waning immunity, especially for diseases such as malaria. Of special importance

are new family members or children who are visiting the area for the first time (see Chapter 8, Immigrants Returning Home to Visit Friends and Relatives [VFRs]).
- Families with young children
- People traveling to adopt children abroad (see Chapter 7, International Adoption)
- The older traveler (aged >60 years)

The importance of the risk assessment may be illustrated by 3 travelers going to the same country: one for a week-long, urban-based business trip; the next on an adventure-seeking, backpack vacation to rural areas over several months; and the third a pregnant VFR traveler. The recommendations and preparation for each of these travelers will vary based on their unique needs and itinerary details.

RISK COMMUNICATION

Risk communication is an integral part of the pre-travel consultation process and relates directly to "who" will be traveling. Risk communication includes the presentation of reliable, evidence-based information in a context appropriate for the individual traveler. Information gathered during the risk assessment interview, including the traveler's baseline knowledge and beliefs about the risks, and his or her understanding and opinions about risk reduction measures, are important to guiding discussions. For risk communication to be effective, adequate time must be allocated for these discussions.

Giving the traveler both verbal and written information helps to guide and focus the discussions and reinforces important traveler-specific issues. Examples include vaccine information statements, disease information pamphlets, and malaria risk maps. During a careful risk assessment and thoughtful risk communication, a risk management plan takes shape (vaccinations, medications, and targeted risk-avoidance education).

RISK MANAGEMENT

The essential elements of risk management include the following:

- Vaccines: selection, administration, and documentation of vaccinations (see Box 2-1)
  > Consider required, recommended, and routine vaccinations (see below)

BOX 2-1. VACCINATIONS FOR CONSIDERATION IN THE PRE-TRAVEL CONSULTATION

A list of vaccines used in the United States (including the manufacturer's vaccine name) can be found on CDC's website at www.cdc.gov/vaccines/vpd-vac/vaccines-list.htm.

Routine Vaccines
The pre-travel consultation is a good opportunity to make sure travelers are up-to-date on their routine vaccines. Clinicians should refer to the age-appropriate immunization schedule published each year by the Advisory Committee for Immunization Practices (ACIP). Current schedules are posted on the CDC website at www.cdc.gov/vaccines/recs/schedules/default.htm.

Depending on the age and risk factors of the patient, the following vaccines may be routinely recommended, regardless of travel:

- Diphtheria
- Hepatitis A
- Hepatitis B
- *Haemophilus influenzae* type b (Hib)
- Herpes zoster (shingles)
- Human papillomavirus (HPV)
- Influenza
- Measles (rubeola)
- Meningococcal
- Mumps
- Pertussis
- Pneumococcal
- Polio
- Rotavirus
- Rubella
- Tetanus
- Varicella (chickenpox)

Travel-Related Vaccines
Recommendations for these vaccines are dependent on many factors, including the travel destination. Refer to the destination-specific web pages on the CDC Travelers' Health website at www.cdc.gov/travel.

The most common vaccines considered for travelers include the following:

- Hepatitis A*
- Hepatitis B*
- Japanese encephalitis (JE)
- Meningococcal*
- Polio (adult booster)
- Rabies*
- Typhoid fever
- Yellow fever

Required Vaccines
Some countries require that travelers carry proof of vaccination on an International Certificate of Vaccination or Prophylaxis (ICVP) to enter the country. Requirements can change at any time, so it is important to check the CDC Travelers' Health website and the US Department of State (embassy or consulate) websites for information about requirements.

- Yellow fever vaccine (see the country-specific requirements in Chapter 3)
- Meningococcal vaccine (for pilgrims entering Saudi Arabia for the Hajj)

* Some travel-related vaccines are routinely recommended for certain travelers based on their age or other risk factors.

> Discuss vaccine indications, contraindications, precautions, and timing of doses
> Offer and discuss vaccine information before vaccines are administered

- Medications:
  > Recommendations and prescriptions as appropriate according to risk, such as antimalarial chemoprophylaxis, travelers' diarrhea self-treatment, and medications for altitude sickness

- Education:
  - > Malaria prevention and adherence to chemoprophylaxis (if indicated by the risk assessment)
  - > Risk and prevention of other insectborne diseases
  - > Methods to reduce foodborne and waterborne illness
  - > Self-management of travelers' diarrhea
  - > Animal avoidance and rabies prevention
  - > Reducing the negative effect of other itinerary risks (such as altitude or pollution)
  - > Activity-specific risks (such as road safety, diving, rafting, and rural road travel)
  - > Personal behavior risks (such as sexually transmitted diseases and illegal drug use)

- General guidance:
  - > Symptoms that may require medical attention during or after travel (such as fever, gastrointestinal symptoms, or dermatologic symptoms)
  - > Preparing a travel health kit (see the Travel Health Kits section later in this chapter)
  - > Accessing medical care abroad and obtaining medical/evacuation insurance (see the Obtaining Health Care Abroad for the Ill Traveler and Travel Health Insurance and Evacuation Insurance sections later in this chapter)

When considering vaccinations, common terms used include "required," "recommended," and "routine." A required vaccine is one a traveler needs to enter a particular destination country for which either proof of vaccination or a medical waiver is mandatory. Recommended vaccines are those vaccines that are medically advised based on the actual disease risks of the itinerary, regardless of the presence or absence of country entry requirements. Routine vaccines refer to those vaccines that are recommended in the United States, regardless of travel. These routine vaccines are an important part of pre-travel care because many of the diseases they protect against are more common in countries outside the United States. In addition, diseases such as measles and mumps continue to cause localized outbreaks even in developed countries.

DOCUMENTATION AND WRITTEN RECORDS

Careful documentation of all vaccinations, medications, and specific recommendations given to the traveler helps to complete the care plan record. Using an electronic record or standardized form facilitates documentation and helps ensure consistency of practice. Travelers should be encouraged to keep a record of their vaccinations and medications, and update it with their health care provider at each visit.

Clinicians who are registered to give yellow fever vaccine must know how to complete the International Certificate of Vaccination or Prophylaxis (ICVP) to ensure that this documentation will be accepted at the borders of destination countries (see Chapter 3, Yellow Fever).

The Immunization Action Coalition (www.immunize.org) gathers essential information on the safety, efficacy, and use of vaccines, including a listing of all the most current vaccine information statements, sample standing orders, forms, storage and handling guidelines, and links to other resources related to vaccines. These may be helpful in developing practice-specific policies and procedures to support the pre-travel consultation process and best practice.

Clinicians should plan to spend an average of 30–45 minutes conducting a complete pre-travel consultation, given the potential complexities in preparing the traveler. Clinicians with limited knowledge and expertise in travel medicine and the pre-travel consultation should consider referring travelers with complex itineraries or special needs (see Chapters 7 and 8) to a travel medicine clinic or travel medicine specialist.

The references for this section will help providers gain a more in-depth perspective on the expectations for providing pre-travel health care, and offer further guidance on the pre-travel consultation process.

BIBLIOGRAPHY

1. Bauer IL. Educational issues and concerns in travel health advice: is all the effort a waste of time? J Travel Med. 2005 Jan–Feb;12(1):45–52.

2. Crockett M, Keystone J. "I hate needles" and other factors impacting on travel vaccine uptake. J Travel Med. 2005 Apr;12 Suppl 1:S41–6.

3. Evans G, Bostrom A, Johnston RB, Fisher BL, Stoto MA, editors. Risk Communication and Vaccination. Washington, DC: National Academies Press; 1997.

4. Hill DR, Ericsson CD, Pearson RD, Keystone JS, Freedman DO, Kozarsky PE, et al. The practice of travel medicine: guidelines by the Infectious Diseases Society of America. Clin Infect Dis. 2006 Dec 15;43(12):1499–539.

5. Immunization Action Coalition. Vaccination information for healthcare professionals. Saint Paul, MN: Immunization Action Coalition; 2010 [cited 2010 Nov 8]. Available from: www.immunize.org.

6. Kozarsky P. The body of knowledge for the practice of travel medicine—2006. J Travel Med. 2006 Sep–Oct;13(5):251–4.

7. Spira A. Setting the standard. J Travel Med. 2003 Jan–Feb;10(1):1–3.

8. Thomson R, Edwards A, Grey J. Risk communication in the clinical consultation. Clin Med. 2005 Sep–Oct;5(5):465–69.

9. Wolfe M, Wolfe Acosta R. Structure and organization of the pre-travel consultation and general advice for travelers. In: Keystone JS, Kozarsky PE, Freedman DO, Nothdurft HD, Connor BA, editors. Travel Medicine. 2nd ed. Philadelphia: Mosby; 2008. p. 35–45.

GENERAL RECOMMENDATIONS FOR VACCINATION & IMMUNOPROPHYLAXIS

Andrew Kroger, William Atkinson

Recommendations for the use of vaccines and other biologic products (such as immune globulin products) in the United States are developed by the Advisory Committee on Immunization Practices (ACIP) and other groups, such as the American Academy of Pediatrics. These recommendations are based on scientific evidence of benefits (immunity to the disease) and risks (vaccine adverse reactions) and, where few or no data are available, on expert opinion. The recommendations include information on general immunization issues and the use of specific vaccines. When these recommendations are issued or revised, they are published in the Morbidity and Mortality Weekly Report (MMWR) (www.cdc.gov/mmwr). This section is based primarily on the ACIP General Recommendations on Immunization.

Vaccinations against diphtheria, tetanus, pertussis, measles, mumps, rubella, varicella, poliomyelitis, hepatitis A, hepatitis B, *Haemophilus influenzae* type b (Hib), rotavirus, human papillomavirus (HPV), and pneumococcal and meningococcal invasive disease are routinely administered in the United States, usually in childhood or adolescence. Influenza vaccine is routinely recommended for all people aged ≥6 months, each year. A dose of herpes zoster (shingles) vaccine is recommended for adults aged ≥60 years. If a person does not have a history of adequate protection against these diseases, immunizations appropriate to age and previous immunization status should be obtained, whether or not international travel is planned. A visit to a clinician for travel-related immunizations should be seen as an opportunity to bring an incompletely vaccinated person up to date on his or her routine vaccinations.

Both the child and adolescent vaccination schedule, and an adult vaccination schedule, are published annually in the MMWR. Vaccine providers should obtain the most current schedules from the CDC Vaccines and Immunization website (www.cdc.gov/vaccines). The text and many tables of this publication present recommendations for the use, number of doses, dose intervals, adverse reactions, precautions, and contraindications for vaccines and toxoids that may be indicated for travelers. Recommendations for travelers are not always the same as routine recommendations. For instance, most adults born after 1956 are recommended to receive 1 dose of MMR vaccine; however, international travelers of this age are recommended to receive 2 doses. For specific vaccines and toxoids, additional details on background, adverse reactions, precautions, and contraindications are found in the respective ACIP statements (see www.cdc.gov/vaccines/recs/acip/default.htm).

SPACING OF IMMUNOBIOLOGICS
Simultaneous Administration
All commonly used vaccines can safely and effectively be given simultaneously (on the same day) at separate sites without impairing antibody responses or increasing rates of adverse reactions. This knowledge is particularly helpful for international travelers, for whom exposure to several infectious diseases might be imminent. Simultaneous administration of all indicated vaccines is encouraged for people who are the recommended age to receive these vaccines and for whom no contraindications exist. If not administered on the same day, an inactivated vaccine may be given at any time before or after a different inactivated vaccine or a live-virus vaccine.

The immune response to an injected or intranasal live-virus vaccine (such as measles, mumps and rubella [MMR], varicella, yellow fever, or live attenuated influenza vaccine) might be impaired if administered within 28 days of another live-virus vaccine (within 30 days for yellow fever vaccine). Whenever possible, injected live-virus vaccines administered on different days should be given ≥28 days apart (≥30 days for yellow fever vaccine). If 2 injected or intranasal live-virus vaccines are not administered on the same day but <28 days apart (<30 days for yellow fever vaccine), the second vaccine should be readministered ≥28 days (≥30 days for yellow fever vaccine) after the second vaccine was administered.

Live-virus vaccines can interfere with the response to tuberculin testing. Tuberculin testing, if otherwise indicated, can be done either on the day that live-virus vaccines are administered or 4–6 weeks later. Tuberculin skin testing is not a prerequisite for administration of any vaccine.

Missed Doses and Boosters
Travelers may forget to return for a booster at the specified time. Occasionally, the demand for a vaccine may exceed its supply, and providers may have difficulty obtaining vaccines. Information on vaccine shortages and recommendations can be found on the CDC Vaccines and Immunization website at www.cdc.gov/vaccines/vac-gen/shortages/default.htm.

It is unnecessary in these cases to restart the interrupted series or to add any extra doses, except for oral typhoid. The next scheduled dose should be given when the patient returns. There are no data for interrupted dosing with oral typhoid vaccine. Advice in this situation would need to be individualized. Information on revaccination (booster) doses of vaccines is listed in Table 2-1.

Antibody-Containing Blood Products
Antibody-containing blood products from the United States do not interfere with the immune response to yellow fever vaccine, and are not believed to interfere with the response to live attenuated influenza, rotavirus, or zoster vaccines. When MMR and varicella vaccines are given shortly before, simultaneously with, or after an antibody-containing blood product, such as immune globulin (IG) or a blood transfusion, response to the vaccine can be diminished. The duration of inhibition of MMR and varicella vaccines is related to the dose of IG in the product. MMR or its components and varicella vaccines either should be administered ≥2 weeks before receipt of a blood product, or should be delayed 3–11 months after receipt of the blood product, depending on the vaccine (Table 2-2).

IG administration may become necessary for another indication after MMR or its individual components or varicella vaccines have been given. In such a situation, the IG may interfere with the immune response to the MMR or varicella vaccines. Vaccine virus replication and stimulation of immunity usually occur 2–3 weeks after vaccination. If the interval between administration of one of these vaccines and the subsequent administration of an IG preparation is ≥14 days, the

Table 2-1. Revaccination (booster) schedules

VACCINE	RECOMMENDATION
Hepatitis A (HAV)	Booster doses not recommended for adults and children who have completed the primary series (2 doses) according to the routine schedule.[1]
Hepatitis B (HBV)	Booster doses not recommended for adults and children who have completed the primary series (3 doses) according to the routine schedule.[1,2]
Influenza	1 annual dose (children aged 6 months to 9 years, and certain incompletely vaccinated children, should receive 2 doses separated by ≥4 weeks the first time that influenza vaccine is administered). Live attenuated influenza vaccine is approved only for healthy, nonpregnant people 2–49 years of age.
Japanese encephalitis	Vero cell formulation (people aged ≥17 years)—a revaccination dose can be considered if it has been 1–2 years since series completion. See the booster dose information in Chapter 3, Japanese Encephalitis.
Measles, mumps, and rubella (MMR)	2 doses of MMR vaccine separated by ≥4 weeks or other evidence of immunity (such as serologic testing) are recommended for people born after 1956 who travel outside the United States. Revaccination is not recommended.
Meningococcal quadrivalent A, C, Y, W-135	Revaccination for people who received meningococcal polysaccharide vaccine or meningococcal conjugate vaccine, and who remain at increased risk for meningococcal disease (including some international travelers): Revaccination with meningococcal conjugate vaccine is recommended after 3 years for children who were previously vaccinated at ages 2–6 years. Revaccination with meningococcal conjugate vaccine is recommended after 5 years for people who were previously vaccinated at ages 7–55 years, and every 5 years thereafter for people who are at continued risk.[3] Revaccination with meningococcal polysaccharide vaccine is recommended for adults >55 years who remain at increased risk.
Pneumococcal (polysaccharide)	1-time revaccination 5 years after original dose for people with certain underlying medical conditions (such as asplenia) or people who were first vaccinated at <65 years of age.

continued

TABLE 2-1. REVACCINATION (BOOSTER) SCHEDULES (continued)

VACCINE	RECOMMENDATION
Polio vaccine (inactivated) or IPV	For adults traveling to areas where poliomyelitis cases are still occurring, a single lifetime booster dose is recommended for those who have documentation of having completed a primary series.
Rabies preexposure vaccine	No serologic testing or boosters recommended for travelers. For people in high-risk groups (such as rabies laboratory workers), serologic testing and booster doses are recommended. See Table 3-15.
Rotavirus	Booster doses not recommended.
Tetanus, diphtheria, and acellular pertussis (Td, Tdap)	Tetanus and diphtheria booster dose is recommended every 10 years. A single dose of adolescent/adult formulation Td that includes acellular pertussis vaccine (Tdap) is recommended to replace 1 Td booster dose for people aged 11–64 years. Adults aged ≥65 years who have or who anticipate having close contact with an infant aged <12 months and who previously have not received Tdap should receive a single dose of Tdap to protect against pertussis and reduce the likelihood of transmission; all other adults aged ≥65 years who have not previously received Tdap may be given a single dose of Tdap instead of Td. See ACIP statement for details.
Typhoid intramuscular	Booster dose every 2 years for those who remain at continued risk.
Typhoid oral	Repeat series every 5 years for those who remain at continued risk.
Varicella	Revaccination is not recommended.
Yellow fever	Repeat vaccination every 10 years for those who remain at risk.

[1] A 3- or 4-dose series of combination hepatitis A-hepatitis B vaccine (HepA-HepB) is also available.
[2] Booster dosing may be appropriate for certain populations, such as hemodialysis patients.
[3] See: CDC. Updated recommendation from the Advisory Committee on Immunization Practices (ACIP) for revaccination of persons at prolonged increased risk for meningococcal disease. MMWR Morb Mortal Wkly Rep. 2009 Sep 25;58(37):1042–3.

Table 2-2. Recommended intervals between administration of antibody-containing products and measles-containing vaccine or varicella-containing vaccine[1]

INDICATION	DOSE	RECOMMENDED INTERVAL BEFORE MEASLES OR VARICELLA VACCINATION
Tetanus (TIG)	250 units (10 mg IgG/kg) IM	3 months
Hepatitis A (IG), duration of international travel		
<3-month stay	0.02 mL/kg (3.3 mg IgG/kg) IM	3 months
≥3-month stay	0.06 mL/kg (10 mg IgG/kg) IM	3 months
Hepatitis B prophylaxis (HBIG)	0.06 mL/kg (10 mg IgG/kg) IM	3 months
Rabies prophylaxis (HRIG)	20 IU/kg (22 mg IgG/kg) IM	4 months
Varicella prophylaxis (VZIG)	125 units/10 kg (60–200 mg IgG/kg) IM (maximum 625 units)	5 months
Measles prophylaxis (IG)		
Immunocompetent contact	0.25 mL/kg (40 mg IgG/kg) IM	5 months
Immunocompromised contact	0.50 mL/kg (80 mg IgG/kg) IM	6 months
Botulism immune globulin, intravenous	1.5 mL/kg (75 mg IgG/kg) IV	6 months
Blood transfusion		
Red blood cells (RBCs), washed	10 mL/kg (negligible IgG/kg) IV	None
RBCs, adenine-saline added	10 mL/kg (10 mg IgG/kg) IV	3 months
Packed RBCs (hematocrit 65%)[2]	10 mL/kg (60 mg IgG/kg) IV	6 months
Whole blood (hematocrit 35%–50%)[2]	10 mL/kg (80–100 mg IgG/kg) IV	6 months
Plasma/platelet products	10 mL/kg (160 mg IgG/kg) IV	7 months
Cytomegalovirus prophylaxis (CMV IGIV)	150 mg/kg maximum	6 months
Respiratory syncytial virus (RSV) monoclonal antibody[3]	15 mg/kg IM	None

continued

TABLE 2-2. RECOMMENDED INTERVALS BETWEEN ADMINISTRATION OF ANTIBODY-CONTAINING PRODUCTS AND MEASLES-CONTAINING VACCINE OR VARICELLA-CONTAINING VACCINE[1] (continued)

INDICATION	DOSE	RECOMMENDED INTERVAL BEFORE MEASLES OR VARICELLA VACCINATION
Intravenous immune globulin (IVIG)		
Replacement therapy	300–400 mg/kg IV	8 months
Immune thrombocytopenic purpura (ITP)	400 mg/kg IV	8 months
Postexposure varicella prophylaxis[4]	400 mg/kg IV	8 months
ITP	1 gm/kg IV	10 months
ITP or Kawasaki disease	1.6–2 gm/kg IV	11 months

Abbreviations: IG, immune globulin; IM, intramuscular; IV, intravenous.

[1] Adapted from Table 5, Kroger AT, Sumaya CV, Pickering LK, Atkinson WL. General recommendations on immunization: recommendations of the Advisory Committee on Immunization Practices (ACIP). MMWR Recomm Rep. 2011 Jan 28;60(RR-2):1–61. This table is not intended for determining the correct indications and dosage for the use of IG preparations. Unvaccinated people may not be fully protected against measles during the entire recommended interval, and additional doses of IG or measles vaccine may be indicated after measles exposure. Concentrations of measles antibody in an IG preparation can vary by manufacturer's lot. For example, more than a 4-fold variation in the amount of measles antibody titers has been demonstrated in different IG preparations. Rates of antibody clearance after receipt of an IG preparation can also vary. Recommended intervals are extrapolated from an estimated half-life of 30 days for passively acquired antibody and an observed interference with the immune response to measles vaccine for 5 months after a dose of 80 mg IgG/kg.

[2] Assumes a serum IgG concentration of 16 mg/mL.

[3] Contains only antibody to respiratory syncytial virus.

[4] IVIG is an alternative to VZIG for postexposure varicella prophylaxis. Both VZIG and IVIG should be administered within 96 hours of varicella exposure. Unlike VZIG, IVIG is a licensed product and in some situations might be obtained more quickly. For pregnant women who cannot obtain VZIG within 96 hours, monitoring for signs and symptoms of varicella disease and instituting treatment with acyclovir are an alternative to IVIG.

vaccine need not be readministered. If the interval is <14 days, the vaccine should be readministered after the interval shown in Table 2-2, unless serologic testing indicates that antibodies have been produced.

If administration of IG becomes necessary, MMR or its components or varicella vaccines can be administered simultaneously with IG, with the recognition that vaccine-induced immunity can be compromised. The vaccine should be administered at a body site different from that chosen for the IG injection. Vaccination should be repeated after the interval noted in Table 2-2, unless serologic testing indicates antibodies have been produced.

When IG is given with the first dose of hepatitis A vaccine, the proportion of recipients who develop a protective level of antibody is not affected, but antibody concentrations are lower. Because the final concentrations of antibody are many times higher than those considered protective, this reduced immunogenicity is not expected to be clinically relevant. IG preparations interact minimally with other inactivated vaccines and toxoids. Other inactivated vaccines may be given simultaneously, or at any time interval before or after an antibody-containing blood product is used. However, such vaccines should be administered at different sites from the IG.

VACCINATION OF PEOPLE WITH ACUTE ILLNESSES

Every opportunity should be taken to provide appropriate vaccinations. The decision to delay vaccination because of a current or recent acute illness depends on the severity of the symptoms and their cause. Although a moderate or severe acute illness is sufficient reason to postpone vaccination, minor illnesses (such as diarrhea, mild upper respiratory infection with or without low-grade fever, other low-grade febrile illness) are not contraindications to vaccination.

People with moderate or severe acute illness, with or without fever, should be vaccinated as soon as the condition improves. This precaution is to avoid superimposing adverse effects from the vaccine on underlying illness, or mistakenly attributing a manifestation of underlying illness to the vaccine. Antimicrobial therapy is not a contraindication to vaccination, with 3 exceptions:

- Antibacterial agents may interfere with the response to oral typhoid vaccine.
- Antiviral agents active against herpesviruses (such as acyclovir) may interfere with the response to varicella-containing vaccines.
- Antiviral agents active against influenza virus (such as zanamivir and oseltamivir) may interfere with the response to live attenuated influenza vaccine.

A physical examination or temperature measurement is not a prerequisite for vaccinating a person who appears to be in good health. Asking if a person is ill, postponing a vaccination for someone with moderate or severe acute illness, and vaccinating someone who does not have contraindications are appropriate procedures for clinic immunizations.

ALTERED IMMUNOCOMPETENCE

Altered immunocompetence is a general term that is often used interchangeably with the terms immunosuppression, immunodeficiency, and a weakened immune system. It can be caused either by a disease (leukemia, HIV infection) or by drugs or other therapies (cancer chemotherapy, prolonged high-dose corticosteroids). It can also include conditions such as asplenia and chronic renal disease.

Determination of altered immunocompetence is important because the incidence or severity of some vaccine-preventable diseases is higher in people with altered immunocompetence. Therefore, certain vaccines (such as inactivated influenza vaccine, pneumococcal vaccines) are recommended specifically for people with altered immunocompetence. Inactivated vaccine may be safely administered to a person with altered immunocompetence, although response to the vaccine may be suboptimal. The vaccine may need to be repeated after immune function has improved.

People with altered immunocompetence may be at increased risk for an adverse reaction after administration of live attenuated vaccines because of reduced ability to mount an effective immune response. Live vaccines should generally be deferred until immune function has improved. This is particularly important when planning to give yellow fever vaccine (see Chapter 3, Yellow Fever). MMR and varicella vaccines are recommended for people with mild or moderate immunosuppression.

For an in-depth discussion, see Chapter 8, Immunocompromised Travelers.

VACCINATION SCHEDULING FOR LAST-MINUTE TRAVELERS

As noted, for people anticipating imminent travel, most vaccine products can be given during the same visit. Unless the vaccines given are booster doses of those typically given during childhood, vaccines may require a month or more to induce a sufficient immune response, depending on the vaccine and the number of doses in the series. Some vaccines require more than 1 dose for best protection. Recommended spacing should be maintained between doses (Table 2-3). Doses given at less than minimum intervals can lessen the antibody response. It is important to note that if a traveler needs yellow fever vaccination to meet a country requirement under the International Health Regulations, the yellow fever vaccine is not considered valid until 10 days after administration.

Administration of a vaccine earlier than the recommended minimum age, or at an interval shorter than the recommended minimum, is discouraged. Table 2-3 lists the minimum age and minimum interval between doses for vaccines routinely recommended in the United States. Because some travelers visit their health care providers at the last minute, studies have been performed to determine whether accelerated scheduling is adequate. This concern is primarily the case for hepatitis B vaccine or the combined hepatitis A and B vaccine. An accelerated schedule for combined hepatitis A and B vaccine has been approved by the Food and Drug

Table 2-3. Recommended and minimum ages and intervals between vaccine doses[1,2]

VACCINE AND DOSE NUMBER	RECOMMENDED AGE FOR THIS DOSE	MINIMUM AGE FOR THIS DOSE	MINIMUM INTERVAL TO NEXT DOSE[3]
Diphtheria and tetanus toxoids and acellular pertussis vaccine, pediatric (6 weeks through 6 years) (DTaP)-1[4]	2 months	6 weeks	4 weeks
DTaP-2	4 months	10 weeks	4 weeks
DTaP-3	6 months	14 weeks	6 months[5,6]
DTaP-4	15–18 months	12 months	6 months[5]
DTaP-5	4–6 years	4 years	NA
Haemophilus influenzae type b (Hib)-1[4,7]	2 months	6 weeks	4 weeks
Hib-2	4 months	10 weeks	4 weeks
Hib-3[8]	6 months	14 weeks	8 weeks
Hib-4	12–15 months	12 months	NA
Hepatitis A (HepA)-1	12–23 months	12 months	6 months[5]
HepA-2	≥18 months	18 months	NA
Hepatitis B (HepB)-1[4]	Birth	Birth	4 weeks
HepB-2	1–2 months	4 weeks	8 weeks
HepB-3[9]	6–18 months	24 weeks	NA
Herpes zoster[10]	≥60 years	60 years	NA
Human papillomavirus (HPV)-1[11]	11–12 years	9 years	4 weeks
HPV-2	2 months after dose 1	9 years, 4 weeks	12 weeks[12]

continued

TABLE 2-3. RECOMMENDED AND MINIMUM AGES AND INTERVALS BETWEEN VACCINE DOSES[1,2] (continued)

VACCINE AND DOSE NUMBER	RECOMMENDED AGE FOR THIS DOSE	MINIMUM AGE FOR THIS DOSE	MINIMUM INTERVAL TO NEXT DOSE[3]
HPV-3[12]	6 months after dose 1	9 years, 24 weeks	NA
Inactivated poliovirus (IPV)-1[4]	2 months	6 weeks	4 weeks
IPV-2	4 months	10 weeks	4 weeks
IPV-3	6–18 months	14 weeks	6 months
IPV-4[13]	4–6 years	4 years	NA
Influenza, inactivated[14]	≥6 months	6 months[15]	4 weeks
Influenza, live attenuated[14]	2–49 years	2 years	4 weeks
Japanese encephalitis, mouse brain (JE-MB)-1[16]	≥1 year	1 year	7 days
JE-MB-2	7 days after dose 1	1 year, 7 days	14 days
JE-MB-3	30 days after dose 1	1 year, 21 days	NA
Japanese encephalitis, Vero cell (JE-VC)-1[16]	≥17 years	≥17 years	28 days
JE-VC-2	28 days after dose 1	≥17 years, 28 days	NA
Measles, mumps, and rubella (MMR)-1[17]	12–15 months	12 months	4 weeks
MMR-2[17]	4–6 years	13 months	NA
Meningococcal conjugate (MenACWY-1)[18]	11–12 years	2 years	8 weeks[19]
MenACWY-2	16 years	11 years, 8 weeks	NA
Meningococcal polysaccharide (MPSV4)-1[18]	NA	2 years	5 years
MPSV4–2	NA	7 years	NA

continued

TABLE 2-3. RECOMMENDED AND MINIMUM AGES AND INTERVALS BETWEEN VACCINE DOSES[1,2] (continued)

VACCINE AND DOSE NUMBER	RECOMMENDED AGE FOR THIS DOSE	MINIMUM AGE FOR THIS DOSE	MINIMUM INTERVAL TO NEXT DOSE[3]
Pneumococcal conjugate (PCV)-1[7]	2 months	6 weeks	4 weeks
PCV-2	4 months	10 weeks	4 weeks
PCV-3	6 months	14 weeks	8 weeks
PCV-4	12–15 months	12 months	NA
Pneumococcal polysaccharide (PPSV)-1	NA	2 years	5 years
PPSV-2[20]	NA	7 years	NA
Rabies-1 (preexposure)	See footnote 21	See footnote 21	7 days
Rabies-2	7 days after dose 1	7 days after dose 1	14 days
Rabies-3	21 days after dose 1	21 days after dose 1	NA
Rotavirus (RV)-1[22]	2 months	6 weeks	4 weeks
RV-2	4 months	10 weeks	4 weeks
RV-3[22]	6 months	14 weeks	NA
Tetanus and reduced diphtheria toxoids (Td)	11–12 years	7 years	5 years
Tetanus toxoid, reduced diphtheria toxoid, and reduced acellular pertussis vaccine (Tdap)[23]	≥11 years	7 years	NA
Typhoid, inactivated (ViCPS)	≥2 years	≥2 years	NA
Typhoid, live attenuated (Ty21a)	≥6 years	≥6 years	See footnote 24
Varicella (Var)-1[17]	12–15 months	12 months	12 weeks[25]
Yellow fever	≥9 months[26]	≥9 months[26]	10 years

continued

[1] Adapted from Table 1, Kroger AT, Sumaya CV, Pickering LK, Atkinson WL. General recommendations on immunization: recommendations of the Advisory Committee on Immunization Practices (ACIP). MMWR Recomm Rep. 2011 Jan 28;60(RR-2):1–61.

[2] Combination vaccines are available. Use of licensed combination vaccines is generally preferred over separate injections of their equivalent component vaccines (CDC. Combination vaccines for childhood immunization. MMWR Recomm Rep. 1999 May 14;48(RR-5):1–14.). When administering combination vaccines, the minimum age for administration is the oldest age for any of the individual components; the minimum interval between doses is equal to the largest interval of any of the individual components.

[3] See Table 2–1 for recommended revaccination (booster) schedules.

[4] Combination vaccines containing the HepB component are available (HepB-Hib, DTaP-HepB-IPV, HepA-HepB). These vaccines should not be administered to infants aged <6 weeks because of the other components (Hib, DTaP, IPV). HepA-HepB is not licensed for children aged <18 years in the United States.

[5] Calendar months.

[6] The minimum recommended interval between DTaP-3 and DTaP-4 is 6 months. However, DTaP-4 need not be repeated if administered ≥4 months after DTaP-3.

[7] For Hib and PCV, children receiving the first dose of vaccine at ≥7 months of age require fewer doses to complete the series (see the current childhood and adolescent immunization schedule at www.cdc.gov/vaccines).

[8] If PRP-OMP (Pedvax-Hib, Merck Vaccine Division) was administered at 2 and 4 months of age, a dose at 6 months of age is not indicated.

[9] HepB-3 should be administered ≥8 weeks after Hep B-2 and ≥16 weeks after Hep B-1; it should not be administered before age 24 weeks.

[10] Herpes zoster (shingles) vaccine is approved as a single dose for people aged ≥60 years.

[11] Bivalent HPV vaccine is approved for girls/women aged 10–25 years. It is recommended to prevent cervical and other anogenital cancers and precursors for girls/women aged 11–26 years. Quadrivalent HPV vaccine is approved for boys/men and girls/women aged 9–26 years. It is recommended to prevent cervical and other anogenital cancers, precursors, and genital warts for girls/women aged 11–26 years. It may be given to girls aged 9–10 years to prevent the same diseases, and to boys/men aged 9–26 years to prevent genital warts.

[12] The third dose of HPV should be administered ≥12 weeks after the second and ≥24 weeks after the first. Dose 3 need not be repeated if administered ≥16 weeks after dose 1.

[13] For people receiving an all-IPV or all-OPV series, if the third dose is given after the fourth birthday, a fourth dose is not needed.

[14] Two doses of influenza vaccine are recommended for children aged <9 years who are receiving the vaccine for the first time, and for certain incompletely vaccinated children (see reference 7). All others need only 1 dose annually. The doses of inactivated influenza vaccine are 0.25 mL for children aged 6–35 months and 0.5 mL for people aged ≥3 years.

[15] The minimum age for inactivated influenza vaccine varies by vaccine manufacturer. See package insert for vaccine-specific minimum ages.

[16] The available supply of JE-Vax should be reserved for children aged 1–16 years. Ixiaro is approved by the Food and Drug Administration for people aged ≥17 years.

[17] Combination MMR-varicella can be used for children aged 12 months through 12 years. Also see footnote 25.

[18] Revaccination with meningococcal vaccine is recommended for people previously vaccinated who remain at high risk for meningococcal disease (see Table 2–1). MenACWY is preferred when revaccinating people aged 2–55 years (Bilukha OO, Rosenstein N. Prevention and control of meningococcal disease. Recommendations of the Advisory Committee on Immunization Practices (ACIP). MMWR Recomm Rep. 2005 May 27;54(RR-7):1–21.).

[19] People aged 2–54 years with persistent complement component deficiency (such as C5–C9, properidin, factor H, or factor D) and functional or anatomic asplenia, and for adolescents with human immunodeficiency virus (HIV) infection should receive a 2-dose primary series administered 2 months apart (CDC. Updated recommendations for use of meningococcal conjugate vaccines—Advisory Committee on Immunization Practices (ACIP), 2010. MMWR 2011;60(03); 72–6).

[20] A second dose of PPSV is recommended for people aged ≥65 years who received a first dose at an age <65 years and at a five year minimum interval. A second dose is also recommended for people aged <65 years at highest risk for serious pneumococcal infection and those who are likely to have a rapid decline in pneumococcal antibody concentration (CDC. Prevention of pneumococcal disease: recommendations of the Advisory Committee on Immunization Practices (ACIP). MMWR Recomm Rep. 1997 Apr 4;46(RR-8):1–24.).

[21] There is no minimum age for preexposure immunization for rabies (Manning SE, Rupprecht CE, Fishbein D, Hanlon CA, Lumlertdacha B, Guerra M, et al. Human rabies prevention—United States, 2008: recommendations of the Advisory Committee on Immunization Practices. MMWR Recomm Rep. 2008 May 23;57(RR-3):1–28.).

[22] The first dose of RV must be administered by 14 weeks and 6 days of age. The vaccine series should not be started at ≥15 weeks of age. The final dose in the series should be administered by age 8 months, 0 days. If Rotarix rotavirus vaccine is administered at 2 and 4 months of age, a dose at 6 months of age is not indicated.

[23] Only 1 dose of Tdap is recommended. Subsequent doses should be given as Td. Children aged 7–10 years who are not fully vaccinated against pertussis and for whom no contraindication to pertussis vaccine exists should receive a single dose of Tdap. If additional doses of tetanus and diphtheria toxoid-containing vaccines are needed, then children aged 7–10 years should be vaccinated according to catch-up guidance, with Tdap preferred as the first dose. Tdap vaccine, when indicated, should be administered regardless of the interval since the last dose of Td vaccine. For management of a tetanus-prone wound, the minimum interval after a previous dose of any tetanus-containing vaccine is 5 years.

[24] Oral typhoid vaccine is recommended to be administered 1 hour before a meal with a cold or lukewarm drink (temperature not to exceed body temperature—98.6°F [37°C]) on alternate days, for a total of 4 doses.

[25] The minimum interval from Var-1 to Var-2 for people beginning the series at ≥13 years of age is 4 weeks.

[26] Yellow fever vaccine may be administered to children aged <9 months in certain situations (Cetron MS, Marfin AA, Julian KG, Gubler DJ, Sharp DJ, Barwick RS, et al. Yellow fever vaccine. Recommendations of the Advisory Committee on Immunization Practices (ACIP), 2002. MMWR Recomm Rep. 2002 Nov 8;51(RR-17):1–11.).

Administration (FDA). It is unclear what level of protection any given traveler will have if he or she does not complete a full series of multidose vaccination.

ALLERGY TO VACCINE COMPONENTS

Vaccine components can cause allergic reactions in some recipients. These reactions can be local or systemic and can include anaphylaxis or anaphylactic-like responses. The vaccine components responsible can include the vaccine antigen, animal proteins, antibiotics, preservatives (such as thimerosal), or stabilizers (such as gelatin). The most common animal protein allergen is egg protein in vaccines prepared by using embryonated chicken eggs (influenza and yellow fever vaccines). Generally, people who can eat eggs or egg products safely may receive these vaccines, while those with histories of anaphylactic allergy (hives, swelling of the mouth and throat, difficulty breathing, hypotension, shock) to eggs or egg proteins ordinarily should not. Screening people by asking whether they can eat eggs without adverse effects is a reasonable way to identify those who might be at risk from receiving yellow fever and influenza vaccines. Recent studies have indicated that other components in vaccines in addition to egg proteins (such as gelatin) may cause allergic reactions, including anaphylaxis in rare instances. Protocols have been developed for testing and vaccinating people with anaphylactic reactions to egg ingestion.

Some vaccines contain a preservative or trace amounts of antibiotics to which people might be allergic. Providers administering the vaccines should carefully review the prescribing information before deciding if the rare person with such an allergy should receive the vaccine. No recommended vaccine contains penicillin or penicillin derivatives. Some vaccines (MMR and its individual component vaccines, inactivated polio vaccine [IPV], varicella, rabies) contain trace amounts of neomycin or other antibiotics; the amount is less than would normally be used for the skin test to determine hypersensitivity. However, people who have experienced anaphylactic reactions to this antibiotic generally should not receive these vaccines. Most often, neomycin allergy is a contact dermatitis—a manifestation of a delayed-type (cell-mediated) immune response rather than anaphylaxis.

A history of delayed-type reactions to neomycin is not a contraindication to receiving these vaccines.

Thimerosal, an organic mercurial compound in use since the 1930s, has been added to certain immunobiologic products as a preservative. Thimerosal is present at preservative concentrations (trace quantities) in multidose vials of some brands of vaccine. Receiving thimerosal-containing vaccines has been postulated to lead to induction of allergy. However, there is limited scientific evidence for this assertion. Allergy to thimerosal usually consists of local delayed-type hypersensitivity reactions. Thimerosal elicits positive delayed-type hypersensitivity patch tests in 1%–18% of people tested, but these tests have limited or no clinical relevance. Most people do not experience reactions to thimerosal administered as a component of vaccines, even when patch or intradermal tests for thimerosal indicate hypersensitivity. A localized or delayed-type hypersensitivity reaction to thimerosal is not a contraindication to receipt of a vaccine that contains thimerosal.

Since mid-2001, vaccines routinely recommended for infants have been manufactured without thimerosal as a preservative. Additional information about thimerosal and the thimerosal content of vaccines is available on the FDA website (www.fda.gov/cber/vaccine/thimerosal.htm).

REPORTING ADVERSE EVENTS AFTER IMMUNIZATION

Modern vaccines are extremely safe and effective. Benefits and risks are associated with the use of all immunobiologics—no vaccine is completely effective or completely free of side effects. Adverse events after immunization have been reported with all vaccines, ranging from frequent, minor, local reactions to extremely rare, severe, systemic illness, such as that associated with yellow fever vaccine. Side effects and adverse events following specific vaccines and toxoids are discussed in detail in each ACIP statement. In the United States, clinicians are required by law to report selected adverse events occurring after vaccination with tetanus vaccine in any combination; pertussis in any combination; measles, mumps, or rubella, alone or in any combination; oral polio vaccine (OPV); IPV; hepatitis A; hepatitis B; varicella; Hib (conjugate);

pneumococcal conjugate; rotavirus vaccines; HPV; and meningococcal vaccines (conjugate and polysaccharide). In addition, CDC strongly recommends that all vaccine adverse events be reported to the Vaccine Adverse Event Reporting System (VAERS), even if a causal relation to vaccination is not certain. VAERS reporting forms and information are available electronically at www.vaers.hhs.gov, or they may be requested by telephone: 800-822-7967. Clinicians are encouraged to report electronically at https://vaers.hhs.gov/esub/step1.

INJECTION ROUTE AND INJECTION SITE

Injectable vaccines are administered by intramuscular and subcutaneous routes. The method of administration of injectable vaccines depends in part on the presence of an adjuvant in some vaccines. The term *adjuvant* refers to a vaccine component distinct from the antigen, which enhances the immune response to the antigen. Vaccines containing an adjuvant (DTaP, DT, HPV, Td, Tdap, pneumococcal conjugate, Hib, hepatitis A, hepatitis B) should be injected into a muscle mass, because administration subcutaneously or intradermally can cause local irritation, induration, skin discoloration, inflammation, and granuloma formation.

Routes of administration are recommended by the manufacturer for each immunobiologic. Deviation from the recommended route of administration may reduce vaccine efficacy or increase local adverse reactions. Detailed recommendations on the appropriate route and site for all vaccines have been published in ACIP recommendations; a compiled list of these publications is available on the CDC website at www.cdc.gov/vaccines/pubs/ACIP-list.htm (also see Table C-1. Travel vaccine summary in Appendix C).

BIBLIOGRAPHY

1. Ball LK, Ball R, Pratt RD. An assessment of thimerosal use in childhood vaccines. Pediatrics. 2001 May;107(5):1147–1154.
2. Bilukha OO, Rosenstein N. Prevention and control of meningococcal disease. Recommendations of the Advisory Committee on Immunization Practices (ACIP). MMWR Recomm Rep. 2005 May 27;54(RR-7):1–21.
3. CDC. Combination vaccines for childhood immunization. MMWR Recomm Rep. 1999 May 14;48(RR-5):1–14.
4. CDC. Prevention of pneumococcal disease: recommendations of the Advisory Committee on Immunization Practices (ACIP). MMWR Recomm Rep. 1997 Apr 4;46(RR-8):1–24.
5. CDC. Updated recommendations for use of meningococcal conjugate vaccines—Advisory Committee on Immunization Practices (ACIP), 2010. MMWR 2011;60(03):72–6.
6. CDC. Updated recommendations for use of tetanus toxoid, reduced diphtheria toxoid and acellular pertussis (Tdap) vaccine from the Advisory Committee on Immunization Practices, 2010. MMWR Morb Mortal Wkly Rep. 2011 Jan 14;60(1):13–5.
7. Cetron MS, Marfin AA, Julian KG, Gubler DJ, Sharp DJ, Barwick RS, et al. Yellow fever vaccine. Recommendations of the Advisory Committee on Immunization Practices (ACIP), 2002. MMWR Recomm Rep. 2002 Nov 8;51(RR-17):1–11; quiz CE1–4.
8. Fiore AE, Shay DK, Broder K, Iskander JK, Uyeki TM, Mootrey G, et al. Prevention and control of influenza: recommendations of the Advisory Committee on Immunization Practices (ACIP), 2008. MMWR Recomm Rep. 2008 Aug 8;57(RR-7):1–60.
9. Kretsinger K, Broder KR, Cortese MM, Joyce MP, Ortega-Sanchez I, Lee GM, et al. Preventing tetanus, diphtheria, and pertussis among adults: use of tetanus toxoid, reduced diphtheria toxoid and acellular pertussis vaccine recommendations of the Advisory Committee on Immunization Practices (ACIP) and recommendation of ACIP, supported by the Healthcare Infection Control Practices Advisory Committee (HICPAC), for use of Tdap among healthcare personnel. MMWR Recomm Rep. 2006 Dec 15;55(RR-17):1–37.
10. Kroger AT, Sumaya CV, Pickering LK, Atkinson WL. General recommendations on immunization: recommendations of the Advisory Committee on Immunization Practices (ACIP). MMWR Recomm Rep. 2011 Jan 28;60(RR-2):1–61.
11. Manning SE, Rupprecht CE, Fishbein D, Hanlon CA, Lumlertdacha B, Guerra M, et al. Human rabies prevention—United States, 2008: recommendations of the Advisory Committee on Immunization Practices. MMWR Recomm Rep. 2008 May 23;57(RR-3):1–28.
12. Plotkin SA. Vaccines: correlates of vaccine-induced immunity. Clin Infect Dis. 2008 Aug 1;47(3):401–99.

13. Varricchio F, Iskander J, Destefano F, Ball R, Pless R, Braun MM, et al. Understanding vaccine safety information from the Vaccine Adverse Event Reporting System. Pediatr Infect Dis J. 2004 Apr;23(4):287–294.

14. Watson JC, Hadler SC, Dykewicz CA, Reef S, Phillips L. Measles, mumps, and rubella—vaccine use and strategies for elimination of measles, rubella, and congenital rubella syndrome and control of mumps: recommendations of the Advisory Committee on Immunization Practices (ACIP). MMWR Recomm Rep. 1998 May 22;47(RR-8):1–57.

15. Wood RA, Berger M, Dreskin SC, Setse R, Engler RJ, Dekker CL, et al. An algorithm for treatment of patients with hypersensitivity reactions after vaccines. Pediatrics. 2008 Sep;122(3):e771–7.

Perspectives

VACCINE RECOMMENDATIONS OF THE ACIP

Amanda Cantor, Jean Clare Smith

The Advisory Committee on Immunization Practices (ACIP) is a federal advisory committee, the purpose of which is to advise and provide guidance to the Secretary of the US Department of Health and Human Services (HHS), the Assistant Secretary for Health (the primary advisor to the Secretary), and the Director of CDC regarding the use of vaccines and related agents to control vaccine-preventable diseases in the civilian population. The committee meets 3 times annually and is made up of 15 members who are selected by the HHS Secretary. These members are considered to be authorities knowledgeable in immunization practices and public health, who have expertise in the use of vaccines and other immunobiologic agents in clinical practice or preventive medicine, have expertise with clinical or laboratory vaccine research, or have expertise in assessing vaccine efficacy and safety.

ACIP advises specifically for the control of diseases for which a vaccine is licensed in the United States. This guidance covers the appropriate use of the licensed vaccine, and can include recommendations for administration of immune globulin preparations or antimicrobial therapy shown to be effective in controlling the same disease. For each recommended vaccine, ACIP advises on population groups or circumstances in which a vaccine or related agent is recommended, and develops guidance on the route, dose, and frequency of administration of the vaccine, immune globulin, or antimicrobial agent. In addition, the committee provides recommendations on contraindications and precautions for use of the vaccine and related agents, as well as information on recognized adverse events. All deliberations on the appropriate use of vaccines include consideration of population-based studies, such as efficacy, cost-benefit, and risk-benefit analyses. As new information becomes available regarding a particular vaccine, or if the risk of disease changes, ACIP can alter or withdraw their recommendations. ACIP recommendations, provisional recommendations, and immunization schedules, along with additional useful information published in Morbidity and Mortality Weekly Report, are listed on the CDC website (www.cdc.gov/vaccines/recs/acip).

In exceptional circumstances, ACIP guidance for use of unlicensed vaccines may be developed. For example, in the late 1980s, the Japanese manufacturer Biken produced an inactivated mouse brain–derived Japanese encephalitis vaccine. The vaccine was not licensed in the United States, but after a US student died in Beijing from Japanese encephalitis, ACIP/CDC formulated recommendations for the use of the Biken vaccine to US travelers and to the military under an investigational new drug application. ACIP/CDC reacted in a flexible way to provide guidance for preventing a serious disease that could affect US citizens.

ACIP also establishes, reviews, and, as appropriate, revises the list of vaccines for administration to children and adolescents who are eligible to receive vaccines through the Vaccines for Children Program. The Vaccines for Children Program is an entitlement program with an annual budget of $3 billion that provides vaccines free of charge to underinsured, uninsured, Medicaid-eligible, and American Indian/Alaska Native children. It also provides schedules regarding the appropriate dose and dosing interval and contraindications to administration of the pediatric vaccines.

Although some of the vaccine recommendations include guidance pertaining to travelers, not all ACIP guidelines specifically address travel. These recommendations are meant to be for the use of vaccines to benefit public health in the most cost-effective manner possible. Many of the routine vaccinations that are considered in the pre-travel consultation do not relate to diseases that are unique to the country of destination, but are included to ensure that travelers are protected against routine vaccine-preventable diseases (such as tetanus or measles). Table 2-4 provides a list of the vaccines listed in the Yellow Book, and a short assessment of the guidance for travelers detailed by ACIP. Instances where ACIP recommendations differ from the prescribing information are indicated.

Other ACIP recommendations are provided for:

- General recommendations on immunizations
- Immunization of health care personnel
- Anthrax
- *Haemophilus influenzae* type B
- Hib and DTP
- Vaccinia (smallpox)
- Herpes zoster (shingles)

For more information regarding the ACIP and to access each ACIP vaccine recommendation, visit www.cdc.gov/vaccines/recs/acip/#recs. To access current prescribing information for FDA-licensed vaccines, visit www.fda.gov/BiologicsBloodVaccines/Vaccines/ApprovedProducts/ucm093830.htm.

Table 2-4. Vaccines described in the CDC Yellow Book and recommendations by ACIP

VACCINE IN THE YELLOW BOOK	BRIEF REVIEW OF TRAVEL ADVICE PROVIDED BY ACIP	DIFFERENCE BETWEEN ACIP GUIDANCE AND FDA LICENSE
Hepatitis A	People traveling to or working in intermediate- to high-endemicity areas	None
Hepatitis B	*Not specific to travelers*	FDA has not approved accelerated schedules in which hepatitis B vaccine is administered more than once in 1 month. If an accelerated schedule (such as doses at 0, 7, and 14 days) is used, the patient also should receive a booster dose ≥6 months after the start of the series to promote long-term immunity.
Human papillomavirus	*Not specific to travelers*	None
Influenza	Any traveler who wants to reduce the risk for influenza infection should consider influenza vaccination, preferably ≥2 weeks before departure. In particular, people at high risk for complications of influenza and who were not vaccinated with influenza vaccine during the preceding fall or winter should consider receiving influenza vaccine before travel if they plan to travel to the tropics, with organized tourist groups at any time of year, or to the Southern Hemisphere during April–September.	None
Japanese encephalitis	Japanese encephalitis vaccine is recommended for travelers who plan to spend ≥1 month in endemic areas during the JEV transmission season. This includes long-term travelers, recurrent travelers, or expatriates who will be based in urban areas but are likely to visit endemic rural or agricultural areas during a high-risk period of JEV transmission. Vaccination should be considered for: • Short-term (<1 month) travelers to endemic areas during the JEV transmission season, if they plan to travel outside an urban area and have an increased risk for JEV exposure • Travelers to an area with an ongoing JEV outbreak • Travelers to endemic areas who are uncertain of specific destinations, activities, or duration of travel	None

continued

VACCINE IN THE YELLOW BOOK	BRIEF REVIEW OF TRAVEL ADVICE PROVIDED BY ACIP	DIFFERENCE BETWEEN ACIP GUIDANCE AND FDA LICENSE
Measles, mumps, and rubella	Protection against measles is especially important for people planning foreign travel, including adolescents and adults who have not had measles and have not been adequately vaccinated, and infants aged 6–11 months. Similarly, protection against rubella is especially important for women of childbearing age who are not immune to the disease. Children who travel or live abroad should be vaccinated at an earlier age than recommended for children remaining in the United States. Parents who travel or reside abroad with infants aged <12 months should have acceptable evidence of immunity to rubella and mumps, as well as measles.	None
Meningococcal	For travelers, vaccination is especially recommended for those visiting the parts of sub-Saharan Africa known as the "meningitis belt" during the dry season (December–June). Vaccination is required by the government of Saudi Arabia for all travelers to Mecca during the annual Hajj. Advisories for travelers to other countries are issued when epidemics of meningococcal disease, caused by vaccine-preventable serogroups, are detected.	On February 19, 2010, FDA licensed a quadrivalent meningococcal conjugate vaccine, MenACWY$_{CRM}$. MenACWY$_{CRM}$ is licensed by FDA as a single dose in people aged 11–55 years.
Pertussis vaccine (acellular)	*Not specific to travelers*	None
Pneumococcal conjugate	*Not specific to travelers*	On February 24, 2010, a 13-valent pneumococcal conjugate vaccine (PCV13) was licensed by FDA to prevent invasive pneumococcal disease caused by the 13 pneumococcal serotypes covered by the vaccine, and to prevent otitis media caused by serotypes in the 7-valent pneumococcal conjugate vaccine formulation. PCV13 is licensed for use among children aged 6 weeks–71 months, and succeeds PCV7, which was licensed by FDA in 2000.
Pneumococcal polysaccharide 23-valent	*Not specific to travelers*	None

continued

TABLE 2-4. VACCINES DESCRIBED IN THE CDC YELLOW BOOK AND RECOMMENDATIONS BY ACIP (continued)

VACCINE IN THE YELLOW BOOK	BRIEF REVIEW OF TRAVEL ADVICE PROVIDED BY ACIP	DIFFERENCE BETWEEN ACIP GUIDANCE AND FDA LICENSE
Polio	IPV is recommended for travelers to areas or countries where polio is epidemic or endemic.	None
Rabies	*Not specific to travelers*	None
Rotavirus	*Not specific to travelers*	None
Tdap vaccine	*Not specific to travelers*	None
Typhoid	Travelers to areas in which there is a risk of exposure to *S.* Typhi. Risk is highest for travelers to developing countries who have prolonged exposure to potentially contaminated food and drink.	None
Varicella (chickenpox)	Adults who might be at increased risk for exposure or transmission and who do not have evidence of immunity should receive special consideration for vaccination, which includes international travelers.	None
Yellow fever	People aged ≥9 months who are traveling to or living in areas at risk for YF virus transmission in South America and Africa. In addition, some countries require proof of YF vaccination for entry.	The manufacturer and FDA state that vaccination of infants aged <9 months is contraindicated because of the risk for encephalitis. ACIP considers ages 6–8 months to be a precaution for YF vaccination. Whenever possible, travel by children ages 6–8 months to YF-endemic countries should be postponed or avoided. If travel is unavoidable, vaccination decisions for these infants need to balance the risk of YF virus exposure with the risk for adverse events following vaccination. (The administration of YF vaccine to infants <6 months is contraindicated by both FDA and ACIP guidelines.)

Abbreviations: ACIP, Advisory Committee on Immunization Practices; FDA, Food and Drug Administration; IPV, inactivated polio vaccine; JEV, Japanese encephalitis virus; OPV, oral polio vaccine; Tdap, tetanus and diphtheria toxoids and acellular pertussis vaccine; YF yellow fever.

BIBLIOGRAPHY

1. CDC. ACIP Charter. Atlanta: CDC; 2010 [updated Apr 6; cited 2010 Nov 8]. Available from: www.cdc.gov/vaccines/recs/acip/charter.htm.

2. CDC. ACIP Recommendations: Advisory Committee on Immunization Practices (ACIP). Atlanta: CDC; 2010 [updated Nov 3; cited 2010 Sep 16]. Available from: http://www.cdc.gov/vaccines/pubs/ACIP-list.htm.

3. Smith J, Snider D, Pickering L. Immunization policy development in the United States: the role of the Advisory Committee on Immunization Practices. Ann Intern Med. 2009 Jan 6;150(1):45–9.

4. Smith JC. The structure, role, and procedures of the US Advisory Committee on Immunization Practices (ACIP). Vaccine. 2010 Apr 19;28 Suppl 1:A68–75.

DRUG-VACCINE & DRUG-DRUG INTERACTIONS

Elizabeth D. Barnett

Vaccines and medications are prescribed frequently in pre-travel consultations, and potential interactions between vaccines and medications, including those already taken by the patient, must be considered. Although a comprehensive list of interactions is beyond the scope of this section, some of the more significant interactions of commonly used vaccines and medications are discussed here.

INTERACTIONS BETWEEN TRAVEL VACCINES AND DRUGS
Oral Typhoid Vaccine

Sulfonamides and antibiotics may be active against the vaccine strain in the oral typhoid vaccine, and prevent an adequate immune response to the vaccine. Therefore, oral typhoid vaccine should not be given to people taking sulfonamides or other antibiotics, including doxycycline. Vaccination with oral typhoid vaccine should be delayed for >72 hours after the administration of any antibacterial agent. Parenteral typhoid vaccine may be a more appropriate choice for these people.

Rabies Vaccine

Concomitant use of chloroquine may reduce antibody response to intradermal rabies vaccine administered for preexposure vaccination. The intramuscular route should be used for people taking chloroquine concurrently (the intradermal route is not approved for use in the United States at this time); ideally, the rabies preexposure vaccination series should be completed before beginning chloroquine.

INTERACTIONS BETWEEN ANTIMALARIALS AND OTHER DRUGS
Mefloquine

Mefloquine may interact with several categories of drugs, including other antimalarials, drugs that alter cardiac conduction, and anticonvulsants. Although the antimalarial halofantrine is not available in the United States, travelers who might be offered treatment with this drug outside the United States should be informed about interactions with mefloquine. Potentially fatal prolongation of the QTc interval may occur if halofantrine is given after mefloquine. Halofantrine should be avoided, if at all possible. If halofantrine is given to treat malaria, mefloquine for prophylaxis should not be resumed until ≥12 hours after the last halofantrine dose. Although no conclusive data are available with regard to coadministration of mefloquine and other drugs that may affect cardiac conduction, these drugs should not be used concurrently with mefloquine. These drugs include antiarrhythmic or β-blocking agents, calcium-channel blockers, antihistamines, H_1-blocking agents, tricyclic antidepressants, or phenothiazines.

Mefloquine used with the anticonvulsants, such as valproic acid, carbamazepine, phenobarbital, or phenytoin, may lower anticonvulsant plasma levels, thus lowering seizure threshold. Monitoring anticonvulsant levels would be appropriate in people for whom mefloquine must be used concomitantly with these drugs.

Chloroquine

Chloroquine absorption may be reduced by antacids or kaolin; ≥4 hours should elapse between doses of these medications. Concomitant use of cimetidine and chloroquine should be avoided, as cimetidine can inhibit the metabolism of chloroquine and may increase drug levels. Chloroquine inhibits bioavailability of ampicillin; 2 hours should elapse between doses.

Atovaquone-proguanil

Tetracycline, rifampin, and rifabutin may reduce plasma concentrations of atovaquone and should not be used concurrently with atovaquone-proguanil. Metoclopramide may reduce bioavailability of atovaquone; unless no other antiemetics are available, this antiemetic should not be used to treat the vomiting that may accompany use of atovaquone at treatment doses. Atovaquone-proguanil should not be used with other medications that contain proguanil. Patients on anticoagulants may need to reduce their anticoagulant doses or monitor their prothrombin time more closely while taking atovaquone-proguanil, although coadministration of these drugs is not contraindicated.

Doxycycline

Phenytoin, carbamazepine, and barbiturates may decrease the half-life of doxycycline. Patients on anticoagulants may need to reduce their anticoagulant doses while taking doxycycline because of its ability to depress plasma prothrombin activity. Absorption of tetracyclines may be impaired by bismuth subsalicylate, preparations containing iron, and antacids containing calcium, magnesium, or aluminum; these preparations should not be taken within 3 hours of doxycycline. Doxycycline may interfere with the bactericidal activity of penicillin, so these drugs, in general, should not be taken together.

INTERACTIONS WITH ANTIDIARRHEAL DRUGS
Fluoroquinolones

Increase in the international normalized ratio has been reported when levofloxacin and warfarin are used concurrently. Concurrent administration of ciprofloxacin and antacids that contain magnesium or aluminum hydroxide may reduce bioavailability of ciprofloxacin. Ciprofloxacin decreases clearance of theophylline and caffeine; theophylline levels should be monitored when ciprofloxacin is used concurrently. Ciprofloxacin should not be used with tizanidine.

Azithromycin

Close monitoring for side effects of azithromycin is recommended when azithromycin is used with nelfinavir. Increased anticoagulant effects have been noted when azithromycin is used with warfarin; monitoring of prothrombin time is recommended for people taking these drugs concomitantly.

Rifaximin

No clinically significant drug interactions have been reported to date with rifaximin. Although the drug induces cytochrome P450 3A4 enzymes, studies of concurrent administration of rifaximin with midazolam, and with a single dose of the oral contraceptive ethinyl estradiol and norgestimate, did not show changes in the pharmacokinetics of these drugs.

INTERACTIONS WITH DRUGS USED FOR TRAVEL TO HIGH ALTITUDES
Acetazolamide

Acetazolamide produces alkaline urine that can increase the rate of excretion of barbiturates and salicylates and may potentiate salicylate toxicity. Decreased excretion of dextroamphetamine, anticholinergics, mecamylamine, ephedrine, mexiletine, or quinidine may also occur. Hypokalemia caused by corticosteroids may be potentiated by concurrent use of acetazolamide.

Dexamethasone

Dexamethasone interacts with multiple classes of drugs. Using this drug to treat altitude illness may, however, be life saving. Interactions may occur with the following drugs and drug classes: macrolide antibiotics, anticholinesterases, anticoagulants, hypoglycemic agents, isoniazid, digitalis preparations, oral contraceptives, and phenytoin.

BIBLIOGRAPHY

1. CDC. Sudden death in a traveler following halofantrine administration—Togo, 2000. MMWR Morb Mortal Wkly Rep. 2001 Mar 9;50(9):169–70, 79.

2. Horowitz H, Carbonaro CA. Inhibition of the *Salmonella typhi* oral vaccine strain, Ty21a, by mefloquine and chloroquine. J Infect Dis. 1992 Dec;166(6):1462–4.

3. Kollaritsch H, Que JU, Kunz C, Wiedermann G, Herzog C, Cryz SJ Jr. Safety and immunogenicity of live oral cholera and typhoid vaccines administered alone or in combination with antimalarial drugs, oral polio

vaccine, or yellow fever vaccine. J Infect Dis. 1997 Apr;175(4):871–5.

4. Matson PA, Luby SP, Redd SC, Rolka HR, Meriwether RA. Cardiac effects of standard-dose halofantrine therapy. Am J Trop Med Hyg. 1996 Mar;54(3):229–31.

5. Pappaioanou M, Fishbein DB, Dreesen DW, Schwartz IK, Campbell GH, Sumner JW, et al. Antibody response to preexposure human diploid-cell rabies vaccine given concurrently with chloroquine. N Engl J Med. 1986 Jan 30;314(5):280–4.

Perspectives

FEAR OF VACCINES
Paul Offit

Pre-travel counseling visits often provide the opportunity to update routine vaccinations for both children and adults. Thus, one of the first topics covered in such sessions is whether the traveler is immune to diseases such as measles and varicella. Unfortunately, in some circumstances, providers may be surprised to find out that the travelers have no interest in being vaccinated or in having their children vaccinated, whether for measles or other potentially life-threatening, travel-related infections, such as yellow fever.

Although vaccines geared for international travelers may not have implications for community health, such as providing herd immunity, they can protect individuals against severe and occasionally fatal illness. For these vaccines, the discussion between clinicians and patients is by nature one of weighing risks and benefits of administering travel-related vaccines for the particular destination. Travelers are often at a higher risk of exposure to diseases for which routine vaccines provide protection, even when traveling to countries in Europe. During this discussion, the travel health provider should seize the opportunity to educate all travelers, and especially parents, about the use of those vaccines. Those providing travel health advice should familiarize themselves with the literature on vaccine safety of both routine and travel-related vaccines, so they can appropriately address any concerns that their clients may have.

The history of the development of vaccination complacency and perhaps, following that, vaccination avoidance is a curious one. During the 1940s, parents in the United States did not hesitate to get the diphtheria, tetanus, and pertussis vaccines; they knew that diphtheria and pertussis were common killers of young children, and they had watched tetanus claim the lives of soldiers in World Wars I and II. During the 1950s, the polio vaccine was a godsend; everyone knew what poliovirus could do. During the 1960s, parents gladly accepted the measles, mumps, and rubella vaccines. They knew that measles caused thousands of hospitalizations and hundreds of deaths every year, mostly from pneumonia; that mumps was a common cause of deafness and a rare cause of sterility; and that rubella caused thousands of children to suffer severe birth defects of the eyes, ears, and heart.

The widespread use of vaccines caused a dramatic decrease—and in some cases a virtual elimination—of several diseases. Parents, no longer compelled by the diseases around them, became complacent. Immunization rates plateaued. Now, the United Sates (as well as many European countries) finds itself in a situation where vaccine safety issues, real or imagined, are a primary concern. Parents confront a flood of misinformation from radio and television programs, magazine and newspaper articles, anti-vaccine blogs, YouTube, and Twitter. Vaccines—considered mankind's greatest lifesaver—are now feared by some to cause a variety of chronic diseases, including autism, diabetes, allergies, asthma, learning disabilities, multiple sclerosis, and attention deficit disorder, among others. As a consequence, many parents are choosing not to immunize their children according to recommended schedules. Travel health providers must be aware of these issues and arm themselves with accurate information to properly educate their clients.

In addition to protecting the health of the vaccinee, vaccination of individuals helps safeguard the health of entire communities, both at home and possibly at travel destinations. Predictably, in communities with clusters of underimmunized children, the incidence of vaccine-preventable diseases has risen. A measles epidemic in 2008 was larger than any measles epidemic in the previous 10 years. Pertussis outbreaks have swept the nation. Increased numbers of cases of *Haemophilus influenzae* type b meningitis have claimed the lives of several children in Minnesota and Pennsylvania, deaths that could have easily been avoided if parents had not feared vaccines more than the diseases they prevent. Some of these outbreaks have been linked to international travel to the United States.

So, where do we go from here? How do we again compel people to vaccinate themselves and their children? One way would be to make parents aware of the impact of vaccine-preventable diseases and to provide the science that exonerates vaccines as a cause of chronic diseases in a manner that is compelling and easily understood. Some of this information is available from CDC (www.cdc.gov/vaccines/recs/acip/default.htm), the American Academy of Pediatrics (www.aap.org), the Immunization Action Coalition (www.immunize.org), the Vaccine Education Center at the Children's Hospital of Philadelphia (www.vaccine.chop.edu), Every Child By Two (www.ecbt.org), the National Network for Immunization Information (www.immunizationinfo.org), the Institute for Vaccine Safety at Johns Hopkins Hospital (www.vaccinesafety.edu), and Parents of Kids with Infectious Diseases (www.pkids.org), among other groups.

But is it enough? As providers whose job it is to protect individuals against vaccine-preventable diseases, whether they be travel-related infections or otherwise, we need to enhance our efforts to educate ourselves and our patients, so that we will not once again be compelled to vaccinate after witnessing the suffering, hospitalization, and death caused by vaccine-preventable diseases—an unwanted return to an earlier phase in history.

BIBLIOGRAPHY

1. CDC. Invasive *Haemophilus influenzae* type B disease in five young children—Minnesota, 2008. MMWR Morb Mortal Wkly Rep. 2009 Jan 30;58(3):58–60.
2. CDC. Pertussis outbreak in an Amish community—Kent County, Delaware, September 2004–February 2005. MMWR Morb Mortal Wkly Rep. 2006 Aug 4;55(30):817–21.
3. CDC. Update: measles—United States, January–July 2008. MMWR Morb Mortal Wkly Rep. 2008 Aug 22;57(33):893–6.
4. Chen RT, Mootrey G, DeStefano F. Safety of routine childhood vaccinations. An epidemiological review. Paediatr Drugs. 2000 Jul–Aug;2(4):273–90.

Self-Treatable Conditions

SELF-TREATABLE CONDITIONS

Alan J. Magill

Despite our best efforts during the pre-travel consultation to help travelers prevent illness, some travelers will become ill while traveling. Obtaining reliable and timely medical care can be problematic in many destinations. As a result, prescribing certain medications in advance can empower the traveler to self-diagnose and treat common health problems. With some activities in remote settings, such as trekking, the only alternative to self-treatment would be no treatment. Appropriate pre-travel counseling may actually result in a more accurate self-diagnosis and treatment than relying on local medical care in some developing countries. In addition, the increasing awareness of substandard and counterfeit drugs in pharmacies in the developing world (as many as 20%–30% of the drugs on the shelves) makes it more important for travelers to bring high-quality drugs with them from a reliable supplier in their own country (see the Perspectives: Counterfeit Drugs section later in this chapter).

Providing education and prescriptions is part of the pre-travel consultation. The key aspect to this strategy is to recognize the conditions for which the traveler may be at risk and to educate the traveler about the diagnosis and treatment of those particular conditions. The keys to successful self-treatment strategies are providing a simple disease or condition definition, providing one choice of treatment, and educating the traveler about the expected outcome of treatment. Using travelers' diarrhea as an example, a practitioner could provide the following advice:

- "Travelers' diarrhea" is the sudden onset of abnormally loose, frequent stools.
- The treatment is ciprofloxacin 500 mg, every 12 hours, for 1 day (2 doses).
- The traveler should feel better within 6–24 hours.
- If symptoms persist for 24–36 hours despite treatment, it may be necessary to seek medical attention.

To minimize the potential negative effects of a self-treatment strategy, the recommendations should follow a few key points:

- Drugs recommended must be safe, well tolerated, and effective for use as self-treatment.
- A drug's toxicity or potential for harm, if used incorrectly or in an overdose situation, should be minimal.

- Simple and clear directions are critical. Consider providing handouts describing how to use the drugs. Keeping the directions simple will increase the effectiveness of the strategy.

The following are some of the most common situations in which people would find self-treatment useful. The extent of self-treatment recommendations offered to the traveler should reflect the remoteness and difficulty of travel and the availability of reliable medical care at the particular destination. The recommended self-treatment options for each disease are provided in the designated section of the Yellow Book.

Travelers' diarrhea (TD) is perhaps the most frequent indication for self-treatment. The success of this strategy is based on the epidemiologic evidence that bacterial pathogens account for more than 90% of TD in short-term travelers. The recognition of antibiotic resistance for certain organisms in specific destinations has made the empiric choice of treatment somewhat more problematic in recent years (see the Travelers' Diarrhea section next in this chapter).

Altitude illness or acute mountain sickness (AMS) is a risk for travelers who ascend rapidly to altitudes >8,000 ft (2,440 m). Certain common travel destinations, such as Cuzco, Peru, or Lhasa, Tibet, involve flying to altitudes of 11,300 ft (3,445 m) or 12,700 ft (3,870 m). The symptoms of headache, anorexia, nausea, fatigue, lassitude, and poor sleep can largely be prevented or treated with acetazolamide (see the Altitude Illness section later in this chapter).

Jet lag affects almost everyone who crosses 3 or more time zones. There is no consensus on the optimal pharmacologic treatment or prevention of the symptoms of jet lag, but sleeping medication taken at the destination may help regularize sleep patterns (see the Jet Lag section later in this chapter).

Motion sickness can be a major deterrent to enjoyment for any susceptible person on a boat or a winding road. Premedication may help alleviate or ameliorate this bothersome syndrome (see the Motion Sickness section later in this chapter).

The self-treatment of suspected **respiratory infections** with empiric antibiotics is controversial. Almost all upper respiratory tract infections are initially caused by viruses. However, these viral infections, under the stress of travel, can lead to bacterial sinusitis, bronchitis, or pneumonia. Respiratory infections that last longer than a week without signs of improvement may require empiric antibiotics for recovery. Prolonged respiratory infections may have more of a negative effect on a trip than diarrheal disease (see the Respiratory Infections section later in this chapter).

Bacterial skin infections are not common among travelers, but when they occur, they can be particularly distressing. Bacterial abscesses or cellulitis can worsen rapidly and be very painful. If the traveler is in a remote area, or even more than a day's travel from medical care, the use of empiric antibiotic treatment can be beneficial (see Chapter 5, Skin and Soft Tissue Infections in Returned Travelers).

Urinary tract infections are common among many women, and carrying an antibiotic for empiric treatment of this condition may be valuable in many circumstances.

Vaginal yeast infections in women can be an annoying and debilitating problem. For women who know they are prone to infections, all sexually active women, and those who may be receiving antibiotics for other reasons, including doxycycline for antimalarial prophylaxis, a self-treatment course of their preferred antifungal medication can be prescribed.

Occupational exposure to HIV is a particular risk to those participating in medical-related activities. Thousands of such people work in areas of sub-Saharan Africa, where the HIV prevalence may be higher than 15%–20%. A needlestick in this setting should prompt immediate wound care and the possible use of antiretroviral medications (see the Occupational Exposure to HIV section later in this chapter).

Malaria self-treatment is often referred to as stand-by emergency treatment (SBET). This strategy asks the traveler to use a therapeutic dose of an appropriate antimalarial drug when the traveler has a significant fever accompanied by systemic illness, and then proceed to reliable medical care within 24 hours. The goal is to prevent death or severe malaria. Since most travelers at risk of malaria should be advised to use prophylactic medication, this strategy is usually discouraged and reserved for a specific type of traveler under certain defined circumstances (see Chapter 3, Malaria).

TRAVELERS' DIARRHEA

Bradley A. Connor

DESCRIPTION

Travelers' diarrhea (TD) is the most predictable travel-related illness. Attack rates range from 30% to 70% of travelers, depending on the destination. Traditionally, it was thought that TD could be prevented by following simple recommendations such as "boil it, peel, it, or forget it," but studies have found that people who follow these rules still get ill. Poor hygiene practice in local restaurants is likely the largest contributor to the risk for TD.

TD is a clinical syndrome that can result from a variety of intestinal pathogens. Bacterial pathogens are the predominant risk, thought to account for 80%–90% of TD. Intestinal viruses have been isolated in studies of TD, but they usually account for 5%–8% of illnesses. Protozoal pathogens are slower to manifest symptoms and collectively account for approximately 10% of diagnoses in longer-term travelers. What is commonly known as "food poisoning" involves the ingestion of preformed toxins in food. In this syndrome, vomiting and diarrhea may both be present, but symptoms usually resolve spontaneously within 12 hours.

INFECTIOUS AGENT

Bacteria are the most common cause of TD. Overall, the most common pathogen is enterotoxigenic *Escherichia coli*, followed by *Campylobacter jejuni*, *Shigella* spp., and *Salmonella* spp. Enteroadherent and other *E. coli* species are also common pathogens in bacterial diarrhea. There is increasing recognition of *Aeromonas* spp. and *Plesiomonas* spp. as causes of travelers' diarrhea as well. Viral diarrhea can be caused by a number of viral pathogens, including norovirus, rotavirus, and astrovirus.

Giardia is the main protozoal pathogen found in TD. *Entamoeba histolytica* is a relatively uncommon pathogen in travelers. *Cryptosporidium* is also relatively uncommon. The risk for *Cyclospora* is highly geographic and seasonal: the most well-known risks are in Nepal, Peru, Haiti, and Guatemala. *Dientamoeba*

fragilis is a low-grade but persistent pathogen that is occasionally diagnosed in travelers. The individual pathogens are each discussed in their own sections in Chapter 3, and persistent diarrhea is discussed in Chapter 5.

OCCURRENCE

The most important determinant of risk is travel destination, and there are regional differences in both the risk for and etiology of diarrhea. The world is generally divided into 3 grades of risk: low, intermediate, and high.

- Low-risk countries include the United States, Canada, Australia, New Zealand, Japan, and countries in Northern and Western Europe.
- Intermediate-risk countries include those in Eastern Europe, South Africa, and some of the Caribbean islands.
- High-risk areas include most of Asia, the Middle East, Africa, Mexico, and Central and South America.

RISK FOR TRAVELERS

TD occurs equally in male and female travelers and is more common in young adults than in older people. In short-term travelers, bouts of TD do not appear to protect against future attacks, and more than 1 episode of TD may occur during a single trip. A cohort of expatriates taking up residence in Kathmandu, Nepal, experienced an average of 3.2 episodes of TD per person in their first year. In more temperate regions, there may be seasonal variations in diarrhea risk. In south Asia, for example, much higher TD attack rates are commonly reported during the hot months preceding the monsoon.

In environments where large numbers of people do not have access to plumbing or outhouses, the amount of stool contamination in the environment will be higher and more accessible to flies. Inadequate electrical capacity may lead to frequent blackouts or poorly functioning refrigeration, which can result in unsafe food storage and an increased risk for disease. Inadequate water supplies can lead to the absence of sinks for handwashing by restaurant staff. Poor training in handling and preparation of food may lead to cross-contamination from meat, and inadequate disinfection of food preparation surfaces and utensils. In destinations in which effective food handling courses have been provided, the risk for TD has been demonstrated to decrease. It should be noted, however, that pathogens that cause TD are not unique to developing countries. The risk of TD is associated with the hygiene practices in specific destinations and the handling and preparation of food in restaurants in developed countries as well.

CLINICAL PRESENTATION

Bacterial diarrhea presents with the sudden onset of bothersome symptoms that can range from mild cramps and urgent loose stools to severe abdominal pain, fever, vomiting, and bloody diarrhea. Viral enteropathogens present in a similar fashion to bacterial pathogens, although with norovirus vomiting may be more prominent. Protozoal diarrhea, such as that caused by *Giardia intestinalis* or E. *histolytica*, generally has a more gradual onset of low-grade symptoms, with 2–5 loose stools per day. The incubation period of the pathogens can be a clue to the etiology of TD:

- Bacterial and viral pathogens have an incubation period of 6–48 hours.
- Protozoal pathogens generally have an incubation period of 1–2 weeks and rarely present in the first few weeks of travel. An exception can be *Cyclospora cayetanensis*, which can present quickly in areas of high risk.

Untreated bacterial diarrhea lasts 3–5 days. Viral diarrhea lasts 2–3 days. Protozoal diarrhea can persist for weeks to months without treatment. An acute bout of gastroenteritis can lead to persistent gastrointestinal symptoms, even in the absence of continued infection (see Chapter 5, Persistent Travelers' Diarrhea). Other postinfectious sequelae may include reactive arthritis and Guillain-Barré syndrome.

PREVENTIVE MEASURES FOR TRAVELERS

For travelers to high-risk areas, several approaches may be recommended that can reduce but never completely eliminate the risk for TD. These include instruction regarding food and beverage selection, use of agents other than antimicrobial drugs for prophylaxis, and use of prophylactic antibiotics. Carrying small containers of alcohol-based hand cleaners (containing at least 60% alcohol) may make it easier for travelers to clean their hands before eating.

Food and Beverage Selection

Care in selecting food and beverages for consumption might minimize the risk for acquiring TD. Travelers should be advised that foods that are freshly cooked and served piping hot are safer than foods that may have been sitting for some time in the kitchen or in a buffet. Care should be taken to avoid beverages diluted with nonpotable water (reconstituted fruit juices, ice, and milk) and foods washed in nonpotable water, such as salads. Other risky foods include raw or undercooked meat and seafood and unpeeled raw fruits and vegetables. Safe beverages include those that are bottled and sealed or carbonated. Boiled beverages and those appropriately treated with iodine or chlorine may also be safely drunk. Although food and water precautions continue to be recommended, travelers may not always be able to adhere to the advice. Furthermore, many of the factors that ensure food safety, such as restaurant hygiene, are out of the traveler's control.

Nonantimicrobial Drugs for Prophylaxis

The primary agent studied for prevention of TD, other than antimicrobial drugs, is bismuth subsalicylate (BSS), which is the active ingredient in Pepto-Bismol. Studies from Mexico have shown this agent (taken daily as either 2 oz of liquid or 2 chewable tablets 4 times per day) reduces the incidence of TD from 40% to 14%. BSS commonly causes blackening of the tongue and stool and may cause nausea, constipation, and rarely tinnitus. BSS should be avoided by travelers with aspirin allergy, renal insufficiency, and gout and by those taking anticoagulants, probenecid, or methotrexate. In travelers taking aspirin or salicylates for other reasons, the use of BSS may result in salicylate toxicity. Caution should be used in administering BSS to children with viral infections, such as varicella or influenza, because of the risk for Reye syndrome. BSS is not recommended for children younger than 3 years of age. Studies have not established the safety of BSS use for periods longer than 3 weeks.

The use of probiotics, such as *Lactobacillus* GG and *Saccharomyces boulardii*, has been studied in the prevention of TD in small numbers of people. Results are inconclusive, partially because standardized preparations of these bacteria are not reliably available. Some people report beneficial outcomes using bovine colostrum as a daily prophylaxis agent for TD. However, commercially sold preparations of bovine colostrum are marketed as dietary supplements that are not Food and Drug Administration (FDA) approved for medical indications. Because no data from rigorous clinical trials demonstrate efficacy in controlled trials, there is insufficient information to recommend the use of bovine colostrum to prevent TD.

Prophylactic Antibiotics

Prophylactic antibiotics are effective in the prevention of TD. Controlled studies have shown that diarrhea attack rates are reduced from 40% to 4% by the use of antibiotics. The prophylactic antibiotic of choice has changed over the past few decades as resistance patterns have evolved. Agents such as trimethoprim-sulfamethoxazole and doxycycline are no longer considered effective antimicrobial agents against enteric bacterial pathogens. The fluoroquinolones have been the most effective antibiotics for the prophylaxis and treatment of bacterial TD pathogens, but increasing resistance to these agents, mainly among *Campylobacter* species, may limit their benefit in the future. A nonabsorbable antibiotic, rifaximin, is being investigated but is not currently approved by the FDA for its potential use in TD prophylaxis. In one study, rifaximin reduced the risk for TD in travelers to Mexico by 77%.

At this time, prophylactic antibiotics should not be recommended for most travelers. In addition to affording no protection against nonbacterial pathogens, the use of antibiotics may be associated with allergic or adverse reactions in a certain percentage of travelers and may potentially contribute to drug resistance. The use of prophylactic antibiotics should be weighed against the result of using prompt, early self-treatment with antibiotics when TD occurs, which can limit the duration of illness to 6–24 hours in most cases. Prophylactic antibiotics may be considered for short-term travelers who are high-risk hosts (such as those who are immunosuppressed) or who are taking critical trips during which even a short bout of diarrhea could affect the trip.

TREATMENT

Antibiotics are the principal element in the treatment of TD. Adjunctive agents used for symptomatic control may also be recommended.

Antibiotics

As bacterial causes of TD far outnumber other microbial causes, empiric treatment with an antibiotic directed at enteric bacterial pathogens remains the best therapy for TD. The benefit of treating TD with antibiotics has been proven in numerous studies. The effectiveness of a particular antimicrobial depends on the etiologic agent and its antibiotic sensitivity. Both as empiric therapy or for treatment of a specific bacterial pathogen, first-line antibiotics include those of the fluoroquinolone class, such as ciprofloxacin or levofloxacin. Increasing microbial resistance to the fluoroquinolones, especially among *Campylobacter* isolates, may limit their usefulness in some destinations such as Thailand, where *Campylobacter* is prevalent. Increasing cases of fluoroquinolone resistance have been reported from other destinations. An alternative to the fluoroquinolones in this situation is azithromycin. Rifaximin has been approved to treat TD caused by noninvasive strains of *E. coli*. However, since it is often difficult for travelers to distinguish between invasive and noninvasive diarrhea, and since they would have to carry a back-up drug in the event of invasive diarrhea, the overall usefulness of rifaximin as empiric self-treatment remains to be determined.

Single-dose or 1-day therapy for TD with a fluoroquinolone is well established, both by clinical trials and clinical experience. The best regimen for azithromycin treatment is not yet established. One study used a single dose of 1,000 mg, but side effects (mainly nausea) may limit the acceptability of this large dose. Azithromycin, 500 mg per day for 1–3 days, appears to be effective in most cases of TD.

Antimotility Agents

Antimotility agents provide symptomatic relief and serve as useful adjuncts to antibiotic therapy in TD. Synthetic opiates, such as loperamide and diphenoxylate, can reduce bowel movement frequency and enable travelers to ride on an airplane or bus while awaiting the effects of antibiotics. Loperamide appears to have antisecretory properties as well. The safety of loperamide when used along with an appropriate antibiotic has been well established, even in cases of invasive pathogens. Loperamide can be used in children, and liquid formulations are available. In practice, however, these drugs are rarely given to small children.

Oral Rehydration Therapy

Fluids and electrolytes are lost in cases of TD, and replenishment is important, especially in young children or adults with chronic medical illness. In adult travelers who are otherwise healthy, severe dehydration resulting from TD is unusual unless prolonged vomiting is present. Nonetheless, replacement of fluid losses remains an adjunct to other therapy and helps the traveler feel better more quickly. Travelers should remember to use only beverages that are sealed or are otherwise known to be purified. For more severe fluid loss, replacement is best accomplished with oral rehydration salts (ORS), such as the World Health Organization ORS, which are widely available at stores and pharmacies in most developing countries (see Table 2-5 for details). ORS is prepared by adding 1 packet to the appropriate volume of boiled or treated water. Travelers may find most ORS formulations to be relatively unpalatable, due to their

saltiness. In most cases, rehydration can be maintained with any palatable liquid.

Treatment of TD Caused by Protozoa

The most common parasitic cause of TD is *G. intestinalis*, and treatment options include metronidazole, tinidazole, and nitazoxanide. Although cryptosporidiosis is usually a self-limited illness in immunocompetent people, nitazoxanide can be considered as a treatment option. Cyclosporiasis is treated with trimethoprim-sulfamethoxazole. Treatment of amebiasis is with metronidazole or tinidazole, followed by treatment with a luminal agent such as paromomycin.

Treatment for Children

Children who accompany their parents on trips to high-risk destinations may be expected to have TD as well. There is no reason to withhold antibiotics from children who contract TD. In older children and teenagers, treatment recommendations for TD follow those for adults, with possible adjustments in the dose of medication. Macrolides such as azithromycin are considered first-line antibiotic therapy in children, although some experts now use short-course fluoroquinolone therapy for travelers aged <18 years. Rifaximin is approved for use starting at 12 years of age.

Infants and younger children with TD are at higher risk for developing dehydration, which is best prevented by the early use of ORS. Breastfed infants should continue to nurse on demand, and bottle-fed infants can

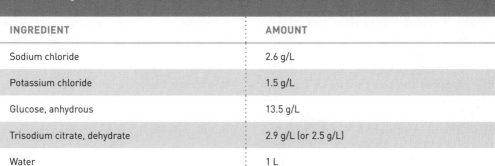

Table 2-5. Composition of the World Health Organization oral rehydration salts for diarrheal illness[1]

INGREDIENT	AMOUNT
Sodium chloride	2.6 g/L
Potassium chloride	1.5 g/L
Glucose, anhydrous	13.5 g/L
Trisodium citrate, dehydrate	2.9 g/L (or 2.5 g/L)
Water	1 L

[1] World Health Organization. Oral rehydration salts (ORS): production of the new ORS. Geneva: WHO; 2006.

continue to drink their formula. Older infants and children may eat a regular diet, depending on the level of their appetite while they are ill. Infants in diapers are at risk for developing a painful, eczematous rash on their buttocks in response to the liquid stool. Hydrocortisone cream will quickly improve this rash. More information about diarrhea and dehydration is discussed in Chapter 7, Traveling Safely with Infants and Children.

BIBLIOGRAPHY

1. Adachi JA, Jiang ZD, Mathewson JJ, Verenkar MP, Thompson S, Martinez-Sandoval F, et al. Enteroaggregative *Escherichia coli* as a major etiologic agent in traveler's diarrhea in 3 regions of the world. Clin Infect Dis. 2001 Jun 15;32(12):1706–9.
2. Black RE. Epidemiology of travelers' diarrhea and relative importance of various pathogens. Rev Infect Dis. 1990 Jan–Feb;12 Suppl 1:S73–9.
3. Connor BA. Sequelae of traveler's diarrhea: focus on postinfectious irritable bowel syndrome. Clin Infect Dis. 2005 Dec 1;41 Suppl 8:S577–86.
4. DuPont HL, Ericsson CD. Prevention and treatment of traveler's diarrhea. N Engl J Med. 1993 Jun 24;328(25):1821–7.
5. DuPont HL, Jiang ZD, Ericsson CD, Adachi JA, Mathewson JJ, DuPont MW, et al. Rifaximin versus ciprofloxacin for the treatment of traveler's diarrhea: a randomized, double-blind clinical trial. Clin Infect Dis. 2001 Dec 1;33(11):1807–15.
6. Hoge CW, Gambel JM, Srijan A, Pitarangsi C, Echeverria P. Trends in antibiotic resistance among diarrheal pathogens isolated in Thailand over 15 years. Clin Infect Dis. 1998 Feb;26(2):341–5.
7. Shah N, DuPont HL, Ramsey DJ. Global etiology of travelers' diarrhea: systematic review from 1973 to the present. Am J Trop Med Hyg. 2009 Apr;80(4):609–14.
8. Shlim DR. Update in traveler's diarrhea. Infect Dis Clin North Am. 2005 Mar;19(1):137–49.
9. Steffen R. Epidemiology of travellers' diarrhoea. Scand J Gastroenterol Suppl. 1983;84:5–17.
10. von Sonnenburg F, Tornieporth N, Waiyaki P, Lowe B, Peruski LF Jr, DuPont HL, et al. Risk and aetiology of diarrhoea at various tourist destinations. Lancet. 2000 Jul 8;356(9224):133–4.

ALTITUDE ILLNESS
Peter H. Hackett, David R. Shlim

OVERVIEW

The stresses of the high-altitude environment include cold, low humidity, increased ultraviolet radiation, and decreased air pressure, all of which can cause problems for travelers. The largest concern, however, is hypoxia. At 10,000 ft (3,000 m), for example, the inspired PO_2 is only 69% of sea-level value. The degree of hypoxic stress depends on altitude, rate of ascent, and duration of exposure. Sleeping at high altitude produces the most hypoxia; day trips to high altitude with return to low altitude are much less stressful on the body. Typical high-altitude destinations include Cuzco (11,000 ft; 3,300 m), La Paz (12,000 ft; 3,640 m), Lhasa (12,100 ft; 3,650 m), Everest Base Camp (17,700 ft; 5,400 m), and Kilimanjaro (19,341ft; 5,895 m).

The human body adjusts very well to moderate hypoxia, but requires time to do so (Box 2-2). The process of acute acclimatization to high altitude takes 3–5 days; therefore, acclimatizing for a few days at 8,000–9,000 ft before proceeding to a higher altitude is ideal. Acclimatization prevents altitude illness, improves sleep, and increases comfort and well-being, although exercise performance will always be reduced compared with low altitude. Increase in ventilation is the most important factor in acute acclimatization; therefore, respiratory depressants must be avoided. Increased red-cell production does not play a role in acute acclimatization.

RISK FOR TRAVELERS

Inadequate acclimatization may lead to altitude illness in any traveler going to 8,000 ft

BOX 2-2. TIPS FOR ACCLIMATIZATION

- Ascend gradually, if possible. Try not to go directly from low altitude to more than 9,000 ft (2,750 m) sleeping altitude in 1 day. Once above 9,000 ft (2,750 m), move sleeping altitude no higher than 1,600 ft (500 m) per day, and plan an extra day for acclimatization every 3,300 ft (1,000 m).
- Consider using acetazolamide to speed acclimatization, if abrupt ascent is unavoidable.
- Avoid alcohol for the first 48 hours.
- Participate in only mild exercise for the first 48 hours.
- Having a high-altitude exposure at more than 9,000 ft (2,750 m) for 2 nights or more, within 30 days before the trip, is useful.

(2,500 m) or higher. Susceptibility and resistance to altitude illness are genetic traits, and no screening tests are available to predict risk. Risk is not affected by training or physical fitness. Children are equally susceptible as adults; people aged >50 years have slightly lower risk. How a traveler has responded to high altitude previously is the most reliable guide for future trips, but is not infallible. However, given certain baseline susceptibility, risk is largely influenced by rate of ascent and exertion (see Table 2-6). Determining an itinerary that will avoid any occurrence of altitude illness is difficult because of variations in individual susceptibility, as well as in starting points and terrain.

CLINICAL PRESENTATION

Altitude illness is divided into 3 syndromes: acute mountain sickness (AMS), high-altitude cerebral edema (HACE), and high-altitude pulmonary edema (HAPE).

Acute Mountain Sickness

AMS is the most common form of altitude illness, affecting, for example, 25% of all visitors sleeping above 8,000 ft (2,500 m) in Colorado. Symptoms are those of an alcohol hangover: headache is the cardinal symptom, sometimes accompanied by fatigue, loss of appetite, nausea, and occasionally vomiting. Headache onset is usually 2–12 hours after arrival at a higher altitude and often during or after the first night. Preverbal children may develop loss of appetite, irritability, and pallor. AMS generally resolves with 24–72 hours of acclimatization.

High-Altitude Cerebral Edema

HACE is a severe progression of AMS and is rare; it is most often associated with HAPE. In addition to AMS symptoms, lethargy becomes profound, with drowsiness, confusion, and ataxia on tandem gait test. A person with HACE requires immediate descent; death from HACE can ensue within 24 hours of developing ataxia, if the person fails to descend.

High-Altitude Pulmonary Edema

HAPE can occur by itself or in conjunction with AMS and HACE; incidence is 1 per 10,000 skiers in Colorado and up to 1 per 100 climbers at more than 14,000 ft (4,270 m). Initial symptoms are increased breathlessness with exertion, and eventually increased breathlessness at rest, associated with weakness and cough. Oxygen or descent is life-saving. HAPE can be more rapidly fatal than HACE.

Preexisting Medical Problems

Travelers with medical conditions, such as heart failure, myocardial ischemia (angina), sickle cell disease, or any form of pulmonary insufficiency, should be advised to consult a physician familiar with high-altitude medical issues before undertaking high-altitude travel. The risk for new ischemic heart disease in previously healthy travelers does not appear to be increased at high altitudes. People with diabetes can travel safely to high altitudes, but they must be accustomed to exercise and carefully monitor their blood glucose. Diabetic ketoacidosis may be triggered by altitude illness and may be more

Table 2-6. Risk categories for acute mountain sickness

RISK CATEGORY	DESCRIPTION	PROPHYLAXIS RECOMMENDATIONS
Low	• People with no prior history of altitude illness and ascending to less than 9,100 ft (2,800 m) • People taking more than 2 days to arrive at 8,200–9,800 ft (2,500–3,000 m), with subsequent increases in sleeping elevation less than 1,600 ft (500 m) per day, and an extra day for acclimatization every 3,200 ft (1,000 m)	Acetazolamide prophylaxis generally not indicated.
Moderate	• People with prior history of AMS and ascending to 8,200–9,100 ft (2,500–2,800 m) in 1 day • No history of AMS and ascending to more than 9,100 ft (2,800 m) in 1 day • All people ascending more than 1,600 ft (500 m) per day (increase in sleeping elevation) at altitudes above 9,800 ft (3,000 m), but with an extra day for acclimatization every 3,200 ft (1,000 m)	Acetazolamide prophylaxis would be beneficial and should be considered.
High	• History of AMS and ascending to more than 9,100 ft (2,800 m) in 1 day • All people with a prior history of HAPE or HACE • All people ascending to more than 11,400 ft (3,500 m) in 1 day • All people ascending more than 1,600 ft (500 m) per day (increase in sleeping elevation) above 9,800 ft (3,000 m), without extra days for acclimatization • Very rapid ascents (such as less than 7-day ascents of Mount Kilimanjaro)	Acetazolamide prophylaxis strongly recommended.

Abbreviations: AMS, acute mountain sickness; HACE, high-altitude cerebral edema; HAPE, high-altitude pulmonary edema.

difficult to treat in those on acetazolamide. Not all glucose meters read accurately at high altitudes.

Most people do not have visual problems at high altitudes. However, at very high altitudes some people who have had radial keratotomy may develop acute farsightedness and be unable to climb by themselves. LASIK and other newer procedures may produce only minor visual disturbances at high altitudes.

There are no studies or case reports of harm to a fetus if the mother travels briefly to high altitudes during pregnancy. However, it may be prudent to recommend that pregnant women do not stay at sleeping altitudes higher than 12,000 ft (3,658 m), if possible. The dangers of having a pregnancy complication in remote, mountainous terrain should also be discussed.

DIAGNOSIS AND TREATMENT
Acute Mountain Sickness/High-Altitude Cerebral Edema

The differential diagnosis of AMS/HACE includes dehydration, exhaustion, hypoglycemia, hypothermia, or hyponatremia. Focal neurologic symptoms, or seizures, are rare in HACE and should lead to suspicion of an intracranial lesion or seizure disorder. Patients with AMS can descend ≥300 m, and symptoms will rapidly abate. Alternatively, supplemental oxygen at 2 L per minute will relieve headache quickly and resolve AMS over hours, but it is rarely available. People with AMS can also safely remain at their current altitude and treat symptoms with nonopiate analgesics and antiemetics, such as ondansetron. They may also take acetazolamide, which speeds acclimatization and effectively treats AMS, but is better for prophylaxis than treatment. Dexamethasone is more effective than acetazolamide at rapidly relieving the symptoms of moderate to severe AMS. **If symptoms are getting worse while the traveler is resting at the same altitude, he or she must descend.**

HACE is a continuation of AMS and is diagnosed when neurologic findings, particularly ataxia, confusion, or altered mental status, are present. HACE may also occur in the presence of HAPE. People developing HACE in populated areas with access to medical care can be treated at altitude with supplemental oxygen and dexamethasone. In remote areas, descent should be initiated in any person suspected of having HACE. If descent is not feasible because of logistical issues, supplemental oxygen or a portable hyperbaric chamber should be used, if available.

High-Altitude Pulmonary Edema

Although the progression of decreased exercise tolerance, increased breathlessness, and breathlessness at rest is almost always recognizable as HAPE, the differential diagnosis includes pneumonia, bronchospasm, myocardial infarction, or pulmonary embolism. Descent in this situation is urgent and mandatory, and should be accomplished with as little exertion as is feasible for the patient. If descent is not immediately possible, supplemental oxygen or a portable hyperbaric chamber should be used. Patients with mild HAPE who have access to oxygen (at a hospital or high-altitude medical clinic, for example) may not need to descend to lower elevation and can be treated with oxygen at the current elevation. In the field setting, where resources are limited and there is a lower margin for error, nifedipine can be used as an adjunct to descent, oxygen, or portable hyperbaric therapy. A phosphodiesterase inhibitor may be used if nifedipine is not available, but concurrent use of multiple pulmonary vasodilators is not recommended.

Medications

In addition to the discussion below, recommendations for the usage and dosing of medications to prevent and treat altitude illness are outlined in Table 2-7.

Acetazolamide

Acetazolamide prevents AMS when taken before ascent and can speed recovery if taken after symptoms have developed. The drug works by acidifying the blood, which causes an increase in respiration and thus aids acclimatization. An effective dose that minimizes the common side effects of increased urination and paresthesias of the fingers and toes is 125 mg every 12 hours, beginning the day before ascent and continuing the first 2 days at altitude, or longer if ascent continues. Allergic reactions to acetazolamide are uncommon, but the drug is related to sulfonamides and should not be used by people allergic to sulfa with history of anaphylaxis. A trial dose taken in a safe environment before travel may be useful for those with a more mild allergic history to sulfonamides. People with history of severe penicillin allergy have occasionally had allergic reactions to acetazolamide. The pediatric dose is 5 mg/kg/day in divided doses, up to 125 mg twice a day.

Dexamethasone

Dexamethasone is effective for preventing and treating AMS and HACE, and perhaps HAPE as well. Unlike acetazolamide, if the drug is discontinued at altitude before acclimatization, rebound can occur. Acetazolamide is preferable to prevent AMS while ascending, with dexamethasone reserved for treatment, as an adjunct to descent. The adult dose is 4 g every 6 hours.

Nifedipine

Nifedipine prevents and ameliorates HAPE in people who are particularly susceptible to the condition. The adult dose is 30 mg of extended release every 12 hours, or 20 mg every 8 hours.

Other Medications

Phosphodiesterase-5 inhibitors can also selectively lower pulmonary artery pressure, with less effect on systemic blood pressure. Tadalafil, 10 mg twice a day, during ascent can prevent HAPE and is being studied for treatment. When taken before ascent, gingko biloba, 100–120 mg twice a day, was shown to reduce AMS in adults in some trials, but it was not effective in others, probably due to variation in ingredients. Gingko biloba has not yet been compared directly with acetazolamide.

Table 2-7. Recommended medication doses to prevent and treat altitude illness

MEDICATION	INDICATION	ROUTE	DOSE
Acetazolamide	AMS, HACE prevention	Oral	125 mg twice a day Pediatrics: 2.5 mg/kg every 12 h
	AMS treatment[1]	Oral	250 mg twice a day Pediatrics: 2.5 mg/kg every 12 h
Dexamethasone	AMS, HACE prevention	Oral	2 mg every 6 h or 4 mg every 12 h Pediatrics: should not be used for prophylaxis
	AMS, HACE treatment	Oral, IV, IM	AMS: 4 mg every 6 h HACE: 8 mg once, then 4 mg every 6 h Pediatrics: 0.15 mg/kg/dose every 6 h
Nifedipine	HAPE prevention	Oral	30 mg SR version every 12 h, or 20 mg SR version every 8 h
	HAPE treatment	Oral	30 mg SR version every 12 h, or 20 mg SR version every 8 h
Tadalafil	HAPE prevention	Oral	10 mg twice a day
Sildenafil	HAPE prevention	Oral	50 mg every 8 h
Salmeterol	HAPE prevention	Inhaled	125 µg twice a day[2]

Abbreviations: AMS, acute mountain sickness; HACE, high-altitude cerebral edema; HAPE, high-altitude pulmonary edema; IM, intramuscular; IV, intravenous; SR, sustained release.
[1] Acetazolamide can also be used at this dose as an *adjunct* to dexamethasone in HACE treatment, but dexamethasone remains the primary treatment for that disorder.
[2] Should not be used as monotherapy and should only be used in conjunction with oral medications.

PREVENTION OF SEVERE ALTITUDE ILLNESS OR DEATH

The main point of instructing travelers about altitude illness is not to eliminate the possibility, but to prevent death or evacuation due to altitude illness. Since the onset of symptoms and the clinical course are sufficiently slow and predictable, there is no reason for someone to die from altitude illness, unless trapped by weather or geography in a situation in which descent is impossible. Three rules can prevent death or serious consequences from altitude illness:

- Know the early symptoms of altitude illness, and be willing to acknowledge when they are present.
- Never ascend to sleep at a higher altitude when experiencing symptoms of altitude illness, no matter how minor they seem.

- Descend if the symptoms become worse while resting at the same altitude.

For trekking groups and expeditions going into remote high-altitude areas, where descent to a lower altitude could be problematic, a pressurization bag (such as the Gamow bag) can be beneficial. A foot pump produces an increased pressure of 2 lb/in², mimicking a descent of 5,000–6,000 ft (1,500–1,800 m) depending on the starting altitude. The total packed weight of bag and pump is about 14 lb (6.5 kg).

BIBLIOGRAPHY

1. Hackett P. High altitude and common medical conditions. In: Hornbein TF, Schoene RB, editors. High Altitude: an Exploration of Human Adaptation. New York: Marcel Dekker; 2001. p. 839–85.
2. Hackett P, Roach R. High-altitude medicine. In: Auerbach PS, editor. Wilderness Medicine. 5th ed. Philadelphia: Mosby Elsevier; 2007. p. 2–36.
3. Hackett PH, Roach RC. High altitude cerebral edema. High Alt Med Biol. 2004 Summer;5(2):136–46.
4. Hackett PH, Roach RC. High-altitude illness. N Engl J Med. 2001 Jul 12;345(2):107–14.
5. Johnson TS, Rock PB, Fulco CS, Trad LA, Spark RF, Maher JT. Prevention of acute mountain sickness by dexamethasone. N Engl J Med. 1984 Mar 15;310(11):683–6.
6. Luks AM, McIntosh SE, Grissom CK, Auerbach PS, Rodway GW, Schoene RB, et al. Wilderness Medical Society consensus guidelines for the prevention and treatment of acute altitude illness. Wilderness Environ Med. 2010 Jun;21(2):146–55.
7. Luks AM, Swenson ER. Medication and dosage considerations in the prophylaxis and treatment of high-altitude illness. Chest. 2008 Mar;133(3):744–55.
8. Maggiorini M, Brunner-La Rocca HP, Peth S, Fischler M, Bohm T, Bernheim A, et al. Both tadalafil and dexamethasone may reduce the incidence of high-altitude pulmonary edema: a randomized trial. Ann Intern Med. 2006 Oct 3;145(7):497–506.
9. Pollard A, Murdoch D. The High Altitude Medicine Handbook. 3rd ed. Abingdon, UK: Radcliffe Medical Press; 2003.
10. Pollard AJ, Niermeyer S, Barry P, Bartsch P, Berghold F, Bishop RA, et al. Children at high altitude: an international consensus statement by an ad hoc committee of the International Society for Mountain Medicine, March 12, 2001. High Alt Med Biol. 2001 Fall;2(3):389–403.

JET LAG
Emad A. Yanni

OVERVIEW

Jet lag is a temporary disorder among air travelers who rapidly travel across 3 or more time zones. Jet lag results from the slow adjustment of the body clock to the destination time, so that daily rhythms and the internal drive for sleep and wakefulness are out of synchronization with the new environment.

The intrinsic body clock resides in the suprachiasmatic nuclei at the base of the hypothalamus, which contains melatonin receptors. Melatonin is manufactured in the pineal gland from tryptophan, and its synthesis and release are stimulated by darkness and suppressed by light; consequently, the secretion of melatonin is responsible for setting our sleep-wake cycle. The body clock is adjusted to the solar day by rhythmic cues in the environment, mainly the light-dark cycle, and the rhythmic secretion of melatonin. Exercise is also believed to exert an effect on the body clock, although with a somewhat weaker effect than other cues.

RISK FOR TRAVELERS

Eastward travel is associated with difficulty falling asleep at the destination bedtime and difficulty arising in the morning. Westward travel is associated with early evening sleepiness and predawn awakening at the travel destination. Travelers flying within the same time zone typically experience the fewest problems, such as nonspecific travel fatigue. Crossing more time zones or traveling eastward generally increases the time required for adaptation. After eastward flights, jet lag lasts for the number of days roughly equal to two-thirds the number of time zones crossed; after westward flights, the number of days is roughly half the number of time zones.

Individual responses to crossing time zones and ability to adapt to a new time zone vary. The intensity and duration of jet lag are related to the number of time zones crossed, the direction of travel, the ability to sleep while traveling, the availability and intensity of local circadian time cues at the destination, and individual differences in phase tolerance.

CLINICAL PRESENTATION

Jet-lagged travelers may experience the following symptoms:

- Poor sleep, including delayed sleep onset (after eastward flight), early awakening (after westward flight), and fractionated sleep (after flights in either direction)
- Poor performance in physical and mental tasks during the new daytime
- Negative subjective changes such as increased fatigue, frequency of headaches and irritability, and decreased ability to concentrate
- Gastrointestinal disturbances and decreased interest in and enjoyment of meals

PREVENTIVE MEASURES FOR TRAVELERS

Travelers can minimize jet lag by doing the following before travel:

- Exercise, eat a healthful diet, and get plenty of rest.
- Begin to reset the body clock by shifting the timing of sleep to 1–2 hours later for a few days before traveling westward and shifting the timing of sleep to 1–2 hours earlier for a few days before traveling eastward.
- Seek exposure to bright light in the evening if traveling westward, in the morning if traveling eastward (although it requires high motivation and strict compliance with the prescribed light–dark schedules).
- Break up a long journey with a stopover, if possible.

Travelers should do the following during travel:

- Avoid large meals, alcohol, and caffeine.
- Drink plenty of water to remain hydrated.
- Move around on the plane to promote mental and physical acuity, as well as protect against deep vein thrombosis.
- Wear comfortable shoes and clothing.
- Sleep, if possible, during long flights.

Travelers should do the following on arrival at the destination:

- Avoid situations requiring critical decision making, such as important meetings, for the first day after arrival.
- Adapt to the local schedule as soon as possible.
- Optimize exposure to sunlight after arrival from either direction.
- Eat meals appropriate to the local time, drink plenty of water, and avoid excess caffeine or alcohol.
- Take short naps (20–30 minutes) to increase energy but not undermine nighttime sleep.

The use of the nutritional supplement melatonin is controversial for preventing jet lag. Some clinicians advocate the use of 0.5–5.0 mg of melatonin during the first few days of travel, and data suggest its efficacy. However, its production is not regulated by the Food and Drug Administration, and contaminants have been found in commercially available products. Current information also does not support the use of special diets to ameliorate jet lag.

TREATMENT

The 2008 American Academy of Sleep Medicine recommendations include the following:

- Remain on home time if the travel period is 2 days or less.
- Promote sleep with hypnotic medication, although the effects of hypnotics on daytime symptoms of jet lag have not been well studied.

- Nonaddictive sedative hypnotics (non-benzodiazepines), such as zolpidem, have been shown in some studies to promote longer periods of high-quality sleep. If a benzodiazepine is preferred, a short-acting one, such as temazepam, is recommended to minimize oversedation the following day. Because alcohol intake is often high during international travel, the risk of interaction with hypnotics should be emphasized with patients.
- Promote daytime alertness with a stimulant such as caffeine, but avoid it after midday.
- Take short naps, shower, and spend time in the afternoon sun.

BIBLIOGRAPHY

1. Daurat A, Benoit O, Buguet A. Effects of zopiclone on the rest/activity rhythm after a westward flight across five time zones. Psychopharmacology (Berl). 2000 Apr;149(3):241–5.
2. Dubocovich ML, Markowska M. Functional MT1 and MT2 melatonin receptors in mammals. Endocrine. 2005 Jul;27(2):101–10.
3. Herxheimer A. Jet lag. Clin Evid. 2005 Jun(13):2178–83.
4. Jamieson AO, Zammit GK, Rosenberg RS, Davis JR, Walsh JK. Zolpidem reduces the sleep disturbance of jet lag. Sleep Med. 2001 Sep;2(5):423–30.
5. Reid KJ, Chang AM, Zee PC. Circadian rhythm sleep disorders. Med Clin North Am. 2004 May;88(3):631–51, viii.
6. Reilly T, Waterhouse J, Edwards B. Jet lag and air travel: implications for performance. Clin Sports Med. 2005 Apr;24(2):367–80, xii.
7. Sack RL. Clinical practice. Jet lag. N Engl J Med. 2010 Feb 4;362(5):440–7.
8. Sack RL, Auckley D, Auger RR, Carskadon MA, Wright KP Jr, Vitiello MV, et al. Circadian rhythm sleep disorders: part I, basic principles, shift work and jet lag disorders. An American Academy of Sleep Medicine review. Sleep. 2007 Nov 1;30(11):1460–83.
9. Waterhouse J, Edwards B, Nevill A, Atkinson G, Reilly T, Davies P, et al. Do subjective symptoms predict our perception of jet-lag? Ergonomics. 2000 Oct;43(10):1514–27.
10. Waterhouse J, Reilly T, Atkinson G, Edwards B. Jet lag: trends and coping strategies. Lancet. 2007 Mar 31;369(9567):1117–29.

MOTION SICKNESS
I. Dale Carroll

RISK FOR TRAVELERS

All people, given sufficient stimulus, will develop motion sickness, although some groups are at higher risk:

- Children aged 2–12 years are especially susceptible, but infants and toddlers seem relatively immune.
- Women, especially when pregnant, menstruating, or on hormones, are more likely to have motion sickness.
- People who get migraine headaches are prone to motion sickness during a migraine and prone to getting a migraine while they are experiencing motion sickness.
- People who expect to be sick are likely to experience symptoms.

TREATMENT

Some providers feel that continued exposure to motions that induce motion sickness will diminish symptoms; however, most people will be reluctant to endure the symptoms and will want medication. Antihistamines are the most commonly used and available medications, although nonsedating ones appear to be the least effective. Sedation is the primary side effect of all the efficacious drugs. Pyridoxine hydrochloride (vitamin B_6) plus doxylamine succinate (an antihistamine) is prescribed under the brand name of Diclectin in Canada, and may be recommended in their separate forms by clinicians in the United States.

Some common prescription medications used by travelers may exacerbate the nausea of motion sickness (see Table 2-8). Other common medications used to treat motion sickness are scopolamine (oral and transdermal), meclizine, cyclizine, antidopaminergic drugs (such as promethazine), metoclopramide, sympathomimetics, benzodiazepines, prochlorperazine, and ondansetron. When recommending any of these medications to travelers, providers should make sure that patients understand the risks and benefits, the adverse event profile of the drugs, and the potential drug interactions, because these medications often have undesirable side effects. Some travelers may need to try the medication before travel to see what effect it may have.

Medications in Children

For children aged 2–12 years, dimenhydrinate (Dramamine), 1–1.5 mg/kg per dose, or diphenhydramine, 0.5–1 mg/kg per dose up to 25 mg, can be given 1 hour before travel and every 6 hours during the trip. Because some children have paradoxical agitation with these medicines, a test dose should be given at home before departure. Scopolamine may cause dangerous adverse effects in children and should not be used; prochlorperazine and metoclopramide should be used with caution in children. Antihistamines are not approved by the Food and Drug Administration to treat motion sickness in children. Caregivers should be reminded to always ask a physician, pharmacist, or other clinician, if they have any questions about how to use or dose antihistamines in children before they administer the medication. Oversedation of young children with antihistamines can lead to life-threatening side effects.

Medications in Pregnancy

Drugs with the most safety data regarding the treatment of the nausea of pregnancy are the logical first choice. Alphabetical scoring of the safety of medications in pregnancy may not be helpful, and clinicians should review the actual safety data or call the patient's obstetric provider for suggestions. Web-based information may be found at the websites www.Motherisk.org and www.Reprotox.org.

Table 2-8. Medications that may increase nausea

MEDICATION CLASS	EXAMPLES
Antibiotics	Azithromycin, metronidazole, erythromycin, trimethoprim-sulfamethoxazole
Antiparasitics	Albendazole, thiabendazole, iodoquinol, chloroquine, mefloquine
Estrogens	Oral contraceptives, estradiol
Cardiovascular	Digoxin, levodopa
Narcotic analgesics	Codeine, morphine, meperidine
Nonsteroidal analgesics	Ibuprofen, naproxen, indomethacin
Antidepressants	Fluoxetine, paroxetine, sertraline
Asthma medication	Aminophylline
Bisphosphonates	Alendronate sodium, ibandronate sodium, risedronate sodium

PREVENTIVE MEASURES FOR TRAVELERS

Nonpharmacologic interventions to treat or manage motion sickness include the following:

- Being aware of situations that tend to trigger symptoms.
- Optimizing positioning—driving a vehicle instead of riding in it, sitting in the front seat of a car or bus, sitting over the wing of an aircraft, or being in the central cabin on a ship.
- Eating before the onset of symptoms, which may hasten gastric emptying, but in some people may aggravate motion sickness.
- Drinking caffeinated beverages along with medications.
- Reducing sensory input by, for example, lying prone, looking at the horizon, or shutting eyes.
- Adding distractions—aromatherapy using mint, lavender, or ginger (oral) helps some; flavored lozenges may help, as well. They may function as placebos or, in the case of oral ginger, may hasten gastric emptying.
- Using acupressure or magnets is advocated by some to prevent or treat nausea (not specifically for motion sickness), although scientific data are lacking.

BIBLIOGRAPHY

1. Benline TA, French J, Poole E. Anti-emetic drug effects on pilot performance: granisetron vs ondansetron. Aviat Space Environ Med. 1997 Nov;68(11):998–1005.
2. Priesol AJ. Motion Sickness. Rose BD, editor. Waltham MA: UpToDate; 2008.
3. Takeda N, Morita M, Horii A, Nishiike S, Kitahara T, Uno A. Neural mechanisms of motion sickness. J Med Invest. 2001 Feb;48(1–2):44–59.

RESPIRATORY INFECTIONS
Regina C. LaRocque, Edward T. Ryan

OVERVIEW

Respiratory infection is a leading cause of seeking medical care in returning travelers and has been reported to occur in up to 20% of all travelers. Thus, respiratory infections may be almost as common as travelers' diarrhea. Upper respiratory infection is more common than lower respiratory infection. In general, the types of respiratory infections that affect travelers are similar to those in nontravelers, and exotic causes are rare.

INFECTIOUS AGENT

Viral pathogens are the most common cause of respiratory infection in travelers; causative agents include coronavirus, adenovirus, rhinovirus, influenza virus, parainfluenza virus, human metapneumovirus, and respiratory syncytial virus. Bacterial pathogens are less common but include *Streptococcus pneumoniae*, *Mycoplasma pneumoniae*, *Haemophilus influenzae*, *Chlamydophila pneumoniae*, and *Legionella* species. Viral pathogens may set the stage for subsequent bacterial sinusitis or bronchitis.

RISK FOR TRAVELERS

Outbreaks are usually associated with common exposure in hotels and cruise ships or among tour groups. A few pathogens have been associated with outbreaks in travelers, including influenza virus, *L. pneumophila*, severe acute respiratory syndrome (SARS) coronavirus, and *Histoplasma capsulatum*. The peak influenza season in the temperate Northern Hemisphere is December through February. In the temperate Southern Hemisphere, the peak influenza season is June through August. Travelers to tropical zones are at risk all year. Exposure to an infected person from another hemisphere, such as on a cruise ship or package tour, can lead to an outbreak of influenza at any time or place.

Air-pressure changes during ascent and descent of aircraft can facilitate the development of sinusitis and otitis media. Intermingling of large numbers of people in airports, travel hubs, transport vehicles, cruise ships, and hotels can also facilitate transmission. Direct airborne transmission aboard aircraft is unusual because of frequent air recirculation and filtration, although sporadic cases of SARS, influenza, tuberculosis, and other diseases have occurred in modern aircraft. Transmission of infection may occur between passengers who are seated near one another, usually through direct contact or droplets.

The air quality at many travel destinations may not be optimal, and exposure to sulfur dioxide, nitrogen dioxide, carbon monoxide, ozone, and particulate matter is associated with a number of health risks, including respiratory tract inflammation, exacerbations of asthma and chronic obstructive pulmonary disease, impaired lung function, bronchitis, and pneumonia. Certain travelers have a higher risk for respiratory tract infection, including children, the elderly, and people with comorbid pulmonary conditions, such as asthma and chronic obstructive pulmonary disease (COPD).

The risk for tuberculosis among travelers is low (see Chapter 3, Tuberculosis).

DIAGNOSIS
Identifying a specific etiologic agent, especially in the absence of pneumonia, is often difficult and not clinically necessary. If indicated, the following methods of diagnosis can be used:

- Molecular methods are available to diagnose a number of respiratory viruses, including influenza virus, parainfluenza virus, adenovirus, human metapneumovirus, and respiratory syncytial virus, and for certain nonviral pathogens, such as L. pneumophila.
- Rapid tests are also available to detect group A streptococcal pharyngitis.
- Microbiologic culturing of sputum and blood, although insensitive, can help identify a causative respiratory pathogen in people with pneumonia.

CLINICAL PRESENTATION
Most respiratory tract infections, especially those of the upper respiratory tract, are mild and not incapacitating. Lower respiratory tract infections, particularly pneumonia, can be more severe. People with influenza commonly have acute onset of fever, myalgia, headache, and cough. Travelers with a viral upper respiratory infection may have persistent symptoms and should consider the possibility of subsequent bacterial sinusitis or bronchitis with symptoms that worsen after 1 week.

TREATMENT
Affected travelers are usually managed similarly to nontravelers, although travelers with progressive or severe illness should be evaluated for illnesses specific to their travel destinations and exposure history. Most respiratory infections in travelers are due to viruses, are mild, and do not require specific treatment or antibiotics. No systematic study of travelers with respiratory infections who self-treat has been reported. Self-treatment with antibiotics during travel can be considered for upper respiratory infections that worsen after 7 days of symptoms, particularly if specific symptoms of sinusitis or bronchitis are present. A respiratory-spectrum fluoroquinolone such as levofloxacin or a macrolide such as azithromycin may be prescribed to the traveler for this purpose before travel.

The rate of influenza among travelers is not known. The difficulty in self-diagnosing influenza makes it problematic to decide whether to provide travelers with a self-treatment dose of a neuraminidase inhibitor. This practice should probably be limited to travelers with a specific underlying condition that may predispose them to severe influenza.

Specific situations that may require medical intervention include the following:

- Pharyngitis without rhinorrhea, cough, or other symptoms that may indicate infection with group A streptococcus.
- Sudden onset of cough, chest pain, and fever that may indicate pneumonia, resulting in a situation where the traveler may be sick enough to seek medical care right away.
- Travelers with underlying medical conditions, such as asthma, pulmonary disease, or heart disease, who may need to seek medical care earlier than otherwise healthy travelers.

PREVENTIVE MEASURES FOR TRAVELERS
Vaccines are available to prevent a number of respiratory diseases, including influenza,

S. pneumoniae infection, *H. influenzae* type B infection (in young children), pertussis, diphtheria, varicella, and measles. Unless contraindicated, travelers should be vaccinated against influenza. Preventing respiratory illness while traveling may not be possible, but common-sense preventive measures include the following:

- Minimizing close contact with people who are coughing and sneezing
- Frequent handwashing, either with soap and water or alcohol-based hand cleaners (containing at least 60% alcohol)
- Using a vasoconstricting nasal spray immediately before air travel, if the traveler has a preexisting eustachian tube dysfunction.

BIBLIOGRAPHY

1. Ansart S, Pajot O, Grivois JP, Zeller V, Klement E, Perez L, et al. Pneumonia among travelers returning from abroad. J Travel Med. 2004 Mar–Apr;11(2):87–91.
2. Cabada MM, Maldonado F, Mozo K, Seas C, Gotuzzo E. Self-reported health problems among travelers visiting Cuzco: a Peruvian airport survey. Travel Med Infect Dis. 2009 Jan;7(1):25–9.
3. Camps M, Vilella A, Marcos MA, Letang E, Munoz J, Salvado E, et al. Incidence of respiratory viruses among travelers with a febrile syndrome returning from tropical and subtropical areas. J Med Virol. 2008 Apr;80(4):711–5.
4. Cobelens FG, van Deutekom H, Draayer-Jansen IW, Schepp-Beelen AC, van Gerven PJ, van Kessel RP, et al. Risk of infection with *Mycobacterium tuberculosis* in travellers to areas of high tuberculosis endemicity. Lancet. 2000 Aug 5;356(9228):461–5.
5. Farhat SC, Paulo RL, Shimoda TM, Conceicao GM, Lin CA, Braga AL, et al. Effect of air pollution on pediatric respiratory emergency room visits and hospital admissions. Braz J Med Biol Res. 2005 Feb;38(2):227–35.
6. Freedman DO, Weld LH, Kozarsky PE, Fisk T, Robins R, von Sonnenburg F, et al. Spectrum of disease and relation to place of exposure among ill returned travelers. N Engl J Med. 2006 Jan 12;354(2):119–30.
7. Leder K, Newman D. Respiratory infections during air travel. Intern Med J. 2005 Jan;35(1):50–5.
8. Leder K, Sundararajan V, Weld L, Pandey P, Brown G, Torresi J. Respiratory tract infections in travelers: a review of the GeoSentinel surveillance network. Clin Infect Dis. 2003 Feb 15;36(4):399–406.
9. Leder K, Tong S, Weld L, Kain KC, Wilder-Smith A, von Sonnenburg F, et al. Illness in travelers visiting friends and relatives: a review of the GeoSentinel Surveillance Network. Clin Infect Dis. 2006 Nov 1;43(9):1185–93.
10. Luna LK, Panning M, Grywna K, Pfefferle S, Drosten C. Spectrum of viruses and atypical bacteria in intercontinental air travelers with symptoms of acute respiratory infection. J Infect Dis. 2007 Mar 1;195(5):675–9.
11. Medina-Ramon M, Zanobetti A, Schwartz J. The effect of ozone and PM10 on hospital admissions for pneumonia and chronic obstructive pulmonary disease: a national multicity study. Am J Epidemiol. 2006 Mar 15;163(6):579–88.
12. Miller JM, Tam TW, Maloney S, Fukuda K, Cox N, Hockin J, et al. Cruise ships: high-risk passengers and the global spread of new influenza viruses. Clin Infect Dis. 2000 Aug;31(2):433–8.
13. Morgan J, Cano MV, Feikin DR, Phelan M, Monroy OV, Morales PK, et al. A large outbreak of histoplasmosis among American travelers associated with a hotel in Acapulco, Mexico, spring 2001. Am J Trop Med Hyg. 2003 Dec;69(6):663–9.
14. Rack J, Wichmann O, Kamara B, Gunther M, Cramer J, Schonfeld C, et al. Risk and spectrum of diseases in travelers to popular tourist destinations. J Travel Med. 2005 Sep–Oct;12(5):248–53.
15. Redman CA, Maclennan A, Wilson E, Walker E. Diarrhea and respiratory symptoms among travelers to Asia, Africa, and South and Central America from Scotland. J Travel Med. 2006 Jul–Aug;13(4):203–11.
16. Schwela D. Air pollution and health in urban areas. Rev Environ Health. 2000 Jan–Jun;15(1–2):13–42.
17. Weitzel EK, McMains KC, Rajapaksa S, Wormald PJ. Aerosinusitis: pathophysiology, prophylaxis, and management in passengers and aircrew. Aviat Space Environ Med. 2008 Jan;79(1):50–3.
18. Zitter JN, Mazonson PD, Miller DP, Hulley SB, Balmes JR. Aircraft cabin air recirculation and symptoms of the common cold. JAMA. 2002 Jul 24–31;288(4):483–6.

OCCUPATIONAL EXPOSURE TO HIV

Eli W. Warnock III, V. Ramana Dhara, Alan G. Czarkowski

RISK FOR HEALTH CARE WORKERS TRAVELING OUTSIDE THE UNITED STATES

The risk of occupational exposure to HIV is most closely related to the activities and duties of the health care worker, but geographic location can also affect the risk of exposure and the quality of postexposure care. Many factors can increase the risk of occupational HIV exposure in developing countries:

- Less stringent safety procedures and standards
- Limited resources for postexposure evaluation and treatment
- High rates of undiagnosed HIV infection
- Limited access to personal protective equipment

MODES OF TRANSMISSION

HIV may be transmitted occupationally to health care workers engaged in routine medical activities and procedures that can result in needlesticks or blood splashes. The routine nature of these procedures may cause health care workers to relax their vigilance and adherence to safety details. Typically exposures occur as a result of percutaneous exposure to contaminated sharps, including needles, lancets, scalpels, and broken glass. Needlesticks from large-bore hollow needles that have contaminated material in the bore are thought to carry a high risk of transmission. Contact between infectious material and mucous membranes or nonintact skin may also transmit HIV.

EPIDEMIOLOGY

The global number of HIV infections among health care workers attributable to sharps injuries has been estimated to be 1,000 cases (range, 200–5,000) per year. In prospective studies, the average risk for HIV transmission after a percutaneous exposure to HIV-infected blood has been estimated to be approximately 0.3% (95% confidence interval [CI], 0.2%–0.5%) and after a mucous membrane exposure, approximately 0.09% (95% CI, 0.006%–0.5%). Although HIV has been transmitted through exposure to nonintact skin, the average risk for transmission by this route has not been quantified but is estimated to be less than the risk for mucous membrane exposures.

PREVENTIVE MEASURES FOR TRAVELERS

People working internationally who will be engaging in high-risk occupational health care activities, such as drawing blood or the other use of sharps during patient care, should consistently follow standard precautions to reduce the risk of occupational exposure to HIV and other bloodborne pathogens. Standard precautions involve the use of protective barriers such as gloves, gowns, aprons, masks, or protective eyewear. Additional information about occupational health and safety standards for bloodborne pathogens can be found at www.osha.gov/pls/oshaweb/owadisp.show_document?p_table=STANDARDS&p_id=10051.

In addition, clinicians working internationally should:

- Always be mindful of the hazards posed by sharps injuries.
- Maintain strict safety standards while working in environments that may have less stringent standards.
- Use devices with safety features and improved work practices (www.cdc.gov/niosh/docs/2000-108/).
- Consider bringing their own protective equipment if they are unsure of its availability at their destination.
- Consider bringing postexposure prophylaxis (PEP) for HIV in the event that they are injured with a potentially contaminated sharp.

POSTEXPOSURE MANAGEMENT

Health care workers who may have been occupationally exposed to HIV should immediately perform the following steps:

- Wash the exposed area with soap and water thoroughly. If mucous membrane exposure has occurred, flush the area with copious amounts of water or saline.

- If possible, assess the HIV status of the source. Rapid HIV testing is preferred. If the source's rapid HIV antibody test result is positive, assume that it is a true positive.
- Seek qualified medical evaluation as soon as possible to guide decisions on postexposure treatment and testing.
- Contact the National Clinicians' Postexposure Prophylaxis Hotline (PEPline) at 1-888-448-4911 (24 hours a day, 7 days per week) for assistance in assessing risk and advice on managing occupational exposures to HIV and other bloodborne pathogens (www.nccc.ucsf.edu/about_nccc/pepline). If the toll-free number is not accessible when calling from another country, the main administrative line for the National HIV/AIDS Clinicians' Consultation Center is 415-206-8700.
- Consider beginning PEP for HIV (see below).

Postexposure Prophylaxis

A number of medication combinations are available for PEP. Since these regimens may change based on new research, refer to MMWR's Updated US Public Health Service Guidelines for the Management of Occupational Exposures to HIV and Recommendations for Postexposure Prophylaxis (http://aidsinfo.nih.gov/Guidelines/GuidelineDetail.aspx?MenuItem=Guidelines&Search=Off&GuidelineID=10&ClassID=3) and the PEPline for more information about PEP recommendations. Specific regimens should be determined by clinicians familiar with the medications and the health care worker's medical history.

If the exposed person chooses to initiate PEP, he or she must do so within hours of the exposure. PEP can be stopped if new information changes the assessment; however, waiting to start PEP until all information is gathered can decrease its efficacy. If indicated, arrange for procurement or shipment of additional PEP from a credible source to complete the recommended 4-week course of treatment.

Consider other potential infectious disease exposures from the source material, including hepatitis B virus or hepatitis C virus (HCV), and manage as appropriate.

Postexposure Testing

People with occupational exposure to HIV should receive HIV antibody testing by enzyme immunoassay as soon as possible after exposure as a baseline, with follow-up testing at 6 weeks, 3 months, and 6 months. Extended HIV follow-up testing for up to 12 months is recommended for those who become infected with HCV after exposure to a source coinfected with HIV and HCV. Postexposure counseling and medical evaluation should be provided, whether or not the exposed person receives PEP (http://aidsinfo.nih.gov/contentfiles/HealthCareOccupExpoGL_PDA.pdf).

Exposed health care workers should be advised to use precautions (avoid blood or tissue donations, breastfeeding, or pregnancy) to prevent secondary transmission, especially during the first 6–12 weeks after exposure. For exposures for which PEP is indicated, exposed people should be counseled regarding possible drug toxicities and interactions, the need for monitoring, and the importance of careful adherence to PEP regimens.

BIBLIOGRAPHY

1. Bell DM. Occupational risk of human immunodeficiency virus infection in healthcare workers: an overview. Am J Med. 1997 May 19;102(5B):9–15.
2. Canadian Centre for Occupation Health and Safety. Needlestick injuries. 2005 [cited 2010 Nov 8]. Available from: http://www.ccohs.ca/oshanswers/diseases/needlestick_injuries.html.
3. CDC. NIOSH alert: preventing needlestick injuries in health care settings. Cincinnati: National Institute for Occupational Safety and Health; 1999 [cited 2010 Nov 8]. Available from: http://www.cdc.gov/niosh/docs/2000-108/.
4. CDC. Notice to readers: updated information regarding antiretroviral agents used as HIV postexposure prophylaxis for occupational HIV exposure. MMWR Recomm Rep. 2007 Dec 14;56(49):1291–2.
5. CDC. Updated US Public Health Service guidelines for the management of occupational exposures to HBV, HCV, and HIV and recommendations for postexposure prophylaxis. MMWR Recomm Rep. 2001 Jun 29;50(RR-11):1–52.
6. Clinical and Laboratory Standards Institute. M29-A3 Protection of Laboratory Workers from Occupationally Acquired Infections: Approved Guideline. 3rd ed. 2005.

7. Gerberding JL. Clinical practice. Occupational exposure to HIV in health care settings. N Engl J Med. 2003 Feb 27;348(9):826–33.

8. International Healthcare Worker Safety Center. EPINet: Exposure Prevention Information Network. Charlottesville, VA: University of Virginia; 2010 [cited 2010 Nov 16]. Available from: http://healthsystem. virginia.edu/internet/epinet/about_epinet.cfm.

9. National HIV/AIDS Clinicians' Consultation Center. PEPline: the national clinicians' post-exposure prophylaxis hotline. San Francisco: University of California, San Francisco; 2010 [cited 2010 Nov 8]. Available from: http://www.nccc.ucsf.edu/about_nccc/pepline/.

10. Occupational Safety and Health Administration. Regulations (standards – 29 CFR): bloodborne pathogens–1910.1030. Washington, DC: Occupational Safety and Health Administration. Available from: http://www.osha.gov/pls/oshaweb/owadisp. show_document?p_table=STANDARDS&p_id=10051.

11. Panlilio AL, Cardo DM, Grohskopf LA, Heneine W, Ross CS. Updated US Public Health Service guidelines for the management of occupational exposures to HIV and recommendations for postexposure prophylaxis. MMWR Recomm Rep. 2005 Sep 30;54(RR-9):1–17.

12. Prüss-Üstün A, Rapiti E, Hutin Y. Estimation of the global burden of disease attributable to contaminated sharps injuries among health-care workers. Am J Ind Med. 2005 Dec;48(6):482–90.

13. Puro V, De Carli G, Petrosillo N, Ippolito G. Risk of exposure to bloodborne infection for Italian healthcare workers, by job category and work area. Studio Italiano Rischio Occupazionale da HIV Group. Infect Control Hosp Epidemiol. 2001 Apr;22(4):206–10.

14. Romea S, Alkiza ME, Ramon JM, Oromi J. Risk for occupational transmission of HIV infection among health care workers. Study in a Spanish hospital. Eur J Epidemiol. 1995 Apr;11(2):225–9.

15. Sagoe-Moses C, Pearson RD, Perry J, Jagger J. Risks to health care workers in developing countries. N Engl J Med. 2001 Aug 16;345(7):538–41.

16. Sepkowitz KA. Occupationally acquired infections in health care workers. Part II. Ann Intern Med. 1996 Dec 1;125(11):917–28.

17. Uslan DZ, Virk A. Postexposure chemoprophylaxis for occupational exposure to human immunodeficiency virus in traveling health care workers. J Travel Med. 2005 Jan–Feb;12(1):14–8.

18. Young TN, Arens FJ, Kennedy GE, Laurie JW, Rutherford G. Antiretroviral post-exposure prophylaxis (PEP) for occupational HIV exposure. Cochrane Database Syst Rev. 2007(1):CD002835.

Counseling & Advice for Travelers

FOOD & WATER PRECAUTIONS

John C. Watson, Michele C. Hlavsa, Patricia M. Griffin

Contaminated food and water often pose a risk for travelers. Among the infectious diseases that travelers can acquire from contaminated food and water are *Escherichia coli* infections, shigellosis or bacillary dysentery, giardiasis, cryptosporidiosis, norovirus infection, hepatitis A, and salmonelloses, including typhoid fever. Contaminated food and water can also pose a risk of cholera, rotavirus infection, and a variety of conditions caused by protozoan and helminthic parasites. Many infectious diseases transmitted through food and water can be acquired directly through the fecal–oral route. Accidental ingestion or contact with recreational water from lakes, rivers, oceans, and inadequately treated swimming pools can also spread many of the above diseases, as well as some infections of the ears, eyes, skin, and respiratory or nervous systems (see Chapter 3 for specific infectious diseases).

FOOD

To avoid illness, travelers should be advised to select food with care. All raw food is subject to contamination. Particularly in areas where hygiene and sanitation are inadequate, travelers should be advised to avoid salads, uncooked vegetables, and unpasteurized milk and milk products, such as cheese. Travelers should eat only food that has been fully cooked and is still hot, and fruit that has been washed in clean water and then peeled by the traveler. Undercooked and raw meat, fish, and shellfish can carry various intestinal pathogens. Cooked food that has been allowed to stand for several hours at ambient temperature can provide a fertile medium for bacterial growth or be recontaminated by food-handling techniques, so it should be thoroughly reheated before serving. These recommendations also apply to eggs, which should be thoroughly cooked, whether they are served alone or used in sauces. Consumption of food and beverages obtained from street vendors has been associated with an increased risk of illness. Travelers should wash their hands or use alcohol-based hand cleaners (with ≥60% alcohol) before eating, after using the bathroom or changing diapers, and after direct contact with preschool children, animals, or feces.

The easiest way to guarantee a safe food source for an infant aged <6 months is to breastfeed the infant. If the infant has already been weaned, formula prepared from commercial powder and boiled water is the safest and most practical food (see Chapter 7, Travel and Breastfeeding).

Travelers should be advised not to bring perishable seafood from high-risk areas upon their return to the United States. Cholera cases have occurred in people who ate crab that had been brought into the United States from Latin America by travelers. Moreover, travelers should not assume that food and water aboard commercial aircraft are safe, since food and water may be obtained in the country of departure, where items may be contaminated.

WATER
Drinking Water

In many parts of the world, particularly where water treatment, sanitation, and hygiene are inadequate, tap water may contain disease-causing contaminants, including viruses, bacteria, and parasites. As a result, tap water in some places may be unsafe for drinking, preparing food and beverages, making ice, cooking, and brushing teeth. Contaminated tap water may also cause illness if inadvertently swallowed or inhaled during showering or bathing. Infants, young children, pregnant women, the elderly, and people whose immune systems are compromised because of AIDS, chemotherapy, or transplant medications may be especially susceptible to illness from some contaminants.

Travelers should avoid drinking or otherwise ingesting tap water unless reasonably certain it is not contaminated. Many people choose to disinfect or filter their water when traveling to destinations where safe tap water may not be available (see the Water Disinfection for Travelers section later in this chapter). Water contaminated with fuel or toxic chemicals, however, will not be made safe by boiling or disinfection; travelers should use a different source of water if they suspect this type of contamination.

In areas where tap water may be contaminated, commercially bottled water from an unopened, sealed container, or water that has been adequately disinfected should be used for brushing teeth and other oral hygiene. Travelers who may be at increased risk for legionellosis, such as elderly or immunocompromised people, may choose to avoid areas such as showers or hot tubs where *Legionella* can be aerosolized and inhaled.

Beverages made with boiled water and served steaming hot (such as tea and coffee) are generally safe to drink. When served in unopened, sealed cans or bottles, carbonated beverages, commercially prepared fruit drinks, water, alcoholic beverages, and pasteurized drinks generally can be considered safe. However, reports exist of apparently sealed bottles or cans from commercial sources that, when opened, contained contaminated products. Because water on the outside of cans and bottles may be contaminated, they should be wiped clean and dried before opening or drinking directly from the container.

Beverages that may not be safe for consumption include fountain drinks, fruit drinks made with tap water, iced tea, and iced coffee. Because ice may be made from contaminated water, travelers should request that beverages be served without ice.

Recreational Water

Pathogens that cause a variety of infections (gastrointestinal, respiratory, dermatologic, aural, ocular, and neurologic) can be transmitted by ingesting, inhaling mists or aerosols of, or having contact with contaminated water while swimming, wading, or participating in other recreational water activities in oceans, lakes, rivers, pools, water parks, fountains, and hot tubs. Water contaminated by sewage, animal waste, wastewater runoff, or human feces from swimmers can appear clear and clean but still contain disease-causing pathogens. Ingesting even small amounts of such water can cause illness. Travelers should avoid ingesting any water in which they are swimming, wading, or participating in other recreational water activities. They also should not swim with open cuts, abrasions, or other wounds that could serve as entry points for pathogens. To protect other swimmers, children and adults with diarrhea should *not* swim or wade in the water to avoid contaminating it.

Travelers should not swim or wade 1) in water that may be contaminated with human or animal feces or sewage; 2) near storm drains; 3) after heavy rainfall; 4) in freshwater streams, canals, and lakes in schistosomiasis-endemic areas of the Caribbean, South America, Africa, and Asia (see Map 3–14); 5) in bodies of water that may be contaminated with urine from animals infected with *Leptospira*; or 6) in seawater, with an open wound or abrasion. When swimming, diving, or participating in similar activities in warm freshwater (including lakes, rivers, ponds, hot springs, or thermally polluted water near power plants and industrial complexes), travelers should prevent water from entering the nose by wearing a nose clip or by not submerging the face or head. *Naegleria fowleri* is found in warm freshwater around the world; infections are rare but often fatal (www.cdc.gov/parasites/naegleria).

Maintaining proper disinfectant (such as chlorine and bromine) and pH levels is necessary to prevent transmission of pathogens in treated recreational water venues such as pools, water parks, fountains, and hot tubs. Travelers should avoid such locations if the water is cloudy. If the water is clear, travelers may choose to use test strips to check chlorine and pH levels. Even if recreational water has been properly disinfected, travelers still should avoid ingesting any water in which they are swimming, wading, or participating in other recreational water activities. Because some pathogens, such as *Cryptosporidium*, can survive even in well-maintained pools, people with diarrhea should *not* swim or enter treated recreational water.

Maintaining disinfectant levels in hot tubs is difficult because the high water temperature depletes disinfectants. *Legionella* (see Chapter 3, Legionellosis) and *Pseudomonas*, which can cause "hot tub rash" and "swimmer's ear," can multiply in recreational water venues in which disinfectant levels are not properly maintained. Travelers can use test strips to check chlorine and pH levels, and may choose to avoid hot tubs where bather limits are not enforced or where the water is visibly cloudy.

BIBLIOGRAPHY

1. Backer H. Water disinfection for international and wilderness travelers. Clin Infect Dis. 2002 Feb 1;34(3):355–64.

2. Cartwright R, Colbourne J. Cryptosporidiosis and hotel swimming pools—a multifaceted challenge. Water Science and Technology: Water Supply. 2002;2(3):47–54.

3. CDC. Drinking water: camping, hiking, travel. Atlanta: CDC; 2010 [cited 2010 Nov 8]. Available from: http://www.cdc.gov/healthywater/drinking/travel/index.html.

4. CDC. For swimmers and hot tub users. Atlanta: CDC; 2010 [cited 2010 Nov 8]. Available from: http://www.cdc.gov/healthywater/swimming/pools/for-swimmers-hot-tub-users.html.

5. CDC. Healthy swimming/recreational water. Atlanta: CDC; 2010 [cited 2010 Nov 8]. Available from: http://www.cdc.gov/healthywater/swimming/index.html.

6. CDC. Legionellosis resource site. Atlanta: CDC; 2009 [cited 2010 Nov 8]. Available from: http://www.cdc.gov/legionella/.

7. CDC. Parasites—*Naegleria*. Atlanta: CDC; 2008 [cited 2010 Nov 8]. Available from: http://www.cdc.gov/parasites/naegleria/.

8. CDC. *Vibrio vulnificus*. Atlanta: CDC National Center for Zoonotic, Vector-Borne, and Enteric Diseases; 2009 [updated 2009 Nov 12; cited 2010 Nov 23]. Available from: http://www.cdc.gov/nczved/divisions/dfbmd/diseases/vibriov/.

9. Eberhart-Phillips J, Besser RE, Tormey MP, Koo D, Feikin D, Araneta MR, et al. An outbreak of cholera from food served on an international aircraft. Epidemiol Infect. 1996 Feb;116(1):9–13.

10. Finelli L, Swerdlow D, Mertz K, Ragazzoni H, Spitalny K. Outbreak of cholera associated with crab brought from an area with epidemic disease. J Infect Dis. 1992 Dec;166(6):1433–5.

PREVENTION OF TRAVELERS' DIARRHEA—IT'S NOT ONLY *WHAT* YOU EAT & DRINK

David R. Shlim

Travel health providers in the 1980s seemed certain that travelers' diarrhea (TD) could be avoided by observing sensible food precautions. A consensus statement published in 1985 concluded, "Data indicate that meticulous attention to food and beverage preparation can decrease the likelihood of developing TD." The experts in the consensus group had 7 studies available to them at that time. In retrospect, it is surprising to note that 6 of the studies concluded that there was no relationship between recommended food and water precautions and the likelihood of developing TD. The seventh article showed a small correlation between eating "mistakes" and the likelihood of developing TD in the first 3 days of a journey.

Overall, the risk of acquiring TD in many countries has not decreased in the >50 years since the syndrome was first characterized in Mexico, despite decades of messages urging travelers to follow food and water precautions. The earliest study that addressed the question of food and water precautions was published in 1973; it concluded that "drinking bottled liquids, and avoiding salads, raw vegetables, and unpeeled fruits failed to prevent illness." In a study of returning travelers from Mexico and Peru published in 1978, in which >70% of travelers reported TD, the author noted that "avoidance of tap water, uncooked foods, and ice cubes did not make a difference in the outcome." In a famous study in 1983, a survey of over 10,000 travelers worldwide found not only that observing food and water precautions failed to prevent TD, but also that people who claimed that they exercised more caution were at increased risk of acquiring TD: "Diarrhea seemed to occur more frequently the more a person tried to elude it!" Although careful travelers are unlikely to have more diarrhea than careless eaters, the authors were not able to confirm what seemed logical—that careful travelers will have *less* diarrhea.

Although these studies do not appear to support the traditional guidance, travelers should not abandon common sense in regard to being careful with food and water. However, the question remains as to why travelers do not seem to decrease their risk of diarrhea even when trying to be scrupulous with food and water precautions. From today's perspective, it is surprising that the consensus statement of 1985 concluded that food and water precautions were an effective way to prevent TD. Since that time, studies have suggested that *where* you eat your food makes more difference than *what* you eat. At least 3 studies have shown that people who eat in restaurants have a significantly higher risk of TD than expatriates who eat in their own homes. Further investigation into the state of restaurant hygiene in several developing countries has demonstrated that many basic health precautions are violated. Some restaurants fail to provide sinks for employees to wash their hands after going to the toilet. Cutting boards may not be washed between cutting raw meat and peeling and cutting vegetables. Foods are cooked but then may be left to sit at ambient temperatures for extended periods of time because of a paucity of refrigerator space or power cuts. Windows may not be screened to keep out flies. Defrosting meat can sit on a refrigerator shelf and drip juices on already cooked foods. In tourist destinations where these restaurant violations were corrected, the rate of TD among the tourists visiting those sites decreased significantly.

How should this information be used in the pre-travel visit? Simply telling travelers to "boil it, cook it, peel it, or forget it" may not prevent diarrhea. A few rules have been proven to help. Food that is served hot is almost always safe to eat. Foods that are cooked earlier in the day and sit out for long periods of time, such as on a buffet, can be unsafe. Dry foods such as cakes, cookies, and bread are usually safe. Beverages that come in factory-sealed containers are safe. All carbonated beverages that come in sealed bottles or cans should be safe because of their high acidity. Travelers should always be counseled on appropriate self-diagnosis and treatment strategies. Future reductions in the rate of TD are likely to be attributable to improved restaurant hygiene in developing countries. Expatriates can control food preparation in their own kitchens, but poor restaurant hygiene in developing countries can create an insurmountable risk of TD in travelers.

BIBLIOGRAPHY

1. Blaser MJ. Environmental interventions for the prevention of travelers' diarrhea. Rev Infect Dis. 1986 May–Jun;8 Suppl 2:S142–50.
2. Ericsson CD, Pickering LK, Sullivan P, DuPont HL. The role of location of food consumption in the prevention of travelers' diarrhea in Mexico. Gastroenterology. 1980 Nov;79(5 Pt 1):812–6.
3. NIH Consensus Development Conference. Travelers' diarrhea. JAMA. 1985 May 10;253(18):2700–4.
4. Shlim DR. Looking for evidence that personal hygiene precautions prevent traveler's diarrhea. Clin Infect Dis. 2005 Dec 1;41 Suppl 8:S531–5.
5. Shlim DR. Update in traveler's diarrhea. Infect Dis Clin North Am. 2005 Mar;19(1):137–49.
6. Tjoa WS, DuPont HL, Sullivan P, Pickering LK, Holguin AH, Olarte J, et al. Location of food consumption and travelers' diarrhea. Am J Epidemiol. 1977 Jul;106(1):61–6.

WATER DISINFECTION FOR TRAVELERS
Howard D. Backer

RISK FOR TRAVELERS

Waterborne disease is a risk for international travelers who visit countries that have poor hygiene and inadequate sanitation, and for wilderness visitors who rely on surface water in any country, including the United States. The list of potential waterborne pathogens is extensive and includes bacteria, viruses, protozoa, and parasitic helminths. Most of the organisms that can cause travelers' diarrhea can be waterborne. Where treated tap water is available, most travelers' intestinal infections are probably transmitted by food, but where untreated surface or well water is used and there is no sanitation infrastructure, the risk of waterborne infection is high. Microorganisms with small infectious doses can even cause illness through recreational water exposure, via inadvertent water ingestion.

Bottled water has become the convenient solution for most travelers, but in some places it may not be superior to tap water. Moreover, the plastic bottles create an ecological problem, since most developing countries do not recycle plastic bottles. All international travelers, especially long-term travelers or expatriates, should become familiar with and use simple methods to ensure safe drinking water. Table 2-9 compares benefits and limitations of different methods.

FIELD TECHNIQUES FOR WATER TREATMENT
Heat

Common intestinal pathogens are readily inactivated by heat. Microorganisms are killed in a shorter time at higher temperatures, whereas temperatures as low as 140°F (60°C) are effective with a longer contact time. Pasteurization uses this principle to kill foodborne enteric pathogens and spoiling organisms at temperatures between 140°F (60°C) and 158°F (70°C), well below the boiling point of water (212°F [100°C]).

Although boiling is not necessary to kill common intestinal pathogens, it is the only easily recognizable point that doesn't require a thermometer. All organisms except bacterial spores, which are not usually waterborne enteric pathogens, are killed in seconds at boiling temperature. Therefore, any water that is boiled for 1 minute (to allow for a margin of safety) should be adequately disinfected. Because the boiling point decreases with increasing altitude, water should be boiled for 3 minutes at altitudes above 6,562 ft (2,000 m). To conserve fuel, the same results can be obtained by bringing water to a boil and then turning off the stove but keeping the container covered for several minutes.

If no other means of water treatment is available, a potential alternative to boiling is to use tap water that is too hot to touch, which is probably at a temperature between 131°F (55°C) and 140°F (60°C). This temperature may be adequate to kill pathogens if the water has been kept hot in the tank for some time. Travelers with access to electricity can bring a small electric heating coil or a lightweight beverage warmer to boil water.

Filtration and Clarification

Filter pore size is the primary determinant of a filter's effectiveness, but microorganisms also adhere to filter media by electrochemical reactions. Microfilters with "absolute" pore sizes of 0.1–0.4 µm are usually effective to remove cysts and bacteria but may not adequately remove viruses, which are a major concern in water with high levels of fecal contamination (Table 2-10). The Environmental Protection Agency (EPA) designation of water "purifier" indicates that company-sponsored testing has substantiated claims for removing 10^6 bacteria, 10^4 (9,999 of 10,000) viruses, and 10^3 *Cryptosporidium* oocysts or *Giardia* cysts, although EPA does not independently test the validity of these claims. NSF International is a nonprofit, nongovernmental organization that develops standards and product certification for public health and safety. They are a designated collaborating center of the World Health Organization (WHO) for Food and Water Safety and Indoor Environment. They are accredited by the American National Standards Institute (ANSI), the International Accreditation Service (IAS), and the Standards Council of Canada (SCC) for third-party certification. Some water filtration units have been evaluated by NSF International under the NSF/ANSI Standard 53. A listing of certified water filtration products can be found at www.nsf.org/consumer.

New portable filter designs include hollow fiber technology, which is a cluster of tiny tubules with variable pore sizes that can remove virus-size particles. Reverse-osmosis filters can both remove microbiologic contamination and desalinate water. The high price and slow output of small hand-pump reverse-osmosis units prohibit use by land-based travelers; however, they are important survival aids for ocean voyagers.

Coagulation-flocculation (CF) removes suspended particles that cause a cloudy appearance and bad taste and do not settle by gravity; this process removes many but not all microorganisms. CF is easily applied in the field. Alum, or one of several other substances, is added to the water, stirred well, allowed to settle, then poured through a coffee filter or fine cloth to remove the sediment. Tablets or packets of powder that combine flocculent and hypochlorite disinfection are available (commercial products such as Chlor-floc or PUR).

Table 2-9. Comparison of water disinfection techniques

TECHNIQUE	ADVANTAGES	DISADVANTAGES
Heat	• Does not impart additional taste or color • Single step that inactivates all enteric pathogens • Efficacy is not compromised by contaminants or particles in the water as for halogenation and filtration	• Does not improve taste, smell, or appearance of water • Fuel sources may be scarce, expensive, or unavailable • Does not prevent recontamination during storage
Filtration	• Simple to operate • Requires no holding time for treatment • Large choice of commercial product designs • Adds no unpleasant taste and often improves taste and appearance of water • Can be combined with halogens to remove or kill all pathogenic waterborne microbes	• Adds bulk and weight to baggage • Many do not reliably remove viruses • Channeling of water or high pressure can force microorganisms through the filter • More expensive than chemical treatment • Eventually clogs from suspended particulate matter and may require some maintenance or repair in the field • Does not prevent recontamination during storage
Halogens (chlorine, iodine)	• Inexpensive and widely available in liquid or tablet forms • Taste can be removed by simple techniques • Flexible dosing • Equally easy to treat large and small volumes	• Corrosive and stains clothing • Imparts taste and odor to water • Flexibility requires understanding of principles • Iodine is physiologically active, with potential adverse effects • Not readily effective against *Cryptosporidium* oocysts • Efficacy decreases with low water temperature and decreasing water clarity
Chlorine dioxide	• Low doses have no taste or color • Simple to use and available in liquid or tablet form • More potent than equivalent doses of chlorine • Effective against all waterborne pathogens	• Volatile and sensitive to sunlight: do not expose tablets to air and use generated solutions rapidly • No persistent residual concentration, so does not prevent recontamination during storage
Ultraviolet (UV)	• Imparts no taste • Portable devices now available • Effective against all waterborne pathogens • Extra doses of UV can be used for added assurance and with no side effects • Moderate benefit from solar UV exposure	• Requires clear water • Does not improve taste or appearance of water • Relatively expensive • Requires batteries or power source • Difficult to know if devices are delivering required UV doses • No persistent residual concentration, so does not prevent recontamination during storage

Table 2-10. Microorganism size and susceptibility to filtration

ORGANISM	AVERAGE SIZE (μm)	MAXIMUM RECOMMENDED FILTER RATING (μm ABSOLUTE)[1]
Viruses	0.03	Not specified (optimally 0.01)
Enteric bacteria (*Escherichia coli*)	0.5 × 3.0–8.0	0.2–0.4
Cryptosporidium oocyst	4–6	1
Giardia cyst	6.0–10.0 × 8.0–15.0	3.0–5.0

[1] NSF 53 rating on a filter certifies for cyst/oocyst removal.

Chemical Disinfection
Halogens

The most common chemical water disinfectants are chlorine and iodine (halogens). Worldwide, chemical disinfection with chlorine is the most commonly used method for improving and maintaining the microbiologic quality of drinking water. Sodium hypochlorite, the active ingredient in common household bleach, is the primary disinfectant promoted by CDC and the WHO Safe Water System at a 1.5% concentration for household use in the developing world. Other chlorine-containing compounds, such as calcium hypochlorite and sodium dichloroisocyanurate, which are both solids, are also effective for household water treatment.

Given adequate concentrations and length of exposure (contact time), chlorine and iodine have similar activity and are effective against bacteria, viruses, and *Giardia* cysts (www.cdc.gov/safewater/about_pages/CTfactor-final.pdf). Because many factors in the field are uncontrolled, extending the contact time adds a margin of safety. However, some common waterborne parasites, such as *Cryptosporidium*, are poorly inactivated by halogen disinfection, even at practical extended contact times. Therefore, chemical disinfection should be supplemented with adequate filtration to remove these microorganisms from drinking water. Cloudy water contains substances that will neutralize disinfectant, so it will require higher concentrations or contact times or, preferably, clarification through settling or filtration before disinfectant is added. Tablets that combine flocculent and disinfectant are available.

Both chlorine and iodine are available in liquid and tablet form. Because iodine has physiologic activity, WHO recommends limiting iodine water disinfection to a few weeks of emergency use. Iodine use is not recommended for people with unstable thyroid disease or known iodine allergy. Iodine should not be used by pregnant women because of the potential effect on the fetal thyroid.

The taste of halogens in water can be improved by several means:

- Reduce concentration and increase contact time proportionately.
- After the required contact time, run water through a filter that contains activated carbon.
- After the required contact time, add a tiny pinch of ascorbic acid.

Iodine Resins

Iodine resins transfer iodine to microorganisms that come into contact with the resin, but leave little iodine dissolved in the water. The resins have been incorporated into many different filter designs available for field use. Most contain a 1-µm cyst filter, which should effectively remove protozoan cysts. Few models are sold in the United States because of inconsistent test results, but some models are still available for international use.

Salt (Sodium Chloride) Electrolysis

Passing a current through a simple brine salt solution generates oxidants, including hypochlorite, which can be used to disinfect microbes.

Chlorine Dioxide

Chlorine dioxide (ClO_2) can kill most water-borne pathogens, including *Cryptosporidium* oocysts, at practical doses and contact times. Tablets and liquid formulations are available to generate chlorine dioxide in the field for small-quantity water treatment.

Ultraviolet (UV) Light

Extensive data show that UV light can kill bacteria, viruses, and *Cryptosporidium* oocysts in water. The effect depends on UV dose and exposure time, and requires clear water because suspended particles can shield microorganisms from UV rays. These units have limited effectiveness in water with high levels of suspended solids and turbidity. They also have no disinfection residual. Portable battery-operated units that deliver a metered, timed dose of UV may be an effective way to disinfect small quantities of clear water in the field; however, more testing is needed for conclusive evidence.

Solar Irradiation and Heating

UV irradiation by sunlight in the UVA range can substantially improve the microbiologic quality of water. Recent work has confirmed the efficacy and optimal procedures of the solar disinfection technique. Transparent bottles (such as clear plastic beverage bottles), preferably lying on a dark surface, are exposed to sunlight for a minimum of 4 hours. UV and thermal inactivation are synergistic for solar disinfection of drinking water. Use of a simple reflector or solar cooker can achieve temperatures of 149°F (65°C), which will pasteurize the water after 4 hours. Solar disinfection is not effective on turbid water. If the headlines in a newspaper can't be read through the bottle of water, then the water must be filtered before solar irradiation is used. If more than half the sky is clouded over, then solar irradiation is not effective and should be repeated before using the water. Solar disinfection of drinking water may be acceptable for austere emergency situations.

Silver and Other Products

Silver ion has bactericidal effects in low doses and some attractive features, including absence of color, taste, and odor. The use of silver as a drinking water disinfectant is popular in Europe, but it is not approved for this purpose in the United States, because silver concentration in water is strongly affected by adsorption onto the surface of the container, and there has been limited testing on viruses and cysts. In the United States, silver is approved for maintaining microbiologic quality of stored water.

Several other common products have antibacterial effects in water and are marketed in commercial products for travelers, including hydrogen peroxide, citrus juice, and potassium permanganate. None have sufficient data to recommend them for water disinfection in the field.

THE PREFERRED TECHNIQUE

The optimal technique for a person or group depends on personal preference, size of the group, water source, and the style of travel. Boiling is the most reliable single-step treatment, but certain filters, UV, and chlorine dioxide are also effective in most situations. Optimal treatment of highly contaminated or cloudy water may require CF followed by chemical disinfection. On long-distance, oceangoing boats where water must be desalinated during the voyage, only reverse-osmosis membrane filters are adequate.

BIBLIOGRAPHY

1. Backer H. Field water disinfection. In: Auerbach PS, editor. Wilderness medicine. 5th ed. Philadelphia: Mosby Elsevier; 2007. p. 1368–417.

2. Backer H, Hollowell J. Use of iodine for water disinfection: iodine toxicity and maximum recommended dose. Environ Health Perspect. 2000 Aug;108(8):679–84.

3. Departments of the Army, Navy, and Air Force. TB MED 577 Technical bulletin: sanitary control and surveillance of field water supplies. Washington, DC: US Army Medical Department; 2010. Available from: http://armypubs.army.mil/med/DR_pubs/dr_a/pdf/tbmed577.pdf.

4. Groh CD, MacPherson DW, Groves DJ. Effect of heat on the sterilization of artificially contaminated water. J Travel Med. 1996 Mar 1;3(1):11–3.

5. Joyce TM, McGuigan KG, Elmore-Meegan M, Conroy RM. Inactivation of fecal bacteria in drinking water by solar heating. Appl Environ Microbiol. 1996 Feb;62(2):399–402.

6. Korich DG, Mead JR, Madore MS, Sinclair NA, Sterling CR. Effects of ozone, chlorine dioxide, chlorine, and monochloramine on *Cryptosporidium parvum* oocyst viability. Appl Environ Microbiol. 1990 May;56(5):1423–8.

7. Lantagne DS. Sodium hypochlorite dosage for household and emergency water treatment. Journal of American Water Works Association. 2008;100(8):106–19.

8. McGuigan KG, Joyce TM, Conroy RM, Gillespie JB, Elmore-Meegan M. Solar disinfection of drinking water contained in transparent plastic bottles: characterizing the bacterial inactivation process. J Appl Microbiol. 1998 Jun;84(6):1138–48.

FOOD POISONING FROM MARINE TOXINS
Vernon E. Ansdell

Seafood poisoning from marine toxins is an underrecognized hazard for travelers, particularly in the tropics and subtropics. Furthermore, the risk is increasing because of factors such as climate change, coral reef damage, and spread of toxic algal blooms.

CIGUATERA FISH POISONING
Ciguatera fish poisoning occurs after eating reef fish contaminated with toxins such as ciguatoxin or maitotoxin. These potent toxins originate from small marine organisms (dinoflagellates) that grow on and around coral reefs. Dinoflagellates are ingested by herbivorous fish. The toxins are then concentrated as they pass up the food chain to large carnivorous fish (usually >6 lb) and finally to humans. Toxins in fish are concentrated in the liver, intestinal tract, roe, and head.

Gambierdiscus toxicus, which produces ciguatoxin, tends to proliferate on dead coral reefs. The risk of ciguatera is likely to increase as more coral reefs die because of climate change, construction, and nutrient runoff.

Risk for Travelers
More than 50,000 cases of ciguatera poisoning occur globally every year. The incidence in travelers to highly endemic areas has been estimated as high as 3 per 100. Ciguatera is widespread in tropical and subtropical waters, usually between the latitudes of 35°N and 35°S; it is particularly common in the Pacific and Indian Oceans and the Caribbean Sea.

Fish that are most likely to cause ciguatera poisoning are carnivorous reef fish, including barracuda, grouper, moray eel, amberjack, sea bass, or sturgeon. Omnivorous and herbivorous fish such as parrot fish, surgeonfish, and red snapper can also be a risk.

Clinical Presentation
Typical ciguatera poisoning results in a gastrointestinal illness, followed by neurologic symptoms and, rarely, cardiovascular collapse. The first symptoms usually appear 1–3 hours after eating contaminated fish and include nausea, vomiting, diarrhea, and abdominal pain.

Neurologic symptoms appear 3–72 hours after the meal and include paresthesias, pain in the teeth or the sensation that the teeth are loose, itching, metallic taste, blurred vision, or even transient blindness. Cold allodynia (dysesthesia when touching cold water or objects) is characteristic and almost pathognomonic of ciguatera poisoning. Neurologic symptoms usually last a few days to several weeks.

Chronic neuropsychiatric symptoms resembling chronic fatigue syndrome may be disabling, last several months, and include malaise, depression, headaches, myalgias, and fatigue. Cardiac manifestations include bradycardia, other arrhythmias, and hypotension.

The overall death rate from ciguatera poisoning is approximately 0.1% but varies according to the toxin dose and availability of medical care to deal with complications. The diagnosis of ciguatera poisoning is based on the clinical signs and symptoms and a history of eating fish that are known to carry ciguatera toxin. Commercial kits are available to test for ciguatera in fish. They are sensitive but expensive. There is no test for ciguatera in humans.

Preventive Measures for Travelers

Travelers can take the following precautions to prevent ciguatera fish poisoning:

- Avoid or limit consumption of the reef fish listed above, particularly when the fish weighs 6 lb or more.
- Never eat high-risk fish such as barracuda or moray eel.
- Avoid the parts of the fish that concentrate ciguatera toxin: liver, intestines, roe, and head.

Remember that ciguatera toxins do not affect the texture, taste, or smell of fish, and they are not destroyed by gastric acid, cooking, smoking, freezing, canning, salting, or pickling. Commercial kits (if available) can be used to check if the fish is safe to eat.

Treatment

There is no specific antidote for ciguatoxin or maitotoxin. Treatment is generally symptomatic and supportive. Intravenous mannitol has been reported to reduce the severity and duration of neurologic symptoms, particularly if given within 48 hours of the appearance of symptoms.

SCOMBROID

Scombroid, one of the most common fish poisonings, occurs worldwide in both temperate and tropical waters. The illness occurs after eating improperly refrigerated or preserved fish containing high levels of histamine, and often resembles a moderate to severe allergic reaction.

Fish that cause scombroid have naturally high levels of histidine in the flesh and include tuna, mackerel, mahimahi (dolphin fish), sardine, anchovy, herring, bluefish, amberjack, and marlin. Histidine is converted to histamine by bacterial overgrowth in fish that has been improperly stored (>20°C) after capture. Histamine and other scombrotoxins are resistant to cooking, smoking, canning, or freezing.

Clinical Presentation

Symptoms of scombroid poisoning resemble an acute allergic reaction and usually appear 10–60 minutes after eating contaminated fish. They include flushing of the face and upper body (resembling sunburn), severe headache, palpitations, itching, blurred vision, abdominal cramps, and diarrhea. Untreated, symptoms usually resolve within 12 hours. Rarely, there may be respiratory compromise, malignant arrhythmias, and hypotension requiring hospitalization. Diagnosis is usually clinical. A clustering of cases helps exclude the possibility of fish allergy.

Preventive Measures for Travelers

Fish contaminated with histamine may have a peppery, sharp, salty, or bubbly taste but may also look, smell, and taste normal. The key to prevention is to make sure that the fish is promptly chilled (below 38°F) after capture. Cooking, smoking, canning, or freezing will not destroy histamine in contaminated fish.

Treatment

Scombroid poisoning usually responds well to antihistamines (H_1-receptor blockers, although H_2-receptor blockers may also be of benefit).

SHELLFISH POISONING

Several forms of shellfish poisoning may occur after ingesting filter-feeding bivalve mollusks (such as mussels, oysters, clams, scallops, and cockles) that contain potent toxins. The toxins originate in small marine organisms (dinoflagellates or diatoms) that are ingested and concentrated by shellfish.

Risk for Travelers

Contaminated shellfish may be found in temperate and tropical waters, typically during or after dinoflagellate blooms or "red tides."

Clinical Presentation

Poisoning results in gastrointestinal and neurologic illness of varying severity. Symptoms typically appear 30–60 minutes after ingesting toxic shellfish but can be delayed for several hours. Diagnosis is usually made clinically in patients who recently ate shellfish.

Paralytic Shellfish Poisoning

This is the most common and most severe form of shellfish poisoning. Symptoms usually appear 30–60 minutes after eating toxic shellfish and include numbness and tingling of the face, lips, tongue, arms, and legs. There may be headache, nausea, vomiting, and diarrhea. Severe cases are associated with ingestion of large doses of toxin and clinical features such as ataxia, dysphagia, mental status changes, flaccid paralysis, and respiratory failure. The case-fatality ratio averages 6%. The death rate may be particularly high in children.

Neurotoxic Shellfish Poisoning

Neurotoxic shellfish poisoning usually presents as gastroenteritis accompanied by minor neurologic symptoms, resembling mild ciguatera poisoning or mild paralytic shellfish poisoning. Inhalation of aerosolized toxin in the sea spray associated with a red tide may cause an acute respiratory illness, rhinorrhea, and bronchoconstriction.

Diarrheic Shellfish Poisoning

This produces chills, nausea, vomiting, abdominal cramps, and diarrhea. No deaths have been reported.

Amnesic Shellfish Poisoning

This is a rare form of shellfish poisoning that produces a gastroenteritis that may be accompanied by headache, confusion, and permanent short-term memory loss. In severe cases, seizures, paralysis, and death may occur.

Preventive Measures for Travelers

Shellfish poisoning can be prevented by avoiding potentially contaminated bivalve mollusks. This is particularly important in areas during or shortly after "red tides." Travelers to developing countries should avoid eating all shellfish because they carry a high risk of viral and bacterial infections. Marine shellfish toxins cannot be destroyed by cooking or freezing.

Treatment

Treatment is symptomatic and supportive. Severe cases of paralytic shellfish poisoning may require mechanical ventilation.

BIBLIOGRAPHY

1. Ansdell V. Food-borne Illness. In: Keystone JS, Kozarsky PE, Freedman DO, Nothdurft HD, Connor BA, editors. Travel Medicine. 2nd ed. Philadelphia: Mosby; 2008. p. 475–84.
2. Isbister GK, Kiernan MC. Neurotoxic marine poisoning. Lancet Neurol. 2005 Apr;4(4):219–28.
3. Palafox NA, Jain LG, Pinano AZ, Gulick TM, Williams RK, Schatz IJ. Successful treatment of ciguatera fish poisoning with intravenous mannitol. JAMA. 1988 May 13;259(18):2740–2.
4. Schnorf H, Taurarii M, Cundy T. Ciguatera fish poisoning: a double-blind randomized trial of mannitol therapy. Neurology. 2002 Mar 26;58(6):873–80.
5. Sobel J, Painter J. Illnesses caused by marine toxins. Clin Infect Dis. 2005 Nov 1;41(9):1290–6.

PROTECTION AGAINST MOSQUITOES, TICKS, & OTHER INSECTS & ARTHROPODS

Emily Zielinski-Gutierrez, Robert A. Wirtz, Roger S. Nasci, William G. Brogdon

Vaccines or chemoprophylactic drugs are available to protect against some vectorborne diseases such as yellow fever and malaria; however, travelers still should be advised to use repellents and other general protective measures against biting arthropods. The effectiveness of malaria chemoprophylaxis is variable, depending on patterns of drug resistance, bioavailability, and compliance with medication, and no similar preventive measures exist for other mosquitoborne diseases such as dengue or chikungunya. There has been a recent resurgence in bed bug infestations worldwide, particularly in developed countries (Box 2-3).

CDC recommends the use of products containing active ingredients that have been registered by the Environmental Protection Agency (EPA) for use as repellents applied to skin and clothing. EPA registration of active ingredients indicates the materials have been reviewed and approved for efficacy and human safety when applied according to the instructions on the label.

GENERAL PROTECTIVE MEASURES

Avoid outbreaks. To the extent possible, travelers should avoid known foci of epidemic disease transmission. The CDC website provides information on regional disease transmission patterns and outbreaks (www.cdc.gov/travel).

Be aware of peak exposure times and places. Exposure to arthropod bites may be reduced if travelers modify their patterns of activity or behavior. Although mosquitoes may bite at any time of day, peak biting activity for vectors of some diseases (such as dengue and chikungunya) is during daylight hours. Vectors of other diseases (such as malaria) are most active in twilight periods (dawn and dusk) or in the evening after dark. Avoiding the outdoors or focusing preventive actions during peak hours may reduce risk. Place also matters; ticks are often found in grasses and other vegetated areas. Local health officials or guides may be able to point out areas with increased arthropod activity.

Wear appropriate clothing. Travelers can minimize areas of exposed skin by wearing long-sleeved shirts, long pants, boots, and hats. Tucking in shirts, tucking pants into socks, and wearing closed shoes instead of sandals may reduce risk. Repellents or insecticides, such as permethrin, can be applied to clothing and gear for added protection.

Check for ticks. Travelers should inspect themselves and their clothing for ticks during outdoor activity and at the end of the day. Prompt removal of attached ticks can prevent some infections.

Bed nets. When accommodations are not adequately screened or air conditioned, bed nets are essential to provide protection and to reduce discomfort caused by biting insects. If bed nets do not reach the floor, they should be tucked under mattresses. Bed nets are most effective when they are treated with a pyrethroid. Pretreated, long-lasting bed nets can be purchased before traveling, or nets can be treated after purchase. Nets treated with a pyrethroid insecticide will be effective for several months if they are not washed. Long-lasting pretreated nets may be effective for much longer.

Insecticides and spatial repellents. An increasing array of products to be used as spatial repellents (containing active ingredients such as metofluthrin and allethrin) is becoming commercially available. These augment the aerosol insecticides, vaporizing mats, and mosquito coils that have been available for some time. Such products can help to clear rooms or areas of mosquitoes (spray aerosols) or repel mosquitoes from a circumscribed area (coils, spatial repellents). Although many of these products appear to have repellent or insecticidal activity under particular conditions, they have not yet been adequately evaluated in

BOX 2-3. BED BUGS AND INTERNATIONAL TRAVEL

A recent resurgence in bed bug infestations worldwide, particularly in developed countries, is thought to be related to the increase in international travel, pest control strategy changes in travel lodgings, and insecticide resistance. Bed bug infestations have been increasingly reported in hotels, theaters, and any locations where people congregate, even in the workplace, dormitories, and schools. Bed bugs may be transported in luggage and on clothing. Transport of personal belongings in contaminated transport vehicles is another means of spread of these insects.

Bed bugs are small, flat insects that are reddish-brown in color, wingless, and range from 1 to 7 mm in length. While bed bugs have not been shown to transmit disease, their bites can produce strong allergic reactions and considerable emotional stress.

Protective Measures against Bed Bugs

Travelers should be encouraged to take the following precautions to avoid or reduce their exposure to bed bugs:

- Inspect the premises of hotels or other unfamiliar sleeping locations for bed bugs on mattresses, box springs, bedding, and furniture, particularly built-in furniture with the bed, desk, and closets as a continuous structural unit. Travelers who observe evidence of bed bug activity—whether it be the bugs themselves or physical signs such as blood-spotting on linens—should seek alternative lodging.
- Keep suitcases closed when they are not in use and try to keep them off the floor.
- It is best in high-risk areas to remove clothing and personal items, such as toiletry bags and shaving kits, from the suitcase only when they are in use.
- Carefully inspect clothing and personal items before returning them to the suitcase.
- Keep in mind that bed bug eggs and nymphs can be very small and are easily overlooked.

Prevention is by far the most effective and inexpensive way to protect oneself from these pests. The costs of ridding a personal residence of these insects are considerable, and efforts at control are often not immediately successful even when conducted by professionals.

peer-reviewed studies for their efficacy in preventing vectorborne disease. As such, travelers should supplement the use of these products with topical or clothing repellents or bed nets in areas with the potential for vectorborne disease transmission or if biting arthropods are noted. Since some products available internationally may contain pesticides that are not registered in the United States, it may be preferable for travelers to bring their own. Insecticides and repellent products should always be used with caution, avoiding direct inhalation of spray or smoke.

Optimum protection can be provided by applying the repellents described in the following sections to clothing and to exposed skin.

REPELLENTS FOR USE ON SKIN AND CLOTHING

CDC has evaluated information published in peer-reviewed scientific literature and data available from EPA to identify several EPA-registered products that provide repellent activity sufficient to help people reduce the bites of disease-carrying mosquitoes. Products containing the following active ingredients typically provide reasonably long-lasting protection:

- **DEET** (chemical name: N,N-diethyl-m-toluamide or N,N-diethyl-3-methyl-benzamide). Products containing DEET include, but are not limited to, Off!, Cutter, Sawyer, and Ultrathon.
- **Picaridin** (KBR 3023 [Bayrepel] and icaridin outside the United States; chemical name: 2-(2-hydroxyethyl)-1-piperidinecarboxylic acid 1-methylpropyl ester). Products containing picaridin include, but are not limited to, Cutter Advanced, Skin So Soft Bug Guard Plus, and Autan (outside the United States).
- **Oil of lemon eucalyptus (OLE)** or **PMD** (chemical name: para-menthane-3,8-diol), the synthesized version of OLE. Products containing

OLE and PMD include, but are not limited to, Repel. This recommendation refers to EPA-registered repellent products containing the active ingredient OLE (or PMD). "Pure" oil of lemon eucalyptus (essential oil) is not the same product; it has not undergone similar, validated testing for safety and efficacy, is not registered with EPA as an insect repellent, and is not covered by this recommendation.

- **IR3535** (chemical name: 3-[N-butyl-N-acetyl]-aminopropionic acid, ethyl ester). Products containing IR3535 include, but are not limited to, Skin So Soft Bug Guard Plus Expedition.

EPA characterizes the active ingredients DEET and picaridin as "conventional repellents" and OLE, PMD, and IR3535 as "biopesticide repellents," which are derived from natural materials.

Repellent Efficacy

Published data indicate that repellent efficacy and duration of protection vary considerably among products and among mosquito species. Product efficacy and duration of protection are also markedly affected by ambient temperature, level of activity, amount of perspiration, exposure to water, abrasive removal, and other factors. In general, higher concentrations of active ingredient provide longer duration of protection, regardless of the active ingredient. Products with <10% active ingredient may offer only limited protection, often 1–2 hours. Products that offer sustained-release or controlled-release (microencapsulated) formulations, even with lower active ingredient concentrations, may provide longer protection times. Studies suggest that concentrations of DEET above approximately 50% do not offer a marked increase in protection time against mosquitoes; DEET efficacy tends to plateau at a concentration of approximately 50%.

Recommendations are based on the summary of peer-reviewed journal articles and scientific studies and data submitted to regulatory agencies. People may experience some variation in protection from different products. Regardless of what product is used, if travelers start to get insect bites they should reapply the repellent according to the label instructions, try a different product, or, if possible, leave the area with biting insects.

Repellents should be purchased before traveling and can be found online or in hardware stores, drug stores, and supermarkets. A wider variety of repellents can be found in camping, sporting goods, and military surplus stores. When purchasing repellents overseas, look for the EPA-registered active ingredients on the product labels; some names of products available internationally have been specified in the list above.

Repellents and Sunscreen

Repellents that are applied according to label instructions may be used with sunscreen with no reduction in repellent activity; however, limited data show a one-third decrease in the sun protection factor (SPF) of sunscreens when DEET-containing insect repellents are used after a sunscreen is applied. Products that combine sunscreen and repellent are not recommended, because sunscreen may need to be reapplied more often and in larger amounts than needed for the repellent component to provide protection from biting insects. In general, the recommendation is to use separate products, applying sunscreen first and then applying the repellent.

Repellents and Insecticides for Use on Clothing

Clothing, hats, shoes, bed nets, mesh jackets, and camping gear can be treated with permethrin for added protection. Products such as Permanone and Sawyer permethrin are registered with EPA specifically for this use.

Permethrin is a highly effective insecticide-acaricide and repellent. Permethrin-treated clothing repels and kills ticks, mosquitoes, and other biting and nuisance arthropods. Clothing and other items must be treated 24–48 hours in advance of travel to allow them to dry. As with all pesticides, follow the label instructions when using permethrin clothing treatments. Alternatively, clothing pretreated with permethrin is commercially available, marketed to consumers in the US as Insect Shield.

Permethrin-treated materials retain repellency or insecticidal activity after repeated laundering but should be retreated, as described on the product label, to provide continued protection. Clothing treated with the other repellent products described above (such as DEET) provides protection from biting arthropods but will not last through washing and will require more frequent reapplications.

Precautions when Using Insect Repellents

Travelers should take the following precautions:

- Apply repellents only to exposed skin or clothing, as directed on the product label.
- Do not use repellents under clothing.
- Never use repellents over cuts, wounds, or irritated skin.
- Do not apply repellents to eyes or mouth, and apply sparingly around ears.
- When using sprays, do not spray directly on face—spray on hands first and then apply to face.
- Wash hands after application to avoid accidental exposure to eyes. Children should not handle repellents. Instead, adults should apply repellents to their own hands first, and then gently spread on the child's exposed skin. Avoid applying directly to children's hands.
- Use just enough repellent to cover exposed skin or clothing. Heavy application and saturation are generally unnecessary for effectiveness. If biting insects do not respond to a thin film of repellent, apply a bit more.
- After returning indoors, wash treated skin with soap and water or bathe. This is particularly important when repellents are used repeatedly in a day or on consecutive days.
- Wash treated clothing before wearing it again. This precaution may vary with different repellents—check the product label.

If a traveler experiences a rash or other reaction, such as itching or swelling, from an insect repellent, the repellent should be discontinued and washed off with mild soap and water, and a local poison-control center should be called for further guidance. Travelers seeking health care because of the repellent should take the repellent to the doctor's office and show the doctor. Permethrin should *never* be applied to skin but only to clothing, bed nets, or other fabrics as directed on the product label.

Children

Most repellents can be used on children aged >2 months. Protect infants aged <2 months from mosquitoes by using an infant carrier draped with mosquito netting with an elastic edge for a tight fit. Products containing OLE specify that they should not be used on children aged <3 years. Other than the safety tips listed above, EPA does not recommend any additional precautions for using registered repellents on children or on pregnant or lactating women.

Useful Links

- Using Insect Repellents Safely (EPA): http://epa.gov/pesticides/insect/safe.htm
- Insect Repellent Use and Safety (CDC): www.cdc.gov/ncidod/dvbid/westnile/qa/insect_repellent.htm
- National Pesticide Information Center: http://npic.orst.edu/index.html

BIBLIOGRAPHY

1. Barnard DR, Bernier UR, Posey KH, Xue RD. Repellency of IR3535, KBR3023, para-menthane-3,8-diol, and DEET to black salt marsh mosquitoes (Diptera: Culicidae) in the Everglades National Park. J Med Entomol. 2002 Nov;39(6):895–9.
2. Barnard DR, Xue RD. Laboratory evaluation of mosquito repellents against Aedes albopictus, Culex nigripalpus, and Ochlerotatus triseriatus (Diptera: Culicidae). J Med Entomol. 2004 Jul;41(4):726–30.
3. Centers for Disease Control and Prevention, Environmental Protection Agency. Joint statement on bed bug control in the United States from the US Centers for Disease Control and Prevention (CDC) and the US Environmental Protection Agency (EPA). Atlanta: US Department of Health and Human Services; 2010 [cited 2010 Nov 24]. Available from: http://www.cdc.gov/nceh/ehs/publications/bed_bugs_cdc-epa_statement.htm.
4. Fradin MS, Day JF. Comparative efficacy of insect repellents against mosquito bites. N Engl J Med. 2002 Jul 4;347(1):13–8.
5. Montemarano AD, Gupta RK, Burge JR, Klein K. Insect repellents and the efficacy of sunscreens. Lancet. 1997 Jun 7;349(9066):1670-1.
6. Murphy ME, Montemarano AD, Debboun M, Gupta R. The effect of sunscreen on the efficacy of insect repellent: a clinical trial. J Am Acad Dermatol. 2000 Aug;43(2 Pt 1):219–22.
7. Thavara U, Tawatsin A, Chompoosri J, Suwonkerd W, Chansang UR, Asavadachanukorn P. Laboratory and field evaluations of the insect repellent 3535 (ethyl butylacetylaminopropionate) and DEET against mosquito vectors in Thailand. J Am Mosq Control Assoc. 2001 Sep;17(3):190–5.

SUNBURN

Vernon E. Ansdell

OVERVIEW

Increased exposure to UV radiation occurs near the equator, during summer months, at high elevation, and between 10 AM and 4 PM. Reflection from the snow, sand, and water increases exposure, a particularly important consideration for beach activities, skiing, swimming, and sailing. In addition, several common medications may cause photosensitivity reactions in travelers:

- Acetazolamide
- Amiodarone
- Antibiotics (fluoroquinolones, sulfonamides, and tetracyclines, especially demeclocycline and doxycycline)
- Furosemide
- Nonsteroidal anti-inflammatory drugs
- Phenothiazines
- Sulfonylureas
- Thiazide diuretics
- Voriconazole

UVA rays are present throughout the day and cause premature aging of the skin. In addition, UVA rays are responsible for photosensitivity reactions and also contribute to skin cancer. UVB rays are intense from 10 AM to 4 PM and are most responsible for sunburn and skin cancer. Serious burns are painful, and the skin may be tender, swollen, and blistered. These sunburns may be accompanied by fever, headache, itching, and malaise. Overexposure to the sun over several years leads to premature aging of the skin, wrinkling, age spots, and an increased risk for skin cancer, including melanoma. Repeated exposure to sunlight can result in pterygium formation, cataracts, and macular degeneration.

PREVENTIVE MEASURES FOR TRAVELERS

Sun Avoidance

Staying indoors or seeking shade between 10 AM and 4 PM is very important in limiting exposure to UV rays, particularly UVB rays. Be aware that sunburn and sun damage can occur even on cloudy days and even when one sits under an umbrella or in the shade.

Protective Clothing

Wide-brimmed hats, long sleeves, and long pants protect against UV rays. Tightly woven clothing and darker fabrics provide additional protection. High-SPF clothing is recommended for travelers at increased risk of sunburn or with a history of skin cancer. This type of clothing contains colorless compounds, fluorescent brighteners, or treated resins that absorb UV rays; this clothing often provides an SPF of 30 or higher. A laundry additive, such as the product SunGuard, can be used to add UV protection to clothing. Sunglasses that provide 100% protection against UV radiation are strongly recommended.

Sun Protection Factor

Sun protection factor (SPF) defines the extra protection against UVB rays that a person receives by using a sunscreen. For example, if a person using SPF 15 sunscreen normally acquires a sunburn in 20 minutes without protection, the benefit will be 20 × 15 minutes (300 minutes; 5 hours) extra protection with sunscreen. SPF does not refer to protection against UVA rays.

Sunscreens

Physical sunscreens contain large particulate substances, such as titanium dioxide or zinc oxide, that reflect and scatter both visible and UV light. They are effective sunscreens but are unpopular because they are opaque and tend to stain clothing. They are recommended for people who burn easily or who take medications that may cause photosensitivity reactions.

Chemical sunscreens absorb rather than reflect UV radiation. A combination of agents is recommended to provide broad-spectrum protection against UVA and UVB rays. Travelers should consider the following key points regarding sunscreens:

- Choose a sunscreen with at least 15 SPF.
- Select a water- and sweat-resistant product.

- Look for a sunscreen with at least 3 different active ingredients to provide broad-spectrum UVA and UVB protection:
  - > PABA derivatives, salicylates (homosalate, octyl salicylate), or cinnamates (octyl methoxycinnamate, cinoxate) for UVB absorption
  - > Benzophenones (oxybenzone, dioxybenzone, sulisobenzone) for shorter-wavelength UVA protection
  - > Avobenzone, ecamsule, titanium dioxide, or zinc oxide for the remaining UVA spectrum
- Apply 30 minutes before exposure to the sun.
- At least 1 oz of sunscreen is needed to cover the entire body.
- Apply to all exposed areas, especially the ears, scalp, lips, back of the neck, tops of the feet, and backs of the hands.
- Use a lip balm with at least 15 SPF.
- Reapply after 1–2 hours and after sweating, swimming, or towel-drying (even on cloudy days).
- Many sunscreens lose potency after 1–2 years. Always check the expiration date.

- Sunscreens should be applied to the skin before insect repellents. (Note: DEET-containing insect repellents may decrease the SPF of sunscreens by one-third. Sunscreens may increase absorption of DEET through the skin.)
- Avoid products that contain both sunscreens and insect repellents, because sunscreen may need to be reapplied more often and in larger amounts than needed for the repellent component to provide protection from biting insects.

TREATMENT

Travelers with sunburn should maintain hydration and stay in a cool, shaded, or indoor environment. Topical and oral non-steroidal anti-inflammatory drugs decrease erythema if used before or soon after exposure to UVB rays and may relieve symptoms such as headache, fever, and local pain. Topical steroids are of limited benefit, and systemic steroids appear to be ineffective. Moisturizing creams, aloe vera, and diphenhydramine may relieve symptoms. In severe cases, narcotic analgesics may be indicated to relieve pain.

BIBLIOGRAPHY

1. Diffey BL, Grice J. The influence of sunscreen type on photoprotection. Br J Dermatol. 1997 Jul;137(1):103–5.
2. Gu X, Wang T, Collins DM, Kasichayanula S, Burczynski FJ. In vitro evaluation of concurrent use of commercially available insect repellent and sunscreen preparations. Br J Dermatol. 2005 Jun;152(6):1263–7.
3. Han A, Maibach HI. Management of acute sunburn. Am J Clin Dermatol. 2004;5(1):39–47.
4. Kaplan L. Exposure to radiation from the sun. In: Auerbach PS, editor. Wilderness Medicine. 5th ed. Philadelphia: Mosby Elsevier; 2007. p. 351–71.
5. McLean DI, Gallagher R. Sunscreens. Use and misuse. Dermatol Clin. 1998 Apr;16(2):219–26.
6. Murphy ME, Montemarano AD, Debboun M, Gupta R. The effect of sunscreen on the efficacy of insect repellent: a clinical trial. J Am Acad Dermatol. 2000 Aug;43(2 Pt 1):219–22.

PROBLEMS WITH HEAT & COLD
Howard D. Backer, David R. Shlim

OVERVIEW

International travelers encounter new environments that may include extremes of climate to which the traveler is not accustomed. Exposure to heat and cold can result in serious injury or death. Travelers should investigate climate extremes that they will face during their journey and prepare with proper clothing, knowledge, and equipment.

PROBLEMS ASSOCIATED WITH A HOT CLIMATE
Risk for Travelers

Many of the most popular travel destinations are tropical or desert areas. Travelers who sit on the beach or by the pool and do only short walking tours incur minimal risk of heat illness. Those who do strenuous hiking or biking in the heat may have significant risk, especially travelers coming from cool or temperate climates who are not in good physical condition and are not acclimatized to the heat.

Clinical Presentations
Physiology of Heat Injuries

Tolerance to heat depends largely on physiologic factors, unlike cold environments where adaptive behaviors are more important. The major means of heat dissipation are radiation while at rest and evaporation of sweat during exercise, both of which become minimal with air temperatures above 95°F (35°C) and high humidity.

The major organs involved in temperature regulation are the skin, where sweating and heat exchange take place, and the cardiovascular system, which must increase blood flow to shunt heat from the core to the surface, while meeting the metabolic demands of exercise. Cardiovascular status and conditioning are the major physiologic variables affecting the response to heat stress at all ages. In addition to environmental conditions and intensity of exercise, dehydration is the most important predisposing factor in heat illness. Dehydration also reduces exercise performance, decreases time to exhaustion, and increases internal heat load; temperature and heart rate increase in direct proportion to the level of dehydration. Sweat is a hypotonic fluid containing sodium and chloride. Sweat rates commonly reach 1–2 L per hour, which may result in significant fluid and sodium loss.

Minor Heat Disorders

Heat cramps are painful muscle contractions following exercise in heat. They begin an hour or more after stopping exercise, most often involving heavily used muscles in the calves, thighs, and abdomen. Rest and passive stretching of the muscle, supplemented by fluids and salt, will rapidly relieve symptoms. Water with a salty snack is sufficient; an oral salt solution, as in rehydration solutions, can be made by adding a half teaspoon of table salt to 1 L of water.

Heat syncope is sudden fainting in heat that occurs in unacclimatized people while standing or after 15–20 minutes of exercise. Consciousness rapidly returns to normal when the patient is supine. Rest, relief from heat, and oral fluids are sufficient treatment.

Heat edema is mild swelling of the hands and feet, more frequent in women during the first few days of heat exposure. It resolves spontaneously and should not be treated with diuretics, which may delay heat acclimatization and cause dehydration.

Prickly heat (such as miliaria or heat rash) manifests as small, red, itchy lesions on the skin caused by obstruction of the sweat ducts. It is best prevented by wearing light, loose clothing and avoiding heavy, continuous sweating.

Major Heat Disorders
Heat exhaustion

Most people who experience acute collapse or other symptoms associated with exercise in the heat are suffering from heat exhaustion, simply defined as the inability to continue exertion in the heat. The presumed cause of heat exhaustion is loss of fluid and electrolytes, but there are no objective markers to define the syndrome, which is a spectrum ranging from minor complaints to a vague boundary shared with heat stroke. Transient mental changes, such as irritability, confusion, or irrational behavior may be present, but neurologic signs, such as seizures or coma, would indicate heat stroke or hyponatremia. Body temperature may be normal or mildly elevated.

Most cases can be treated with supine rest in the shade or other cool place, and oral water or fluids containing glucose and salt. Spontaneous cooling occurs, and patients recover within hours without progression to more serious illness. An oral solution for treating heat exhaustion can be made by adding one-fourth teaspoon or two 1-g salt tablets to 1 L of water, plus 4–8 teaspoons of sugar, if desired, for taste. Commercial sports-electrolyte drinks or water with snacks are also effective. Subacute heat exhaustion may develop over several days and is often misdiagnosed as "summer flu" because of findings of weakness, fatigue, headache, dizziness, anorexia, nausea, vomiting, and diarrhea. Treatment is as described for acute heat exhaustion.

Exercise-associated hyponatremia

Hyponatremia due to excessive water intake occurs in both endurance athletes and recreational hikers, particularly if the sodium lost through sweating is only replaced with plain water. Sports-electrolyte drinks do not contain sufficient amounts of sodium to prevent hyponatremia.

In the field setting, altered mental status with normal body temperature and a history of large volumes of water intake are highly suggestive of hyponatremia. The vague and nonspecific symptoms are the same as those described for hyponatremia in other settings (for example, anorexia, nausea, emesis, headache, muscle weakness, lethargy, confusion, and seizures). Symptoms of heat exhaustion and early hyponatremia are similar. Hyponatremia can be distinguished by persistent alteration of mental status. Delay in onset of major neurologic symptoms (confusion, seizures, or coma) or deterioration after cessation of exercise and heat exposure strongly suggest hyponatremia.

The recommendation of forcing fluid during prolonged exercise and the attitude that "you can't drink too much" are the main contributors to exercise-associated hyponatremia. Prevention includes drinking as one desires to relieve thirst and to maintain urine output. During prolonged exercise or heat exposure, supplemental sodium can be taken. For hikers, food is the most efficient vehicle for salt replacement. Trail snacks should include salty foods (such as trail mix, crackers, pretzels, and jerky) and not just sweets.

Heat stroke

Heat stroke is an extreme medical emergency requiring aggressive cooling measures and hospitalization for support. Damage is related to duration, as well as peak elevation of body temperature. Heat stroke is the only form of heat illness in which the mechanisms for thermal homeostasis have failed. As a result of uncontrolled fever and circulatory collapse, organ damage can occur in the brain, liver, kidneys, and heart. The onset of heat stroke may be acute (exertional heat stroke) or gradual (nonexertional heat stroke, also referred to as classic or epidemic).

Early symptoms are similar to heat exhaustion, with confusion or change in personality, loss of coordination, dizziness, headache, and nausea. A presumptive diagnosis of heat stroke is made in the field when people have elevation of body temperature (hyperpyrexia) and marked alteration of mental status,

including delirium, convulsions, and coma. Body temperatures in excess of 106°F (41°C) can be observed; even without a thermometer, people will feel hot to the touch. If a thermometer is available, a rectal temperature is the safest and most reliable way to check the temperature of someone who may have heat stroke.

In the field, immediately institute measures by one of several simple methods:

- Use evaporative cooling by maximizing skin exposure, spraying tepid water on the skin, and maintaining air movement over the body by fanning.
- Apply ice or cold packs to the neck, axillas, and groin. Vigorously massage the skin to prevent constriction of blood vessels and try to avoid shivering, which will increase body temperature.
- Immerse the person in water (such as a nearby pool or natural body of water).

Unless the recovery is rapid, the person should be evacuated to a hospital. If that is not possible, encourage rehydration for those able to take oral fluids, and monitor closely for several hours for temperature swings. Delayed complications in the first 24–48 hours may include liver or kidney damage and bleeding.

Prevention of Heat Disorders
Heat Acclimatization
Heat acclimatization is a process of physiologic adaptation to a hot environment that occurs in both residents and visitors. The result of acclimatization is an increase in sweating with less salt content, and decreased energy expenditure with lower rise in body temperature for a given workload. Only partial adaptation occurs by passive exposure to heat. Full acclimatization, especially cardiovascular response, requires 1–2 hours of exercise in the heat each day. Most acclimatization changes occur within 10 days, provided a suitable amount of exercise is taken each day in the heat. After this time, only increased physical fitness will result in further exercise tolerance. Decay of acclimatization occurs within days to weeks if there is no heat exposure.

Physical Conditioning and Acclimatization
Higher levels of physical fitness improve exercise tolerance and capacity in heat, but not as

much as acclimatization. If possible, travelers should acclimatize before leaving by exercising at least 1 hour daily in the heat. If this is not possible before departing, exercise in heat during the first week of travel should be limited in intensity and duration (30- to 90-minute periods) with rest in between. It is a good idea to conform to the local practice in most hot regions and avoid strenuous activity during the hottest part of the day.

Clothing

Clothing should be lightweight, loose, and light-colored to allow maximum air circulation for evaporation yet give protection from the sun. A wide-brimmed hat markedly reduces radiant heat exposure.

Fluid and Electrolyte Replacement

During exertion, fluid intake improves performance and decreases the likelihood of illness. Reliance on thirst alone is not sufficient to prevent significant dehydration, bearing in mind the potential danger of hyponatremia. During mild to moderate exertion, electrolyte replacement offers no advantage over plain water. However, for those exercising many hours in heat, a weak solution similar to commercial electrolyte drinks is recommended. Eating salty snacks or lightly salting mealtime food or fluids is the most efficient way to replace salt losses. Salt tablets, when swallowed whole, may cause gastrointestinal irritation and vomiting, but 2 tablets can be dissolved in 1 L of water. Urine volume and color are readily available means to monitor fluid needs.

PROBLEMS ASSOCIATED WITH A COLD CLIMATE
Risk for Travelers

Travelers do not have to be in an arctic or high-altitude environment to encounter problems with the cold. Humidity, rain, and wind can produce hypothermia even with temperatures around 50°F (10°C). Reports of severe hypothermia in international travelers are rare. Many high-altitude destinations are not wilderness areas, and villages offer an escape from extreme weather. In Nepal, trekkers almost never experience hypothermia, except in the rare instance in which they get lost in a storm. Even in a temperate climate, a traveler in a small boat that overturns in very cold water can rapidly become hypothermic.

Clinical Presentations
Hypothermia

Hypothermia can be defined, in general terms, as having a core body temperature below 95°F (35°C). When people are faced with an environment in which they cannot keep warm, they first feel chilled, then begin to shiver, and eventually stop shivering as their metabolic reserves are exhausted. At that point, body temperature continues to decrease, depending on the ambient temperatures. As the core temperature falls, neurologic functioning decreases until almost all hypothermic people with a core temperature of 86°F (30°C) or lower are comatose. The record low core body temperature in an adult who survived is 56°F (13°C). Travelers headed to a cold climate should be encouraged to ask questions and research appropriate clothing and equipment.

Travelers who will be engaging in recreational activities or working around cold water face a different sort of risk. Immersion hypothermia can render a person unable to swim or keep floating within 30–60 minutes. In these cases, a personal flotation device is critical, as is knowledge about self-rescue and righting a capsized boat.

The other medical conditions associated with cold affect mainly the skin and the extremities. These can be divided into nonfreezing cold injuries and freezing injuries (frostbite).

Nonfreezing Cold Injury

The nonfreezing cold injuries are trench foot, pernio (chilblains), and cold urticaria. **Trench foot** (immersion foot) is caused by prolonged immersion of the feet in cold water (32°F–59°F, 0°C–15°C). The damage is mainly to nerves and blood vessels, and the result is pain that is aggravated by heat and a dependent position of the limb. Severe cases can take months to resolve. Unlike the treatment for frostbite, immersion foot should not be rapidly rewarmed, which can make the damage much worse.

Pernio are localized, inflammatory lesions that occur mainly on the hands of susceptible people. They can occur with exposure to only moderately cold weather. The bluish-red lesions are thought to be caused by prolonged, cold-induced vasoconstriction. As with trench foot, rapid rewarming should be avoided, as it makes the pain worse. Nifedipine may be an effective treatment.

Cold urticaria involves the formation of localized or general wheals and itching after exposure to cold. It is not the absolute temperature that induces this form of urticaria but the rate of change of temperature in the skin.

Freezing Cold Injury
Categories of frostbite
Frostbite is the term that is used to describe tissue damage from direct freezing of the skin. Modern equipment and clothing have decreased the risk of frostbite resulting from adventure tourism, and frostbite occurs mainly during an accident, severe unexpected weather, or as a result of poor planning.

Once frostbite injury has occurred, little can be done to reverse the changes. Therefore, taking great care to prevent frostbite is crucial. Frostbite is usually graded like burns. First-degree frostbite involves reddening of the skin without deeper damage. The prognosis for complete healing is virtually 100%. Second-degree frostbite involves blister formation. Blisters filled with clear fluid have a better prognosis than blood-tinged blisters. Third-degree frostbite represents full-thickness injury to the skin, and possibly the underlying tissues. No blister forms, the skin darkens over time and may turn black, and if the tissue is completely devascularized, amputation will be necessary.

Management of frostbite
Frostbitten skin is numb and appears whitish or waxy. The generally accepted method for treating a frozen digit or limb is through rapid rewarming in water heated to 104°F–108°F (40°C–42°C). The frozen area should be completely immersed in the warm water. A thermometer is needed to maintain the water at the correct temperature. Rewarming can be associated with severe pain, and analgesics can be given if needed. Once the area is rewarmed, it must be safeguarded against freezing again. It is thought to be better to keep digits frozen a little longer, and rapidly rewarm them, than to allow them to thaw out slowly or to thaw and refreeze. A cycle of freeze-thaw-refreeze is devastating to tissue and leads more directly to the need for amputation.

Once the area has rewarmed, it can be examined. If blisters are present, note whether they extend to the end of the digit. Proximal blisters usually mean that the tissue distal to the blister has suffered full-thickness damage. Treatment consists of avoiding further mechanical trauma to the area and preventing infection. Reasonable field treatment consists of washing the area thoroughly with a disinfectant such as povidone-iodine, putting dressings between the toes or fingers to prevent maceration, using fluffs (expanded gauze sponges) for padding, and covering with a roller gauze bandage. These dressings can safely be left on for up to 3 days at a time. By leaving the dressings on longer, the traveler can preserve what may be limited supplies of bandages. Prophylactic antibiotics are not needed in most situations.

Once the patient has reached a definitive medical setting, there should be no rush to do surgery. The usual time from injury to surgery is 4–5 weeks. By that time the dead tissue has begun to separate from viable tissue, and the surgeon can plan surgery that maximizes the remaining digits.

BIBLIOGRAPHY

1. Armstrong LE, Casa DJ, Millard-Stafford M, Moran DS, Pyne SW, Roberts WO. American College of Sports Medicine position stand. Exertional heat illness during training and competition. Med Sci Sports Exerc. 2007 Mar;39(3):556–72.
2. Epstein Y, Moran DS. Extremes of temperature and hydration. In: Keystone JS, Kozarsky PE, Freedman DO, Nothdurft HD, Connor BA, editors. Travel Medicine. 2nd ed. Philadelphia: Mosby; 2008. p. 413–22.
3. McCauley RL, Killyon GW, Smith DJ. Frostbite. In: Auerbach PS, editor. Wilderness Medicine. 5th ed. Philadelphia: Mosby Elsevier; 2007.
4. Moran DS, Gaffin SL. Clinical management of heat-related illnesses. In: Auerbach PS, editor. Wilderness Medicine. 5th ed. Philadelphia: Mosby Elsevier; 2007.
5. Rogers IR, Hew-Butler T. Exercise-associated hyponatremia: overzealous fluid consumption. Wilderness Environ Med. 2009 Summer;20(2):139–43.

INJURIES & SAFETY

David A. Sleet, Michael F. Ballesteros

OVERVIEW

According to the World Health Organization (WHO), injuries are among the leading causes of death and disability in the world, and they are the leading cause of preventable death in travelers. Worldwide, among people aged 5–44 years, injuries account for 7 of the 15 leading causes of death. Tourists are 10 times more likely to die as the result of an injury than from an infectious disease; injuries cause 23% of tourist deaths compared with only 2% caused by infectious diseases. Contributing to the injury toll while traveling are exposure to unfamiliar and perhaps risky environments, differences in language and communications, less stringent product safety and vehicle standards, unfamiliar rules and regulations, a carefree holiday or vacation spirit leading to more risk-taking behavior, and overreliance on travel and tour operators to protect one's safety and security.

From 2007 through 2009, an estimated 2,352 US citizens died from injuries and violence while in foreign countries (excluding deaths occurring in the wars in Iraq and Afghanistan). Motor vehicle crashes—not crime or terrorism—are the number one killer of healthy US citizens traveling in foreign countries. From 2007 through 2009, road traffic crashes accounted for 32% of tourist deaths due to injuries, followed by homicide (18%) and drowning (14%) (Figure 2-1).

Depending on the travel destination, duration, and planned activities, other common injury and safety concerns include natural hazards and disasters, civil unrest, terrorism, falls, burns, poisoning, drug overdose, and suicide. If a traveler is seriously injured, emergency care may not be available or acceptable by US standards. Trauma centers capable of providing optimal trauma care are uncommon outside urban areas.

Men are more likely than women to die from injuries while traveling internationally. Acquaintance rape and sexual assault are risks to women travelers. Travelers should be aware of the increased risk of certain injuries while traveling abroad, particularly in low-income countries, and be prepared to take preventive steps to avoid them. Injuries are the primary reason for US travelers to be transported back to the United States by air medical transport; the main nonfatal causes are motor vehicle traffic crashes (45%), falls (8%), aircraft crashes (2.5%), and burns and electrical shocks (1%).

ROAD TRAFFIC INJURIES

An estimated 3,500 people are killed each day, including 1,000 children, around the world in road traffic crashes involving cars, buses, motorcycles, bicycles, trucks, or pedestrians. Annually, 1.3 million are killed and at least 50 million are injured each year from traffic injuries—a number likely to double by 2020. More than 85% of these casualties (and 96% of child deaths) occur in low- and middle-income countries. Table 2-11 lists the countries with the highest death rates from road traffic crashes.

International efforts to combat road deaths command a tiny fraction of the resources deployed to fight other diseases like malaria and tuberculosis, yet the burden of road traffic injuries is comparable. In response to this crisis, in March 2010 the 64th General Assembly of the United Nations described the global road safety crisis as "a major public health problem" and proclaimed 2011–2020 as "The Decade of Action for Road Safety."

According to Department of State data, road traffic crashes are also the leading cause of injury death to US citizens while traveling internationally (Figure 2-1) and the leading cause of death to healthy US travelers. Recent estimates show that 745 US citizens were killed in road traffic crashes from 2007 through 2009. Approximately 13% of these road traffic deaths involved motorcycles and 5% involved pedestrians. A study from Bermuda reported that the rate of motorbike injuries is much higher in tourists than in the local population, and the rate is highest in

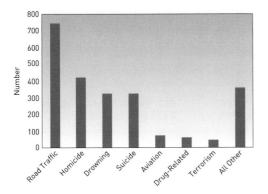

FIGURE 2-1. LEADING CAUSES OF INJURY DEATH FOR US CITIZENS IN FOREIGN COUNTRIES, 2007–2009[1,2]

[1] Data from US Department of State. Death of US citizens abroad by non-natural causes. Washington, DC: US Department of State; 2010. Available from: http://travel.state.gov/law/family_issues/death/death_600.html.
[2] Excludes deaths of US citizens fighting wars in Afghanistan or Iraq.

people aged 50–59 years. As noted in Chapter 4, The Caribbean, motor vehicle rentals in Bermuda and some other small Caribbean islands are typically limited to motorbikes for tourists, possibly contributing to the higher rates of motorbike injuries. Loss of vehicular control, unfamiliar equipment, and inexperience with motorized 2-wheelers contributed to crashes and injuries, even at speeds less than 30 miles per hour. Road traffic crashes are also a leading cause of nonfatal injuries among US citizens who require emergency transport back to the United States.

Road traffic crashes are common in foreign tourists for a number of reasons: lack of familiarity with the roads, driving on the opposite side of the road, poorly made or maintained vehicles, travel fatigue, poor road surfaces without shoulders, unprotected curves and cliffs, and poor visibility due to lack of adequate lighting, both on the road and on the vehicle. In many low-income areas of the world, unsafe roads and vehicles and an inadequate transportation infrastructure contribute to the traffic injury problem. In many of these countries, motor vehicles often share the road with vulnerable road users, such as pedestrians, bicyclists, and motorbike users. The mix of traffic involving cars, buses, taxis, rickshaws, large trucks, and even animals (on one road or in a single travel lane) increases the risk for crashes and injuries.

Traffic death rates in the 20 countries most frequented by US travelers are listed in Table 2-12. These data show that travelers should be particularly concerned in Mexico. In 2008, 20.3 million travelers visited Mexico. From 2007 through 2009, over 280 US travelers lost their lives in motor vehicle crashes in Mexico, the nation most frequently visited by US citizens.

Strategies to reduce the risk of traffic injury are shown in Table 2-13. The Association for International Road Travel (www.asirt.org) and Make Roads Safe (www.makeroadssafe.org) have useful safety information for international travelers, including road safety checklists and country-specific driving risks. The Department of State has safety information useful to international travelers, including road safety and security, international driving permits, and insurance (www.travel.state.gov).

WATER AND AQUATIC INJURIES

Drowning accounts for 14% of deaths of US citizens abroad. The risk factors have not been clearly defined but are most likely related to unfamiliarity with local water currents and water conditions. Rip tides can be especially dangerous, as are sea animals, such as urchins, jellyfish, coral, and sea lice. Alcohol also contributes to drowning and boating mishaps.

Drowning was the leading cause of injury death to US travelers visiting countries where water recreation is a major activity, such as Fiji, The Bahamas, Jamaica, and Costa Rica. Young men are particularly at risk of head and spinal cord injuries from diving into shallow water, and alcohol is a factor in some cases.

Boating can be a hazard, especially if boaters are unfamiliar with boats, do not know boating etiquette, or are new to the water environment in a foreign country. Many boating fatalities result from inexperience or failure to wear lifejackets.

Scuba diving is a frequent pursuit of travelers in coastal destinations (see the Scuba Diving section later in this chapter). Travelers should either be experienced divers or dive with a reliable dive shop and instructors. They should be reminded not to dive on the same day they arrive by airplane. The death rate among all divers, worldwide, is thought to be 15–20 deaths per 100,000 divers per year.

Table 2-11. Countries with the highest estimated traffic death rates[1,2]

COUNTRY	REPORTED NUMBER OF TRAFFIC DEATHS	ESTIMATED TRAFFIC DEATH RATE PER 100,000
Eritrea	81	48.4
Cook Islands (New Zealand)	6	45.0
Egypt	15,983	41.6
Libya	2,138	40.5
Afghanistan	1,179	39.0
Iraq	1,932	38.1
Angola	2,358	37.7
Niger	570	37.7
United Arab Emirates	1,056	37.1
The Gambia	54	36.6
Iran	22,918	35.8
Mauritania	262	35.5
Ethiopia	2,441	35.0
Sudan	2,227	34.7
Mozambique	1,952	34.7
Tunisia	1,497	34.5
Kenya	3,760	34.4
Guinea-Bissau	512	34.4
Tanzania	2,595	34.3
Chad	814	34.3

[1] Data from World Health Organization. Global Status Report on Road Safety: Time for Action. Geneva: WHO; 2009. Available from: http://whqlibdoc.who.int/publications/2009/9789241563840_eng.pdf.
[2] Deaths reported in the local population in 2007. For comparison, the reported number of traffic deaths in the United States was 42,642, with an estimated traffic death rate of 13.9 per 100,000.

Table 2-12. Estimated traffic death rates in the 20 countries most frequently traveled by US residents[1,2]

COUNTRY	REPORTED NUMBER OF TRAFFIC DEATHS	ESTIMATED TRAFFIC DEATH RATE PER 100,000
Mexico	22,103	20.7
Thailand	12,492	19.6
India	105,725	16.8
China	96,611	16.5
Greece	1,657	14.9
South Korea	6,166	12.8
Jamaica	350	12.3
Colombia	5,409	11.7
Italy	5,669	9.6
Spain	4,104	9.3
Canada	2,889	8.8
Ireland	365	8.5
Australia	1,616	7.8
France	4,620	7.5
Germany	4,949	6.0
Israel	398	5.7
United Kingdom	3,298	5.4
Japan	6,639	5.0
Switzerland	370	4.9
The Netherlands	791	4.8

[1] Data from the US Department of Commerce. 2008 United States resident travel abroad. Washington, DC: US Department of Commerce; 2010. Available from: http://tinet.ita.doc.gov/outreachpages/download_data_table/2008_US_Travel_Abroad.pdf. and World Health Organization. Global Status Report on Road Safety: Time for Action. Geneva: WHO; 2009. Available from: http://whqlibdoc.who.int/publications/2009/9789241563840_eng.pdf.
[2] Deaths reported in the local population in 2007. For comparison, the number of reported traffic deaths in the United States was 42,642, with an estimated traffic death rate of 13.9 per 100,000.

Table 2-13. Recommended strategies to reduce injuries while traveling internationally

MECHANISM OR TYPE OF INJURY	PREVENTION STRATEGIES
Road Traffic Crashes	
Seat belts and child safety seats	Always use safety belts and child safety seats. Rent vehicles with seat belts; when possible, ride in taxis with seat belts and sit in the rear seat; bring child safety seats and booster seats from home for children to ride properly restrained.
Driving hazards	When possible, avoid driving in low-income countries at night; always pay close attention to the correct side of the road when driving in countries that drive on the left.
Country-specific driving hazards	Check the Association for International Road Travel website for driving hazards or risks by country (www.asirt.org).
Motorcycles, motor bikes, and bicycles	Always wear helmets (bring a helmet from home, if needed). When possible, avoid driving or riding on motorcycles or motorbikes, especially motorbike taxis. Traveling overseas is a bad time to learn to drive a motorbike.
Alcohol-impaired driving	Alcohol increases the risk for all causes of injury. Do not drive, swim, or pilot a boat after drinking, and avoid riding with someone who has been drinking.
Cellular telephones	Do not use a cellular telephone or text while driving. To date, at least 32 countries have enacted laws banning cellular telephone use while driving, and Portugal has made using any kind of telephone, including hands-free, illegal while driving.
Taxis or hired drivers	Ride only in marked taxis and try to ride in those that have safety belts. Hire drivers familiar with the area.
Bus travel	Avoid riding in overcrowded, overweight, or top-heavy buses or minivans.
Pedestrians	Be alert when crossing streets, especially in countries where motorists drive on the left side of the road. Walk with a companion or someone from the host country.
Other Tips	
Airplane travel	Avoid using local, unscheduled aircraft. If possible, fly on larger planes (more than 30 seats), in good weather, and during the daylight hours.
Drowning	Avoid swimming alone or in unfamiliar waters. Wear life jackets while boating or during water recreation activities.

continued

TABLE 2-13. RECOMMENDED STRATEGIES TO REDUCE INJURIES WHILE TRAVELING INTERNATIONALLY (continued)

MECHANISM OR TYPE OF INJURY	PREVENTION STRATEGIES
Violence	
Country-specific	The Department of State provides useful safety information for international travelers. Read the consular information sheets, travel warnings, and any public announcements for country-specific personal security risks and safety tips (www.travel.state.gov).
Assault	When in low-income countries or high-poverty areas, avoid traveling at night in unfamiliar environments. Use alcohol in moderation, and do not travel alone. If confronted, give up all valuables, and do not resist attackers.

OTHER UNINTENTIONAL INJURIES

From 2007 through 2009, aviation incidents, drug-related incidents, and other unintentional injuries accounted for more than one-third of all injury deaths to US travelers in foreign countries (Figure 2-1). Fires can be a substantial risk in low-income countries where building codes are not present or not enforced, there are no smoke alarms, there is no emergency access to 9-1-1 services, and the fire department's focus is on putting out fires rather than on fire prevention or victim rescue.

Travel by local commercial air carriers in many countries can be risky. From 2007 through 2009, an estimated 74 US travelers were killed in airplane crashes in foreign countries. Travel on unscheduled flights, in small aircraft, at night, in inclement weather, and with inexperienced pilots carries the highest risk.

Travel health providers and travelers should consider the following:

- Travelers should consider purchasing special health and evacuation insurance if their destinations include countries where there may not be access to good medical care (see the Travel Health Insurance and Evacuation Insurance section later in this chapter).
- Because trauma care is poor in many countries, victims of injuries can die before reaching a hospital, and there may be no coordinated ambulance services. In remote areas, medical assistance and modern drugs may be unavailable, and travel to the nearest medical facility can take a long time.
- Adventure travel activities, such as mountain climbing, whitewater rafting, and kayaking, are popular in foreign countries. Risks include the lack of rapid emergency trauma response when injured, inadequate trauma care in remote locations, and sudden, unexpected weather changes that compromise safety and hamper rescue efforts.
- Travelers should avoid using local, unscheduled, small aircraft. If available, choose larger aircraft (more than 30 seats), as they have most likely undergone more strict and regular safety inspections. Larger aircraft also provide more protection in the event of a crash. For country-specific airline crash events, see www.airsafe.com.
- To prevent fire-related injuries, travelers should select accommodations no higher than the sixth floor (fire ladders generally cannot reach higher than the sixth floor). Hotels should be checked for smoke alarms and preferably sprinkler systems. Two escape routes from buildings should always be identified. Crawling low under smoke and covering one's mouth with a wet cloth are helpful in escaping a fire.
- Improperly vented heating devices may cause poisoning from carbon monoxide. Carbon monoxide at the back of boats near the

engine can be especially dangerous. Travelers may carry a personal detector that can alert to the presence of this lethal gas.

- Travelers should consider learning basic first aid and CPR before travel overseas with another person. Travelers should bring a travel health kit, which should be customized to the anticipated itinerary and activities (see the Travel Health Kits section later in this chapter).

VIOLENCE-RELATED INJURIES

Violence is a leading worldwide public health problem and a growing concern of travelers. In 2000, about 1.6 million people lost their lives to violence, and only one-fifth were casualties of armed conflicts. Rates of violent deaths in low- to middle-income countries are more than 3 times those in higher-income countries, although there are variations within countries.

Homicide was the second-leading cause of injury death among US travelers in foreign countries, accounting for over 400 deaths from 2007 through 2009 (Figure 2-1). For some low-income countries, such as Honduras, Colombia, Guatemala, and Haiti, homicide was the leading cause of injury death for US travelers, accounting for 38%–52% of all injury deaths.

US travelers are viewed by many criminals as wealthy, naïve targets, who are inexperienced, unfamiliar with the culture, and inept at seeking assistance once victimized. Traveling in high-poverty areas, civil unrest, alcohol or drug use, and traveling in unfamiliar environments at night increase the likelihood that a US traveler will be the victim of planned or random violence.

To avoid violence while traveling, travelers should limit travel at night, travel with a companion, and vary routine travel habits. Travelers should not wear expensive clothing or accessories. Since criminals are less likely to victimize upper floors, travelers should avoid accommodations on the ground floor of hotels and avoid rooms immediately next to the stairs. It is important to lock all doors and windows. Travelers may even consider carrying and using a door intruder alarm, a smoke alarm, and a rubber doorstop that can be used as a supplemental door lock. If confronted, travelers should give up all valuables and not resist attackers. Victims of a crime overseas should contact the nearest US embassy, consulate, or consular agency for assistance.

Suicide is the fourth-leading cause of injury death to US citizens traveling abroad. For longer-term travelers (such as missionaries and volunteers), social isolation and substance abuse, particularly in the face of living in areas of poverty and rigid gender roles, may increase the risk of depression and suicide.

BIBLIOGRAPHY

1. Association for Safe International Road Travel. Association for Safe International Road Travel. Rockville, MD: ASIRT; 2010 [updated Nov 9; cited 2010 Apr 29]. Available from: www.asirt.org.
2. Balaban V, Sleet D. Prevention of injuries to children traveling. In: Kamat D, Fischer P, editors. Textbook of Child Global Health. Elk Grove Village, IL: American Academy of Pediatrics; 2011.
3. Ball DJ, Machin N. Foreign travel and the risk of harm. Int J Inj Contr Saf Promot. 2006 Jun;13(2):107–15.
4. Carey MJ, Aitken ME. Motorbike injuries in Bermuda: a risk for tourists. Ann Emerg Med. 1996 Oct;28(4):424–9.
5. Cortes LM, Hargarten SW, Hennes HM. Recommendations for water safety and drowning prevention for travelers. J Travel Med. 2006 Jan–Feb;13(1):21–34.
6. Dinh-Zarr TB, Hargarten SW. Road crash deaths of American travelers: the Make Roads Safe report. An analysis of US State Department data on unnatural causes of death to US citizens abroad (2004–2006). 2007 [cited 2010 May 18]. Available from: www.fiafoundation.org.
7. FIA Foundation for the Automobile and Society. Make roads safe report: a decade of action for road safety. FIA Foundation for the Automobile and Society; 2009 [cited 2010 Nov 16]. Available from: http://www.fiafoundation.org/publications/Pages/PublicationHome.aspx.
8. Guse CE, Cortes LM, Hargarten SW, Hennes HM. Fatal injuries of US citizens abroad. J Travel Med. 2007 Sep–Oct;14(5):279–87.
9. Hargarten SW, Bouc GT. Emergency air medical transport of US-citizen tourists: 1988 to 1990. Air Med J. 1993 Oct;12(10):398–402.
10. Krug EG, Mercy JA, Dahlberg LL, Zwi AB. The world report on violence and health. Lancet. 2002 Oct 5;360(9339):1083–8.
11. Leggat PA, Fischer PR. Accidents and repatriation. Travel Med Infect Dis. 2006 May–Jul;4(3–4):135–46.

12. McInnes RJ, Williamson LM, Morrison A. Unintentional injury during foreign travel: a review. J Travel Med. 2002 Nov–Dec;9(6):297–307.

13. Peden MM. World Report on Road Traffic Injury Prevention. Geneva: World Health Organization; 2004.

14. US Department of Commerce. 2008 United States resident travel abroad. Washington, DC: US Department of Commerce; 2010 [updated 2010 Nov 9]. Available from: http://tinet.ita.doc.gov/outreachpages/download_data_table/2008_US_Travel_Abroad.pdf.

15. US Department of State. Death of US citizens abroad by non-natural causes. Washington, DC: US Department of State; 2010 [cited 2010 Apr 28]. Available from: http://travel.state.gov/law/family_issues/death/death_600.html.

16. US Department of State. Tips for traveling abroad. Washington, DC: US Department of State; 2010 [cited 2010 Apr 29]. Available from: http://www.travel.state.gov/travel/tips/tips_1232.html.

ANIMAL-ASSOCIATED HAZARDS
Nina Marano, G. Gale Galland

HUMAN INTERACTION WITH ANIMALS: A RISK FACTOR FOR INJURY AND ILLNESS

Animals tend to avoid humans, but they can attack if they perceive threat, are protecting their young or territory, or are injured or ill. Although attacks by wild animals are more dramatic, attacks by domestic animals are far more common, and secondary infections of wounds may result in serious systemic disease. In addition, animals can transmit zoonotic infections such as rabies. Of the estimated 35,000–55,000 rabies deaths every year worldwide, more than 95% occur as a result of dog bites in the developing countries of Africa and Asia. A recent 10-year retrospective review of dog bites in Austria showed that 75% of the bites were preventable because the person had intentionally interacted with the dog.

BITE OR SCRATCH WOUNDS

Animal bites present a risk for rabies, tetanus, and other bacterial infections. Animals' saliva can be so heavily contaminated with bacteria that a bite may not even be necessary to cause infection if the animal licks a preexisting cut or scratch. Young children are more likely to be bitten by animals and to sustain more severe injuries from animal bites.

Prevention

Before departure, travelers should have a current tetanus vaccination or documentation of having received a booster vaccination within the previous 5–10 years. Travel health providers should assess a traveler's need for preexposure rabies immunization according to the guidelines in Table 3-15. While traveling, people should never try to pet, handle, or feed unfamiliar animals (whether domestic or wild), particularly in areas where rabies is endemic. To mitigate the risk of exposure to rabies, dogs and other mammals should be avoided.

Management

In order to prevent infection, all wounds should be promptly cleaned with soap and water, and the wound promptly debrided, if necrotic tissue, dirt, or other foreign material is present. These steps of wound care are especially important for tetanus- or rabies-prone wounds (see the Rabies and Tetanus sections in Chapter 3). Travelers who might have been exposed to rabies should contact a reliable health care provider for advice about rabies postexposure prophylaxis. Travelers who received their most recent tetanus toxoid-containing vaccine more than 5 years previously, or who have not received at least 3 doses of tetanus toxoid–containing vaccines, may require a dose of tetanus toxoid–containing vaccine (Tdap, Td, or DTaP) according to the guidelines in Table 3-18.

MONKEYS

Macaques are native to Asia and North Africa. They are also housed in research facilities, zoos, and wildlife or amusement parks and are kept as pets in private homes throughout the world. Monkey bites occasionally occur in certain urban sites, such as temples in Nepal or India, and can transmit herpes B virus.

Herpes B virus is related to the herpes simplex viruses that cause oral and genital ulcers. Herpes B infection is rare in humans. The virus was discovered in 1933, and since that time approximately 50 cases have been reported in humans, with an 80% case-fatality ratio. No cases of herpes B infection have been reported in people exposed to monkeys in the wild. Most documented cases have resulted from occupational exposures. However, travelers to areas where macaques range freely should be aware of the potential risk. A monkey infected with herpes B may appear completely healthy.

Documented routes of human infection with herpes B virus include animal bites and scratches, exposure to infected tissue or body fluids from splashes, and in one instance, human-to-human transmission. Even minor scratches or bites should be considered potential exposures, because, experimentally, herpes B virus has been isolated from surfaces for up to 2 weeks after it was applied. The incubation period ranges from <1 week to a month or longer. Neurologic symptoms develop as the virus infects the central nervous system and may lead to ascending paralysis and respiratory failure. Increased public and clinician awareness about the risks associated with an injury from a macaque, improved first aid after exposure, the availability of better diagnostic tests, and improved antiviral therapeutics have decreased the case-fatality ratio to 20% in treated people. As a result, from 1987 through 2004 only 5 infections were fatal.

Although only macaque bites pose a herpes B virus threat, any monkey bite may pose a threat for rabies.

Prevention

Travelers should never attempt to feed, pet, or otherwise handle any monkeys.

Management

After a monkey bite or scratch, travelers should be advised to thoroughly clean the wound and seek medical care immediately to be evaluated for possible rabies and herpes B postexposure prophylaxis. Additional information and photos of macaques can be found at the website for the National B Virus Resource Center at the Georgia State University Viral Immunology Center (www2.gsu.edu/~wwwvir).

BATS

Bats can be found almost anywhere in the world except the polar regions and extreme deserts. Bats are reservoir hosts for viruses that can cross species barriers to infect humans and other domestic and wild mammals. Viruses such as rabies and viral hemorrhagic fevers can be transmitted from bats to people. It is not possible to tell if a bat has rabies; however, any bat that is active by day, is found where bats are not usually seen (for example, indoors or outdoors in areas near humans), or is unable to fly is far more likely to be rabid. A recent example of an imported case of Marburg fever in a tourist who had visited a "python cave" in western Uganda illustrates the risk of acquiring diseases from contact with cave-dwelling bats. This same cave was the source of a fatal case of Marburg hemorrhagic fever in a Dutch tourist in 2008. Exposure to bats can occur during adventure activities such as caving or spelunking, and can include bites, scratches, and mucosal or cutaneous exposure to bat saliva. Like any other wild animal, bats, whether sick or healthy, will bite in self-defense if handled.

Prevention

Bats should never be handled. Travelers should be discouraged from going into caves or mines that have large bat infestations. Depending on the country being visited, preexposure rabies vaccination may be recommended for people engaged in activities such as caving.

Management

If a bite occurs or if infectious material (such as saliva) from a bat gets into the eyes, nose, mouth, or a wound, the traveler should wash the affected area thoroughly and get medical advice immediately. Any suspected or documented bite or scratch from a bat should be grounds for seeking postexposure rabies immunoprophylaxis in any destination in the world.

People usually know when they have been bitten by a bat. However, bats have tiny teeth, and not all wounds may be apparent. Travelers should seek medical advice even in the absence of an obvious bite wound if they wake up to find a bat in the room or see a bat in the room of a sleeping child.

RODENTS

Rodents carry a variety of viral, bacterial, and parasitic agents that may pose a threat to human health. Human exposure can occur directly by a bite or scratch, or indirectly by exposure to surfaces or water contaminated with urine or feces. Rodents should never be handled. Travelers should avoid places that have evidence of infestation with rodents and should avoid contact with rodent feces. Travelers should not eat or drink anything that is suspected to be contaminated by rodent feces or urine.

Management

Wild rodents are unlikely to have rabies; however, each exposure needs to be evaluated as follows:

- If the bite was provoked (such as through feeding, petting, or playing with the animal) and the animal appeared healthy, the animal was probably not rabid at the time of the bite. Most experts would not recommend postexposure prophylaxis in this situation.
- If the bite was unprovoked or the animal appeared unhealthy and is unavailable for testing, rabies postexposure prophylaxis should be considered.

Travelers who were exposed to rodents and who develop febrile illness shortly after returning home should be evaluated by a clinician. Depending on the history and symptoms, diseases such as yersinia, plague, leptospirosis, hantavirus and rickettsial infections, Lyme disease, tickborne encephalitis, poxvirus, and bartonellosis (all discussed in further detail in Chapter 3) should be included in the list of diagnostic differentials.

SNAKES

Poisonous snakes are hazards in many locations, although deaths from snakebites are rare. Snakebites usually occur in areas where dense human populations coexist with dense snake populations, such as Southeast Asia, sub-Saharan Africa, and tropical areas in the Americas.

Prevention

Common sense is the best precaution. Most snake bites are the direct result of startling, handling, or harassing snakes. Therefore, all snakes should be left alone. Travelers should be aware of their surroundings, especially at night and during warm weather when snakes tend to be more active. For extra precaution, when practical, travelers should wear heavy, ankle-high or higher boots and long pants when walking outdoors in areas possibly inhabited by venomous snakes.

Management

Travelers should be advised to seek immediate medical attention any time a bite wound breaks the skin or when snake venom is ejected into their eyes or mucous membranes. Immobilization of the affected limb and application of a pressure bandage that does not restrict blood flow are recommended first-aid measures while the victim is moved as quickly as possible to a medical facility. Incision of the bite site and tourniquets that restrict blood flow to the affected limb are not recommended. Specific therapy for snakebites is controversial and should be left to the judgment of local emergency medical personnel. Specific antivenoms are available for some snakes in some areas, so trying to ascertain the species of snake that bit the victim may be critical.

ARTHROPODS AND INSECTS

Bites and stings from spiders and scorpions can be painful and can result in illness and death, particularly among infants and children. Other insects and arthropods, such as mosquitoes and ticks, can transmit communicable diseases; these diseases are discussed in more detail in Chapter 3. Bites and stings can occur without the traveler's awareness of the bite, particularly when camping or staying in rustic accommodations.

There has been a recent resurgence in bed bug infestations worldwide, particularly in developed countries, thought to be related to the increase in international travel and insecticide resistance. Bed bug infestations have been increasingly reported in hotels. Bed bugs may be transported in luggage and on clothing.

Prevention

Insect bites can be avoided by using repellents and insecticides, wearing long sleeves and pants while hiking, sleeping under mosquito nets, and shaking clothing and shoes before putting them on (see the Protection against Mosquitoes, Ticks, and Other Insects and Arthropods earlier in this chapter). Exposure to bed bugs can be avoided by inspecting the premises of hotels or other unfamiliar sleeping locations for bed bugs on mattresses, box springs, bedding, and furniture. Keep suitcases closed when they are not in use and try to keep them off the floor when traveling (see Box 2-3).

Management

Travelers should seek medical attention if a bite or sting causes redness, swelling, bruising, rash, or persistent pain or fever. Travelers who have a history of severe allergic reactions to insect bites or stings should also ask their physician to evaluate them for the need to carry an epinephrine auto-injector (such as an EpiPen) to use, in case of recurrence (both in general and especially while traveling).

MARINE ANIMALS

Venomous injuries from marine fish and invertebrates are increasing with the popularity of surfing, scuba diving, and snorkeling. Most species responsible for human injuries live in tropical coastal waters, including stingrays, jellyfish, stonefish, sea urchins, and scorpionfish.

Prevention

Travelers should be advised to use protective footwear and maintain vigilance while engaging in recreational water activities.

In case of injury, identifying the species involved can help determine the best course of treatment.

Management

Symptoms of venomous injuries can range from mild swelling and redness at the site to more severe symptoms, such as difficulty breathing or swallowing, chest pain, or intense pain at the site of the sting, for which immediate medical treatment should be sought. Management will vary according to the severity of symptoms and can include medications, such as diphenhydramine, steroids, pain medication, and antibiotics.

BIRDS

Ill birds have been associated with outbreaks of highly pathogenic avian influenza in people. When traveling in an area that is experiencing an outbreak of avian influenza, travelers should avoid all contact with live poultry (such as chickens, ducks, geese, pigeons, turkeys, and quail) or any wild birds and should avoid settings where avian influenza A (H5N1)-infected poultry may be present, such as commercial or backyard poultry farms and live poultry markets. Travelers should not eat uncooked or undercooked poultry or poultry products, including dishes made with uncooked eggs or poultry blood. Other zoonotic diseases from birds may potentially infect humans through infected feces or by aerosol. These would include diseases such as histoplasmosis (see the Histoplasmosis section in Chapter 3), salmonella, psittacosis, or avian mycobacteriosis. Travelers should avoid contact with ill birds and should wash their hands if they come in contact with bird feces.

BIBLIOGRAPHY

1. Callahan M. Bites, stings, and envenoming injuries. In: Keystone JS, Kozarsky PE, Freedman DO, Nothdurft HD, Connor BA, editors. Travel Medicine. 2nd ed. Philadelphia: Mosby; 2008. p. 463–74.

2. CDC. Dog-bite-related fatalities—United States, 1995–1996. MMWR Morb Mortal Wkly Rep. 1997 May 30;46(21):463–7.

3. CDC. Nonfatal dog bite-related injuries treated in hospital emergency departments—United States, 2001. MMWR Morb Mortal Wkly Rep. 2003 Jul 4;52(26):605–10.

4. Cohen JI, Davenport DS, Stewart JA, Deitchman S, Hilliard JK, Chapman LE. Recommendations for prevention of and therapy for exposure to B virus (cercopithecine herpesvirus 1). Clin Infect Dis. 2002 Nov 15;35(10):1191–203.

5. Diaz JH. The global epidemiology, syndromic classification, management, and prevention of spider bites. Am J Trop Med Hyg. 2004 Aug;71(2):239–50.

6. Feldman KA, Trent R, Jay MT. Epidemiology of hospitalizations resulting from dog bites in California, 1991–1998. Am J Public Health. 2004 Nov;94(11):1940–1.

7. Gibbons RV. Cryptogenic rabies, bats, and the question of aerosol transmission. Ann Emerg Med. 2002 May;39(5):528–36.

8. Gold BS, Dart RC, Barish RA. Bites of venomous snakes. N Engl J Med. 2002 Aug 1;347(5):347–56.

9. Huff JL, Barry PA. B-virus (cercopithecine herpesvirus 1) infection in humans and macaques: potential for zoonotic disease. Emerg Infect Dis. 2003 Feb;9(2):246–50.

10. Löe J, Röskaft E. Large carnivores and human safety: a review. Ambio. 2004 Aug;33(6):283–8.

11. Meerburg BG, Singleton GR, Kijlstra A. Rodent-borne diseases and their risks for public health. Crit Rev Microbiol. 2009;35(3):221–70.

12. Pan American Health Organization. Rabies. In: Acha PN, Szyfres B, editors. Zoonoses and Communicable Diseases Common to Man and Animals. 3rd ed. Washington, DC: Pan American Health Organization; 2003. p. 246–76.

13. Schalamon J, Ainoedhofer H, Singer G, Petnehazy T, Mayr J, Kiss K, et al. Analysis of dog bites in children who are younger than 17 years. Pediatrics. 2006 Mar;117(3):e374–9.

14. Warrell DA. Treatment of bites by adders and exotic venomous snakes. BMJ. 2005 Nov 26;331(7527):1244–7.

15. World Health Organization. WHO Expert Consultation on rabies. World Health Organ Tech Rep Ser. 2005;931:1–88.

NATURAL DISASTERS & ENVIRONMENTAL HAZARDS

Josephine Malilay, Dahna Batts, Armin Ansari, Charles W. Miller, Clive M. Brown

NATURAL DISASTERS

Travelers should be aware of the potential for natural phenomena such as hurricanes, floods, tsunamis, tornadoes, or earthquakes. Natural disasters can contribute to the transmission of some diseases, especially since water supplies and sewage systems may be disrupted, sanitation and hygiene may be compromised by population displacement and overcrowding, and normal public health services may be interrupted.

When arriving at a destination, travelers should be familiar with local risks for seismic, flood-related, landslide-related, tsunami-related, and other hazards, as well as warning systems, evacuation routes, and shelters in areas of high risk.

Disease Risks

The risk for infectious diseases among travelers to affected areas is minimal unless a disease is endemic in an area before the disaster, since transmission cannot take place unless the causative agent is present. Although typhoid can be endemic in developing countries, natural disasters have seldom led to epidemic levels of disease. Floods have been known to prompt outbreaks of leptospirosis and cholera in areas where the organism is found in water sources (see the Leptospirosis and Cholera sections in Chapter 3).

When water and sewage systems have been disrupted, safe water and food supplies are of great importance in preventing enteric disease transmission. If contamination is suspected, water should be boiled and appropriately disinfected (see the Water Disinfection for Travelers section earlier in this chapter). Travelers who are injured during a natural disaster should have a medical evaluation to determine what additional care may be required for wounds potentially contaminated with feces, soil, or saliva, or that have been exposed to fresh or sea water that may contain parasites or bacteria. Tetanus booster status should always be kept current.

Various vaccine-preventable diseases have been eliminated or are near elimination in some developing countries. However, if someone who has the disease travels to the country, there is a risk of reintroducing those diseases, leading to an outbreak. Therefore, it is very important that people traveling to offer relief or other services in countries affected by natural disasters be protected against such diseases.

Injuries

After a natural disaster, deaths are rarely due to infectious diseases and are most often due to blunt trauma, crush-related injuries, or drowning. Travelers should thus be aware of the risks for injury during and after a natural disaster. In floods, people should avoid driving through swiftly moving water. Travelers should exercise caution during clean-up, particularly when encountering downed power lines, water-affected electrical outlets, interrupted gas lines, and stray or frightened animals. During natural disasters, technological malfunctions may release hazardous materials (such as release of toxic chemicals from a point source displaced by strong winds, seismic motion, or rapidly moving water).

Environmental Risks

Natural disasters often lead to wide-ranging air pollution in large cities. Uncontrolled forest fires have caused widespread pollution over vast expanses. Natural or manmade disasters resulting in massive structural collapse or dust clouds can cause the release of chemical or biologic contaminants (such as asbestos or the arthrospores that lead to coccidioidomycosis). Health risks associated with these environmental occurrences have not been fully studied. Travelers with chronic pulmonary disease may be more susceptible to adverse effects from these exposures.

Event-Specific Information

Typically, after natural disasters of a magnitude that may affect travelers, current information about the disaster, as well as travel health information specific to those needing to travel to the affected area, is provided on the CDC Travelers' Health website (www.cdc.gov/travel). Recommendations may include specific immunizations or cautions regarding unique hazards in the affected area.

ENVIRONMENTAL HAZARDS
Air

Air pollution may be found in large cities throughout the world; its sources are often attributed to automobile exhaust and industrial emissions and may be aggravated by climate and geography. Specifically, particulate matter (PM), or particle pollution, consisting of fine particles 2.5 µm or smaller in diameter may enter the lungs and cause serious health problems. Travelers should be aware that global long-term average PM2.5 concentrations have been estimated to exceed the World Health Organization's Air Quality PM2.5 Interim Target-1 (35 µg/m3 annual average) in eastern and central Asia and North Africa.

The harmful effects of air pollution are difficult to avoid when visiting some cities; limiting strenuous activity and not smoking can help. Any risk to healthy short-term travelers to such areas is probably small, but people with preexisting health conditions (such as asthma, chronic obstructive pulmonary disease, or heart disease) could be more susceptible. Avoiding dust clouds and areas of heavy dust or haze is wise.

Water

Rivers, lakes, and the ocean may be contaminated with organic or inorganic chemical compounds (such as heavy metals or other toxins), harmful algal blooms (cyanobacteria) that can be toxic both to fish and to people who eat the fish, or who swim or bathe in the water, and pathogens from human and animal waste that may cause disease in swimmers. Such hazards may not be immediately apparent in a body of water.

Extensive water damage after major hurricanes and floods increases the likelihood of mold contamination in buildings. Travelers may visit flooded areas overseas as part of emergency, medical, or humanitarian missions. Mold is a more serious hazard for people with conditions such as impaired host defenses or mold allergies. To prevent exposure that could result in adverse health effects from disturbed mold, people should adhere to the following recommendations:

- Avoid areas where mold contamination is obvious.
- Use personal protective equipment (PPE), such as gloves, goggles, or a tight-fitting approved N-95 respirator. Travelers should take sufficient PPE with them, as these may be scarce in the countries visited.
- Keep hands, skin, and clothing clean and free from mold-contaminated dust.
- Review the CDC guidance, Mold Prevention Strategies and Possible Health Effects in the Aftermath of Hurricanes and Major Floods (www.cdc.gov/mmwr/preview/mmwrhtml/rr5508a1.htm), which provides

recommendations for dealing with mold in these settings.

Radiation

Natural background radiation levels can vary substantially from region to region, but these natural variations are not a health concern for either the traveler or resident population. Travelers should be aware of regions known to have been contaminated with radioactive materials, such as the area surrounding the Chernobyl nuclear power station, 100 km (62 miles) northwest of Kiev, Ukraine. This unprecedented radiation emergency and subsequent contamination primarily affected regions in 3 republics—Ukraine, Belarus, and Russia—with the highest radioactive ground contamination within 30 km (19 miles) of Chernobyl.

In most countries, known areas of radioactive contamination are fenced or marked with signs. These areas should not be trespassed.

Any traveler seeking long-term (more than a few months) residence near a known or suspected contaminated area should consult with staff of the nearest US embassy and inquire about any applicable advisories in that area regarding drinking water quality or purchase of meat, fruit, and vegetables from local farmers. Radiation emergencies are rare events. In case of such an emergency, however, travelers should follow instructions provided by local emergency and public health authorities. If such information is not forthcoming, US travelers should immediately seek advice from the nearest US embassy.

Natural disasters (such as floods) may also displace industrial or clinical radioactive sources. In all circumstances, travelers should exercise caution when they encounter unknown objects or equipment, especially if they bear the radioactive symbol. Travelers who encounter a questionable object should notify appropriate authorities.

BIBLIOGRAPHY

1. Brandt M, Brown C, Burkhart J, Burton N, Cox-Ganser J, Damon S, et al. Mold prevention strategies and possible health effects in the aftermath of hurricanes and major floods. MMWR Recomm Rep. 2006 Jun 9;55(RR-8):1–27.
2. Eisenbud M, Gesell TF. Environmental Radioactivity: from Natural, Industrial, and Military Sources. 4th ed. San Diego: Academic Press; 1997.
3. FDA Center for Devices and Radiological Health. Accidental radioactive contamination of human food and animal feeds: recommendations for state and local agencies. Rockville, MD: US Department of Health and Human Services; 1998 [updated 1998 Aug 13]. Available from: http://www.fda.gov/downloads/MedicalDevices/DeviceRegulationandGuidance/GuidanceDocuments/UCM094513.pdf.
4. National Council on Radiation Protection and Measurements. Ionizing radiation exposure of the population of the United States: recommendations of the National Council on Radiation Protection and Measurements. Bethesda, MD: National Council on Radiation Protection and Measurements; 2009. Available from: http://www.knovel.com/knovel2/Toc.jsp?BookID=2562.
5. Noji EK. The Public Health Consequences of Disasters. New York: Oxford University Press; 1997.
6. Nukushina J. Japanese earthquake victims are being exposed to high density of asbestos. We need protective masks desperately. Epidemiol Prev. 1995 Jun;19(63):226–7.
7. PAHO. Natural Disasters: Protecting the Public's Health. Washington, DC: PAHO Emergency Preparedness Program; 2000. Available from: http://www.paho.org/English/dd/ped/SP575.htm.
8. Schneider E, Hajjeh RA, Spiegel RA, Jibson RW, Harp EL, Marshall GA, et al. A coccidioidomycosis outbreak following the Northridge, Calif, earthquake. JAMA. 1997 Mar 19;277(11):904–8.
9. Scientific Committee on the Effects of Atomic Radiation. Annex J: exposure and effects of the Chernobyl accident. Sources and Effects of Ionizing Radiation. New York: United Nations; 2000. p. 451–556.
10. van Donkelaar A, Martin RV, Brauer M, Kahn R, Levy R, Verduzco C, et al. Global estimates of ambient fine particulate matter concentrations from satellite-based aerosol optical depth: development and application. Environ Health Perspect. 2010 Jun;118(6):847–55.
11. Watson JT, Gayer M, Connolly MA. Epidemics after natural disasters. Emerg Infect Dis. 2007 Jan;13(1):1–5.
12. Young S, Balluz L, Malilay J. Natural and technologic hazardous material releases during and after natural disasters: a review. Sci Total Environ. 2004 Apr 25;322(1–3):3–20.

SCUBA DIVING

Daniel A. Nord

OVERVIEW

An estimated 3 million people participate in recreational diving in the United States, and many travel to tropical areas of the world to dive. Traveling divers can face a variety of medical challenges, but because dive injuries are generally rare, few clinicians are trained in their diagnosis and treatment. Therefore, the recreational diver must be able to recognize the signs of injury and find qualified dive medicine help when needed.

PREPARING FOR DIVE TRAVEL

Planning for dive-related travel should take into account any recent changes in health, including injuries or surgery, and medication use. Respiratory disorders (such as asthma), disorders that affect higher function and consciousness (such as diabetes or seizures), psychological problems (such as anxiety), cardiovascular disease, and pregnancy raise special concerns about diving fitness.

DIVING DISORDERS

Barotrauma

Ear and sinus

Ear barotrauma is the most common injury in divers. On descent, failure to equalize pressure changes in the middle ear space creates a pressure gradient across the eardrum. This pressure change must be controlled through proper equalization techniques to avoid bleeding or fluid accumulation in the middle ear, and stretching or rupture of the eardrum and the membranes covering the windows of the inner ear. Symptoms of barotrauma include the following:

- pain
- tinnitus (ringing in the ears)
- vertigo (dizziness or sensation of spinning)
- sensation of fullness
- effusion (fluid accumulation in the ear)
- decreased hearing

Paranasal sinuses, because of their relatively narrow connecting passageways, are especially susceptible to barotrauma, generally on descent. With small changes in pressure (depth), symptoms are usually mild and subacute but can be exacerbated by continued diving. Larger pressure changes, especially with forceful attempts at equilibration (Valsalva maneuver), can be more injurious. Additional risk factors for ear and sinus barotrauma include the following:

- earplugs
- medications
- ear or sinus surgery
- nasal deformity
- disease

A diver who may have sustained ear or sinus barotrauma should discontinue diving and seek medical attention.

Pulmonary

A scuba diver must reduce the risk of lung overpressure problems by breathing normally and ascending slowly when breathing compressed gas. Overinflation of the lungs can result if a scuba diver ascends toward the surface without exhaling, which may happen, for example, when a novice diver panics. During ascent, compressed gas trapped in the lung increases in volume until the expansion exceeds the elastic limit of lung tissue, causing damage and allowing gas bubbles to escape into 1 or more of 3 possible locations:

- Gas entering the pleural space can cause lung collapse or pneumothorax.
- Gas entering the space around the heart, trachea, and esophagus (the mediastinum) causes mediastinal emphysema and frequently tracks under the skin (subcutaneous emphysema) or into the tissue around the larynx, sometimes precipitating a change in voice characteristics.
- Gas rupturing the alveolar walls can enter the pulmonary capillaries and pass via the pulmonary veins to the left side of the heart, where it

is distributed according to relative blood flow, resulting in arterial gas embolism (AGE).

While mediastinal or subcutaneous emphysema usually resolves spontaneously, pneumothorax generally requires specific treatment to remove the air and reinflate the lung. AGE is a medical emergency, requiring appropriate intervention, which includes recompression treatment with hyperbaric oxygen.

Lung overinflation injuries from scuba diving can range from dramatic and life threatening to mild symptoms of chest pain and dyspnea. Although pulmonary barotrauma is relatively uncommon in divers, prompt medical evaluation is necessary, and evidence for this condition should always be considered in the presence of respiratory or neurologic symptoms following a dive.

Decompression Illness

Decompression illness (DCI) is an all-inclusive term that describes the dysbaric injuries (AGE) and decompression sickness (DCS). Because the 2 diseases are considered to result from separate causes, they are described here separately. However, from a clinical and practical standpoint, distinguishing between them in the field may be impossible and unnecessary, since the initial treatment is the same for both. Decompression illness can occur even in divers who have carefully followed the standard decompression tables and the principles of safe diving. Serious permanent injury may result from either AGE or DCS.

Arterial Gas Embolism

Gas entering the arterial blood through ruptured pulmonary vessels can distribute bubbles into the body tissues, including the heart and brain, where they disrupt circulation. AGE may cause minimal neurologic symptoms, dramatic symptoms that require immediate attention, or death. Common signs and symptoms include the following:

- numbness
- weakness
- tingling
- dizziness
- blurred vision
- chest pain
- personality change

- paralysis or seizures
- loss of consciousness

In general, any scuba diver who surfaces unconscious or loses consciousness within 10 minutes after surfacing should be assumed to have AGE. Intervention with basic life support is indicated, including the administration of 100% oxygen, followed by rapid evacuation to a hyperbaric oxygen treatment facility.

Decompression Sickness

Breathing air under pressure causes excess inert gas (usually nitrogen) to dissolve in body tissues. The amount dissolved is proportional to and increases with depth and time. As the diver ascends to the surface, the excess dissolved gas must be cleared through respiration via the bloodstream. Depending on the amount dissolved and the rate of ascent, some gas can supersaturate tissues, where it separates from solution to form bubbles, interfering with blood flow and tissue oxygenation and causing the following signs and symptoms of DCS:

- joint aches or pain
- numbness or tingling
- mottling or marbling of skin
- coughing spasms or shortness of breath
- itching
- unusual fatigue
- dizziness
- weakness
- personality changes
- loss of bowel or bladder function
- staggering, loss of coordination, or tremors
- paralysis
- collapse or unconsciousness

FLYING AFTER DIVING

The risk of developing decompression sickness is increased when divers are exposed to increased altitude too soon after a dive. The cabin pressure of commercial aircraft may be the equivalent of 6,000–8,000 ft (1,829–2,438 m). Thus, divers should avoid flying or an altitude exposure higher than 2,000 ft (610 m) for:

- a minimum of 12 hours after surfacing from a single no-decompression dive
- a minimum of 18 hours after repetitive dives or multiple days of diving
- substantially longer than 18 hours after dives where decompression stops were required

These recommended preflight surface intervals do not eliminate risk of DCS, and longer surface intervals will further reduce this risk.

PREVENTING DIVING DISORDERS

Recreational divers should dive conservatively and well within the no-decompression limits of their dive tables or computers. Risk factors for DCI are primarily dive depth, dive time, and rate of ascent. Additional factors such as repetitive dives, strenuous exercise, dives to depths more than 60 ft (18.3 m), altitude exposure soon after a dive, and certain physiological variables also increase risk. Divers should be cautioned to stay hydrated and rested and dive within the limits of their training. Diving is a skill that requires training and certification and should be done with a companion.

TREATMENT OF DIVING DISORDERS

Definitive treatment of DCI begins with early recognition of symptoms, followed by recompression with hyperbaric oxygen. A high concentration (100%) of supplemental oxygen is recommended. Surface-level oxygen given for first aid may relieve the signs and symptoms of decompression illness and should be administered as soon as possible. Divers are often dehydrated, either because of incidental causes, immersion, or DCI itself, which can cause capillary leakage. Administration of isotonic glucose-free intravenous fluid is recommended in most cases. Oral rehydration fluids may also be helpful, provided they can be safely administered (for example, if the diver is conscious). The definitive treatment of DCI is recompression and oxygen administration in a hyperbaric chamber.

Divers Alert Network (DAN) maintains 24-hour emergency consultation and evacuation assistance at 919-684-9111 (collect calls are accepted). DAN will help with managing the injured diver, help decide if recompression is needed, provide the location of the closest recompression facility, and help arrange patient transport. DAN can also be contacted for routine, nonemergency consultation by telephone at 919-684-2948, extension 222, or by accessing the DAN website (www.diversalertnetwork.org).

Travelers who plan to scuba dive may want to ascertain whether there are recompression facilities at their destination before embarking on their trip.

BIBLIOGRAPHY

1. Brubakk AO, Neuman TS, Bennett PB, Elliott DH. Bennett and Elliott's Physiology and Medicine of Diving. 5th ed. London: Saunders; 2003.
2. Dear G, Pollock N. DAN America Dive and Travel Medical Guide. 5th ed. Durham, NC: Divers Alert Network; 2009.
3. McAniff JJ. An analysis of recreational, technical, and occupational populations and fatality rates in the United States, 1970–1994. 1995. Available from: http://archive.rubicon-foundation.org/8401.
4. Moon RE. Treatment of decompression illness. In: Bove AA, Davis JC, editors. Bove and Davis' Diving Medicine. 4th ed. Philadelphia: WB Saunders; 2004. p. 195–223.
5. Sheffield P, Vann R. Flying after recreational diving, workshop proceedings of the Divers Alert Network 2002 May 2. Durham, NC: Divers Alert Network; 2004 [cited 2008 Nov 25]. Available from: http://www.diversalertnetwork.org/research/projects/fad/workshop/FADWorkshopProceedings.pdf.

MEDICAL TOURISM
C. Virginia Lee, Victor Balaban

OVERVIEW

"Medical tourism" is the term commonly used to describe people traveling outside their home country for medical treatment. Traditionally, international medical travel involved patients from less-developed countries traveling to a medical center in a developed country for treatment that was not available in their home country. In the United States, the term "medical tourism" generally refers to people traveling to less-developed countries for medical care. Medical tourism is a worldwide, multibillion-dollar phenomenon that is expected to grow substantially in the next 5–10 years. However, little reliable epidemiologic data on medical tourism exist. Studies using different definitions and methods have estimated anywhere from 60,000 to 750,000 medical tourists annually.

The most common categories of procedures that people pursue during medical tourism trips are cosmetic surgery, dentistry, cardiology (cardiac surgery), and orthopedic surgery. Common destinations include Thailand, Mexico, Singapore, India, Malaysia, Cuba, Brazil, Argentina, and Costa Rica. The type of procedure and the destination need to be considered when reviewing the risk of travel for medical care.

Most medical tourists rely on private companies or "medical concierge" services to identify foreign health care facilities, and they pay for their care out of pocket. Some insurers and large employers have alliances with overseas hospitals to control health care costs, and several major medical schools in the United States have developed joint initiatives with overseas providers, such as the Harvard Medical School Dubai Center, the Johns Hopkins Singapore International Medical Center, and the Duke-National University of Singapore. Whether these joint ventures will increase the number of US citizens who go overseas for health care is unknown.

Travel health providers should advise prospective medical tourists to determine if health care facilities they are considering are accredited by the Joint Commission International (JCI). JCI is the international division of the Joint Commission Resources, a US-based not-for-profit affiliate of the Joint Commission that certifies health care facilities in the United States. As of 2009, JCI has accredited more than 300 international hospitals. As more facilities are accredited, more providers will likely offer incentives for their patients to travel overseas for care.

PRE-TRAVEL ADVICE FOR MEDICAL TOURISTS

As discussed in Chapter 1, Planning for Healthy Travel, patients who elect to travel for medical reasons should consult a travel health provider for advice tailored to individual health needs, preferably at least 4–6 weeks before travel. In addition to other considerations for healthy travel related to their destination, medical tourists should consider the risks associated with surgery and travel, either while ill or while recovering from treatment. Air pressure in an aircraft is equivalent to the pressure at an altitude of 6,000–8,000 ft (1,829–2,438 m). Patients should not travel for 10 days after chest or abdominal surgery to avoid risks associated with this change in pressure. Flying and surgery both increase the risk of the development of blood clots and the formation of pulmonary embolus. The American Society of Plastic Surgeons advises people who have had cosmetic procedures of the face, eyelids, or nose, or who have had laser treatments, to wait 7–10 days before flying. Patients are also advised to avoid "vacation" activities such as sunbathing, drinking alcohol, swimming, taking long tours, and engaging in strenuous activities or exercise after surgery. The Aerospace Medical Association has published medical guidelines for airline travel that provide useful information on the risks of travel with certain medical conditions (www.asma.org/pdf/publications/medguid.pdf).

TRANSPLANT TOURISM

One controversial form of medical tourism is "transplant tourism," which is travel for the purpose of receiving an organ purchased from an unrelated donor for transplant. An estimated 5%–10% of all kidney transplants in 2007 were from commercial living donors or vendors (although most of these were not transplant tourism). In 2004, the World Health Assembly Resolution 57.18 encouraged member countries to "take measures to protect the poorest and vulnerable groups from 'transplant tourism' and the sale of tissues and organs." A meeting in 2008 in Istanbul addressed the issue of transplant tourism and organ trafficking, which resulted in a call for these activities to be prohibited. In view of those events, the World Health Organization revised the Guiding Principles on Human Cell, Tissue and Organ Transplantation and released those revised principles in March 2009. A 2007 report on the international organ trade found that China, the Philippines, and Pakistan were the largest organ-exporting countries. Several studies have indicated potential problems that travelers and clinicians need to be aware of when considering transplantation overseas: the donor and the procedures lacked documentation, most patients received fewer immunosuppressive drugs than is current practice to use in the United States, and most patients did not receive antibiotic prophylaxis. However, it is not clear if these issues are representative of the issues faced by all patients who travel for transplants.

GUIDELINES FOR TRAVELERS SEEKING MEDICAL CARE ABROAD

Several professional organizations have developed guidelines that include questions useful for travelers when discussing medical or dental care abroad, either with the facility providing the care or with the group facilitating the trip. When considering a trip overseas for medical care, travelers should be aware of the guiding principles developed by the American Medical Association (Box 2-4). For cosmetic surgery, the American Society for Plastic Surgery (ASPS) developed a briefing paper that includes a patient safety checklist (Box 2-5). Similarly, the American Dental Association provides informational documents, including "Traveler's Guide to Safe Dental Care" through the Global Dental Safety Organization for Safety and Asepsis Procedures (Box 2-6). Although the dental guidelines were not developed for medical tourists, they provide useful information for travelers to consider when selecting a facility or planning a trip for medical or dental care. These 3 guides are targeted for specific groups; however, they provide an indication of the types of questions that people considering travel for medical care should discuss with their regular health care provider.

BOX 2-4. GUIDING PRINCIPLES ON MEDICAL TOURISM[1]

The American Medical Association advocates that employers, insurance companies, and other entities that facilitate or promote medical care outside the United States adhere to the following principles:

(a) Medical care outside the United States must be voluntary.

(b) Financial incentives to travel outside the United States for medical care should not limit the diagnostic and therapeutic alternatives that are offered to patients, or restrict treatment or referral options.

(c) Patients should be referred for medical care only to institutions that have been accredited by recognized international accrediting bodies (e.g., the Joint Commission International or the International Society for Quality in Health Care).

(d) Prior to travel, local follow-up care should be coordinated and financing should be arranged to ensure continuity of care when patients return from medical care outside the United States.

(e) Coverage for travel outside the United States for medical care must include the costs of necessary follow-up care upon return to the United States.

(f) Patients should be informed of their rights and legal recourse prior to agreeing to travel outside the United States for medical care.

(g) Access to physician licensing and outcome data, as well as facility accreditation and outcomes data, should be arranged for patients seeking medical care outside the United States.

(h) The transfer of patient medical records to and from facilities outside the United States should be consistent with Health Insurance Portability and Accountability Action (HIPAA) guidelines.

(i) Patients choosing to travel outside the United States for medical care should be provided with information about the potential risks of combining surgical procedures with long flights and vacation activities.

---

[1] From American Medical Association. New AMA guidelines on medical tourism. Chicago: AMA; 2008. Available from: http://www.ama-assn.org/ama1/pub/upload/mm/31/medicaltourism.pdf.

BOX 2-5. PATIENT SAFETY CHECKLIST FOR COSMETIC SURGERY[1]

To help ensure optimal results and to limit risks and complications, the American Society for Plastic Surgery (ASPS) offers the following tips to anyone considering cosmetic surgery in the United States.

Do Your Homework: Research the procedure, the benefits, and the risks. Refer to www.plasticsurgery.org for the latest information on plastic surgery procedures.

Have Realistic Expectations: Ask your plastic surgeon questions about how the surgery will work for you: identify expectations and understand side effects and recovery time.

Be Informed: Talk to patients who have had your procedure so you know what to expect.

Require a Medical Evaluation: Consult with your plastic surgeon for an evaluation and discuss your full medical history to determine the most appropriate treatment.

Choose an ASPS Member Surgeon: Why? ASPS Member Surgeons are qualified, trained, properly certified, experienced in your procedure, and operate only in accredited facilities.

Ask Questions:

- Are you an ASPS Member Surgeon?
- Are you certified by the American Board of Plastic Surgery?
- Do you have hospital privileges to perform this procedure? If so, at which hospitals?
- How many procedures of this type have you performed?
- Am I a good candidate for this procedure? What will be expected of me to get optimal results?
- Where and how will you perform my procedure?
- Is the surgical facility accredited?
- What are the risks involved with my procedure?
- How long of a recovery period can I expect, and what kind of help will I need during my recovery?
- Will I need to take time off work? If so, how long?
- How much will my procedure cost? Are financing options available?
- How are complications handled?

[1] Excerpt from American Society of Plastic Surgeons. Cosmetic surgery tourism briefing paper. Arlington Heights, IL: American Society of Plastic Surgeons; 2010. Available from: http://www.plasticsurgery.org/Media/Briefing_Papers/Cosmetic_Surgery_Tourism.html.

BOX 2-6. PATIENT CHECKLIST FOR OBTAINING SAFE DENTAL CARE DURING INTERNATIONAL TRAVEL[1]

Before you leave:

- Visit your dentist for a check-up to reduce the chances you will have a dental emergency.
- See a health care provider to receive any needed vaccinations, medications, and advice related to your travel destination.

When seeking treatment for a dental emergency during your trip:

- Consult hotel staff or the American Embassy or consulate for assistance in finding a dentist.
- If possible, consider recommendations from Americans living in the area or from other trusted sources.

continued

BOX 2-6. PATIENT CHECKLIST FOR OBTAINING SAFE DENTAL CARE DURING INTERNATIONAL TRAVEL[1] (continued)

If the answers to any of the asterisked (*) items below are "No," you should have reservations about the office's infection control standards. If the answer to a two-star item (**) is "No," consider making a swift but gracious exit.

When making the appointment, ask:

- Do you use new gloves for each patient?*
- Do you use an autoclave (steam sterilizer) or dry heat oven to sterilize your instruments between patients?**
- Do you sterilize your handpieces (drills)?* (If not, do you disinfect them?)**
- Do you use new needles for each patient?**
- Is sterile (or boiled) water used for surgical procedures?** (In areas where drinking water is unsafe, the water also may cause illness if used for dental treatment.)

Upon arriving at the office, observe the following:

- Is the office clean and neat?
- Do staff wash their hands, with soap, between patients?**
- Do they wear gloves for all procedures?**
- Do they clean and disinfect or use disposable covers on surfaces touched during treatment?

[1] Excerpt from Organization for Safety and Asepsis Procedures. Traveler's guide to safe dental care. Annapolis, MD: Organization for Safety and Asepsis Procedures; 2001. Available from: http://www.osap.org/?page=TravelersGuide.

BIBLIOGRAPHY

1. Aerospace Medical Association. Medical Guidelines for Airline Travel. 2nd ed. Alexandria, VA: Aerospace Medical Association; 2003.

2. American Medical Association. New AMA Guidelines on Medical Tourism. Chicago: AMA; 2008 [cited 2010 Nov 23]. Available from: http://www.ama-assn.org/ama1/pub/upload/mm/31/medicaltourism.pdf.

3. American Society of Plastic Surgeons. Cosmetic Surgery Tourism Briefing Paper. Arlington Heights: American Society of Plastic Surgeons; 2010 [cited 2010 Nov 23]. Available from: http://www.plasticsurgery.org/Media/Briefing_Papers/Cosmetic_Surgery_Tourism.html.

4. Bookman MZ, Bookman KR. Medical Tourism in Developing Countries. New York: Palgrave MacMillan; 2007.

5. Budiani-Saberi DA, Delmonico FL. Organ trafficking and transplant tourism: a commentary on the global realities. Am J Transplant. 2008 May;8(5):925–9.

6. Ehrbeck T, Guevara C, Mango PD. Mapping the market for medical travel. McKinsey Quarterly. 2008(May).

7. Einhorn B, Arnst C. Outsourcing the patients: more US health insurers are slashing costs by sending policyholders overseas for pricey procedures. Businessweek News. 2008 Mar 13.

8. Galland Z. Medical tourism: the insurance debate: most insurers balk at covering medical procedures performed overseas, but some are exploring the option Businessweek News. 2008 Nov 9.

9. Gill J, Madhira BR, Gjertson D, Lipshutz G, Cecka JM, Pham PT, et al. Transplant tourism in the United States: a single-center experience. Clin J Am Soc Nephrol. 2008 Nov;3(6):1820–8.

10. Horowitz MD, Rosensweig JA, Jones CA. Medical tourism: globalization of the healthcare marketplace. MedGenMed. 2007;9(4):33.

11. Joint Commission Organization. Joint Commission International. 2009 [cited 2010 Nov 9]. Available from: http://www.jointcommissioninternational.org/.

12. Keckley PH, Underwood HR. Medical Tourism: Consumers in Search of Value. Washington, DC: Deloitte Center for Health Solutions; 2008.

13. Merion RM, Barnes AD, Lin M, Ashby VB, McBride V, Ortiz-Rios E, et al. Transplants in foreign countries among patients removed from the US transplant waiting list. Am J Transplant. 2008 Apr;8(4 Pt 2):988–96.

14. Organization for Safety and Asepsis Procedures. Traveler's Guide to Safe Dental Care. Annapolis, MD: Organization for Safety and Asepsis Procedures; 2001 [cited 2010 Nov 23]. Available from: http://www.osap.org/?page=TravelersGuide.

15. Reed CM. Medical tourism. Med Clin North Am. 2008 Nov;92(6):1433–46, xi.

16. Sajjad I, Baines LS, Patel P, Salifu MO, Jindal RM. Commercialization of kidney transplants: a systematic review of outcomes in recipients and donors. Am J Nephrol. 2008;28(5):744–54.

17. Sanford C, Merck. Air travel. Whitehouse Station, NJ: Merck Sharp & Dohme Corp; 2009 [updated 2009 Feb; cited 2010 Nov 9]. Available from: http://www.merck.com/mmpe/sec22/ch333/ch333b.html#CBBIEDEH.

18. Shimazono Y. The state of the international organ trade: a provisional picture based on integration of available information. Bull World Health Organ. 2007 Dec;85(12):955–962.

19. US Department of Commerce. 2008 United States resident travel abroad. Washington, DC: US Department of Commerce; 2008. Available from: http://tinet.ita.doc.gov/outreachpages/download_data_table/2008_US_Travel_Abroad.pdf.

20. US Department of Health and Human Services. 2007 annual report of the US Organ Procurement and Transplantation Network and the Scientific Registry of Transplant Recipients: transplant data 1997–2006. Rockville, MD: US Department of Health and Human Services; 2007 [cited 2008 Jul 22]. Available from: http://www.ustransplant.org/annual_reports/current/ar_archives.htm.

21. World Health Organization. Guiding principles on human organ transplantation. Geneva: World Health Organization; 2010 [cited 2010 Nov 9]. Available from: http://www.who.int/ethics/topics/transplantation_guiding_principles/en/index1.html.

22. World Health Organization. Human organ and tissue transplantation. Geneva: World Health Organization; 2009 [updated 2010 Nov 9]. Available from: http://apps.who.int/gb/ebwha/pdf_files/A62/A62_15-en.pdf.

DEEP VEIN THROMBOSIS & PULMONARY EMBOLISM

Deborah Nicolls Barbeau

BACKGROUND

Venous thromboembolism (VTE) consists of 2 related conditions: 1) deep vein thrombosis (DVT) and 2) pulmonary embolism (PE). DVT occurs when a deep vein is partially or completely blocked by a blood clot, most commonly in the legs. The clot may break off and travel to the vessels in the lung, causing a life-threatening PE.

VTE associated with air travel was first described in the early 1950s. Previous studies have shown a 2- to 4-fold increased risk of VTE after air travel. In 2001, the World Health Organization (WHO) set up the WHO Research into Global Hazards of Travel (WRIGHT) Project, a large collaborative research study to confirm the association between VTE and air travel. The results of phase I of the WRIGHT Project were published in June 2007 and are discussed below. Several epidemiologic and pathophysiologic studies were performed during phase I to determine the magnitude of the risk of VTE due to air travel, the effect of other factors on the association, and the mechanism by which air travel leads to VTE. Studies into the effect of preventive measures on VTE risk during travel were deferred to phase II of the project.

RISK FOR TRAVELERS

Several factors have been associated with an increased risk for developing VTE (Box 2-7). Combined effects have been observed between these established risk factors and different forms of travel. A population-based case-control study of adults receiving treatment for their first VTE (performed as part of the WRIGHT Project) found that long-distance travel longer than 4 hours increased the risk of VTE 2-fold compared with not traveling. The effect was largest in the first week after travel but remained elevated for 2 months.

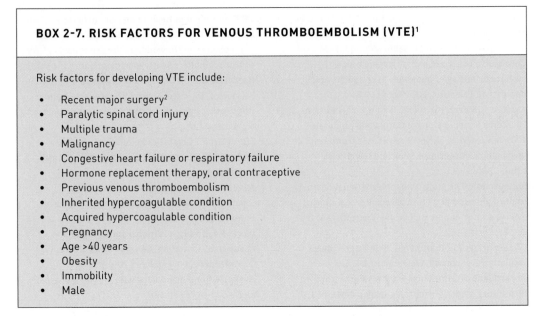

BOX 2-7. RISK FACTORS FOR VENOUS THROMBOEMBOLISM (VTE)[1]

Risk factors for developing VTE include:

- Recent major surgery[2]
- Paralytic spinal cord injury
- Multiple trauma
- Malignancy
- Congestive heart failure or respiratory failure
- Hormone replacement therapy, oral contraceptive
- Previous venous thromboembolism
- Inherited hypercoagulable condition
- Acquired hypercoagulable condition
- Pregnancy
- Age >40 years
- Obesity
- Immobility
- Male

[1] Adapted from Anderson FA Jr, Spencer FA. Risk factors for venous thromboembolism. Circulation. 2003 Jun 17;107(23 Suppl 1):I9–16.
[2] Especially cardiothoracic, abdominal, major orthopedic surgery.

Travel by air increased the risk to the same extent as travel by bus, train, or car, suggesting that the increased risk of air travel is due primarily to prolonged immobility. Synergistic effects were noted with factor V Leiden mutations, women who used oral contraceptives, body mass index (BMI) more than 30 kg/m², and height more than 1.9 m (approximately 6 ft 3 in). Some of these effects were largest after air travel compared with other forms of travel. Furthermore, people shorter than 1.6 m (approximately 5 ft, 3 in) had an increased risk of VTE only after prolonged air travel. These findings suggest that additional factors related to air travel may be involved in the increased risk for VTE.

OCCURRENCE

A recent meta-analysis investigating the association between travel and VTE found a 2-fold higher risk for VTE in travelers compared with nontravelers. Significant variability was noted in the outcomes of the studies included in the review. This variability was directly related to the method used to select the comparison group in each study. When studies that used people referred for VTE evaluation as comparisons were excluded from the meta-analysis, the remaining studies showed a 3-fold higher risk of VTE associated with travel. The risk

for VTE increased with travel duration. Each 2-hour increase in travel duration resulted in an 18% higher risk for VTE.

Two retrospective cohort studies (performed as part of the WRIGHT Project) address the issue of air travel–associated VTE incidence. The first was a cohort of 2,499 healthy Dutch commercial pilots. The incidence of VTE in this group was 0.3 per 1,000 person-years. When the data were adjusted for age and sex, the rate was not different from that in the general Dutch population. There was no association between the number of hours flown.

The second study was among 8,755 employees of several international companies and organizations. The overall incidence of VTE after air travel was 1.4 per 1,000 person-years. The incidence of VTE within 8 weeks of a long-haul flight (>4 hours) was 3.2 per 1,000 person-years compared with an incidence of 1.0 per 1,000 person-years in employees who did not fly. The absolute risk of VTE per flight more than 4 hours was 1 per 4,656 flights. The rates of VTE were higher in women, especially those using oral contraceptives. Incidence was also higher in employees with a BMI more than 25 kg/m² and those with height less than 1.65 m (5 ft 5 in) or more than 1.85 m (6 ft 1 in). The risk of VTE increased with flight duration and with the number of times the employee flew during an 8-week period; the risk of VTE tripled in employees who went on 5 or more long-haul (>4 hours) flights. Each extra flight increased the risk of VTE 1.4-fold. The risk of VTE was highest in the first 2 weeks after a long-haul flight and gradually decreased to baseline after 8 weeks.

Both these studies were performed among populations that were younger (mean age 35–40 years) and healthier than the general population and are not, therefore, generalizable to a higher-risk population.

CLINICAL PRESENTATION

Symptoms of DVT include swelling, redness, pain, or tenderness and increased warmth over the skin. It may be difficult to distinguish from muscle strain, injury, or skin infection. Prospective studies have shown that many leg DVTs are asymptomatic; therefore, the first symptoms may be due to a PE.

Symptoms of PE range from mild and nonspecific to acute, resembling heart attack or stroke. Once a clot has traveled to the lungs, common symptoms of PE are chest pain and shortness of breath. Other symptoms include dizziness, fainting, anxiety, and malaise. PE can occur in the absence of overt signs of DVT.

DIAGNOSIS

Specialized imaging tests (duplex venous ultrasound, venography, CT scans, and MRI) are needed to make a definitive diagnosis of DVT. Helical CT or ventilation-perfusion scans are commonly used to diagnose PE.

PREVENTIVE MEASURES FOR TRAVELERS

Although results are not available for phase II of the WRIGHT Project, several randomized controlled trials have been performed to assess the effect of prophylactic measures on VTE risk after air travel. All studies examined the risk of asymptomatic DVT in travelers making flights ≥7 hours. All travelers were encouraged to do regular exercises and to drink nonalcoholic beverages during the flight. DVT was diagnosed by venous ultrasound from 90 minutes to 48 hours after the flight. Interventions that were studied include compression stockings, aspirin, low-molecular weight heparin,

and various natural extracts with anticoagulant properties. Compression stockings (10–20 mm Hg and 20–30 mm Hg) were shown to significantly reduce the risk of asymptomatic DVT; however, 4 travelers wearing compression stockings in one study developed superficial thrombophlebitis. Symptomatic DVT and PE were not observed in any of the travelers enrolled in the studies.

The LONFLIT3 study was a randomized trial conducted to compare the effects of aspirin and a low-molecular-weight heparin (enoxaparin) versus no treatment in the prevention of VTE in 300 high-risk patients (such as previous DVT, coagulation disorders, severe obesity, limitation of mobility due to bone or joint problems, neoplastic disease within the previous 2 years, or large varicose veins). Aspirin (400 mg daily for 3 days, starting 12 hours before air travel) did not reduce the frequency of DVT compared with controls (4.8% in people not on prophylaxis; 3.6% in people taking aspirin). No DVT and one superficial thrombosis were identified in people using enoxaparin prophylaxis (1 dose at 1,000 IU per 10 kg of body weight injected 2–4 hours before the flight). Although these results are encouraging for the use of low-molecular-weight heparin to prevent VTE in high-risk patients, the study size and number of patients with DVT were small. Currently no convincing data suggest that pharmacologic interventions reduce the risk of significant VTE in low-risk travelers.

The American College of Chest Physicians (ACCP) published the eighth edition of their Antithrombotic and Thrombolytic Therapy Evidence-Based Clinical Practice Guidelines in a June 2008 supplement to the journal CHEST. Recommendations for long-distance travel associated VTE are the following:

- For travelers who are taking flights >8 hours, the following general measures are recommended: avoidance of constrictive clothing around the lower extremities or waist, maintenance of adequate hydration, and frequent calf muscle contraction (ACCP grade 1C: strong recommendation, low-quality evidence).
- For long-distance travelers with additional risk factors for VTE, the general measures listed above are recommended. If active thromboprophylaxis is considered because

of a perceived high risk of VTE, the use of properly fitted, below-knee graduated compression stockings, providing 15–30 mm Hg of pressure at the ankle (ACCP grade 2C: modest recommendation, low-quality evidence) or a single prophylactic dose of low-molecular-weight heparin, injected before departure (ACCP grade 2C: modest recommendation, low-quality evidence) are suggested.

- For long-distance travelers, the use of aspirin to prevent VTE is not recommended (ACCP grade 1B: strong recommendation, moderate-quality evidence).

BIBLIOGRAPHY

1. Anderson FA Jr, Spencer FA. Risk factors for venous thromboembolism. Circulation. 2003 Jun 17;107(23 Suppl 1):I9–16.
2. Cannegieter SC, Doggen CJ, van Houwelingen HC, Rosendaal FR. Travel-related venous thrombosis: results from a large population-based case control study (MEGA study). PLoS Med. 2006 Aug;3(8):e307.
3. Cesarone MR, Belcaro G, Nicolaides AN, Incandela L, De S, Geroulakos G, et al. Venous thrombosis from air travel: the LONFLIT3 study—prevention with aspirin vs low-molecular-weight heparin (LMWH) in high-risk subjects: a randomized trial. Angiology. 2002 Jan–Feb;53(1):1–6.
4. Chandra D, Parisini E, Mozaffarian D. Meta-analysis: travel and risk for venous thromboembolism. Ann Intern Med. 2009 Aug 4;151(3):180–90.
5. Clarke M, Hopewell S, Juszczak E, Eisinga A, Kjeldstrom M. Compression stockings for preventing deep vein thrombosis in airline passengers. Cochrane Database Syst Rev. 2006(2):CD004002.
6. Geerts WH, Bergqvist D, Pineo GF, Heit JA, Samama CM, Lassen MR, et al. Prevention of venous thromboembolism: American College of Chest Physicians evidence-based clinical practice guidelines (8th edition). Chest. 2008 Jun;133(6 Suppl):381S–453S.
7. Goodacre S, Sutton AJ, Sampson FC. Meta-analysis: the value of clinical assessment in the diagnosis of deep venous thrombosis. Ann Intern Med. 2005 Jul 19;143(2):129–39.
8. Kuipers S, Cannegieter SC, Middeldorp S, Robyn L, Buller HR, Rosendaal FR. The absolute risk of venous thrombosis after air travel: a cohort study of 8,755 employees of international organisations. PLoS Med. 2007 Sep;4(9):e290.
9. Kuipers S, Schreijer AJ, Cannegieter SC, Buller HR, Rosendaal FR, Middeldorp S. Travel and venous thrombosis: a systematic review. J Intern Med. 2007 Dec;262(6):615–34.
10. World Health Organization. WHO Research Into Global Hazards of Travel (WRIGHT) project: final report of phase I. Geneva: World Health Organization; 2007 [cited 2010 Nov 9]. Available from: http://www.who.int/cardiovascular_diseases/wright_project/phase1_report/en/index.html.

MENTAL HEALTH & TRAVEL

Victor Balaban

DESCRIPTION

Although most travelers complete their journeys with a manageable amount of stress, foreign travel can produce a wide range of psychiatric, behavioral, and neurologic issues in travelers. Any journey can produce challenges, but longer journeys to more remote and strange environments can increase the psychological stresses for travelers.

RISK FACTORS

Certain drugs can increase the risk of a psychiatric reaction. People with underlying psychiatric disorders should not receive the antimalarial medication mefloquine (Lariam). The neuropsychiatric side effects associated with mefloquine may become pronounced in these patients. Neuropsychiatric side effects may also be compounded when mefloquine is administered concurrently with the antiretroviral medication efavirenz (Sustiva), which also carries the risk of neurologic toxicity. Elderly travelers and travelers with memory or cognitive deficits may be more prone to develop delirium in flight, particularly when combined with dehydration, alcohol, or the use of sleep aids such as zolpidem (Ambien). The use of recreational drugs has also been found to be a trigger for psychiatric symptoms in travelers.

Stress can trigger or exacerbate psychiatric reactions in travelers with preexisting psychiatric or behavioral conditions. Even in travelers with no history of psychiatric problems, stressful events during travel, such as loneliness, a feeling of loss of control, financial difficulties, or a traumatic event, such as a serious illness or viewing disturbing sights, can have behavioral and psychosocial consequences.

OCCURRENCE AND RISK FOR TRAVELERS

Data are limited on the prevalence of travel-related psychiatric and neurologic disorders:

- Hartjes et al. conducted a web survey of 318 US study-abroad students and found that psychological distress was the second most commonly perceived travel health risk before travel and that 10% of students reported experiencing psychological distress during their travel, primarily loneliness, depression, or anxiety.
- In Potasman et al., a study of 2,500 Israeli long-term travelers to Southeast Asia found that 11% reported psychiatric or neurologic symptoms during travel, most commonly sleep disturbances, fatigue, and dizziness. Most symptoms were short-lived and transient, but 3% of travelers reported severe psychiatric or neurologic symptoms, and 1% had symptoms that lasted longer than 2 months.
- Patel et al. conducted a study of urgent repatriation of British diplomats and found that 41% of evacuations for nonphysical causes were due to depression.
- Adventure travelers in extreme settings, such as high-altitude mountain climbs and polar expeditions, may undergo psychiatric changes, including disturbed sleep, impaired cognitive ability, negative affect, and interpersonal tension and conflict. Studies of polar expeditions have found that approximately 5% of travelers meet criteria for psychiatric disorders (including substance-related and sleep disorders). Fagenholz et al. described 6 foreign trekkers treated at a rescue clinic in Nepal with an anxiety-related primary diagnosis and no history of anxiety-related disorders or other psychiatric disorders.

PRE-TRAVEL MENTAL HEALTH EVALUATION

Although it is not practical or appropriate to screen all travelers for potential mental health problems, the travel health provider should be alert for the following conditions and recommend follow-up or further screening, especially for long-term travel, people taking up residence overseas, or rescue workers. The following factors should be assessed:

- Preexisting psychiatric diagnoses, such as depression or anxiety disorders
- History of psychosis in the traveler or a close family member
- History of suicide attempts
- Evidence of depressed mood at assessment
- Exposure to prior traumas (such as disasters, severe injury, abuse, assault), particularly before travel that could involve reexposure to traumatic events or situations
- Recent major life stressors or emotional strain
- Use of medications that may have psychiatric or neurologic side effects
- Pre-travel anxieties and phobias that are severe enough to interfere with a patients' ability to function or to prepare for and enjoy their travel

Long-term travelers, aid workers, military personnel, and other travelers likely to be exposed to stressful situations should be advised that the stresses and challenges they may face, particularly if combined with long hours of work, lack of sleep, or fatigue, can contribute to stress and anxiety. Long-term travelers should be encouraged to:

- Learn how to recognize signs of stress, exhaustion, depression, and anxiety in themselves.
- Take care of themselves physically by eating and exercising regularly.
- Use their full allotment of time off or annual vacation time, particularly if they recognize signs of stress or exhaustion in themselves.

DURING TRAVEL

Severe mental illness occurring abroad can be extremely stressful for travelers, their families, and people who try to care for them. Acute psychosis, leading to disruptive behavior, can land a traveler in jail in a developing country. Inpatient psychiatric facilities may be nonexistent or inadequate for a foreigner. It can be difficult to repatriate a psychotic person until the symptoms have been brought under control with medication. Someone will most often have to accompany the person home. Many evacuation insurance plans specifically exclude psychiatric illness from their coverage.

POST-TRAVEL MENTAL HEALTH EVALUATION

Returning travelers may have experienced physical illnesses, personal difficulties, or traumas that could result in psychiatric reactions. Travel-related injuries and diseases that affect quality of life can also have profound and long-term psychiatric effects. Even in the absence of trauma, some returning long-term travelers report experiencing "reverse culture shock" after their return, characterized by feelings of disorientation, unfamiliarity, and loss of confidence. Approximately 36% of aid workers report depression shortly after returning home, and as many as 60% of returned aid workers have reported feeling predominantly negative emotions on returning home, even though many reported that their time overseas was positive and fulfilling.

Post-travel evaluations should assess:

- Behavioral and psychiatric symptoms, including:
  > Experiences during or soon after travel that have been painful or hard to reconcile

or that still cause distress, anxiety, or avoidance
  > Persistent sleep disturbance or unusual fatigue
  > Excessive use of alcohol or drugs
  > Behavioral or interpersonal difficulties at home, school, or work, or in friendships or relationships

- Somatic symptoms that can also be indications of distress, including:
  > Unexplained somatic symptoms, such as headaches, backaches, or abdominal pain, and somatic disorders, such as fibromyalgia, chronic fatigue syndrome, temporomandibular disorder, and irritable bowel syndrome
  > Rashes, itching, and skin diseases, such as psoriasis, atopic dermatitis, and urticaria, which can be exacerbated by stress

Clinicians should be aware that some travelers may be reluctant to acknowledge psychiatric symptoms or distress. For example, many cultures have stigmas associated with experiencing or disclosing behaviors associated with mental illness, as well as different culturally appropriate ways of expressing grief, pain, and loss. In addition, some travelers may fear being penalized or stigmatized at work if they have psychiatric diagnoses noted on their medical records.

Regardless of the type or duration of travel and whether or not travelers appear to meet criteria for a psychiatric diagnosis, returned travelers who are having difficulties functioning or who appear to be unduly depressed or distressed should be encouraged to seek appropriate treatment or counseling.

BIBLIOGRAPHY

1. Balaban V. Psychological assessment of children in disasters and emergencies. Disasters. 2006 Jun;30(2):178–98.
2. Beny A, Paz A, Potasman I. Psychiatric problems in returning travelers: features and associations. J Travel Med. 2001 Sep–Oct;8(5):243–6.
3. Bhadelia N, Klotman M, Caplivski D. The HIV-positive traveler. Am J Med. 2007 Jul;120(7):574–80.
4. Bor R. Psychological factors in airline passenger and crew behaviour: a clinical overview. Travel Med Infect Dis. 2007 Jul;5(4):207–16.
5. Crofford LJ. Violence, stress, and somatic syndromes. Trauma Violence Abuse. 2007 Jul;8(3):299–313.
6. Espino CM, Sundstrom SM, Frick HL, Jacobs M, Peters M. International business travel: impact on families and travellers. Occup Environ Med. 2002 May;59(5):309–22.
7. Fagenholz PJ, Murray AF, Gutman JA, Findley JK, Harris NS. New-onset anxiety disorders at high altitude. Wilderness Environ Med. 2007 Winter;18(4):312–6.

8. Hartjes LB, Baumann LC, Henriques JB. Travel health risk perceptions and prevention behaviors of US study abroad students. J Travel Med. 2009 Sep–Oct;16(5):338–43.

9. Hochedez P, Vinsentini P, Ansart S, Caumes E. Changes in the pattern of health disorders diagnosed among two cohorts of French travelers to Nepal, 17 years apart. J Travel Med. 2004 Nov–Dec;11(6):341–6.

10. Lankester T. Health care of the long-term traveller. Travel Med Infect Dis. 2005 Aug;3(3):143–55.

11. Palinkas LA, Suedfeld P. Psychological effects of polar expeditions. Lancet. 2008 Jan 12;371(9607):153–63.

12. Patel D, Easmon CJ, Dow C, Snashall DC, Seed PT. Medical repatriation of British diplomats resident overseas. J Travel Med. 2000 Mar–Apr; 7(2):64–9.

13. Potasman I, Beny A, Seligmann H. Neuropsychiatric problems in 2,500 long-term young travelers to the tropics. J Travel Med. 2000 Jan;7(1):5–9.

14. Reed CM. Travel recommendations for older adults. Clin Geriatr Med. 2007 Aug;23(3):687–713, ix.

15. Rolfe M, Tang CM, Sabally S, Todd JE, Sam EB, Hatib N'Jie AB. Psychosis and cannabis abuse in The Gambia. A case-control study. Br J Psychiatry. 1993 Dec;163:798–801.

16. Urpe M, Buggiani G, Lotti T. Stress and psychoneuroimmunologic factors in dermatology. Dermatol Clin. 2005 Oct;23(4):609–17.

TRAVEL HEALTH KITS
Amanda D. Whatley, Candace M. Marshall

OVERVIEW

An important step in preparing for international travel is for travelers to assemble a travel health kit. The contents of a travel health kit should be tailored to the traveler's needs, type of travel, length of travel, and destination. A travel health kit can help to ensure travelers have supplies they need to:

- Manage preexisting medical conditions and treat any exacerbations of these conditions
- Prevent illness related to traveling
- Take care of minor health problems as they occur

Travel health kits can be assembled at home or purchased at a local store, pharmacy, or online.

TRAVELING WITH MEDICATIONS

All medications should be carried in their original containers with clear labels, so the contents are easily identified. When carrying prescription medications, the patient's name and dose regimen should be on the container. Although many travelers prefer placing medications into small containers or packing them in daily-dose containers, officials at ports of entry may require proper identification of medications.

Travelers should carry copies of all prescriptions, including their generic names. For controlled substances and injectable medications, travelers should carry a note from the prescribing physician or from the travel clinic on letterhead stationery. Certain medications are not permitted in certain countries. If there is a question about these restrictions, particularly with controlled substances, travelers should contact the embassy or consulate of the destination country.

A travel health kit is useful only when it is available. It should be carried with the traveler at all times (such as in a carry-on bag), although sharp objects must remain in checked luggage. Travelers should make sure that any liquid or gel-based items packed in the carry-on bags do not exceed the size limits. They can consult with the airline for all air-related travel restrictions.

SUPPLIES FOR PREEXISTING MEDICAL CONDITIONS

Travelers with preexisting medical conditions should carry enough medication for the duration of their trip and an extra supply, in case the trip is extended for any reason. If additional supplies or medications are needed to manage exacerbations of existing medical conditions, these should be carried as well. The clinician managing a traveler's preexisting medical conditions should be consulted for the best plan of action (see Chapter 8, Travelers with Chronic Illnesses).

People with preexisting conditions, such as diabetes or allergies, should consider wearing an alert bracelet (such as those available from www.medicalert.org) and making sure this information is on a card in their wallet and with their other travel documents.

GENERAL TRAVEL HEALTH KIT SUPPLIES

Although this is not a comprehensive list, basic items that should be considered for a travel health kit are listed below. See Chapters 7 and 8 for additional suggestions that may be useful in planning the contents of a kit for travelers with specific needs.

Medications

- Destination-related, if applicable:
  > Antimalarial medications
  > Medication to prevent or treat high-altitude illness

- Pain or fever (one or more of the following, or an alternative):
  > Acetaminophen
  > Aspirin
  > Ibuprofen

- Stomach upset or diarrhea:
  > Over-the-counter antidiarrheal medication (such as loperamide [Imodium] or bismuth subsalicylate [Pepto-Bismol])
  > Antibiotics for self-treatment of moderate to severe diarrhea
  > Packets of oral rehydration salts for dehydration
  > Mild laxative
  > Antacid

- Throat and respiratory discomfort:
  > Antihistamine
  > Decongestant, alone or in combination with antihistamine
  > Cough suppressant or expectorant

  > Throat lozenges

- Anti-motion sickness medication
- Epinephrine auto-injector (such as an EpiPen), especially if history of severe allergic reaction; smaller-dose packages are available for children
- Any medications, prescription or over the counter, taken on a regular basis at home

Basic First Aid

- Disposable gloves (≥2 pairs)
- Adhesive bandages, multiple sizes
- Gauze
- Adhesive tape
- Elastic bandage wrap for sprains and strains
- Antiseptic
- Cotton swabs
- Tweezers*
- Scissors*
- Antifungal and antibacterial ointments or creams
- 1% hydrocortisone cream
- Anti-itch gel or cream for insect bites and stings
- Aloe gel for sunburns
- Moleskin or molefoam for blisters
- Digital thermometer
- Saline eye drops
- First aid quick reference card

Other Important Items

- Insect repellent (see the Protection against Mosquitoes, Ticks, and Other Insects and Arthropods section earlier in this chapter for recommended types)
- Sunscreen (≥15 SPF)
- Antibacterial hand wipes or an alcohol-based hand cleaner, containing at least 60% alcohol
- Useful items in certain circumstances:
  > Extra pair of contact lenses, prescription glasses, or both, for people who wear corrective lenses
  > Mild sedative (such as zolpidem [Ambien]), other sleep aid, or antianxiety medication
  > Latex condoms
  > Water purification tablets

*Note: If traveling by air, travelers should pack these sharp items in checked baggage, since they could be confiscated by airport or airline security if packed in carry-on bags.

> Commercial suture or syringe kits to be used by a local clinician. (These items will require a letter from the prescribing physician on letterhead stationery.)

Contact Card

Travelers should carry a contact card with the addresses and phone numbers of the following:

- Family member or close contact remaining in the United States
- Place of lodging at the destination
- Health care provider(s) at home
- Medical insurance information
- Travel insurance and medical evacuation insurance information
- Area hospitals or clinics, including emergency services
- US embassy or consulate in the destination country or countries

See the Obtaining Health Care Abroad for the Ill Traveler section later in this chapter for information about how to locate local health care and embassy or consulate contacts.

Travelers should also leave a copy of this contact card with a family member or close contact who will remain in the United States, in case of an emergency.

COMMERCIAL MEDICAL KITS

Commercial medical kits are available for a wide range of circumstances, from basic first aid to advanced emergency life support. Many pharmacy, grocery, retail, and outdoor sporting goods stores sell their own basic first aid kits. Travelers who choose to purchase a health kit should review the contents of the kit carefully to ensure that it has everything needed. Additional items may be necessary and can be added to the purchased kit.

For more adventurous travelers, a number of companies produce advanced medical kits and will even customize kits based on specific travel needs. In addition, specialty kits are available for managing diabetes, dealing with dental emergencies, and handling aquatic environments. Below is a list of websites supplying a wide range of medical kits. There are many suppliers, and this list is not meant to be all-inclusive.

- American Red Cross: www.redcrossstore.org
- Adventure Medical Kits: www.adventuremedicalkits.com
- Chinook Medical Gear: www.chinookmed.com
- International Medical Center: www.traveldoc.com/products/kits.aspx
- Travel Medicine, Inc.: www.travmed.com
- Wilderness Medicine Outfitters: www.wildernessmedicine.com

BIBLIOGRAPHY

1. Rose SR, Keystone JS. Chapter 2, trip preparation. In: Rose SR, Keystone JS, editors. International Travel Health Guide. 14th ed. Northampton: Travel Medicine, Inc; 2008.
2. Weiss EA, Franco-Paredes C. Travel health and medical kits. In: Keystone JS, Kozarsky PE, Freedman DO, Nothdurft HD, Connor BA, editors. Travel Medicine. 2nd ed. Philadelphia: Mosby; 2008. p. 69–74.
3. World Health Organization. WHO guidelines on hand hygiene in health care. Geneva: World Health Organization; 2009 [updated 2010 Nov 9]. Available from: http://whqlibdoc.who.int/publications/2009/9789241597906_eng.pdf.

2

COUNTERFEIT DRUGS

Michael D. Green

GENERAL INFORMATION

Counterfeit and substandard drugs are an international problem contributing to illness, death, toxicity, and drug resistance. A counterfeit medicine is a compound that is not made by an authorized manufacturer but is presented to the consumer as if it were. Both the packaging and pill construction of counterfeit drugs are often virtually identical to the authentic medication. Regulatory agencies in the United States, such as the Food and Drug Administration (FDA), protect citizens from products that are inherently unsafe. In developing countries, regulatory controls are much less effective or even nonexistent, leading to conditions that allow for proliferation of counterfeit and substandard medicines. Overall, global estimates of drug counterfeiting are ambiguous, depending on region, but proportions range from 1% of sales in developed countries to more than 10% in developing countries. In specific regions in Africa, Asia, and Latin America, chances of purchasing a counterfeit drug may be higher than 30%.

Since counterfeit drugs are not made by the legitimate manufacturer and are produced under unlawful circumstances, toxic contaminants or lack of proper ingredients may result in serious harm. For example, the active pharmaceutical ingredient may be completely lacking, present in small quantities, or substituted by a less-effective compound. In addition, the wrong inactive ingredients (excipients) can contribute to poor drug dissolution and bioavailability. As a result, a patient may not respond to treatment or may have adverse reactions to unknown substituted or toxic ingredients.

Before international departure, travel health providers should alert travelers to the dangers of counterfeit and substandard drugs and provide suggestions on how to avoid them.

HOW TO AVOID COUNTERFEIT DRUGS WHEN TRAVELING

The best way to avoid counterfeit drugs is to reduce the need to purchase medications abroad. Anticipated amounts of medications for chronic conditions such as hypertension, sinusitis, arthritis, and hay fever; medications for gastroenteritis (travelers' diarrhea); and prophylactic medications for infectious diseases such as malaria (depending on the destination) should all be purchased before traveling.

Before departure, travelers should do the following:

- Purchase in advance all the medicines they will need for the trip. Prescriptions written in the United States usually cannot be filled overseas, and over-the-counter medicines may not be available in many foreign countries. Checked baggage can get lost; therefore, travelers should pack as much as possible in a carry-on bag and bring extra medicine in case of travel delays.

- Make sure medicines are in their original containers. If the drug is a prescription, the patient's name and dose regimen should be on the container.
- Bring the "patient prescription information" sheet. This sheet provides information on common generic and brand names, use, side effects, precautions, and drug interactions.

If travelers run out and require additional medications, they should take steps to ensure the medicines they buy are safe:

- Purchase medicines from a legitimate pharmacy. Patients should not buy from open markets, street vendors, or suspicious-looking pharmacies, and they should request a receipt when making the purchase. The US embassy may be able to help find a legitimate pharmacy in the area.
- Do not buy medicines that are significantly cheaper than the typical price. Although generics are usually less expensive, many counterfeited brand names are sold at prices significantly below the normal price for that particular brand.
- Make sure the medicines are in their original packages or containers. If travelers receive medicines as loose tablets or capsules supplied in a plastic bag or envelope, they should ask the pharmacist to see the container from which the medicine was originally dispensed. The traveler should record the brand, batch number, and expiration date. Sometimes a wary consumer will prompt the seller into supplying quality medicine.
- Be familiar with medications. The size, shape, color, and taste of counterfeit medicines may be different from the authentic. Discoloration, splits, cracks, spots, and stickiness of the tablets or capsules are indications of a possible counterfeit. Travelers should keep examples of authentic medications to compare if they purchase the same brand.
- Be familiar with the packaging. Different color inks, poor-quality print or packaging material, and misspelled words are clues to counterfeit drugs. Travelers should keep an example of packaging for comparison, and observe the expiration date to make sure the medicine has not expired.

USEFUL WEBSITES
General Information about Counterfeit Drugs
- CDC: wwwn.cdc.gov/travel/contentCounterfeitDrugs.aspx
- World Health Organization:
  > www.who.int/mediacentre/factsheets/fs275/en
  > www.who.int/medicines/services/counterfeit/overview/en
- Food and Drug Administration: www.fda.gov//Drugs/DrugSafety/ucm170314.htm
- US Pharmacopeia: www.usp.org/worldwide

Traveling and Customs Guidelines
Researching what travelers can pack and bring back into the United States, especially for travelers with disabilities and medical conditions, is helpful in preparing for travel.

- Transportation Security Administration: www.tsa.gov/travelers/airtravel/specialneeds/editorial_1059.shtm
- Customs and Border Protection: www.cbp.gov/xp/cgov/travel/clearing/restricted/medication_drugs.xml

Reporting Counterfeit Cases

- World Health Organization: www.who.int/medicines/services/counterfeit/report/en/

BIBLIOGRAPHY

1. Newton P, Fernandez F, Green M. Counterfeit and substandard antimalarial drugs. In: Schlagenhauf-Lawlor P, editor. Travelers' Malaria. 2nd ed. Hamilton, ON: BC Decker; 2008. p. 331–42.
2. Newton PN, Green MD, Fernandez FM, Day NP, White NJ. Counterfeit anti-infective drugs. Lancet Infect Dis. 2006 Sep;6(9):602–13.
3. World Health Organization. Medicines: counterfeit medicines. Fact sheet no. 275. Geneva: World Health Organization; 2010 [updated 2010 Jan; cited 2008 Jun 6]. Available from: http://www.who.int/mediacentre/factsheets/fs275/en/.

OBTAINING HEALTH CARE ABROAD FOR THE ILL TRAVELER

Theresa E. Sommers

LOCATING A HEALTH CARE PROVIDER ABROAD

It is important for travelers to develop a plan before departure for where and how they will obtain medical assistance during their trip, should the need arise. Several resources provide lists of health care providers and medical facilities that will provide care to travelers. When searching these lists, travelers should consider the languages in which that provider or clinic is proficient.

- The Department of State (www.usembassy.gov) can help travelers locate medical services and notify friends, family, or employer of an emergency.
- The International Society of Travel Medicine (ISTM) (www.istm.org) maintains a directory of health care professionals with expertise in travel medicine in almost 50 countries worldwide.
- The American Society of Tropical Medicine and Hygiene (ASTMH) (www.astmh.org) lists few clinicians outside the United States, so travelers looking for physicians in their destination should also consult other sources. Travelers in need of specialized post-travel care upon return, however, will find this directory useful in finding a tropical medicine expert.
- The International Association for Medical Assistance to Travelers (IAMAT) (www.iamat.org) maintains an international network of physicians, hospitals, and clinics who have agreed to provide care to members while abroad. Membership is free, although donations are suggested.
- Travelers can search the Joint Commission International website (www.jointcommissioninternational.org) to find accredited health care facilities at their destination.
- Travel Health Online (https://www.tripprep.com) maintains a list of travel health providers worldwide. Information is obtained from a variety of sources, so the quality of services and the expertise of the providers cannot be guaranteed.

Travelers may also get information about local health care from embassies and consulates of other countries, hotel doctors, and credit card companies. Travelers who obtain evacuation insurance before travel will have access to a 24-hour hotline that can direct them to medical care or arrange emergency transportation (see the next section in this chapter, Travel Health Insurance and Evacuation Insurance).

PREPARATION BEFORE A TRIP

The quality and availability of medical care abroad may be variable. Travelers should prepare for the possibility of a medical emergency abroad and are encouraged to:

- Evaluate their health prior to the trip to ensure that they are healthy enough to travel and carry out their proposed itinerary.
- Consider travel health or evacuation insurance for their trip.
- Register with the US embassy in their destinations. Travelers can register their trip at https://travelregistration.state.gov/ibrs/ui/.
- Carry a card that identifies, in the local language, blood type, any chronic conditions, serious allergies, and generic names of any medications.
- If appropriate, wear medical identification jewelry (such as a MedicAlert bracelet) for serious medical conditions.
- Find the names of health providers and medical facilities in each location they plan to visit and carry this list with them during travel.

DRUGS AND OTHER PHARMACEUTICALS

The quality of drugs and medical products abroad may not meet US standards or could be counterfeit (see Perspectives: Counterfeit Drugs earlier in this chapter). Travelers should bring with them all the drugs and medicines that they might need, including pain relievers, antidiarrheal medication, and, if applicable, antimalarials. Travelers who may require injections abroad should bring their own injection supplies (see the Travel Health Kits section earlier in this chapter). Travelers who need an injection but do not have their own supplies should insist that a new needle and syringe be used.

BLOOD SAFETY

The safety of blood products in many countries cannot be guaranteed. Not all countries have accurate, reliable, and systematic screening of blood donations for infectious agents, which increases the risk of transfusion-related transmission of disease. Because of the increased risk of bloodborne pathogens, travelers in developing countries should receive a blood transfusion only in life-or-death situations. When a situation requires blood transfusion, travelers should make every effort to ascertain whether the blood has been screened for transmissible diseases, including HIV. Doing so is difficult at the point of service, but travelers who locate medical services before traveling may increase their chances of obtaining higher quality care abroad.

The limited storage period of blood and the need for special equipment negate the feasibility of independent blood banking for individual travelers or small groups. Shipping blood internationally is practical only when handled by agreement between responsible organizations, such as national blood transfusion services. This mechanism is not useful for the emergency needs of individual travelers and should not be attempted by private travelers or organizations not operating recognized blood programs.

BIBLIOGRAPHY

1. Kolars JC. Rules of the road: a consumer's guide for travelers seeking health care in foreign lands. J Travel Med. 2002 Jul–Aug;9(4):198–201.

TRAVEL HEALTH INSURANCE & EVACUATION INSURANCE

Katherine J. Johnson, Theresa E. Sommers

INTRODUCTION

Travelers must consider the financial consequences of a severe illness or injury abroad. Basic accident or travel insurance may even be required for travelers to certain destinations. A growing number of people do not have health insurance at home, and these travelers must consider both travel health and evacuation insurance, which can be purchased together or in separate packages. People who have domestic health insurance policies need to determine if any needed medical care abroad will be covered adequately or if supplemental travel health insurance policies are needed. Travelers whose domestic policies provide adequate health insurance abroad should look for potential gaps in coverage: domestic health insurance policies may not cover medical evacuation from a resource-poor area to a hospital where definitive care can be obtained, or the insurance company may not have the resources to help organize such an evacuation. Evacuation-only policies are available to fill this gap. Evacuation by air ambulance can cost $50,000–$100,000 and must be paid in advance by people who do not have insurance.

PAYING FOR HEALTH SERVICES ABROAD

Travelers who receive medical care in other countries will usually be required to pay in cash or with a credit card at the point of service, even if they have insurance coverage in their home country. This could result in a large out-of-pocket expenditure of perhaps thousands of dollars for medical care. Travelers should also remember that the existence of nationalized health care services in a given destination does not ensure that nonresidents will be given full coverage.

When traveling abroad, travelers with any insurance coverage should always carry copies of their insurance policy identity card and an insurance claim form. Travelers should be reminded to locate medical services in areas they plan to visit and carry this information with them (see Obtaining Medical Care Abroad for the Ill Traveler earlier in this chapter). In the event that they must pay out of pocket for care, travelers should obtain copies of all bills and receipts. If necessary, the US consular office can assist US citizens with transferring funds from the United States.

Medical evacuation insurance may only cover the cost to the nearest destination where definitive care can be obtained. Some policies will cover eventual repatriation to one's home country. The traveler should be sure to understand what coverage is purchased.

EVALUATING DOMESTIC HEALTH INSURANCE POLICIES

Some health insurance carriers in the United States may provide coverage for emergencies that occur while traveling abroad. Travelers should carefully examine their present coverage and planned itinerary to determine exactly which medical services, if any, will be covered abroad and what supplemental insurance is needed. The following is a list of things to consider:

- Exclusions for treating exacerbations of preexisting medical conditions
- The company's policy for "out-of-network" services
- Coverage for complications of pregnancy
- Exclusions for high-risk activities such as skydiving, scuba diving, and mountain climbing
- Exclusions regarding psychiatric emergencies or injuries related to terrorist attacks or acts of war
- Whether preauthorization is needed for treatment, hospital admission, or other services

- Whether a second opinion is required before obtaining emergency treatment
- Whether there is a 24-hour physician-backed support center

Medicare and Medicaid will not cover services outside the United States, except in limited circumstances.

SUPPLEMENTAL TRAVEL HEALTH AND MEDICAL EVACUATION INSURANCE

Travelers need to evaluate their existing health insurance policies using the list above to see whether they have adequate coverage. Short-term supplemental policies that cover health care costs on a trip can be purchased. Evacuation coverage can be sold separately or in conjunction with travel health insurance. Evacuation companies often have better resources and experience in some parts of the world than others; travelers may want to ask about a company's resources in a given area before purchase, especially if planning a trip to remote destinations. In general, travelers should purchase a policy that provides the following:

- Arrangements with hospitals to guarantee payments directly.
- Assistance via a 24-hour physician-backed support center (critical if the traveler is going to pay for evacuation insurance).
- Emergency medical transport, including repatriation. Medical evacuation without insurance can be costly, ranging from a few thousand dollars to over $100,000.
- Any specific medical services that may apply to their circumstances, such as coverage of high-risk activities.

Although travel health and medical evacuation insurance are considerations for all travelers, they are particularly important for travelers who will be outside the United States for an extended period of time, have underlying health conditions (travelers should make certain that complications will be covered), and participate in high-risk activities. Even if an insurance provider is selected carefully, travelers should be aware that unexpected delays in care may still arise, especially in remote destinations. In special circumstances, travelers may be advised to postpone or cancel international trips if the health risks are too high.

FINDING A TRAVEL HEALTH AND MEDICAL EVACUATION INSURANCE PROVIDER

The following resources, while not all-inclusive, provide information about purchasing travel health and medical evacuation insurance:

- Department of State (www.travel.state.gov)
- International SOS (www.internationalsos.com)
- MEDEX (www.medexassist.com)
- International Association for Medical Assistance to Travelers (www.iamat.org)
- American Association of Retired Persons (www.aarp.org) (for information about Medicare supplement plans, see below)

SPECIAL CONSIDERATIONS FOR TRAVELERS WITH UNDERLYING MEDICAL CONDITIONS

Travelers with underlying medical conditions may want to take extra precautions in preparing for travel. These travelers should choose a medical assistance company that allows customers to store their medical history before departure, so it can be accessed from anywhere in the world, if needed. Travelers should carry a letter from their physician listing underlying medical conditions and all current medications (including their generic names). They should also pack all medications in their original bottles, checking beforehand with the appropriate international embassy to ensure that none are considered illegal narcotics in the destination country. If possible, travelers may want to carry with them the name of their medical condition and medications written in the local languages of the areas they plan to visit.

SPECIAL CONSIDERATIONS FOR MEDICARE BENEFICIARIES

The Social Security Medicare program does not provide coverage for medical costs outside the United States, except in limited circumstances. Medicare beneficiaries can purchase supplemental travel health insurance to cover medical expenses outside the United States. Some Medigap plans may provide limited coverage for emergency care abroad. As with all travelers, Medicare beneficiaries should examine their coverage carefully to know exactly what will be covered abroad, and supplement with additional travel health insurance as appropriate.

BIBLIOGRAPHY

1. Centers for Medicare and Medicaid Services. Medicare coverage outside the United States. Baltimore: CMS; 2010 [updated 2010 Sep; cited 2008 Jun 30]. Available from: http://www.medicare.gov/Publications/Pubs/pdf/11037.pdf.

2. US Department of State. Medical information for Americans abroad. Washington, DC: US Department of State; 2010 [cited 2010 Nov15]. Available from: http://travel.state.gov/travel/tips/brochures/brochures_1215.html.

3. US Department of State. Medical insurance. Washington, DC: US Department of State; 2010 [cited 2010 Nov 15]. Available from: http://travel.state.gov/travel/cis_pa_tw/cis/cis_1470.html.

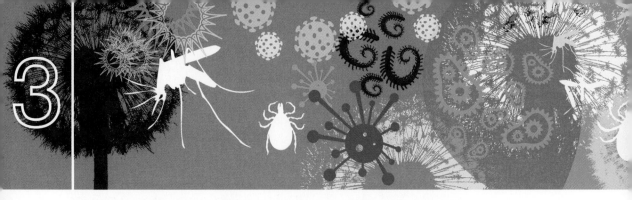

Infectious Diseases Related to Travel

AMEBIASIS

Sharon L. Roy

INFECTIOUS AGENT

Amebiasis is caused by the protozoan parasite *Entamoeba histolytica*.

MODE OF TRANSMISSION

Transmission occurs via the fecal-oral route, either directly by person-to-person contact (such as by diaper-changing or sexual practices) or indirectly by eating or drinking fecally contaminated food or water.

EPIDEMIOLOGY

Amebiasis occurs worldwide, particularly in the tropics, and is more common in areas of poor sanitation where barriers between human feces and food and water (including ice) are inadequate. From 1996 through 2005, 14 per 1,000 returned travelers seeking medical care at GeoSentinel-associated medical centers around the world were diagnosed with *E. histolytica*. Amebiasis was most commonly diagnosed in travelers returning from South Asia, South America, and the Middle East, although travelers returning from all regions were affected. Rates were highest among missionaries and volunteers, although tourists, business travelers, travelers visiting friends and relatives, and people traveling for education or research were also diagnosed with the disease. Long-term travelers (duration >6 months) were significantly more likely than short-term travelers (duration <1 month) to develop *E. histolytica* diarrhea.

Only an estimated 10%–20% of people infected with *E. histolytica* become symptomatic. While the specific effect of amebiasis on travel is not well understood, travelers' diarrhea in general incapacitates about 40% of ill travelers, who have to alter their travel plans for a mean of 2–3 days. Approximately 50 million cases of invasive *E. histolytica* disease occur each year, with as many as 100,000 deaths. People at high risk for severe disease include pregnant women, immunocompromised people, and patients receiving corticosteroids. Associations with diabetes and alcohol use have also been reported.

CLINICAL PRESENTATION

Amebic colitis tends to present with more insidious symptoms than bacterial dysentery. Often patients have a 1- to 4-week history of cramps, watery or bloody diarrhea, and weight loss; approximately one-third of patients have fever. Most patients do not have grossly bloody stools, but almost all patients with amebic colitis have stools that test positive for occult blood. Complications of amebic colitis can include acute necrotizing colitis, bowel perforation, toxic megacolon, amebomas, and perianal ulcers with fistula formation.

Occasionally, the parasite may spread to other organs (extraintestinal amebiasis), most commonly the liver. Amebic liver abscesses may be asymptomatic, but most patients present with fever and right upper quadrant abdominal pain, usually in the absence of diarrhea.

DIAGNOSIS

Microscopy does not distinguish between the amebas E. *histolytica* (pathogenic) and E. *dispar* (nonpathogenic). EIA or PCR is needed to confirm the diagnosis of E. *histolytica*. Clinicians should contact their state health department reference laboratory for recommendations on E. *histolytica*–specific testing. The sensitivity of serologic tests varies depending on clinical presentation (approximately 90% extraintestinal and 70% intestinal) and cannot distinguish between current and past infection.

TREATMENT

Travelers with either asymptomatic E. *histolytica* infection or symptomatic E. *histolytica* disease should be treated if the organism can be proven to be E. *histolytica*. Otherwise, asymptomatic travelers do not need to be treated. For asymptomatic infection, iodoquinol or paromomycin are the drugs of choice. For symptomatic intestinal infection and extraintestinal disease, treatment with metronidazole or tinidazole should be followed by treatment with iodoquinol or paromomycin.

PREVENTIVE MEASURES FOR TRAVELERS

No vaccine is available to prevent amebiasis, and there is no recommended chemoprophylaxis. To prevent infection, travelers should be advised to follow food and water precautions (including those for ice) described in Chapter 2, Food and Water Precautions. Additionally, travelers should practice good hygiene (including frequent handwashing) and avoid fecal exposure during sexual activity.

BIBLIOGRAPHY

1. Abramowicz M. Drugs for Parasitic Infections. New Rochelle (NY): The Medical Letter, Inc; 2007.
2. Bercu TE, Petri WA, Behm JW. Amebic colitis: new insights into pathogenesis and treatment. Curr Gastroenterol Rep. 2007 Oct;9(5):429–33.
3. Bruni M, Steffen R. Impact of travel-related health impairments. J Travel Med. 1997 Jun 1;4(2):61–4.
4. Chen LH, Wilson ME, Davis X, Loutan L, Schwartz E, Keystone J, et al. Illness in long-term travelers visiting GeoSentinel clinics. Emerg Infect Dis. 2009 Nov;15(11):1773–82.
5. Freedman DO, Weld LH, Kozarsky PE, Fisk T, Robins R, von Sonnenburg F, et al. Spectrum of disease and relation to place of exposure among ill returned travelers. N Engl J Med. 2006 Jan 12;354(2):119–30.
6. Greenwood Z, Black J, Weld L, O'Brien D, Leder K, Von Sonnenburg F, et al. Gastrointestinal infection among international travelers globally. J Travel Med. 2008 Jul–Aug;15(4):221–8.
7. McIntosh IB, Reed JM, Power KG. Travellers' diarrhoea and the effect of pre-travel health advice in general practice. Br J Gen Pract. 1997 Feb;47(415):71–5.
8. Okhuysen PC. Current concepts in travelers' diarrhea: epidemiology, antimicrobial resistance and treatment. Curr Opin Infect Dis. 2005 Dec;18(6):522–6.
9. Petri WA Jr, Singh U. Diagnosis and management of amebiasis. Clin Infect Dis. 1999 Nov;29(5):1117–25.
10. Petri WA Jr, Singh U. Enteric amoebiasis. In: Guerrant RL, Walker DH, Weller PF, editors. Tropical Infectious Diseases: Principles, Pathogens, & Practice. 2nd ed. Philadelphia: Churchill Livingstone; 2006. p. 967–83.
11. Ravdin JI, Stauffer WM. *Entamoeba histolytica* (amoebiasis). In: Mandell GL, Bennett JE, Dolin R, editors. Mandell, Bennet, & Dolin: Principles and Practice of Infectious Diseases. 6th ed. Philadelphia: Churchill Livingstone; 2005. p. 3097–111.
12. Stanley SL Jr. Amoebiasis. Lancet. 2003 Mar 22;361(9362):1025–34.
13. Swaminathan A, Torresi J, Schlagenhauf P, Thursky K, Wilder-Smith A, Connor BA, et al. A global study of pathogens and host risk factors associated with infectious gastrointestinal disease in returned international travellers. J Infect. 2009 Jul;59(1):19–27.
14. World Health Organization. Amoebiasis. Wkly Epidemiol Rec. 1997 Apr 4;72(14):97–9.

ANGIOSTRONGYLIASIS (*ANGIOSTRONGYLUS CANTONENSIS* INFECTION, NEUROLOGIC ANGIOSTRONGYLIASIS)

Barbara L. Herwaldt

INFECTIOUS AGENT

Angiostrongyliasis is caused by *Angiostrongylus cantonensis*, a nematode parasite that is considered the most common infectious cause of eosinophilic meningitis in humans.

MODE OF TRANSMISSION

Various species of rats are the **definitive hosts** of the parasite, also known as the rat lungworm. The mature (adult) form of the parasite is found only in rats, not in humans or other hosts. Infected rats shed first-stage larvae, which are infective for snails and slugs but not for humans or for transport hosts (defined below), in their feces.

Snails and slugs are **intermediate hosts**. They become infected by ingesting first-stage larvae in rat feces. These immature larvae mature to third-stage larvae, which are infective for rats (in which they develop to adult worms), other animals, and humans. Humans become infected by eating snails or slugs, whether for cultural reasons, "on a dare," or accidentally, such as by ingesting contaminated raw produce, including lettuce and vegetable juices.

Infective larvae have been found in various **transport (paratenic) hosts**, such as freshwater shrimp or prawns, crabs, and frogs (fish are not known to transmit the parasite). The parasite does not mature in paratenic hosts, but they can transport infective larvae. Some transport hosts (for example, raw frogs) have been associated with human infection; however, the importance of transport hosts in transmitting the parasite is unclear.

EPIDEMIOLOGY

Most of the described cases have occurred in Asia and the Pacific Basin (such as in parts of Thailand, Taiwan, mainland China, the Hawaiian Islands, and other Pacific Islands). However, cases have been reported in many areas of the world, including the Caribbean. The geographic range of the parasite is expanding, probably facilitated by infected shipborne rats and the diversity of snail species that can be intermediate hosts.

Both individual and outbreak-associated cases have been described. An outbreak of *A. cantonensis*–associated eosinophilic meningitis occurred among a group of US travelers exposed in Jamaica in 2000, before angiostrongyliasis was known to be endemic there. The presumptive vehicle was the lettuce in a salad.

CLINICAL PRESENTATION

Ingested larvae can migrate to the central nervous system and cause eosinophilic meningitis. Typically, the incubation period is about 1–3 weeks but has ranged from approximately 1 day to >6 weeks. Common manifestations include headache, photophobia, stiff neck, nausea, vomiting, fatigue, and body aches. Abnormal skin sensations (such as tingling or painful feelings) are more common than in other types of meningitis. A low-grade fever might be noted. The symptoms and signs may persist for weeks or months but are usually self-limited. Severe cases can be associated with sequelae such as paralysis or blindness or death.

DIAGNOSIS

Typically, the diagnosis is presumptive, on the basis of clinical and epidemiologic criteria, in people with otherwise unexplained eosinophilic meningitis. If lumbar punctures are done early or late in the course of infection, few, if any, eosinophils may be found in the cerebrospinal fluid. Peripheral blood eosinophilia is occasionally noted. Parasitologic confirmation of the diagnosis—by detecting A. cantonensis larvae in the cerebrospinal fluid—is unusual in most settings. Serologic assays and other diagnostic modalities are considered investigational but might provide supportive evidence for the diagnosis.

TREATMENT

The larvae die spontaneously, and supportive care usually suffices. The use of corticosteroid or antiparasitic therapy should be individualized, with expert consultation. The utility of such therapy may differ among A. cantonensis-endemic areas. Clinicians may consult with CDC about evaluation and treatment of patients (770-488-7775; parasites@cdc.gov).

Additional information can be found at www.cdc.gov/parasites/angiostrongylus.

PREVENTIVE MEASURES FOR TRAVELERS

No vaccine is available. Preventive measures are aimed at reducing the risk of ingesting the parasite. In particular, travelers are advised to follow standard food and water precautions (see Chapter 2, Food and Water Precautions) and particularly to:

- Avoid eating raw or undercooked snails, slugs, and other possible hosts.
- Eat raw produce, such as lettuce, only if it has been thoroughly washed or treated with bleach.
- Wear gloves (and wash hands) if snails or slugs are handled.

BIBLIOGRAPHY

1. Hochberg NS, Park SY, Blackburn BG, Sejvar JJ, Gaynor K, Chung H, et al. Distribution of eosinophilic meningitis cases attributable to Angiostrongylus cantonensis, Hawaii. Emerg Infect Dis. 2007 Nov;13(11):1675–80.
2. Lai CH, Yen CM, Chin C, Chung HC, Kuo HC, Lin HH. Eosinophilic meningitis caused by Angiostrongylus cantonensis after ingestion of raw frogs. Am J Trop Med Hyg. 2007 Feb;76(2):399–402.
3. Slom TJ, Cortese MM, Gerber SI, Jones RC, Holtz TH, Lopez AS, et al. An outbreak of eosinophilic

meningitis caused by Angiostrongylus cantonensis in travelers returning from the Caribbean. N Engl J Med. 2002 Feb 28;346(9):668–75.
4. Tsai HC, Lee SS, Huang CK, Yen CM, Chen ER, Liu YC. Outbreak of eosinophilic meningitis associated with drinking raw vegetable juice in southern Taiwan. Am J Trop Med Hyg. 2004 Aug;71(2):222–6.
5. Wang QP, Lai DH, Zhu XQ, Chen XG, Lun ZR. Human angiostrongyliasis. Lancet Infect Dis. 2008 Oct;8(10):621–30.

ANTHRAX

Sean V. Shadomy

INFECTIOUS AGENT

Anthrax is caused by the aerobic, gram-positive, encapsulated, spore-forming, nonmotile, nonhemolytic, rod-shaped bacterium, Bacillus anthracis.

MODE OF TRANSMISSION

B. anthracis is primarily transmitted by direct contact with infected animals or with contaminated products from infected animals, including carcasses, meat, hides, wool, or

items made with those products, such as drums or wool clothing.

Anthrax presents in 3 forms: cutaneous, gastrointestinal, and inhalational. Introduction of the spores through the skin can result in cutaneous anthrax; abrasion of the skin increases susceptibility. Eating meat from infected animals can result in gastrointestinal anthrax. Inhalational anthrax typically occurs when a person inhales spores aerosolized by industrial processing of contaminated materials, such as hides or wool; it can also result from bioterrorism. Anthrax in humans is not generally considered to be contagious; person-to-person transmission of cutaneous anthrax has rarely been reported.

EPIDEMIOLOGY

Anthrax is a zoonotic disease that primarily affects herbivores such as cattle, sheep, goats, antelope, and deer, which become infected by ingesting contaminated vegetation, water, or soil; humans are generally incidental hosts.

Anthrax is most common in agricultural regions in Central and South America, sub-Saharan Africa, central and southwestern Asia, and southern and Eastern Europe. Anthrax is now rare in the United States and Canada; however, sporadic outbreaks occur every year in livestock and wild herbivores in these countries. Travelers to endemic areas have acquired anthrax through either direct or indirect contact with carcasses of animals that died from anthrax. Cases of cutaneous and inhalation anthrax have been reported among people who have handled or played drums made with contaminated goat hide from countries endemic for anthrax. Cases have also been reported among people making drums from contaminated goat hides imported from countries endemic for anthrax, as well as members of their households exposed to environments contaminated by the drum-making process.

CLINICAL PRESENTATION

Cutaneous anthrax usually develops 1–7 days after exposure. The case-fatality ratio is as high as 20% if untreated but typically is <1% with appropriate antimicrobial therapy. Cutaneous anthrax is characterized by localized itching, followed by the development of a painless papule, which turns vesicular and enlarges, ulcerates, and develops into a depressed black eschar within 7–10 days of the initial lesion. The head, neck, forearms, and hands are the most commonly affected sites. Edema usually surrounds the lesion, sometimes with secondary vesicles, hyperemia, and regional lymphadenopathy. Patients may have associated fever, malaise, and headache.

Gastrointestinal anthrax usually develops 1–7 days after consumption of contaminated meat and can present in either intestinal or oropharyngeal forms. Shock and death may occur within 2–5 days of onset;

estimates of the case-fatality ratio for gastro-intestinal anthrax are >50% if untreated, but <40% with treatment.

Inhalational anthrax usually develops within a week after exposure, but the incubation period may be prolonged (up to 2 months). Estimates for the case-fatality ratio are >85%; even with aggressive treatment, this ratio can be as high as 45%. Initial symptoms are nonspecific and may mimic those of influenza, including myalgia, fever, nonproductive cough, malaise, nausea, and vomiting; upper respiratory tract symptoms are rare. The patient's condition dramatically worsens 2–3 days after symptom onset, with the development of severe respiratory distress, diaphoresis, cyanosis, and shock.

Hemorrhagic meningitis may develop with any form of anthrax from hematogenous spread. Anthrax meningitis is nearly always fatal.

DIAGNOSIS

Laboratory diagnosis depends on bacterial culture and isolation of B. anthracis, or the detection of bacterial DNA or antigens. Serologic testing of host antibody responses requires acute- and convalescent-phase sera for diagnosis. Confirmatory testing, including isolate identification, antigen detection in tissues, or quantitative serology, should be performed in the United States by the state health department or Laboratory Response Network laboratories, or internationally by the relevant national reference laboratory. Guidelines for collecting and submitting clinical specimens for testing and algorithms for laboratory diagnosis can be found at www.bt.cdc.gov/agent/anthrax/lab-testing. Specimens for culture should be collected before antimicrobial therapy is initiated. Diagnostic procedures for inhalational anthrax include thoracic imaging studies to detect a widened mediastinum or pleural effusion.

TREATMENT

Ciprofloxacin is the drug of choice. Because of intrinsic resistance, neither cephalosporins nor trimethoprim-sulfamethoxazole should be used. Localized or uncomplicated naturally occurring cutaneous anthrax can be treated for 7–10 days with ciprofloxacin (500 mg orally, 2 times/day) or oral doxycycline (100 mg orally, 2 times/day), except in children aged <2 years. If susceptibility testing is supportive, oral penicillin V or amoxicillin may be used to complete the regimen. Therapeutic treatment recommendations for severe systemic or life-threatening disease (such as inhalational anthrax; gastrointestinal anthrax; anthrax meningitis; severe cutaneous anthrax with systemic involvement, extensive edema, or head and neck lesions; treatment of children aged <2 years; or cutaneous anthrax associated with aerosol exposure) are found at www.cdc.gov/mmwr/preview/mmwrhtml/mm5042a1.htm.

PREVENTIVE MEASURES FOR TRAVELERS

Vaccination against anthrax is not recommended for travelers and is not available for civilian travelers. Travelers should not have direct or indirect contact with carcasses of animals found in anthrax-endemic regions or eat meat from animals that were not healthy at the time of slaughter. The risk of acquiring anthrax from playing with or handling an animal hide drum is low. Since 2006, 6 cases of anthrax (including all 3 forms: cutaneous, gastrointestinal, and inhalational) in the United States and United Kingdom have been associated with making animal-hide drums or participating in drumming workshops or events where animal-hide drums were played. Some of these cases were fatal. Travelers who wish to bring back animal hides from anthrax-endemic regions to make drums should strongly consider the health risks before importing the hides.

No tests are available to determine if animal products are contaminated with B. anthracis spores. Animal-hide drum owners or players should report any unexplained fever or new skin lesions to their health care provider and describe their recent contact with animal-hide drums.

The importation of goat-hide souvenirs, such as goat-hide drums, from Haiti is prohibited by CDC (see Chapter 6, Taking Animals and Animal Products Across International Borders). Importation of animal products, including processed or unprocessed cattle and goat hides, is regulated by the US Department of Agriculture (USDA). Animal products, trophies, or souvenirs from anthrax-endemic regions must be accompanied by a certificate saying they are from animals that were free of anthrax. Cattle or goat hides that have been tanned, pickled in a solution of salt and mineral acid, or treated with lime are considered to pose less of a risk for infectious diseases and may be imported under certain conditions. For more information, consult the USDA website (www.aphis.usda.gov/import_export/animals/animal_import/animal_imports.shtml).

BIBLIOGRAPHY

1. Anaraki S, Addiman S, Nixon G, Krahe D, Ghosh R, Brooks T, et al. Investigations and control measures following a case of inhalation anthrax in east London in a drum maker and drummer, October 2008. Euro Surveill. 2008 Dec 18;13(51).

2. Bales ME, Dannenberg AL, Brachman PS, Kaufmann AF, Klatsky PC, Ashford DA. Epidemiologic response to anthrax outbreaks: field investigations, 1950–2001. Emerg Infect Dis. 2002 Oct;8(10):1163–74.

3. CDC. Cutaneous anthrax associated with drum making using goat hides from West Africa—Connecticut, 2007. MMWR Morb Mortal Wkly Rep. 2008 Jun 13;57(23):628–31.

4. CDC. Gastrointestinal anthrax after an animal-hide drumming event—New Hampshire and Massachusetts, 2009. MMWR Morb Mortal Wkly Rep. 2010 Jul 23;59(28):872–7.

5. CDC. Inhalation anthrax associated with dried animal hides—Pennsylvania and New York City, 2006. MMWR Morb Mortal Wkly Rep. 2006 Mar 17;55(10):280–2.

6. Eurosurveillance editorial team. Probable human anthrax death in Scotland. Euro Surveill. 2006;11(8):E060817.2.

7. Inglesby TV, O'Toole T, Henderson DA, Bartlett JG, Ascher MS, Eitzen E, et al. Anthrax as a biological weapon, 2002: updated recommendations for management. JAMA. 2002 May 1;287(17):2236–52.

8. Van den Enden E, Van Gompel A, Van Esbroeck M. Cutaneous anthrax, Belgian traveler. Emerg Infect Dis. 2006 Mar;12(3):523–5.

BARTONELLA-ASSOCIATED INFECTIONS

Alicia Anderson, Jennifer McQuiston

INFECTIOUS AGENT

At least a dozen bacterial species in the genus *Bartonella* cause several different diseases, but few are significant causes of human illness. Cat-scratch disease (CSD) is caused by *Bartonella henselae*. Bartonellosis (Carrión disease) results from infection with *B. bacilliformis*. This disease has 2 distinct phases: an acute febrile illness (Oroya fever) and an eruptive phase, manifesting as cutaneous lesions (verruga peruana). Trench fever is caused by *B. quintana*. A variety of *Bartonella* spp. have been associated with culture-negative endocarditis.

MODE OF TRANSMISSION

CSD is contracted through scratches and bites from domestic or feral cats, particularly kittens. The disease occurs most frequently in children aged <10 years. Cats acquire the organism from infected fleas. Infected flea dirt is harbored in their claws when they scratch themselves and may then be transmitted to a person or another cat.

Bartonellosis is transmitted by sand flies (genus *Lutzomyia*) that are infected with the organism. Much is still unknown regarding the existence of other competent arthropod vectors and the identification of a natural, nonhuman, vertebrate reservoir. Trench fever is transmitted by the human body louse. Because of its association with body louse infestations, trench fever is most commonly associated with homeless populations or areas of high population density and poor sanitation.

EPIDEMIOLOGY

CSD occurs worldwide and may be present wherever cats are found. Stray cats may be more likely than pets to carry *Bartonella*. In the United States, most cases occur in the fall and winter. Bartonellosis has limited geographic distribution; cases occur in the Andes Mountains in western South America, including Peru, Colombia, and Ecuador. Most cases are reported in Peru. A few cases of Oroya fever and verruga peruana (Peruvian wart) have been reported in travelers who returned from the Andean highlands in South America, but the risk is low. In 2007, a newly recognized species of *Bartonella* (*B. melophagi*) was identified in an ill traveler returning from Peru. Trench fever has a worldwide distribution; cases have been reported from Europe, North America, Africa, and China.

CLINICAL PRESENTATION

The symptoms of CSD include fever; enlarged, tender lymph nodes that develop 1–2 weeks after exposure; and a papule or pustule at the inoculation site. Unusual manifestations such as granulomatous conjunctivitis, neuroretinitis, atypical pneumonia, or endocarditis may occur in a small percentage of patients. The manifestations of Oroya fever include fever, myalgia, headache, and anemia. The case-fatality ratio may exceed 40% in untreated people. Verruga peruana is characterized by red-to-purple nodular skin lesions. The symptoms of trench fever include fever, headache, a transient rash, and bone pain, mainly in the shins, neck, and back.

Bacillary angiomatosis (caused by *B. henselae* or *B. quintana*) and peliosis hepatis (caused by *B. henselae*) occur primarily in people infected with HIV. They may present as skin, subcutaneous, or bone lesions. Many *Bartonella* spp. can cause signs and symptoms of subacute endocarditis, which is often culture-negative.

DIAGNOSIS

Diagnosis of CSD can be made by detection of *B. henselae* DNA by PCR, or in culture of pus or lymph node aspirates by using special techniques. CSD is usually confirmed by serology. Oroya fever is typically diagnosed via blood culture or direct observation of the bacilli in peripheral blood smears. Diagnosis of trench fever can be made by isolation of *B. quintana* from blood cultured on blood or chocolate agar under 5% CO_2. Microcolonies can be seen after 1–3 weeks of incubation at

3

37°C. Trench fever can also be confirmed by serology. PCR technology is improving the diagnosis of disseminated *Bartonella* infections. Endocarditis remains difficult to diagnose. Sometimes serology is helpful, or PCR may be done on valve tissue.

TREATMENT

Most cases of CSD eventually resolve without treatment, but a small percentage of people will develop disseminated disease with severe complications. The use of antibiotics to shorten the course of disease is controversial, although azithromycin administered for 5 days has been shown to decrease lymph node volume (500 mg on day 1, followed by 250 mg for 4 days for patients weighing >45.5 kg; or 10 mg/kg on day 1, followed by 5 mg/kg for 4 days for those weighing <45.5 kg).

A wide range of antibiotics is effective against *Bartonella* infections, including penicillins, tetracyclines, cephalosporins, aminoglycosides, and fluoroquinolones. Often, with serious infections, more than one antibiotic is used. Physicians should consult with an expert in infectious diseases.

PREVENTIVE MEASURES FOR TRAVELERS

For CSD, travelers should avoid rough play with cats, particularly strays, to prevent scratches or bites and should wash hands promptly after handling cats. Preventive measures for Oroya fever include protecting against sand flies via clothing, repellents, and reduced outdoor activities when sand flies are most active (dusk and dawn). Preventive measures for trench fever include avoiding exposures to human body lice.

BIBLIOGRAPHY

1. Bass JW, Freitas BC, Freitas AD, Sisler CL, Chan DS, Vincent JM, et al. Prospective randomized double blind placebo-controlled evaluation of azithromycin for treatment of cat-scratch disease. Pediatr Infect Dis J. 1998 Jun;17(6):447–52.

2. Chamberlin J, Laughlin LW, Romero S, Solorzano N, Gordon S, Andre RG, et al. Epidemiology of endemic *Bartonella bacilliformis*: a prospective cohort study in a Peruvian mountain valley community. J Infect Dis. 2002 Oct 1;186(7):983–90.

3. Fournier PE, Thuny F, Richet H, Lepidi H, Casalta JP, Arzouni JP, et al. Comprehensive diagnostic strategy for blood culture-negative endocarditis: a prospective study of 819 new cases. Clin Infect Dis. 2010 Jul 15;51(2):131–40.

4. Guptill L, Wu CC, HogenEsch H, Slater LN, Glickman N, Dunham A, et al. Prevalence, risk factors, and genetic diversity of *Bartonella henselae* infections in pet cats in four regions of the United States. J Clin Microbiol. 2004 Feb;42(2):652–9.

5. Maguina C, Gotuzzo E. Bartonellosis. New and old. Infect Dis Clin North Am. 2000 Mar;14(1):1–22, vii.

6. Margileth AM. Cat scratch disease. Adv Pediatr Infect Dis. 1993;8:1–21.

BRUCELLOSIS

Marta A. Guerra, Barun K. De

INFECTIOUS AGENT

Brucella is a genus of facultative, intracellular, gram-negative coccobacilli. Ten species of Brucella are defined by phenotypic and antigenic differences, in addition to differential host specificity. Known human pathogens include *Brucella abortus*, *B. melitensis*, *B. suis*, and *B. canis*. Pathogenicity to humans of several other species is not well known: *B. ovis*, *B. neotomae*, *B. ceti*, *B. pinnipedialis*, *B. microti*, and *B. inopinata*.

MODE OF TRANSMISSION

Eating or drinking contaminated milk products is the most common route of infection for *Brucella* spp. *Brucella* can enter the body via skin wounds, mucous membranes, or inhalation. Person-to-person transmission is rare.

EPIDEMIOLOGY

High-risk regions include the Mediterranean basin, South and Central America, Eastern Europe, Asia, Africa, and the Middle East. Brucellosis is primarily an occupational disease among people working with infected livestock or handling the organism in laboratory settings. The infection is present in wildlife and in domestic animals such as goats, sheep, pigs, and cattle. Brucellosis is common in countries that have poorly developed public health systems and no standardized brucellosis-control programs for livestock.

Risk is mainly associated with the consumption of unpasteurized milk and other dairy products in countries where brucellosis is endemic or enzootic. Unpasteurized soft goat cheeses are frequently contaminated with Brucella and associated with the development of brucellosis. People exposed to contaminated fluids and tissue while helping animals give birth, slaughtering and dressing of infected animals, or preparing foods from infected animals are at increased risk of infection. Eating undercooked infected meat is another route of infection.

CLINICAL PRESENTATION

The incubation period is 2–4 weeks (range, 5 days to 5 months). The initial presentation is nonspecific, including fever, muscle aches, fatigue, headache, and night sweats. The fever may be continuous or intermittent (undulant). Systemic infection may localize in the liver, spleen, bone marrow, joints, heart, or reproductive organs. When it occurs, endocarditis is a primary cause of death. Neuropsychiatric symptoms, such as depression or sleep disturbance, may occur rarely. More severe symptoms are generally associated with B. melitensis or B. suis infections than with infections from other Brucella spp.

DIAGNOSIS

Blood culture is the diagnostic gold standard but is not always positive. If blood or bone marrow culture is used, the laboratory must be informed that Brucella is suspected, so that they will process the sample for a longer period of time and protect laboratory personnel. A serum agglutination test is the most common serologic approach, but other serology, ELISA testing, and PCR have been used to make a diagnosis.

TREATMENT

The optimum antimicrobial therapy for brucellosis includes a minimum 6- to 8-week course of a combination of antimicrobial agents. Antimicrobials most commonly used are doxycycline, rifampin, and streptomycin. Relapses may occur with late initiation or premature discontinuation of therapy.

PREVENTIVE MEASURES FOR TRAVELERS

No vaccine is available for humans. Antimicrobial prophylaxis is not recommended. People traveling to countries where brucellosis is endemic or enzootic should avoid ingesting unpasteurized dairy products. In addition, travelers should avoid eating undercooked meat.

BIBLIOGRAPHY

1. American Public Health Association. Control of communicable diseases manual: an official report of the American Health Association. 15th ed. Heyman D, editor. Washington DC: American Public Health Association; 2004.

2. Ariza J, Bosilkovski M, Cascio A, Colmenero JD, Corbel MJ, Falagas ME, et al. Perspectives for the treatment of brucellosis in the 21st century: the Ioannina recommendations. PLoS Med. 2007 Dec;4(12):e317.

3. CDC. Update: potential exposures to attenuated vaccine strain Brucella abortus RB51 during a laboratory proficiency test—United States and Canada, 2007. MMWR Morb Mortal Wkly Rep. 2008 Jan 18;57(2):36–9.

4. Live I, Wolf B. Response of individuals to injection with ether-killed Brucella abortus. Am J Public Health Nations Health. 1960 Jul;50:966–75.

5. Pappas G, Papadimitriou P, Akritidis N, Christou L, Tsianos EV. The new global map of human brucellosis. Lancet Infect Dis. 2006 Feb;6(2):91–9.

6. Snyder JW. Sentinel laboratory guidelines for suspected agents of bioterrorism: Brucella species. Washington, DC: American Society for Microbiology; 2004. Available from: http://www.asm.org/asm/images/pdf/Brucella101504.pdf.

7. World Health Organization. Brucellosis. Geneva: World Health Organization [cited 2008 Nov 30]. Available from: http://www.who.int/zoonoses/diseases/brucellosis/en/.

CAMPYLOBACTER ENTERITIS

Melissa Viray, Michael Lynch

INFECTIOUS AGENT

Infection is caused by gram-negative, spiral-shaped microaerophilic bacteria of the family Campylobacteraceae. Most infections are caused by *Campylobacter jejuni*; other species, including *C. coli*, also cause infection. *C. jejuni* and *C. coli* are carried normally in the intestinal tracts of many domestic and wild animals.

MODE OF TRANSMISSION

The major modes of transmission include eating contaminated foods (especially undercooked chicken and foods contaminated by raw chicken), drinking contaminated water or raw (unpasteurized) milk, or having contact with animals, particularly farm animals such as cattle and poultry, as well as cats and dogs.

EPIDEMIOLOGY

Campylobacter is a leading cause of bacterial diarrheal disease worldwide; in the United States, it is estimated to affect 2.4 million people every year. Campylobacteriosis is a common cause of travelers' diarrhea. The percentage of bacterial travelers' diarrhea caused by *Campylobacter* ranges from 1%–2% in Mexico to 28% in Thailand. The infectious dose is thought to be small, typically fewer than 500 organisms.

The geographic distribution of cases is worldwide; risk for infection is higher in the developing world, especially in areas with poor restaurant hygiene and inadequate sanitation.

CLINICAL PRESENTATION

Incubation period is typically 2–4 days. Campylobacteriosis is characterized by diarrhea (frequently bloody), abdominal pain, fever, and occasionally, nausea and vomiting. More severe presentations can occur, including bloodstream infection and disease mimicking acute appendicitis or ulcerative colitis. *Campylobacter* infection can trigger Guillain-Barré syndrome. Additional information can be found on the CDC website (www.cdc.gov/nczved/divisions/dfbmd/diseases/campylobacter).

DIAGNOSIS

Diagnosis is based on isolation of the organism from stools by using selective media and reduced oxygen tension. Most laboratories also combine this with incubation at 42°C (107.6°F). Visualization of motile and curved, spiral, or S-shaped rods by stool phase-contrast or dark-field microscopy can provide rapid presumptive evidence for *Campylobacter* enteritis.

TREATMENT

The disease is generally self-limited and may last up to a week. Antibiotic therapy decreases the duration of symptoms if administered early in the course of disease. Because it is generally not possible to distinguish campylobacteriosis from other causes of travelers' diarrhea without a diagnostic test, the use of empiric antibiotics in travelers should follow the guidelines for travelers' diarrhea.

Rates of antibiotic resistance have been on the rise in the past 20 years, in particular for fluoroquinolones; travel abroad has been associated with infection with resistant *Campylobacter*. Clinicians should have a high degree of suspicion for resistant infection in returning travelers who may have failed empiric fluoroquinolone treatment. Documented fluoroquinolone resistance has been highest among travelers to Thailand. When fluoroquinolone resistance is proven or suspected, azithromycin is usually the next choice of treatment.

PREVENTIVE MEASURES FOR TRAVELERS

No vaccine is available. Antibiotic prophylaxis, as used for travelers' diarrhea, is likely to be effective, although antibiotic prophylaxis is not routinely recommended. Preventive measures are aimed at avoiding foods at high risk for contamination and taking safe water precautions while traveling (see Chapter 2, Food and Water Precautions).

BIBLIOGRAPHY

1. Altekruse SF, Stern NJ, Fields PI, Swerdlow DL. *Campylobacter jejuni*—an emerging foodborne pathogen. Emerg Infect Dis. 1999 Jan–Feb;5(1):28–35.

2. Coker AO, Isokpehi RD, Thomas BN, Amisu KO, Obi CL. Human campylobacteriosis in developing countries. Emerg Infect Dis. 2002 Mar;8(3):237–44.

3. Friedman CR, Hoekstra RM, Samuel M, Marcus R, Bender J, Shiferaw B, et al. Risk factors for sporadic *Campylobacter* infection in the United States: a case-control study in FoodNet sites. Clin Infect Dis. 2004 Apr 15;38 Suppl 3:S285–96.

4. Gupta A, Nelson JM, Barrett TJ, Tauxe RV, Rossiter SP, Friedman CR, et al. Antimicrobial resistance among *Campylobacter* strains, United States, 1997–2001. Emerg Infect Dis. 2004 Jun;10(6):1102–9.

5. Humphrey T, O'Brien S, Madsen M. Campylobacters as zoonotic pathogens: a food production perspective. Int J Food Microbiol. 2007 Jul 15;117(3):237–57.

6. Moore JE, Barton MD, Blair IS, Corcoran D, Dooley JS, Fanning S, et al. The epidemiology of antibiotic resistance in *Campylobacter*. Microbes Infect. 2006 Jun;8(7):1955–66.

7. Moore JE, Corcoran D, Dooley JS, Fanning S, Lucey B, Matsuda M, et al. *Campylobacter*. Vet Res. 2005 May–Jun;36(3):351–82.

8. Tribble DR, Sanders JW, Pang LW, Mason C, Pitarangsi C, Baqar S, et al. Traveler's diarrhea in Thailand: randomized, double-blind trial comparing single-dose and 3-day azithromycin-based regimens with a 3-day levofloxacin regimen. Clin Infect Dis. 2007 Feb 1;44(3):338–46.

CHIKUNGUNYA

J. Erin Staples, Susan L. Hills, Ann M. Powers

INFECTIOUS AGENT

Infection is caused by the chikungunya virus (CHIKV), a single-stranded RNA virus that belongs to the family Togaviridae, genus *Alphavirus*.

MODE OF TRANSMISSION

Transmission occurs via the bite of an infected mosquito of the *Aedes* spp., predominantly *Aedes aegypti* and *Ae. albopictus*. Nonhuman and human primates are likely the main reservoirs of the virus with anthroponotic (human-to-vector-to-human) transmission occurring during outbreaks of the disease. Bloodborne transmission is possible; cases have been documented among laboratory personnel handling infected blood and a health care worker drawing blood from an infected patient.

The risk of a person transmitting the virus to a biting mosquito or through blood is highest when the patient is viremic during the first 2–6 days of illness. Maternal-fetal transmission has been documented during pregnancy. The highest risk occurs when a woman is viremic at the time of delivery, with a vertical transmission rate of 49%. CHIKV does not appear to be transmitted through breast milk.

EPIDEMIOLOGY

CHIKV has been identified in many countries in Africa and Asia and is responsible for numerous epidemics in these areas. Since the disease reemerged in 2004, millions of cases have occurred and continue to occur throughout countries in and around the Indian Ocean. Transmission has also been documented periodically in temperate areas, such as in Italy in 2007. Given the large CHIKV epidemics, high level of viremia in humans, and the worldwide distribution of *Ae. aegypti* and *Ae. albopictus*, there is a risk of importation of chikungunya virus into new areas by infected travelers.

Risk for travelers is highest with travel to areas experiencing ongoing epidemics of the disease. Most epidemics occur during the tropical rainy season and abate during the dry season. However, outbreaks in Africa have occurred after periods of drought, where open water containers served as vector-breeding sites. Risk of CHIKV infection exists throughout the day, as the primary vector, *Ae. aegypti*, aggressively bites during the daytime. *Ae. aegypti* mosquitoes bite indoors or outdoors near a dwelling. They typically breed in domestic containers that hold water, including buckets and flower pots.

Both adults and children can become infected and symptomatic with the disease. From 2006 through 2009, 105 cases of chikungunya fever were identified among US travelers. Most cases were travelers returning from areas with ongoing disease activity.

CLINICAL PRESENTATION

Approximately 3%–28% of people infected with CHIKV will remain asymptomatic. For people who develop symptomatic illness, the incubation period is typically 3–7 days (range, 2–12 days). Disease is most often characterized by sudden onset of high fever (temperature typically higher than 39°C [102°F]) and severe joint pain or stiffness. Other symptoms may include rash, headache, fatigue, nausea, vomiting, and myalgias. Fevers typically last from several days up to 1 week; the fever can be biphasic. Joint symptoms are severe and often debilitating. They are usually symmetric and occur most commonly in hands and feet, but they can affect more proximal joints. Rash usually occurs after onset of fever. It is typically maculopapular, involving the trunk and extremities, but can also include palms, soles, and face.

Abnormal laboratory findings can include thrombocytopenia, leukopenia, and elevated liver function tests. Rare but serious complications of the disease can occur, including myocarditis, ocular disease (uveitis, retinitis), hepatitis, acute renal disease, severe bulbous lesions, and neuroinvasive disease, such as meningoencephalitis, Guillain-Barré syndrome, paresis, or palsies. Fatalities related to CHIKV infection are rare. Older age and comorbidities are likely risk factors for poor outcomes.

After the acute illness, some patients have prolonged fatigue lasting several weeks. Additionally, some patients have reported incapacitating joint pain, stiffness, or tenosynovitis, which may last for weeks or months. Some studies have reported joint symptoms more than a year after the initial infection.

Pregnant women have symptoms and outcomes similar to those of other people, and most CHIKV infections that occur during pregnancy will not result in the virus being transmitted to the fetus. However, when intrapartum transmission occurs, it can result in complications for the baby, including neurologic disease, hemorrhagic symptoms, and myocardial disease. There are also rare reports of spontaneous abortions after maternal CHIKV infection.

DIAGNOSIS

Preliminary diagnosis is based on the patient's clinical features, places and dates of travel, and activities. Laboratory diagnosis is generally accomplished by testing serum to detect virus, viral nucleic acid, or virus-specific IgM and neutralizing antibodies. During the first week after onset of symptoms, CHIKV infection can often be diagnosed by using viral culture or nucleic acid amplification on serum. CHIKV-specific IgM and neutralizing antibodies normally develop toward the end of the first week of illness. Therefore, to definitively rule out the diagnosis, convalescent-phase samples should be obtained from patients whose acute-phase samples test negative.

Testing for CHIKV IgM and IgG is commercially available. However, confirmatory neutralizing antibody testing is only available through CDC (970-221-6400) and a few state health laboratories. Although reporting CHIKV infections is not mandatory in the United States, all clinicians are encouraged to notify their state or local health department of suspected CHIKV cases to mitigate the risk of local (anthroponotic) transmission.

TREATMENT

No specific antiviral treatment is available for chikungunya fever. Treatment is for symptoms and can include rest, fluids, and use of analgesics and antipyretics. Infected people should be protected from further mosquito exposure (staying indoors in areas with screens or under a mosquito net) during the first few days of the illness, so they do not contribute to the transmission cycle.

PREVENTIVE MEASURES FOR TRAVELERS

No vaccine or preventive drug is available. Caution should be used when advising travelers at increased risk for more severe disease, including travelers with significant comorbidities and pregnant women whose unborn infants are at increased risk, about travel to areas with ongoing outbreaks of the disease. The best way to prevent chikungunya virus infection is to avoid mosquito bites (see Chapter 2, Protection against Mosquitoes, Ticks, and Other Insects and Arthropods).

BIBLIOGRAPHY

1. Brighton SW, Prozesky OW, de la Harpe AL. Chikungunya virus infection. A retrospective study of 107 cases. S Afr Med J. 1983 Feb 26;63(9):313–5.
2. CDC. Chikungunya distribution and global map. Atlanta: CDC; 2010 [updated Oct 22 2010; cited 2010 Apr 26]. Available from: http://www.cdc.gov/ncidod/dvbid/Chikungunya/CH_GlobalMap.html.
3. CDC. Chikungunya fever diagnosed among international travelers—United States, 2005–2006. MMWR Morb Mortal Wkly Rep. 2006 Sep 29;55(38):1040–2.
4. Chretien JP, Anyamba A, Bedno SA, Breiman RF, Sang R, Sergon K, et al. Drought-associated chikungunya emergence along coastal East Africa. Am J Trop Med Hyg. 2007 Mar;76(3):405–7.
5. Jupp PG, McIntosh BM. Chikungunya virus disease. In: Monath TP, editor. The Arboviruses: Epidemiology and Ecology. Boca Raton, FL: CRC; 1988. p. 137–57.
6. Kularatne SA, Gihan MC, Weerasinghe SC, Gunasena S. Concurrent outbreaks of chikungunya and dengue fever in Kandy, Sri Lanka, 2006–07: a comparative analysis of clinical and laboratory features. Postgrad Med J. 2009 Jul;85(1005):342–6.
7. Lanciotti RS, Kosoy OL, Laven JJ, Panella AJ, Velez JO, Lambert AJ, et al. Chikungunya virus in US travelers returning from India, 2006. Emerg Infect Dis. 2007 May;13(5):764–7.
8. Moro ML, Gagliotti C, Silvi G, Angelini R, Sambri V, Rezza G, et al. Chikungunya virus in northeastern Italy: a seroprevalence survey. Am J Trop Med Hyg. 2010 Mar;82(3):508–11.
9. Panning M, Grywna K, van Esbroeck M, Emmerich P, Drosten C. Chikungunya fever in travelers returning to Europe from the Indian Ocean region, 2006. Emerg Infect Dis. 2008 Mar;14(3):416–22.
10. Powers AM, Logue CH. Changing patterns of chikungunya virus: re-emergence of a zoonotic arbovirus. J Gen Virol. 2007 Sep;88(Pt 9):2363–77.
11. Queyriaux B, Simon F, Grandadam M, Michel R, Tolou H, Boutin JP. Clinical burden of chikungunya virus infection. Lancet Infect Dis. 2008 Jan;8(1):2–3.
12. Rajapakse S, Rodrigo C, Rajapakse A. Atypical manifestations of chikungunya infection. Trans R Soc Trop Med Hyg. 2010 Feb;104(2):89–96.
13. Ramful D, Carbonnier M, Pasquet M, Bouhmani B, Ghazouani J, Noormahomed T, et al. Mother-to-child transmission of chikungunya virus infection. Pediatr Infect Dis J. 2007 Sep;26(9):811–5.
14. Renault P, Solet JL, Sissoko D, Balleydier E, Larrieu S, Filleul L, et al. A major epidemic of chikungunya virus infection on Reunion Island, France, 2005–2006. Am J Trop Med Hyg. 2007 Oct;77(4):727–31.
15. Rezza G, Nicoletti L, Angelini R, Romi R, Finarelli AC, Panning M, et al. Infection with chikungunya virus in Italy: an outbreak in a temperate region. Lancet. 2007 Dec 1;370(9602):1840–6.
16. Soumahoro MK, Fontenille D, Turbelin C, Pelat C, Boyd A, Flahault A, et al. Imported chikungunya virus infection. Emerg Infect Dis. 2010 Jan;16(1):162–3.
17. Staples JE, Breiman RF, Powers AM. Chikungunya fever: an epidemiological review of a re-emerging infectious disease. Clin Infect Dis. 2009 Sep 15;49(6):942–8.
18. Touret Y, Randrianaivo H, Michault A, Schuffenecker I, Kauffmann E, Lenglet Y, et al. [Early maternal-fetal transmission of the Chikungunya virus]. Presse Med. 2006 Nov;35(11 Pt 1):1656–8.
19. World Health Organization. Outbreak and spread of chikungunya. Wkly Epidemiol Rec. 2007 Nov 23;82(47):409–15.

CHOLERA

Kashmira Date, Eric Mintz

INFECTIOUS AGENT

Cholera is an acute bacterial, intestinal infection caused by toxigenic *Vibrio cholerae* O-group 1 or O-group 139. Many other serogroups of *V. cholerae*, with or without the cholera toxin gene (including the non-toxigenic strains of the O1 and O139 serogroups), can cause a cholera-like illness. Only toxigenic strains of serogroups O1 and O139 have caused widespread epidemics and are reportable to the World Health Organization (WHO) as "cholera."

V. cholerae O1 has 2 biotypes, classical and El Tor, and each biotype has 2 distinct serotypes, Inaba and Ogawa. The symptoms of infection are indistinguishable, although more people infected with the El Tor biotype remain asymptomatic or have only a mild illness. In recent years, infections with the classical biotype of V. cholerae O1 have become rare and are limited to parts of Bangladesh and India.

MODE OF TRANSMISSION

Toxigenic V. cholerae O1 and O139 are free-living bacterial organisms found in fresh and brackish water, often in association with copepods or other zooplankton, shellfish, and aquatic plants. Cholera infections are most commonly acquired from drinking water in which V. cholerae is found naturally or into which it has been introduced from the feces of an infected person. Other common vehicles include contaminated fish and shellfish, produce, or leftover cooked grains that have not been properly reheated. Transmission from person to person, even to health care workers during epidemics, is rarely documented.

EPIDEMIOLOGY

Since 1961, the seventh pandemic of cholera, caused by V. cholerae serogroup O1, biotype El Tor, has spread from Indonesia through most of Asia into Eastern Europe and Africa, and from North Africa to the Iberian Peninsula. In 1991, an extensive epidemic began in Peru and spread to neighboring countries in the Western Hemisphere. Although few cases of cholera occur in South or Central America, V. cholerae O1 remains endemic in much of Africa and South and Southeast Asia. V. cholerae O139 spread rapidly through Asia in the early 1990s but has since remained localized to a few areas in Bangladesh and India.

In 2009, 45 countries reported 221,226 cholera cases and 4,946 cholera deaths (case-fatality ratio, 2.24%) to WHO. Resource-poor areas report the most cases; 98% of cases and 99% of deaths were reported from Africa. Cholera has the potential to emerge in dramatic epidemics, as was seen with the massive outbreaks that affected Zimbabwe in 2008 and 2009, with close to 100,000 cases and over 4,000 deaths reported. More recently, in October 2010, a cholera outbreak was confirmed in Haiti, within months of the devastating earthquake that destroyed the Haitian capital of Port-au-Prince and surrounding areas. As of early November 2010, nearly 17,000 hospitalized cases and more than 1,000 deaths had been reported. Consequent to the lack of safe water infrastructure in Haiti and additional destruction caused by the earthquake, the number of cases and deaths is expected to continue to increase in Haiti, and travel-associated cases may appear in other Caribbean nations and in the United States.

From 1999 through 2008, 60 confirmed cases of cholera in the United States were acquired abroad. Travelers who follow the usual tourist itineraries and who observe safe food and water recommendations and hygiene precautions while in countries reporting cholera have virtually no risk. The risk is increased for those who drink untreated water, do not follow proper hygiene recommendations, or eat poorly cooked or raw food, especially seafood, in endemic or outbreak settings.

Two reports of cholera have been associated with food served on board international flights, most recently in 1992, during the Latin American epidemic, on a flight from Argentina to Los Angeles. CDC consequently advised the International Air Transport Association that oral rehydration solutions should be carried on international flights and that certain food items prepared in cities with cholera epidemics should not be served. Airline flights have not been implicated in any subsequent cases of cholera.

CLINICAL PRESENTATION

Cholera infection is most often asymptomatic or results in a mild gastroenteritis. Severe cholera is characterized by acute, profuse watery diarrhea, described as "rice-water stools," and often vomiting, leading to volume depletion. Signs and symptoms include tachycardia, loss of skin turgor, dry mucous membranes, hypotension, and thirst. Additional symptoms, including muscle cramps, are secondary to the resulting electrolyte imbalances. If untreated, volume depletion can rapidly lead to hypovolemic shock and death.

DIAGNOSIS

Cholera is confirmed through culture of a stool specimen or rectal swab. Cary-Blair medium is ideal for transport, and the selective thiosulfate-citrate-bile salts (TCBS) agar is ideal for isolation and identification. Reagents for serogrouping *V. cholerae* isolates are available in all state health department laboratories. Commercially available rapid test kits do not yield an isolate for antimicrobial susceptibility testing and subtyping and should not be used for routine diagnosis. All isolates should be sent to CDC via state health department laboratories for cholera toxin testing and subtyping. Cholera is a nationally reportable disease.

TREATMENT

Rehydration is the cornerstone of therapy. Oral rehydration salts and, when necessary, intravenous fluids and electrolytes, if administered in a timely manner and in adequate volumes, will reduce case-fatality ratios to well under 1%. Antibiotics reduce fluid requirements and duration of illness. Antimicrobial therapy is indicated for severe cases, which can be treated with tetracycline, doxycycline, furazolidone, erythromycin, or ciprofloxacin. When possible, antimicrobial susceptibility testing should inform treatment choices.

PREVENTIVE MEASURES FOR TRAVELERS

Safe food and water precautions and frequent handwashing are critical in preventing cholera (see Chapter 2, Food and Water Precautions). Chemoprophylaxis is not indicated.

No cholera vaccine is available in the United States. Two oral vaccines are available outside the United States: Dukoral (Crucell, the Netherlands) and Shanchol (Shantha Biotechnics, India)/mORCVAX (Vabiotech, Vietnam). Shanchol and mORCVAX are similar vaccines produced by different manufacturers. These vaccines appear to be safe, provide better immunity, and have fewer adverse effects than the previously licensed injectable vaccine. However, CDC does not recommend these vaccines for most travelers because of the low risk of cholera to US travelers and the incomplete immunity that the vaccines confer. No country or territory requires vaccination against cholera as a condition for entry.

Further information on Dukoral can be obtained from Crucell (www.crucell.com). Information on Shanchol can be obtained from Shantha Biotechnics (www.shanthabiotech.com, 516-859-3010 [United States], 91-40-23234136 [India], info@shanthabiotech.co.in). Information on mORCVAX can be obtained from Vabiotech (www.vabiotechvn.com/english, 84-4-9717710 [Vietnam]).

BIBLIOGRAPHY

1. CDC. Cholera associated with an international airline flight, 1992. MMWR Morb Mortal Wkly Rep. 1992 Feb 28;41(8):134–5.
2. CDC. Cholera outbreak—Haiti, October 2010. MMWR Morb Mortal Wkly Rep. 2010 Nov 5;59(43):1411.
3. CDC. Two cases of toxigenic *Vibrio cholerae* O1 infection after Hurricanes Katrina and Rita—Louisiana, October 2005. MMWR Morb Mortal Wkly Rep. 2006 Jan 20;55(2):31–2.
4. CDC. Update: cholera outbreak—Haiti, 2010. MMWR Morb Mortal Wkly Rep. 2010 Nov 19;59(45):1473–9.
5. Gaffga NH, Tauxe RV, Mintz ED. Cholera: a new homeland in Africa? Am J Trop Med Hyg. 2007 Oct;77(4):705–13.
6. Griffith DC, Kelly-Hope LA, Miller MA. Review of reported cholera outbreaks worldwide, 1995–2005. Am J Trop Med Hyg. 2006 Nov;75(5):973–7.
7. Sack DA, Sack RB, Nair GB, Siddique AK. Cholera. Lancet. 2004 Jan 17;363(9404):223–33.
8. Sutton RG. An outbreak of cholera in Australia due to food served in flight on an international aircraft. J Hyg (Lond). 1974 Jun;72(3):441–51.

COCCIDIOIDOMYCOSIS

Loretta S. Chang, Tom M. Chiller

INFECTIOUS AGENT

Coccidioidomycosis, or "valley fever," is a disease caused by the fungi *Coccidioides immitis* and *C. posadasii*.

MODE OF TRANSMISSION

The disease is acquired by inhalation of fungal conidia from dust found in ambient air or generated by soil-disrupting human activities or natural disasters. Coccidioidomycosis is not transmitted from person to person.

EPIDEMIOLOGY

Coccidioides spp. are endemic in arid regions. In the United States, the areas with the highest incidence are primarily in the Sonoran Desert in Arizona (Phoenix and Tucson metropolitan areas) and the San Joaquin Valley in California. Other endemic areas in the United States include parts of New Mexico, western Texas, and parts of Utah. Outside the United States, coccidioidomycosis is endemic in parts of Argentina, Brazil, Colombia, Guatemala, Honduras, Mexico, Nicaragua, Paraguay, and Venezuela.

Up to 29% of community-acquired pneumonias in endemic areas may be due to *Coccidioides* infection. In disease-endemic areas, people may be at increased risk for disease if they participate in, or are present during, activities that disturb the ground and result in exposure to dust, including construction, landscaping, mining, agriculture, archaeologic excavation, military maneuvers, and recreational pursuits such as dirt biking. Natural events such as earthquakes or windstorms that generate dust clouds increase the risk of exposure. However, cases may also occur after travel to an endemic area in the absence of these exposures.

CLINICAL PRESENTATION

The incubation period ranges from 7 to 21 days. Most infections (60%) are asymptomatic. Symptomatic people will generally have disease ranging from a self-limited influenzalike illness, characterized by fever, headache, rash, muscle aches, dry cough, weight loss, and malaise, to primary pulmonary coccidioidomycosis, characterized by pneumonia with changes on chest radiography.

In rare instances, severe lung disease (such as cavitary pneumonia) or dissemination to the central nervous system, joints, bones, or skin may develop. People at increased risk for severe pulmonary disease are the elderly, those with diabetes or recent smoking history, and people of low socioeconomic status. People at increased risk for disseminated disease include African Americans and Filipinos, those with immunocompromising conditions (such as HIV), and women in the third trimester of pregnancy. Once infected with *Coccidioides*, a person is immune to reinfection. People with no prior exposure to coccidioidomycosis are more likely to become infected.

DIAGNOSIS

Coccidioidomycosis is best diagnosed by using serologic, histopathologic, and culture methods. Serologic tests are useful to confirm diagnoses and provide prognostic information. Because clinical laboratories use different diagnostic test kits, positive results should be confirmed in a reference laboratory.

Spherules can be visualized in infected body fluid specimens (pleural fluid, bronchoalveolar lavage) and biopsy specimens of skin lesions or organs. The presence of a mature spherule with endospores is pathognomonic of infection. An EIA antigen assay for testing urine, serum, plasma, bronchoalveolar lavage, cerebrospinal fluid, or other sterile body fluids is commercially available. Positive levels of antigen in urine have a sensitivity of 71% to diagnose more severe forms of coccidioidomycosis. Cross-reaction occurs in about 10% of patients with other endemic mycoses.

TREATMENT

The benefit of treating people with uncomplicated, acute primary coccidioidomycosis is not well studied. Although some experts feel that people without risk for severe or disseminated disease do not require treatment because the illness is self-limited, others propose treatment to reduce the intensity or duration of symptoms.

People at high risk for dissemination should receive antifungal therapy when diagnosed with acute coccidioidomycosis. Additionally, people with severe acute pulmonary disease, chronic pulmonary infection, or disseminated disease should receive antifungal therapy. Depending on the clinical situation, azole antifungal agents (such as fluconazole or itraconazole) or amphotericin B may be used for treatment. All patients with clinical disease consistent with coccidioidomycosis should be tested for primary infection and followed closely to monitor the course of disease and to document improvement. An infectious diseases specialist should manage these patients.

PREVENTIVE MEASURES FOR TRAVELERS

No vaccine is available. It is not possible to completely prevent infection with *Coccidioides* spp., because the spores are aerosolized in endemic areas. However, travelers, especially those at increased risk for severe and disseminated disease, can decrease their risk by limiting their exposure to outdoor dust in disease-endemic areas, especially during dust storms. Dust-control measures, such as wetting soil before disturbing the earth, may be effective. Other protective measures aimed at reducing exposure to dust, such as wearing well-fitted dust masks capable of filtering particles as small as 0.4 µm and using vehicles with enclosed, air-conditioned cabs can provide added protection for those with high risk of occupational exposure to dust.

BIBLIOGRAPHY

1. Ampel NM. Coccidioidomycosis: a review of recent advances. Clin Chest Med. 2009 Jun;30(2):241–51.

2. Ampel NM, Giblin A, Mourani JP, Galgiani JN. Factors and outcomes associated with the decision to treat primary pulmonary coccidioidomycosis. Clin Infect Dis. 2009 Jan 15;48(2):172–8.

3. Blair JE. Coccidioidal meningitis: update on epidemiology, clinical features, diagnosis, and management. Curr Infect Dis Rep. 2009 Jul;11(4):289–95.

4. Cairns L, Blythe D, Kao A, Pappagianis D, Kaufman L, Kobayashi J, et al. Outbreak of coccidioidomycosis in Washington state residents returning from Mexico. Clin Infect Dis. 2000 Jan;30(1):61–4.

5. Chiller TM, Galgiani JN, Stevens DA. Coccidioidomycosis. Infect Dis Clin North Am. 2003 Mar;17(1):41–57, viii.

6. Crum NF, Lederman ER, Stafford CM, Parrish JS, Wallace MR. Coccidioidomycosis: a descriptive survey of a reemerging disease. Clinical characteristics and current controversies. Medicine (Baltimore). 2004 May;83(3):149–75.

7. Crum-Cianflone NF. Coccidioidomycosis in the US military: a review. Ann N Y Acad Sci. 2007 Sep;1111:112–21.

8. Durkin M, Connolly P, Kuberski T, Myers R, Kubak BM, Bruckner D, et al. Diagnosis of coccidioidomycosis with use of the *Coccidioides* antigen enzyme immunoassay. Clin Infect Dis. 2008 Oct 15;47(8):e69–73.

9. Fisher FS, Bultman MW, Pappagianis D. Operational guidelines for geological fieldwork in areas endemic for coccidioidomycosis (valley fever). Reston (VA): US Geological Survey; 2000. Available from: http://geopubs.wr.usgs.gov/open-file/of00-348/of00-348.pdf

10. Galgiani JN, Ampel NM, Catanzaro A, Johnson RH, Stevens DA, Williams PL. Practice guideline for the treatment of coccidioidomycosis. Infectious Diseases Society of America. Clin Infect Dis. 2000 Apr;30(4):658–61.

11. Hooper JE, Lu Q, Pepkowitz SH. Disseminated coccidioidomycosis in pregnancy. Arch Pathol Lab Med. 2007 Apr;131(4):652–5.

12. Johnson RH, Einstein HE. Amphotericin B and coccidioidomycosis. Ann N Y Acad Sci. 2007 Sep;1111:434–41.

13. Kwok HK, Chan JW, Li IW, Chu SY, Lam CW. Coccidioidomycosis as a rare cause of pneumonia in non-endemic areas: a short exposure history should not be ignored. Respirology. 2009 May;14(4):617–20.

14. Panackal AA, Hajjeh RA, Cetron MS, Warnock DW. Fungal infections among returning travelers. Clin Infect Dis. 2002 Nov 1;35(9):1088–95.

15. Petersen LR, Marshall SL, Barton-Dickson C, Hajjeh RA, Lindsley MD, Warnock DW, et al. Coccidioidomycosis among workers at an archeological site, northeastern Utah. Emerg Infect Dis. 2004 Apr;10(4):637–42.

16. Rosenstein NE, Emery KW, Werner SB, Kao A, Johnson R, Rogers D, et al. Risk factors for severe pulmonary and disseminated coccidioidomycosis: Kern County, California, 1995–1996. Clin Infect Dis. 2001 Mar 1;32(5):708–15.

17. Smith CE, Beard RR, et al. Effect of season and dust control on coccidioidomycosis. J Am Med Assoc. 1946 Dec 7;132(14):833–8.

18. Stern NG, Galgiani JN. Coccidioidomycosis among scholarship athletes and other college students, Arizona, USA. Emerg Infect Dis. 2010 Feb;16(2):321–3.

19. Valdivia L, Nix D, Wright M, Lindberg E, Fagan T, Lieberman D, et al. Coccidioidomycosis as a common cause of community-acquired pneumonia. Emerg Infect Dis. 2006 Jun;12(6):958–62.

CRYPTOSPORIDIOSIS
Sharon L. Roy, Michele C. Hlavsa

INFECTIOUS AGENT

Cryptosporidiosis is a diarrheal illness caused by the protozoan parasite *Cryptosporidium*. Many species of *Cryptosporidium* exist that infect humans and a wide range of animals. The most common species infecting humans are *Cryptosporidium* hominis and C. *parvum*.

MODE OF TRANSMISSION

Transmission occurs by ingesting fecally contaminated food or water, including water swallowed while swimming. Infection can also occur after exposure to fecally contaminated environmental surfaces and objects and from person-to-person contact, such as diaper changing, caring for an infected person, and sexual contact. Humans can also be infected after contact with infected animals, particularly cows.

EPIDEMIOLOGY

Cryptosporidiosis transmission occurs worldwide. From 1996 through 2005, 1.2 per 1,000 returned travelers seeking medical care at GeoSentinel-associated medical centers around the world were diagnosed with cryptosporidiosis. This proportion likely underestimates the disease incidence, because *Cryptosporidium* requires special staining techniques for diagnosis that are not routinely available in many laboratories. Cryptosporidiosis was most commonly diagnosed in travelers returning from the Middle East, Central America, and South America, although travelers returning from South Asia, sub-Saharan Africa, and the Caribbean were also affected.

Cryptosporidiosis was diagnosed most frequently in missionaries and volunteers but was also diagnosed in tourists, business travelers, and travelers visiting friends and relatives. Overall, however, cryptosporidiosis is a small contributor to travelers' diarrhea in the relatively few detailed etiologic studies that have been done in travelers.

CLINICAL PRESENTATION

Symptoms usually begin 3–14 days after infection with the parasite and are generally self-limited. The most common symptom is watery diarrhea. Other symptoms can include abdominal cramps, vomiting, dehydration, fever, and weight loss. In immunocompetent people, symptoms usually last 1–2 weeks but may persist for a month or, rarely, up to 4 months. Some people may experience a recurrence of symptoms after a brief period of recovery before the illness resolves; symptoms that come and go generally resolve within 1 month. In immunosuppressed people, such as those with AIDS or patients taking immunosuppressive medications, cryptosporidiosis can become chronic and occasionally is fatal. Some people infected with *Cryptosporidium* have no symptoms at all.

DIAGNOSIS

Tests for *Cryptosporidium* are not routinely included in ova and parasite testing in most laboratories. Therefore, clinicians should specifically request testing for this parasite, when suspected. Because *Cryptosporidium* can be difficult to detect, patients may need to submit more than one specimen over several days. Diagnostic techniques include microscopy after modified acid-fast staining or direct fluorescent antibody (considered the gold standard). Enzyme immunoassays to detect *Cryptosporidium* antigens are commercially available. Molecular methods (such as PCR) are increasingly used in reference diagnostic laboratories, since they can be used to identify *Cryptosporidium* at the species level.

TREATMENT

Most immunocompetent people will recover without treatment. Diarrhea should be managed with adequate fluid replacement to prevent dehydration. Nitazoxanide has been approved by the Food and Drug Administration to treat diarrhea caused by *Cryptosporidium* in immunocompetent people and is available for patients aged ≥1 year. However, the effectiveness of nitazoxanide in immunosuppressed people is unclear.

PREVENTIVE MEASURES FOR TRAVELERS

No vaccine is available to prevent cryptosporidiosis, and there is no recommended chemoprophylaxis. Food and water precautions are the main preventive measures (see Chapter 2, Food and Water Precautions). More detailed information about cryptosporidiosis can be found on the CDC website (www.cdc.gov/parasites/crypto). *Cryptosporidium* is poorly inactivated by chlorine or iodine disinfection. Water can be treated effectively by boiling or filtration with an absolute 1-µm filter. Specific information on preventing cryptosporidiosis through filtration can be found in Cryptosporidiosis: A Guide to Water Filters (www.cdc.gov/parasites/crypto/gen_info/filters.html).

BIBLIOGRAPHY

1. American Public Health Association. Cryptosporidiosis. In: Heymann DL, editor. Control of communicable disease manual. Washington, DC: American Public Health Association; 2004. p. 138–42.
2. Greenwood Z, Black J, Weld L, O'Brien D, Leder K, Von Sonnenburg F, et al. Gastrointestinal infection among international travelers globally. J Travel Med. 2008 Jul–Aug;15(4):221–8.
3. Kosek M, Alcantara C, Lima AA, Guerrant RL. Cryptosporidiosis: an update. Lancet Infect Dis. 2001 Nov;1(4):262–9.
4. Roy SL, DeLong SM, Stenzel SA, Shiferaw B, Roberts JM, Khalakdina A, et al. Risk factors for sporadic cryptosporidiosis among immunocompetent persons in the United States from 1999 to 2001. J Clin Microbiol. 2004 Jul;42(7):2944–51.
5. Smith H. Diagnostics. In: Fayer R, Xiao L, editors. Cryptosporidium and Cryptosporidiosis. 2nd ed. Boca Raton, FL: CRC; 2008. p. 173–207.
6. Swaminathan A, Torresi J, Schlagenhauf P, Thursky K, Wilder-Smith A, Connor BA, et al. A global study of pathogens and host risk factors associated with infectious gastrointestinal disease in returned international travellers. J Infect. 2009 Jul;59(1):19–27.
7. Warren CA, Guerrant RL. Clinical disease and pathology. In: Fayer R, Xiao L, editors. Cryptosporidium and Cryptosporidiosis. 2nd ed. Boca Raton, FL: CRC; 2008. p. 235–53.
8. White CA Jr. Nitazoxanide: a new broad spectrum antiparasitic agent. Expert Rev Anti Infect Ther. 2004 Feb;2(1):43–9.

CUTANEOUS LARVA MIGRANS

Susan Montgomery

INFECTIOUS AGENT

Infection is caused by the larval stages of dog and cat hookworms (*Ancylostoma* spp.). Although other worms, such as *Strongyloides* and *Gnathostoma* spp., can migrate through the skin, this section will describe infections with *Ancylostoma* spp.

MODE OF TRANSMISSION

Infection occurs by contact of skin with contaminated soil or beach sand. Eggs shed in the feces of infected hosts hatch in the soil and develop into third-stage larvae, which penetrate the skin and migrate through the epidermis. In humans, larvae are generally confined to the dermis and only rarely penetrate deeper. Deeper penetration is thought to be species specific (such as *A. caninum*).

EPIDEMIOLOGY

Dog hookworms are found worldwide and are the species most commonly associated with cutaneous larva migrans (CLM). Cat hookworms are less commonly implicated. Infection is more likely to occur in tropical and semitropical countries where skin exposure is common and environmental conditions are conducive to larval development in the soil. For tourists, beach environments are the most likely source of infection due to walking and sitting in the sand with bare skin. Most cases are reported in travelers to the Caribbean, Africa, Asia, and South America. Patients without travel history may have acquired the infection in the United States. CLM can occur during summer months in northern areas when warmth and moisture are adequate for development of infective larvae in soil.

CLINICAL PRESENTATION

CLM is typically characterized by a serpiginous, erythematous track that appears in the skin, associated with intense itchiness, redness, and mild swelling. The larvae causing the tracks can migrate a few millimeters to several centimeters per day, depending on parasite species. Typical locations are the bottom or top of the foot or the buttocks.

Itching can occur as the larvae penetrate the skin. Creeping eruption usually appears 1–5 days later, but the incubation period may be up to a month or longer. Infection usually heals spontaneously within weeks to months but has been reported to persist for years in rare cases. Bacterial secondary infection can occur.

DIAGNOSIS

CLM is diagnosed clinically on the basis of characteristic skin lesions. Eosinophilia may not be present, and total IgE is usually normal. Serologic tests are not helpful in CLM except to rule out other causes of larva migrans syndromes such as toxocariasis or strongyloidiasis. Biopsy is not recommended since the track does not usually correlate with larva location.

TREATMENT

Albendazole, 400 mg orally, daily for 3 days, is considered the treatment of choice. Ivermectin (200 µg/kg orally, daily for 1–2 days) is effective but not approved by the Food and Drug Administration for this indication. Additional information can be found on the CDC website (www.cdc.gov/parasites/hookworm).

PREVENTIVE MEASURES FOR TRAVELERS

Infective larvae take about 7 days to develop from eggs passed in dog feces and can survive for weeks in warm, moist soil. Preventive measures include reducing contact with contaminated soil by wearing shoes and protective clothing and using barriers when seated on the ground.

BIBLIOGRAPHY

1. Ansart S, Perez L, Jaureguiberry S, Danis M, Bricaire F, Caumes E. Spectrum of dermatoses in 165 travelers returning from the tropics with skin diseases. Am J Trop Med Hyg. 2007 Jan;76(1):184–6.
2. Bowman DD, Montgomery SP, Zajac AM, Eberhard ML, Kazacos KR. Hookworms of dogs and cats as agents of cutaneous larva migrans. Trends Parasitol. 2010 Apr;26(4):162–7.
3. Caumes E. Treatment of cutaneous larva migrans. Clin Infect Dis. 2000 May;30(5):811–4.
4. Feldmeier H, Heukelbach J. Epidermal parasitic skin diseases: a neglected category of poverty-associated plagues. Bull World Health Organ. 2009 Feb;87(2):152–9.
5. Gillespie SH. Cutaneous larva migrans. Curr Infect Dis Rep. 2004 Feb;6(1):50–3.
6. Heukelbach J, Feldmeier H. Epidemiological and clinical characteristics of hookworm-related cutaneous larva migrans. Lancet Infect Dis. 2008 May;8(5):302–9.
7. Hochedez P, Caumes E. Hookworm-related cutaneous larva migrans. J Travel Med. 2007 Sep-Oct;14(5):326–33.

CYCLOSPORIASIS
David R. Shlim, Barbara L. Herwaldt

INFECTIOUS AGENT

Cyclosporiasis is caused by *Cyclospora cayetanensis*, which is a protozoan (unicellular), coccidian parasite; oocysts (rather than cysts) are shed in the feces of infected people.

MODE OF TRANSMISSION

Infection results from ingestion of mature (infective) *Cyclospora* oocysts, such as in contaminated food or water. Direct person-to-person transmission is unlikely, because the oocysts shed in feces must mature in the environment (outside the host) to become infective to someone else. Limited data indicate that the maturation process requires from days to weeks in favorable conditions.

EPIDEMIOLOGY

Cyclosporiasis appears to be most common in tropical and subtropical regions of the world. Outbreaks in the United States and Canada have been linked to various types of imported fresh produce. People of all ages are at risk for infection, and travelers to developing countries can be at increased risk. In some regions where cyclosporiasis has been studied, the risk for infection is seasonal. However, no consistent pattern has been discerned with respect to time of year or environmental conditions.

CLINICAL PRESENTATION

Cyclospora infects the small intestine. Asymptomatic infection has been documented, particularly in settings where cyclosporiasis is endemic. Among symptomatic people, the incubation period averages 1 week (range, 2 days to more than 2 weeks). Onset of symptoms is often abrupt but can be gradual; some people have an influenzalike prodrome. The most common symptom is watery diarrhea, which can be profuse. Other common symptoms include anorexia, weight loss, abdominal cramps, bloating, nausea, and body aches. Vomiting and low-grade fever may be noted. If untreated, the illness can last for several weeks or months, with a remitting-relapsing course and prolonged fatigue and malaise.

DIAGNOSIS

Infection is diagnosed by detecting *Cyclospora* oocysts (8–10 μm in diameter) in stool specimens. Stool examinations for ova and parasites usually do not include methods for detecting *Cyclospora*. Therefore, clinicians should specifically request testing for this parasite. *Cyclospora* oocysts commonly are shed at low levels, even by people with profuse diarrhea. This constraint underscores the utility of repeated stool examinations, sensitive recovery methods (particularly concentration procedures), and detection methods that highlight the organism. *Cyclospora* oocysts autofluoresce when viewed by UV fluorescence microscopy and can be stained with modified acid-fast or modified ("hot") safranin techniques; these techniques can be used as detection methods for *Cyclospora*. For more information about these and other laboratory methods, visit the CDC website at www.dpd.cdc.gov/dpdx/HTML/Cyclosporiasis.htm. Diagnostic assistance is also available from CDC (see contact information below).

TREATMENT

The treatment of choice is trimethoprim-sulfamethoxazole (TMP-SMX). The typical regimen for immunocompetent adults is TMP 160 mg plus SMX 800 mg (1 double-strength tablet), orally, twice per day for 7–10 days. No highly effective alternatives have been identified for people allergic to (or intolerant of) TMP-SMX. Clinicians may consult CDC about possible approaches for such people (CDC Parasitic Diseases Public Inquiries, 770-488-7775; parasites@cdc.gov). Additional information about clinical issues can be found at www.cdc.gov/parasites/cyclosporiasis.

PREVENTIVE MEASURES FOR TRAVELERS

No vaccine is available. Travelers to developing countries should follow the precautions described in Chapter 2, Food and Water Precautions. Disinfection with chlorine or iodine is unlikely to be effective against *Cyclospora* oocysts.

BIBLIOGRAPHY

1. Herwaldt BL. *Cyclospora cayetanensis*: a review, focusing on the outbreaks of cyclosporiasis in the 1990s. Clin Infect Dis. 2000 Oct;31(4):1040–57.

2. Shlim DR. *Cyclospora cayetanensis*. Clin Lab Med. 2002 Dec;22(4):927–36.

CYSTICERCOSIS
Caryn Bern, Susan Montgomery

INFECTIOUS AGENT

Cysticercosis is caused by infection with the cestode parasite *Taenia solium* in the larval stage.

MODE OF TRANSMISSION

Cysticercosis is acquired by ingesting eggs excreted by a human carrier of the pork tapeworm, *T. solium*. Eating undercooked pork with cysticerci results in tapeworm infection (taeniasis), not human cysticercosis. Fecally contaminated food can transmit the disease, but epidemiologic studies suggest that close (such as household) contact with a tapeworm carrier is the most common risk factor. Tapeworm carriers can be infected by ingestion of eggs they themselves have excreted; patients with cysticercosis and their household contacts should have stool specimens examined for eggs.

EPIDEMIOLOGY

Cysticercosis is common in all countries where sanitary conditions are poor or where pigs are raised with access to human feces (Latin America, Asia, and Africa). Cysticercosis is uncommon in returning travelers; 3 case reports have been published.

CLINICAL PRESENTATION

The latent period (before symptoms) is a median of 5 years (range, 1–30 years). Cysticercosis symptoms depend on the number, location, and stage of cysts. The most common location is brain parenchyma, with late-onset seizures. Other presentations include increased intracranial pressure, encephalitis, symptoms of space-occupying lesion, and hydrocephalus. Cysticercosis should be ruled out in any adult with first-onset seizures who comes from an endemic area.

DIAGNOSIS

Diagnosis is based on neuroimaging studies (CT or MRI) and confirmatory serologic testing. The most reliable serologic test is the enzyme-linked immunotransfer blot, but even this test may be negative in up to 30% of patients with a single parenchymal lesion. The test is more sensitive in serum than in cerebrospinal fluid.

TREATMENT

Neurocysticercosis is uncommon in the United States, and the inexperienced clinician is advised to consult an infectious disease or tropical medicine specialist for diagnosis and treatment. Physicians can consult with CDC's Division of Parasitic Diseases and Malaria to obtain information about diagnosis and treatment (dpdx@cdc.gov; www.dpd.cdc.gov/dpdx). Albendazole and dexamethasone are some of the drugs used for treatment. For some lesions, surgical intervention may be the treatment of choice.

Antiparasitic treatment should **not** be initiated in patients with heavy infections, cysticercotic encephalitis, or increased intracranial pressure, because dying cysts can worsen symptoms and cause increased inflammation and edema. In these cases, the priority is neurologic management (steroids, mannitol), neurosurgical management, or both.

PREVENTIVE MEASURES FOR TRAVELERS

No vaccine is available. No drugs for preventing infection are available. Preventive measures are aimed at avoiding consumption of fecally contaminated food.

BIBLIOGRAPHY

1. Garcia HH, Del Brutto OH. Neurocysticercosis: updated concepts about an old disease. Lancet Neurol. 2005 Oct;4(10):653–61.

2. Garcia HH, Del Brutto OH, Nash TE, White AC, Jr., Tsang VC, Gilman RH. New concepts in the diagnosis and management of neurocysticercosis (*Taenia solium*). Am J Trop Med Hyg. 2005 Jan;72(1):3–9.

DENGUE FEVER & DENGUE HEMORRHAGIC FEVER

Kay M. Tomashek

INFECTIOUS AGENT

The 4 dengue viruses (DENV) are immunologically related, positive-strand RNA viruses of the genus *Flavivirus*, family Flaviviridae. These viruses cause both dengue fever (DF) and dengue hemorrhagic fever (DHF). Asymptomatic infection also occurs. Infection with 1 DENV produces lifelong immunity against reinfection with that DENV type but no long-term cross-protection against the other 3 DENV types (any cross-protection is ≤2 months).

MODE OF TRANSMISSION

Transmission occurs principally from the bite of an infected *Aedes aegypti* (and, less commonly, *Ae. albopictus* or *Ae. polynesiensis*) mosquito. Female mosquitoes acquire DENV by biting viremic humans and become infective after an extrinsic incubation period of 8–12 days. The infected mosquito can then transmit DENV for the rest of its life (the mosquito lifespan is approximately 1 month).

Less common modes of DENV transmission include through exposure to DENV-infected blood, organs, or other tissues via blood transfusion, solid organ or bone marrow transplantation, and nosocomial injury (needlestick or mucous membrane contact with spilled blood). DENV can be vertically transmitted from an infected woman to her fetus in utero or to the infant during childbirth. Direct person-to-person transmission has not been documented.

EPIDEMIOLOGY

DENV infections have been reported in over 100 countries in Africa, the Americas, the Caribbean, Eastern Mediterranean, Southeast Asia and the Western Pacific regions (Maps 3-1 and 3-2). The World Health Organization (WHO) estimates that 50 million cases of dengue occur every year, and 500,000 (1%) require hospitalization. The geographic spread of dengue is similar to that of malaria, but unlike malaria, dengue is often found in populated urban and residential areas of tropical nations. Travelers are advised to consult CDC (www.cdc.gov/dengue/travelOutbreaks/index.html) and WHO (www.who.int/topics/dengue/en/) websites to determine if dengue is endemic in the country they plan to visit and if an outbreak is ongoing.

Several dengue outbreaks have been detected in the continental United States since 1980, including 7 outbreaks in southern Texas along the United States-Mexico border, one outbreak in Hawaii in 2001, and 2 outbreaks in southern Florida in 2009 and 2010. Several southeastern states have a nearly year-round *Aedes* population, a susceptible human population, and ample opportunity for viral introduction from international visitors and returning US travelers. Differences in housing (use of air conditioning and screens, for example) and lifestyle, however, may prevent dengue from becoming endemic in these states.

Cases of DF and DHF are confirmed every year among travelers returning to the United States. However, it was not until June 2009 that DENV infections became nationally reportable in the United States, so case reporting among travelers before January 2010 is limited. Infection rates (based on serology) among febrile travelers returning from dengue-endemic areas in the tropics are 3%–8%. In a recent study of 17,353 ill travelers seen at GeoSentinel surveillance network clinics, dengue was the leading cause of systemic febrile illness among travelers returning from the Caribbean, South America, south-central Asia, and Southeast Asia. In some case studies, dengue is the second most common cause of hospitalization (malaria is the most common) among travelers returning from the tropics.

Published data are limited on the health outcomes associated with DENV infection among pregnant women and the effects of maternal DENV infection on a developing fetus. Vertical transmission can occur, and peripartum maternal infections may increase the likelihood of symptomatic disease in the newborn. Of the 24 vertical transmission cases described in the literature, average time of onset between maternal and neonatal onset of fever was 7 days (range, 5–13 days). All cases presented with fever and thrombocytopenia, and many also had hepatomegaly and hemorrhage. Transplacental transfer of maternal IgG anti-DENV (from a previous maternal infection) may place infants at higher risk for DHF if they acquire DENV infection during the second half of their first year of life.

CLINICAL PRESENTATION

Dengue should be considered in the differential diagnosis of all febrile patients with a history of travel to the tropics and subtropics in the 2 weeks before symptom onset. The incubation period is typically 4–7 days (range, 3–14 days). A mild febrile infection with DENV may not be identified as DF. Many travelers infected with DENV for the first time have mild, undifferentiated febrile illness or are asymptomatic. However, subsequent infections with DENV are usually associated with more severe disease. DF is defined clinically by WHO as an acute febrile illness with 2 or more of the following: headache, retroorbital pain, muscle aches, joint pain, rash, hemorrhagic manifestation, or leukopenia. The rash usually appears as the fever subsides and lasts 2–4 days. The rash is either macular or maculopapular and generalized, often confluent with small patches of normal skin, and it may become scaly and pruritic. Other signs and symptoms include flushed skin (usually during the first 24–48 hours), nausea, and vomiting. Approximately 1% of patients with DF develop DHF as the fever subsides (usually 3–8 days after the onset of fever). Subsequent infection with a different DENV is usually associated with more severe disease.

Increased vascular permeability and plasma leakage differentiates DHF from DF. DHF is characterized by all of the following: fever or history of fever lasting 2–7 days, evidence of hemorrhagic manifestation or a positive tourniquet test, thrombocytopenia ($\leq$100,000 cells/mm^3), evidence of plasma leakage including hemoconcentration (an increase in hematocrit $\geq$20% above average for age or a decrease in hematocrit $\geq$20% of baseline after fluid replacement therapy), pleural effusion, ascites, or hypoproteinemia. Thrombocytopenia by itself does not indicate DHF. Dengue shock syndrome (DSS) is defined as a syndrome in a patient who meets the criteria for DHF and has hypotension, narrow pulse pressure ($\leq$20 mm Hg), or frank shock.

DIAGNOSIS

A suspected case of dengue can be laboratory confirmed by using a combination of the following in a single serum specimen: detection of DENV genomic sequences or detection of DENV antigens (nonstructural protein 1; NS1 antigen) and serologic testing for IgM anti-DENV. Detection of DENV genomes or NS1 antigen is used primarily in the acute febrile stage of the illness ($\leq$5 days after symptom onset), and testing for IgM anti-DENV is used primarily >5 days after fever onset.

Although DENV can be isolated in cell culture from serum, cerebrospinal fluid, or autopsy tissue specimens, this method is not particularly useful in this era of molecular diagnostic testing. Specific DENV genomes can be routinely identified by RT-PCR from serum or plasma, cerebrospinal fluid, or autopsy tissue specimens. NS1 antigen circulates in blood during the period of viremia, and several immunoassays are available. DENV antigens can be identified in tissue specimens by immunofluorescence or immunohistochemical analysis. The primary serologic test for DENV in patients with acute illness is IgM anti-DENV, which becomes positive >5 days after symptom onset.

Other approaches to laboratory confirmation include the following:

- Seroconversion (negative to positive) to IgM anti-DENV from acute-phase (<5 days after fever onset) specimens to convalescent-phase (>5 days after symptom onset) specimens
- ≥4-fold rise in reciprocal IgG anti-DENV titer or hemagglutination inhibition titer to DENV antigens in acute- and convalescent-phase serum samples
- IgM anti-DENV in cerebrospinal fluid

In combination with a compatible travel history and symptom profile, IgM anti-DENV in a single serum sample suggests a probable recent DENV infection. However, IgG anti-DENV in a single serum sample can indicate either a recent or past DENV infection. Caution should be exercised when using only antibody testing results (IgM or IgG anti-DENV) from a single specimen, because DENV antibodies cross-react with antibodies from other flaviviruses, such as West Nile, yellow fever, and Japanese encephalitis viruses. Previous infection or vaccination with another flavivirus may result in false-positive IgG or IgM anti-DENV results.

There are several commercially available diagnostic tests for dengue; however, none have been approved by the Food and Drug Administration. Testing is available at some state laboratories. Testing is also available through CDC (see "Requesting Dengue Laboratory Testing and Reporting" at www.cdc.gov/Dengue/clinicalLab/index.html). Acute- and convalescent-phase serum samples should be sent through state or territorial health department laboratories to CDC at 1324 Calle Cañada, San Juan, Puerto Rico 00920-3860. Serum samples should be accompanied by clinical and epidemiologic information, including the date of disease onset and sample collection and the patient's detailed recent travel history. For additional information, contact the CDC Dengue Branch (787-706-2399) or see www.cdc.gov/dengue.

TREATMENT

No specific therapeutic agents exist for dengue virus infections. Encourage bed rest and maintenance of fluids to prevent dehydration while the patient is febrile. Control fever with acetaminophen. Headache, eye pain, joint pain, and muscle ache may require narcotics. Aspirin, aspirin-containing drugs, and other nonsteroidal anti-inflammatory drugs (such as ibuprofen) should be avoided because of their anticoagulant properties. Aspirin and other salicylates should be especially avoided in children because of the association with Reye syndrome.

Ask patients to watch for warning signs of DHF or DSS as the fever declines, and instruct them to go to the hospital if they develop any of the following warning signs: abrupt change from fever to hypothermia, severe abdominal pain, persistent vomiting, bleeding, difficulties breathing, or altered mental status (such as irritability, confusion, lethargy). Prompt and judicious intravenous administration of isotonic crystalloids and colloids in patients with DHF or DSS can improve outcomes. In patients with DHF or DSS, hospitalization with close monitoring of vital signs, fluid balance, and hematologic parameters (hematocrit, platelet count) is indicated, as well as additional supportive measures.

PREVENTIVE MEASURES FOR TRAVELERS

Neither vaccine nor drugs for preventing infection are available. The bite of one infected mosquito can result in infection. The risk of being bitten is highest during the early morning, several hours after daybreak, and in the late afternoon before sunset. However, mosquitoes may feed at any time during the day. *Aedes* mosquitoes typically live indoors and are often found in dark, cool places such as in closets, under beds, behind curtains, and in bathrooms. Travelers should be advised to use insecticides to get rid of mosquitoes in these areas and to select accommodations with well-screened windows or air conditioning when possible. Additionally, travelers should take measures to avoid being bitten by mosquitoes (see Chapter 2, Protection against Mosquitos, Ticks, and Other Arthropods). Long-term travelers and expatriates can take extra precautions to reduce mosquito-breeding sites around their accommodations by emptying and cleaning or covering any standing water (such as in water storage tanks and flowerpot trays).

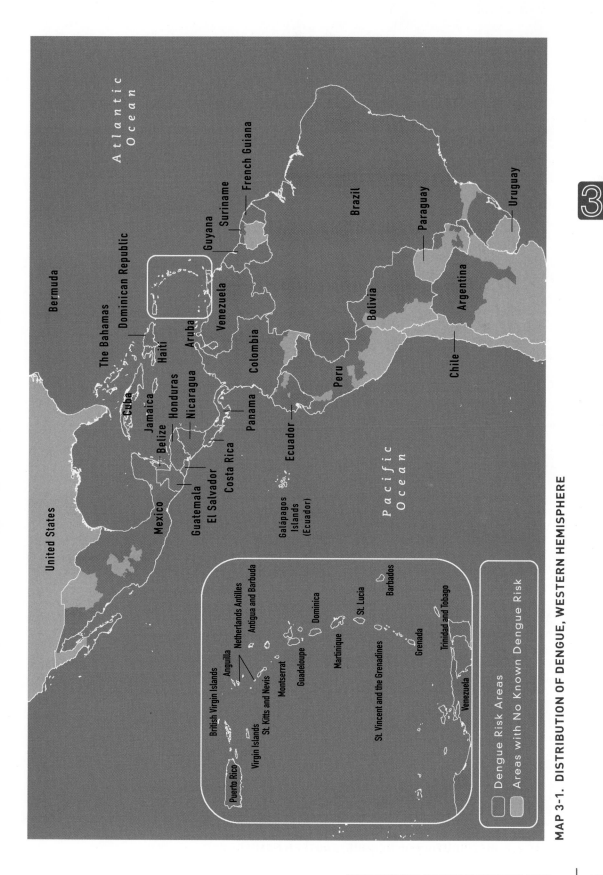

MAP 3-1. DISTRIBUTION OF DENGUE, WESTERN HEMISPHERE

Dengue Risk Areas

Areas with No Known Dengue Risk

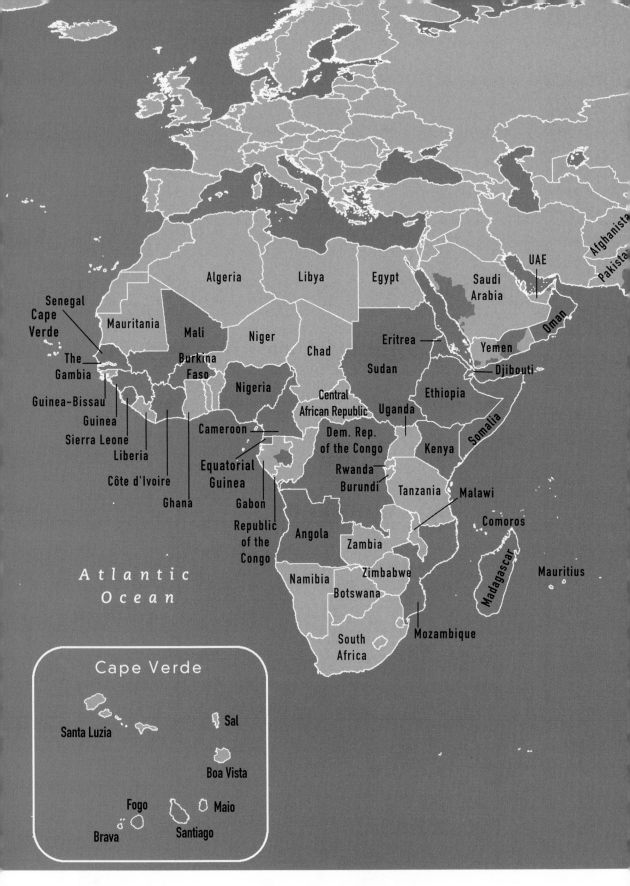

MAP 3-2. DISTRIBUTION OF DENGUE, EASTERN HEMISPHERE

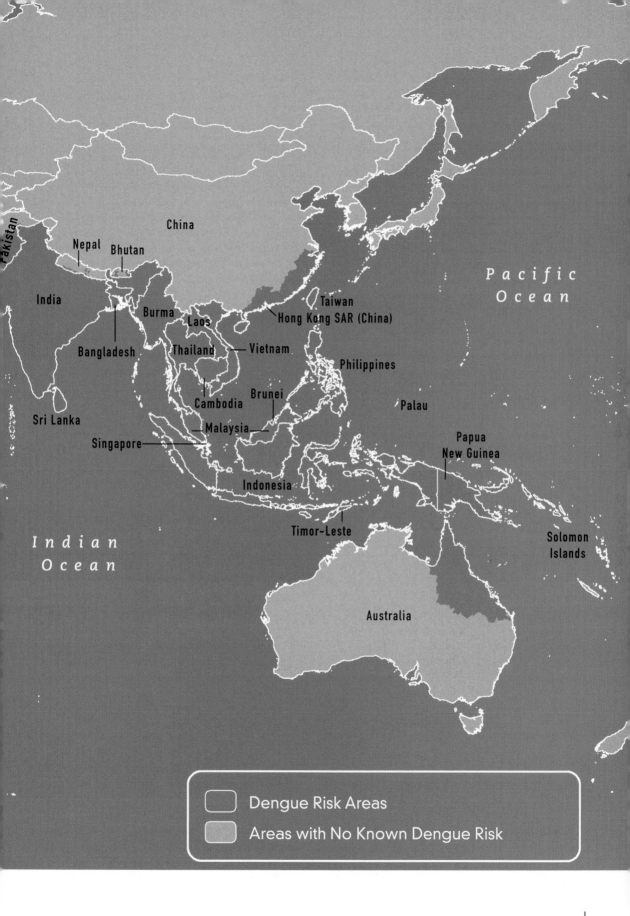

BIBLIOGRAPHY

1. Cobelens FG, Groen J, Osterhaus AD, Leentvaar-Kuipers A, Wertheim-van Dillen PM, Kager PA. Incidence and risk factors of probable dengue virus infection among Dutch travellers to Asia. Trop Med Int Health. 2002 Apr;7(4):331–8.

2. Freedman DO, Weld LH, Kozarsky PE, Fisk T, Robins R, von Sonnenburg F, et al. Spectrum of disease and relation to place of exposure among ill returned travelers. N Engl J Med. 2006 Jan 12;354(2):119–30.

3. Gubler DJ. The global emergence/resurgence of arboviral diseases as public health problems. Arch Med Res. 2002 Jul–Aug;33(4):330–42.

4. Hunsperger EA, Yoksan S, Buchy P, Nguyen VC, Sekaran SD, Enria DA, et al. Evaluation of commercially available anti-dengue virus immunoglobulin M tests. Emerg Infect Dis. 2009 Mar;15(3):436–40.

5. Jelinek T, Dobler G, Holscher M, Loscher T, Nothdurft HD. Prevalence of infection with dengue virus among international travelers. Arch Intern Med. 1997 Nov 10;157(20):2367–70.

6. Lindback H, Lindback J, Tegnell A, Janzon R, Vene S, Ekdahl K. Dengue fever in travelers to the tropics, 1998 and 1999. Emerg Infect Dis. 2003 Apr;9(4):438–42.

7. O'Brien D, Tobin S, Brown GV, Torresi J. Fever in returned travelers: review of hospital admissions for a 3-year period. Clin Infect Dis. 2001 Sep 1;33(5):603–9.

8. Potasman I, Srugo I, Schwartz E. Dengue seroconversion among Israeli travelers to tropical countries. Emerg Infect Dis. 1999 Nov-Dec;5(6):824–7.

9. Schwartz E, Mendelson E, Sidi Y. Dengue fever among travelers. Am J Med. 1996 Nov;101(5):516–20.

10. Wichmann O, Lauschke A, Frank C, Shu PY, Niedrig M, Huang JH, et al. Dengue antibody prevalence in German travelers. Emerg Infect Dis. 2005 May;11(5):762–5.

11. Wilder-Smith A, Schwartz E. Dengue in travelers. N Engl J Med. 2005 Sep 1;353(9):924–32.

12. World Health Organization. Dengue haemorrhagic fever: diagnosis, treatment, prevention and control. 3rd ed. Geneva: World Health Organization; 2008.

DIPHTHERIA

Tejpratap S. P. Tiwari

INFECTIOUS AGENT

Diphtheria is caused by toxigenic strains of *Corynebacterium diphtheriae* biotype *mitis, gravis, intermedius,* or *belfanti.* The bacteria produce an exotoxin that, if absorbed in the bloodstream, may damage nerves and organs such as the heart and kidneys.

MODE OF TRANSMISSION

Humans are the only known reservoir of *C. diphtheriae.* Person-to-person transmission occurs through oral or respiratory droplets, close physical contact, and rarely, by fomites. Cutaneous diphtheria is common in tropical countries, and contact with discharge from skin lesions may transmit infection in these environments.

EPIDEMIOLOGY

Diphtheria is found worldwide; countries with endemic diphtheria are shown in Table 3-1.

During the 1990s, large epidemics occurred in the newly independent states of the former Soviet Union. More recently in the Americas, diphtheria outbreaks have occurred in Haiti and the Dominican Republic. Diphtheria is uncommon in industrialized countries because of longstanding routine use of DTP (diphtheria and tetanus toxoids and pertussis vaccine). Diphtheria is rare in the United States; the last case occurred in an elderly traveler returning from Haiti in 2003. Diphtheria causes significant illness and death in developing countries where vaccination coverage is low.

Symptomatic infection is extremely rare in adequately immunized people, even though active immunization with diphtheria toxoid does not prevent colonization or transient carriage of *C. diphtheriae.* Higher risk of acquiring disease and potentially life-threatening

Table 3-1. Countries with endemic diphtheria

REGION	COUNTRIES
Africa	Algeria, Angola, Egypt, Eritrea, Ethiopia, Guinea, Niger, Nigeria, Sudan, Zambia, and other sub-Saharan countries
Americas	Bolivia, Brazil, Colombia, Dominican Republic, Ecuador, Haiti, and Paraguay
Asia/South Pacific	Bangladesh, Bhutan, Burma (Myanmar), Cambodia, China, India, Indonesia, Laos, Malaysia, Mongolia, Nepal, Pakistan, Papua New Guinea, Philippines, Thailand, and Vietnam
Middle East	Afghanistan, Iran, Iraq, Saudi Arabia, Syria, Turkey, and Yemen
Europe	Albania, Armenia, Azerbaijan, Belarus, Estonia, Georgia, Kazakhstan, Kyrgyzstan, Latvia, Lithuania, Moldova, Russia, Tajikistan, Turkmenistan, Ukraine, and Uzbekistan

complications are possible in inadequately immunized or unimmunized travelers to countries with endemic diphtheria.

CLINICAL PRESENTATION

The incubation period is 2–5 days (range, 1–10 days). Affected anatomic sites include the mucous membrane of the upper respiratory tract (nose, pharynx, tonsils, larynx, and trachea [respiratory diphtheria]), skin (cutaneous diphtheria), or rarely, mucous membranes at other sites (eye, ear, vulva). Nasal diphtheria can be asymptomatic or mild, with a blood-tinged discharge.

Respiratory diphtheria has a gradual onset and is characterized by a mild fever (rarely >101°F [38.3°C]), sore throat, difficulty swallowing, malaise, loss of appetite, and if the larynx is involved, hoarseness. The hallmark of respiratory diphtheria is a pseudomembrane that appears within 2–3 days of illness over the mucous lining of the tonsils, pharynx, larynx, or nares and that can extend into the trachea. The pseudomembrane is firm, fleshy, grey, and adherent, and it will bleed after attempts to remove or dislodge it. Fatal airway obstruction can result if the pseudomembrane extends into the larynx or trachea, or if a piece of it becomes dislodged.

In severe respiratory diphtheria, cervical lymphadenopathy and soft-tissue swelling in the neck give rise to a "bull-neck" appearance. Systemic complications, including myocarditis and polyneuropathies, can result from absorption of diphtheria toxin from the infection site. However, cutaneous and nasal diphtheria are localized and rarely associated with systemic toxicity. The case-fatality ratio of respiratory diphtheria is 5%–10%.

DIAGNOSIS

A presumptive diagnosis is usually based on clinical features. Diagnosis is confirmed by isolating C. diphtheriae from culture of nasal or throat swabs or membrane tissue. Toxin production is confirmed by performing a modified Elek test. PCR assays can also be performed on isolates, swabs, or membrane specimens to rapidly confirm the presence of the tox gene responsible for production of diphtheria toxin, but the test is available only in research or reference laboratories.

TREATMENT

Patients with respiratory diphtheria require hospitalization to monitor response to treatment and manage complications. Equine diphtheria antitoxin (DAT) is the mainstay of treatment and is administered after specimen testing, without waiting for laboratory confirmation. In the United States, DAT is available to physicians under a Food and Drug Administration–approved investigational new drug protocol by contacting CDC at 770-488-7100.

An appropriate antibiotic (erythromycin or penicillin) should be used to eliminate the causative organisms, stop exotoxin production, and reduce communicability. Supportive care (airway, cardiac monitoring) is required. Antimicrobial prophylaxis (erythromycin or penicillin) is recommended for close contacts of patients.

PREVENTIVE MEASURES FOR TRAVELERS

Vaccine

For protection against diphtheria, all travelers should be up to date with diphtheria toxoid vaccine before departure. Diphtheria toxoid is not manufactured as a monovalent vaccine but is available in pediatric (D) and adult formulations (d) that are combined with other vaccines such as tetanus toxoid (DT, Td), tetanus toxoid and acellular or whole-cell pertussis antigens (DTaP, DTwP, Tdap), or as a DTwP/DTaP combination with other antigens (such as hepatitis B, inactivated poliovirus vaccines, or *Haemophilus influenzae* type b vaccine).

In the United States, infants and children aged <7 years are vaccinated with diphtheria toxoid in combination with tetanus toxoid and acellular pertussis vaccine (DTaP) according to the routine childhood immunization schedule recommended by the ACIP (see Chapter 7, Vaccine Recommendations for Infants and Children). Immunization for infants and children aged <7 years consists of 5 doses of DTaP vaccine. The first 3 doses are usually given at ages 2, 4, and 6 months, followed by booster doses at ages 12–18 months and 4–6 years (see Table 7-2).

Adolescents aged 11–18 years should receive a dose of Tdap instead of Td for booster immunization against tetanus, diphtheria, and pertussis if they have completed the recommended childhood DTwP/DTaP vaccination series (see Table 7-3). Adults aged 19–64 years who have not previously received Tdap should receive a single dose of age-appropriate Tdap to replace a single dose of Td for active booster immunization against tetanus, diphtheria and pertussis. Adults aged ≥65 years who have or who anticipate having close contact with an infant aged <12 months and who have not previously received Tdap should receive a single dose of Tdap to protect against pertussis and reduce the likelihood of transmission; all other adults aged ≥65 years who have not previously received Tdap may be given a single dose of Tdap instead of Td. Thereafter, routine booster doses with Td should be given to all adults every 10 years to maintain seroprotection against diphtheria, as well as tetanus. This booster is particularly important for travelers who will live or work with local populations in countries where diphtheria is endemic.

Adolescents and adults who have never been immunized against pertussis, tetanus, or diphtheria, who have incomplete immunization, or whose immunity is uncertain should follow the catch-up schedule established for Td/Tdap. Tdap can be substituted for any of the Td doses in the series.

BIBLIOGRAPHY

1. American Academy of Pediatrics. Diphtheria. In: Pickering LK, Baker CJ, Long SS, McMillan JA, editors. Red Book: 2009 Report of the Committee on Infectious Diseases. 28th ed. Elk Grove Village, IL: American Academy of Pediatrics; 2009. p. 280–83.

2. Bisgard KM, Hardy IR, Popovic T, Strebel PM, Wharton M, Chen RT, et al. Respiratory diphtheria in the United States, 1980 through 1995. Am J Public Health. 1998 May;88(5):787–91.

3. CDC. Availability of diphtheria antitoxin through an investigational new drug protocol. MMWR Morb Mortal Wkly Rep. 2004;53(19):413.

4. CDC. Diphtheria acquired by US citizens in the Russian Federation and Ukraine—1994. MMWR Morb Mortal Wkly Rep. 1995 Mar 31;44(12):237, 43–4.

5. CDC. Fatal respiratory diphtheria in a US traveler to Haiti—Pennsylvania, 2003. MMWR Morb Mortal Wkly Rep. 2004 Jan 9;52(53):1285–6.

6. CDC. Updated recommendations for use of tetanus toxoid, reduced diphtheria toxoid and acellular pertussis (Tdap) vaccine from the Advisory Committee on Immunization Practices, 2010. MMWR Morb Mortal Wkly Rep. 2011 Jan 14;60(1):13–5.

7. Farizo KM, Strebel PM, Chen RT, Kimbler A, Cleary TJ, Cochi SL. Fatal respiratory disease due to

Corynebacterium diphtheriae: case report and review of guidelines for management, investigation, and control. Clin Infect Dis. 1993 Jan;16(1):59–68.

8. Galazka A. The changing epidemiology of diphtheria in the vaccine era. J Infect Dis. 2000 Feb;181 Suppl 1:S2–9.

9. Kretsinger K, Broder KR, Cortese MM, Joyce MP, Ortega-Sanchez I, Lee GM, et al. Preventing tetanus, diphtheria, and pertussis among adults: use of tetanus toxoid, reduced diphtheria toxoid and acellular pertussis vaccine recommendations of the Advisory Committee on Immunization Practices (ACIP) and recommendation of ACIP, supported by the Healthcare Infection Control Practices Advisory Committee (HICPAC), for use of Tdap among health-care personnel. MMWR Recomm Rep. 2006 Dec 15;55(RR-17):1–37.

10. Wharton M, Vitek CR. Diphtheria toxoid. In: Plotkin SA, Orenstein WA, editors. Vaccines. 4th ed. Philadelphia: WB Saunders; 2004. p. 211–28.

11. World Health Organization. WHO vaccine-preventable diseases monitoring system: 2009 global summary. Geneva: WHO; 2009. Available from: http://www.who.int/immunization/documents/WHO_IVB_2009/en/index.html.

ECHINOCOCCOSIS

Pedro L. Moro, Peter M. Schantz

INFECTIOUS AGENT

Echinococcosis (hydatid disease) is the infection of humans by the larval stages of taeniid cestodes of the genus *Echinococcus*. Of 6 species recognized, 4 are of public health concern: *Echinococcus granulosus*, causing cystic echinococcosis; *E. multilocularis*, causing alveolar echinococcosis; and *E. vogeli* and *E. oligarthrus*, both causing polycystic echinococcosis.

E. shiquicus in small mammals from the Tibetan plateau and *E. felidis* in African lions are 2 recently identified species whose zoonotic transmission potential is unknown.

MODE OF TRANSMISSION

The life cycle of *Echinococcus* species involves carnivores as final hosts and herbivores as intermediate hosts. Certain human activities (such as the widespread rural practice of feeding viscera of home-butchered sheep to dogs) facilitate transmission of the parasite, and consequently raise the risk that humans will become infected. Dogs infected with *Echinococcus* tapeworms pass eggs in their feces, and humans become infected through fecal-oral contact, particularly in the course of playful and close contact between children and dogs. Indirect transfer of eggs, either through contaminated water and uncooked food or through the intermediary of flies and other arthropods, can also result in infection of humans.

EPIDEMIOLOGY

E. granulosus is prevalent in broad regions of Eurasia, several South American countries, and Africa. In North America, most cases are diagnosed in immigrants from endemic countries. The disease seems to have reemerged in Bulgaria, where the incidence of cystic echinococcosis in children increased from 0.7 to 5.4 per 100,000 population per year between the 1970s and the mid-1990s, after the collapse of control efforts. In Wales, the prevalence of infected dogs more than doubled between 1993 (3.4%) and 2002 (8.1%), after the implementation of policy changes favoring health education over weekly dosing of dogs with praziquantel. E. multilocularis is endemic in the central part of Europe, parts of the Near East, Russia, the Central Asian Republics, China, northern Japan, and Alaska. Recent findings show major endemic areas for *E. granulosis* and *E. multilocularis* in China. E. vogeli is indigenous to the humid tropical forests in central and northern South America. In endemic areas, hunting dogs are often fed the raw viscera of pacas; dogs thus infected may then expose humans. A small number of polycystic echinococcosis cases in these geographic areas are caused by *E. oligarthrus*.

CLINICAL PRESENTATION

Cystic Echinococcosis or Cystic Hydatid Disease

In humans, hydatid cysts of E. *granulosus* are slowly enlarging masses comparable to benign neoplasms; most human infections remain asymptomatic. The clinical manifestations are variable and are determined by the site, size, and condition of the cysts. Hydatid cysts in the liver and the lungs together account for 90% of affected localizations.

Alveolar Echinococcosis or Alveolar Hydatid Disease

The embryo of E. *multilocularis* seems to localize invariably in the liver of the intermediate host. The hepatic parenchyma is gradually invaded and replaced by fibrous tissue in which great numbers of vesicles, many microscopic, are embedded. Patients eventually succumb to hepatic failure, invasion of contiguous structures, or less frequently, metastases to the brain.

Polycystic Echinococcosis or Polycystic Hydatid Disease

Relatively large cysts develop over years and are primarily found in the liver and occasionally in the thorax or abdominal cavity. Those who are symptomatic may present with a painful right hypochondrial mass, progressive jaundice, or as in the other forms of disease, with liver abscess(es).

DIAGNOSIS

A presumptive diagnosis can be made on the basis of imaging studies, such as a CT scan, and sometimes lesions are found incidentally in an asymptomatic person. Serologic assays may also be performed, and newer ones are under development. Additional information and diagnostic assistance is available through CDC's Division of Parasitic Diseases and Malaria (www.dpd.cdc.gov/dpdx).

TREATMENT

Travelers should consult an infectious disease or tropical medicine specialist for diagnosis and treatment. Surgical removal of hydatid cysts remains the treatment of choice in many countries, and it is the preferred treatment when liver cysts are large (>10 cm in diameter), secondarily infected, or located in certain organs (brain, lung, or kidney). Puncture, aspiration, injection, reaspiration (PAIR) is a minimally invasive technique used to treat liver cysts and other abdominal locations. It is less risky and less expensive than surgery. Approximately 30% of patients treated with albendazole become cured after 3–6 months (complete and permanent disappearance of cysts), and even higher proportions (30%–50%) demonstrate significant regression of cyst size and alleviation of symptoms. However, 20%–40% of cases do not respond favorably. Albendazole should be given orally at a dose of 10–15 mg/kg/day, in 2 divided doses, with a fat-rich meal to increase bioavailability. It should be administered continuously. An intermittent treatment schedule has been recommended in the past, but evidence suggests that continuous treatment may be equally effective. Benzimidazoles (albendazole, mebendazole) should be given to prevent recurrence after surgery or PAIR. With or without surgery, alveolar hydatid disease has a high case-fatality rate. Long-term treatment with a benzimidazole inhibits growth of larval E. *multilocularis*, reduces metastasis, and enhances both the quality and length of survival; prolonged therapy may eventually be larvicidal in some patients. The principles of management for cystic and alveolar echinococcoses also apply to polycystic echinococcosis.

PREVENTIVE MEASURES FOR TRAVELERS

No vaccine is available for humans, and no drugs are recommended as chemoprophylactic agents. Travelers should avoid contact with dogs or wild canids while in endemic areas. Untreated water from streams, canals, lakes, and rivers may contain Echinococcus eggs. Heating potentially contaminated food and water at >140°F (60°C) for at least 30 minutes destroys the eggs.

BIBLIOGRAPHY

1. Brunetti E, Kern P, Vuitton DA. Expert consensus for the diagnosis and treatment of cystic and alveolar echinococcosis in humans. Acta Trop. 2010 Apr;114(1):1–16.

2. D'Alessandro A. Polycystic echinococcosis in tropical America: *Echinococcus vogeli* and E. *oligarthrus*. Acta Trop. 1997 Sep 15;67(1–2):43–65.

3. Eckert J, Gottstein B, Heath D, Liu FJ. Prevention of echinococcosis in humans and safety precautions. In: Eckert J, Gemmell MA, Meslin FX, Pawlowski ZS, editors. WHO/OIE Manual on Echinococcosis in Humans and Animals: a Public Health Problem of Global Concern. Paris: World Organization for Animal Health; 2001. p. 238–45.

4. Filippou D, Tselepis D, Filippou G, Papadopoulos V. Advances in liver echinococcosis: diagnosis and treatment. Clin Gastroenterol Hepatol. 2007 Feb;5(2):152–9.

5. Moro P, Schantz PM. Hydatid disease (echinococcosis). In: Wallace R, editor. Public Health and Preventive Medicine. 15th ed. New York: McGraw-Hill 2008. p. 448–60.

6. Moro PL, Schantz PM. Echinococcosis: historical landmarks and progress in research and control. Ann Trop Med Parasitol. 2006 Dec;100(8):703–14.

7. Romig T, Dinkel A, Mackenstedt U. The present situation of echinococcosis in Europe. Parasitol Int. 2006;55 Suppl:S187–91.

8. Schantz PM. Progress in diagnosis, treatment and elimination of echinococcosis and cysticercosis. Parasitol Int. 2006;55 Suppl:S7–S13.

9. Siqueira NG, de Almeida FB, Chalub SR, Machado-Silva JR, Rodrigues-Silva R. Successful outcome of hepatic polycystic echinococcosis managed with surgery and chemotherapy. Trans R Soc Trop Med Hyg. 2007 Jun;101(6):624–6.

10. Smego RA Jr, Sebanego P. Treatment options for hepatic cystic echinococcosis. Int J Infect Dis. 2005 Mar;9(2):69–76.

11. Wilson JF, Rausch RL. Alveolar hydatid disease. A review of clinical features of 33 indigenous cases of *Echinococcus multilocularis* infection in Alaskan Eskimos. Am J Trop Med Hyg. 1980 Nov;29(6):1340–55.

12. Yang YR, Craig PS, Ito A, Vuitton DA, Giraudoux P, Sun T, et al. A correlative study of ultrasound with serology in an area in China co-endemic for human alveolar and cystic echinococcosis. Trop Med Int Health. 2007 May;12(5):637–46.

FILARIASIS, LYMPHATIC

LeAnne M. Fox

INFECTIOUS AGENT

Lymphatic filariasis is caused by the filarial nematodes *Wuchereria bancrofti*, *Brugia malayi*, and *B. timori*.

MODE OF TRANSMISSION

Vectorborne transmission occurs through the bite of infected *Aedes*, *Culex*, *Anopheles*, and *Mansonia* mosquito species.

EPIDEMIOLOGY

Lymphatic filariasis affects an estimated 120 million people in tropical areas of the world. Lymphatic filariasis is found in sub-Saharan Africa, Egypt, southern Asia, the western Pacific Islands, the northeastern coast of Brazil, Guyana, Haiti, and the Dominican Republic. Since most infections are asymptomatic, many go unrecognized. Short-term travelers to endemic areas are at low risk for this infection. Travelers who visit endemic areas for extended periods of time (generally >3 months) and who are intensively exposed to infected mosquitoes are at higher risk of infection. Most infections seen in the United States are in immigrants from endemic countries.

A recent report from the GeoSentinel Surveillance Network showed only 0.62% (271 of 43,722) of medical conditions reported from 1995 through 2004 were caused by any filarial infection, and of these, only 68 (25%) were caused by *W. bancrofti* and were acquired worldwide: 32% from South America, 12% from sub-Saharan Africa, 22% from south-central Asia, and 14% from the Caribbean. As expected, most cases (62%) were seen in immigrants or refugees. In the few nonresident visitors with a known trip duration who acquired *W. bancrofti*, the stay was >180 days.

CLINICAL PRESENTATION

Most infections are asymptomatic, but living adult worms cause progressive lymphatic vessel dilation and dysfunction. Lymphatic dysfunction may lead to lymphedema of the leg, scrotum, penis, arm, or breast, which can increase in severity as a result of recurrent secondary bacterial infections. Tropical pulmonary eosinophilia is a potentially serious progressive lung disease that presents with nocturnal cough, wheezing, and fever, resulting from immune hyperresponsiveness to microfilariae in the pulmonary capillaries.

DIAGNOSIS

The standard for diagnosis is microscopic detection of microfilariae on a thick blood film. In most endemic areas, the highest concentration of microfilariae in the peripheral blood occurs at night; therefore, blood specimens should be collected between 10 PM and 2 AM. Determination of serum antifilarial IgG is also a diagnostically useful test. This assay is available through the Parasitic Diseases Laboratory at the National Institutes of Health or through CDC's Division of Parasitic Diseases and Malaria.

TREATMENT

Diethylcarbamazine (DEC) is the drug of choice to treat travelers with *W. bancrofti*, *B. malayi*, or *B. timori* infection. DEC, which is available to physicians licensed in the United States for this purpose, can be obtained

from the CDC Parasitic Disease Drug Service under an investigational new drug protocol (404-639-3670; www.cdc.gov/laboratory/drugservice/index.html). DEC kills circulating microfilariae and is partially effective against the adult worms. DEC is also used to treat tropical pulmonary eosinophilia.

Although ivermectin kills microfilariae, it does not kill the adult worms. Many patients with lymphedema are no longer infected with the filarial parasite and do not benefit from antifilarial drug treatment. For chronic manifestations of lymphatic filariasis, such as lymphedema and hydrocele, specific lymphedema treatment—including hygiene, skin care, physiotherapy, and in some cases, antibiotics—and surgical repair are recommended. To ensure correct diagnosis and treatment, travelers should consult an infectious disease or tropical medicine specialist.

PREVENTIVE MEASURES FOR TRAVELERS

No vaccine is available. No drugs for preventing infection are available. Protective measures include avoidance of mosquito bites through the use of personal protection measures against biting insects (see Chapter 2, Protection against Mosquitoes, Ticks and Other Insects and Arthropods).

BIBLIOGRAPHY

1. Abramowicz M. Drugs for Parasitic Infections. New Rochelle (NY): The Medical Letter, Inc; 2007.
2. Dreyer G, Addiss D, Dreyer P, Noroes J. Basic lymphoedema management: treatment and prevention of problems associated with lymphatic filariasis. Hollis (NH): Hollis Publishing Co; 2002.
3. Dreyer G, Addiss D, Noroes J, Amaral F, Rocha A, Coutinho A. Ultrasonographic assessment of the adulticidal efficacy of repeat high-dose ivermectin in bancroftian filariasis. Trop Med Int Health. 1996 Aug;1(4):427–32.
4. Dreyer G, Addiss D, Roberts J, Noroes J. Progression of lymphatic vessel dilatation in the presence of living adult *Wuchereria bancrofti*. Trans R Soc Trop Med Hyg. 2002 Mar–Apr;96(2):157–61.
5. Dreyer G, Medeiros Z, Netto MJ, Leal NC, de Castro LG, Piessens WF. Acute attacks in the extremities of persons living in an area endemic for bancroftian filariasis: differentiation of two syndromes. Trans R Soc Trop Med Hyg. 1999 Jul–Aug;93(4):413–7.
6. Eberhard ML, Lammie PJ. Laboratory diagnosis of filariasis. Clin Lab Med. 1991 Dec;11(4):977–1010.

7. Gardner A, Hardy L, Bell SK. Eosinophilia in a returned traveler. Clin Infect Dis. 2010 Mar 1;50(5):745–6; 92–4.
8. Lipner EM, Law MA, Barnett E, Keystone JS, von Sonnenburg F, Loutan L, et al. Filariasis in travelers presenting to the GeoSentinel Surveillance Network. PLoS Negl Trop Dis. 2007;1(3):e88.
9. Michael E, Bundy DA, Grenfell BT. Re-assessing the global prevalence and distribution of lymphatic filariasis. Parasitology. 1996 Apr;112 (Pt 4):409–28.
10. Nutman TB, editor. Lymphatic Filariasis. London: Imperial College Press; 2000.
11. Ottesen EA. Efficacy of diethylcarbamazine in eradicating infection with lymphatic-dwelling filariae in humans. Rev Infect Dis. 1985 May–Jun;7(3):341–56.
12. Shenoy RK, Suma TK, Rajan K, Kumaraswami V. Prevention of acute adenolymphangitis in brugian filariasis: comparison of the efficacy of ivermectin and diethylcarbamazine, each combined with local treatment of the affected limb. Ann Trop Med Parasitol. 1998 Jul;92(5):587–94.

GIARDIASIS

Sharon L. Roy, Michele C. Hlavsa

INFECTIOUS AGENT

Giardiasis is a diarrheal illness caused by the protozoan parasite *Giardia intestinalis* (formerly known as *G. lamblia* or *G. duodenalis*).

MODE OF TRANSMISSION

Transmission occurs by ingesting fecally contaminated food or water, including water swallowed while swimming. Infection can also occur after contact with fecally contaminated environmental surfaces and objects or during person-to-person contact, such as diaper changing, caring for an infected person, or sexual contact.

EPIDEMIOLOGY

Giardiasis transmission occurs worldwide. Risk of infection increases with duration of travel. From 1996 through 2005, 31.3 per 1,000 returned travelers seeking medical care at GeoSentinel-associated medical centers around the world were diagnosed with giardiasis. Giardiasis was most commonly diagnosed in travelers returning from south Asia, the Middle East, and South America, although travelers returning from all other regions were also affected. Long-term travelers (duration >6 months) were significantly more likely than short-term travelers (duration <1 month) to develop giardiasis. In studies of travelers and expatriates in Nepal, *Giardia* is found in about 10% of stool samples submitted by patients with diarrhea.

CLINICAL PRESENTATION

Symptoms usually begin 1–2 weeks after infection and are generally self-limiting within 2–4 weeks. Giardiasis can cause a variety of intestinal symptoms or signs, which include diarrhea (often with foul-smelling, greasy stools), abdominal cramps, bloating, flatulence, fatigue, anorexia, and nausea. Typically, a patient presents with the gradual onset of 2–5 loose stools per day and gradually increasing fatigue. Weight loss may occur over time. Fever and vomiting are uncommon. Rarely, reactive arthritis has occurred after infection with *Giardia*.

DIAGNOSIS

Giardia cysts or trophs are not consistently seen in the stools of infected patients. Diagnostic yield can be increased by examining up to 3 stool samples over several days. Enzyme immunoassays can also be used to detect *Giardia* antigen, but it is unclear if they increase the diagnostic sensitivity.

TREATMENT

Several antimicrobial drugs, including tinidazole, metronidazole, nitazoxanide, paromomycin, furazolidone, and quinacrine are known to treat giardiasis (see Table 5-5). Because of the difficulty of making a definitive diagnosis, empiric treatment can be used in patients with the appropriate history and typical symptoms.

PREVENTIVE MEASURES FOR TRAVELERS

No vaccine is available to prevent giardiasis, and there is no recommended chemoprophylaxis. To prevent infection, travelers should be advised to follow food and water precautions described in Chapter 2, Food and Water Precautions.

BIBLIOGRAPHY

1. Chen LH, Wilson ME, Davis X, Loutan L, Schwartz E, Keystone J, et al. Illness in long-term travelers visiting GeoSentinel clinics. Emerg Infect Dis. 2009 Nov;15(11):1773–82.
2. Freedman DO, Weld LH, Kozarsky PE, Fisk T, Robins R, von Sonnenburg F, et al. Spectrum of disease and relation to place of exposure among ill returned travelers. N Engl J Med. 2006 Jan 12;354(2):119–30.
3. Greenwood Z, Black J, Weld L, O'Brien D, Leder K, Von Sonnenburg F, et al. Gastrointestinal infection among international travelers globally. J Travel Med. 2008 Jul–Aug;15(4):221–8.

4. Hill DR, Nash TE. Intestinal flagellate and ciliate infections. In: Guerrant RL, Walker DH, Weller PF, editors. Tropical Infectious Diseases. Philadelphia: Churchill Livingstone; 2006. p. 984–1002.

5. Hill Gaston JS, Lillicrap MS. Arthritis associated with enteric infection. Best Pract Res Clin Rheumatol. 2003 Apr;17(2):219–39.

6. Okhuysen PC. Traveler's diarrhea due to intestinal protozoa. Clin Infect Dis. 2001 Jul 1;33(1):110–4.

7. Swaminathan A, Torresi J, Schlagenhauf P, Thursky K, Wilder-Smith A, Connor BA, et al. A global study of pathogens and host risk factors associated with infectious gastrointestinal disease in returned international travellers. J Infect. 2009 Jul;59(1):19–27.

8. Taylor DN, Houston R, Shlim DR, Bhaibulaya M, Ungar BL, Echeverria P. Etiology of diarrhea among travelers and foreign residents in Nepal. JAMA. 1988 Sep 2;260(9):1245–8.

HELICOBACTER PYLORI

Ezra J. Barzilay, Ryan P. Fagan

INFECTIOUS AGENT

Helicobacter pylori is a small, curved, microaerophilic, gram-negative, rod-shaped bacterium.

MODE OF TRANSMISSION

Exact transmission is unknown, but it is thought to be fecal-oral or possibly oral-oral.

EPIDEMIOLOGY

H. pylori infection is one of the most common bacterial infections in the world. Estimated prevalence is 70% in developing countries and 30%–40% in the United States and other industrialized countries. Infection usually occurs during childhood and may persist lifelong unless treated. Humans are the only known reservoir. No increased risk of *H. pylori* seroconversion has been documented among residents of industrialized countries who traveled to developing countries for up to 16 months. Among missionaries and long-term travelers to developing countries, the annual incidence of seroconversion is 1.9%, which is higher than the annual incidence of seroconversion (0.3%–1.0%) in industrialized countries.

CLINICAL PRESENTATION

Most people infected with *H. pylori* never develop symptoms. *H. pylori* is the major cause of peptic ulcer disease and gastritis, which most commonly presents as gnawing or burning epigastric pain. Less commonly, symptoms include nausea, vomiting, loss of appetite, or bleeding. Rarely, and primarily in older adults, *H. pylori* is associated with a gastric lymphoma of the mucosal-associated lymphoid tissue.

DIAGNOSIS

Testing is recommended for patients with active gastric or duodenal ulcers, gastric mucosa–associated lymphoid tissue lymphomas, or those who have undergone resection of early-stage gastric cancer. Esophago-gastroduodenal endoscopic biopsy is performed to obtain tissue samples for histologic identification of organisms, culture, urease test, antibiotic susceptibility testing, and PCR. Active infection can also be diagnosed with a [13]C- or ^{14}C-labeled urea breath test or with a fecal antigen detection assay. *H. pylori*–specific IgG (serum or salivary antibody) is a useful marker for epidemiologic studies of past or current infection, but its sensitivity is suboptimal. A positive antibody screen should be confirmed by a different test (such as fecal antigen, urea breath test, or endoscopy).

TREATMENT

In the United States, the recommended primary therapies are 14 days of clarithromycin-based triple therapy (proton pump inhibitor [PPI] + clarithromycin + amoxicillin or metronidazole) or 10–14 days of bismuth quadruple therapy (PPI or H_2-blocker + bismuth + metronidazole + tetracycline). Detailed information about these and other recommended treatment regimens is available in the American College of Gastroenterology Guideline on the Management of *Helicobacter pylori* Infection (www.acg.gi.org/physicians/guidelines/ManagementofHpylori.pdf).

PREVENTIVE MEASURES FOR TRAVELERS

Because the mode of transmission is not known, there are no specific recommendations to prevent *H. pylori* infection. No vaccine is available, and no drugs for preventing infection are recommended.

BIBLIOGRAPHY

1. Becker SI, Smalligan RD, Frame JD, Kleanthous H, Tibbitts TJ, Monath TP, et al. Risk of *Helicobacter pylori* infection among long-term residents in developing countries. Am J Trop Med Hyg. 1999 Feb;60(2):267–70.
2. CDC. *Helicobacter pylori* fact sheet for health care providers. Atlanta: CDC; 1998 [updated 2010 Oct 22; cited 2008 Nov 30]. Available from: http://www.cdc.gov/ulcer/files/hpfacts.PDF.
3. Chey WD, Wong BC. American College of Gastroenterology guideline on the management of *Helicobacter pylori* infection. Am J Gastroenterol. 2007 Aug;102(8):1808–25.
4. Gold BD, Colletti RB, Abbott M, Czinn SJ, Elitsur Y, Hassall E, et al. *Helicobacter pylori* infection in children: recommendations for diagnosis and treatment. J Pediatr Gastroenterol Nutr. 2000 Nov;31(5):490–7.
5. Lindkvist P, Wadstrom T, Giesecke J. *Helicobacter pylori* infection and foreign travel. J Infect Dis. 1995 Oct;172(4):1135–6.
6. Peterson WL, Fendrick AM, Cave DR, Peura DA, Garabedian-Ruffalo SM, Laine L. *Helicobacter pylori*-related disease: guidelines for testing and treatment. Arch Intern Med. 2000 May 8;160(9):1285–91.
7. Potasman I, Yitzhak A. *Helicobacter pylori* serostatus in backpackers following travel to tropical countries. Am J Trop Med Hyg. 1998 Mar;58(3):305–8.

HELMINTHS, INTESTINAL
Els Mathieu

INFECTIOUS AGENTS

Ascaris lumbricoides (roundworm), *Ancylostoma duodenale* (hookworm), *Necator americanus* (hookworm), and *Trichuris trichiura* (whipworm) cause infection in humans. Two other helminths cause infections in humans *Enterobius vermicularis* (pinworm) and parasites of the genus *Schistosoma*; these infections are discussed specifically in the Pinworm (Enterobiasis, Oxyuriasis, Threadworm) and Schistosomiasis sections later in this chapter.

MODE OF TRANSMISSION

Adult female worms in the intestine of infected people produce eggs that are excreted in the stool. Defecation on the ground and use of stool to fertilize crops allow eggs to reach soil—the necessary environment for the next phase of their development. Infection with *Ascaris* and *Trichuris* occurs when eggs in soil have become infective and are ingested.

Hookworm eggs are not infective; they release larvae in soil that can penetrate skin. Hookworm infection primarily occurs when skin comes in contact with contaminated soil (by walking barefoot, for example) but can also occur through the ingestion of larvae. *Ascaris* larvae, after they have hatched from eggs in the small intestine, and hookworm larvae, after they have penetrated the skin, migrate through the lungs before they become adult worms in the intestine.

EPIDEMIOLOGY

Helminths are widespread; the prevalence is highest in tropical, developing countries. In 2002, an estimated 1.5 billion, 1.3 billion, and

1.1 billion people were infected with *Ascaris*, hookworm, and *Trichuris*, respectively. The risk of infection in travelers is low. Since adult worms do not multiply in the body, travelers who are diagnosed with intestinal worms generally have few worms. Sporadic exposure to infection is less likely to produce symptomatic disease. Because eggs must pass through a developmental phase in soil before becoming infective or releasing infective larvae, soil-transmitted helminth infections are not transmitted person to person.

CLINICAL PRESENTATION

Most infections are asymptomatic, especially when few worms are present. Heavy infections with intestinal helminths almost never occur in travelers.

In developing countries, moderate to heavy *Ascaris* infections can impair the nutritional status of children. The most serious complication is intestinal obstruction, usually of the small intestine. Pulmonary symptoms occur in a small percentage of patients when *Ascaris* larvae pass through the lungs. These symptoms include cough, fever, and chest discomfort. Hookworm infection can lead to anemia and protein deficiency due to blood loss. *Trichuris* infection can cause blood loss as well as dysentery and rectal prolapse. However, travelers are almost never at risk for these more severe manifestations of intestinal helminths.

DIAGNOSIS

Diagnosis is made by identifying the eggs of soil-transmitted helminths in the microscopic examination of a stool specimen. Adult *Ascaris* worms may occasionally be coughed up or found in stool or vomit.

TREATMENT

Soil-transmitted helminth infections are usually treated with albendazole or mebendazole, drugs that are effective and well tolerated.

PREVENTIVE MEASURES FOR TRAVELERS

No vaccine is available. Drugs are not used to prevent infection. In addition to usual food precautions (see Chapter 2, Food and Water Precautions), travelers should avoid walking barefoot on soil that may be contaminated with sewage, where human feces may have been used as fertilizer, or where people may have defecated.

BIBLIOGRAPHY

1. Bethony J, Brooker S, Albonico M, Geiger SM, Loukas A, Diemert D, et al. Soil-transmitted helminth infections: ascariasis, trichuriasis, and hookworm. Lancet. 2006 May 6;367(9521):1521–32.
2. Brooker S, Bethony J, Hotez PJ. Human hookworm infection in the 21st century. Adv Parasitol. 2004;58:197–288.
3. Brooker S, Clements AC, Bundy DA. Global epidemiology, ecology and control of soil-transmitted helminth infections. Adv Parasitol. 2006;62:221–61.
4. Cooper E. Trichuriasis. In: Guerrant RL, Walker DH, Weller PF, editors. Tropical Infectious Diseases: Principles, Pathogens & Practice. 2nd ed. Philadelphia: Elsevier; 2006. p. 1252–56.
5. Crompton DW. Ascaris and ascariasis. Adv Parasitol. 2001;48:285–375.
6. Gilles HM. Soil-transmitted helminths (geohelminths). In: Cook GC, Zumla A, editors. Manson's Tropical Diseases. 21st ed. London: Saunders; 2003. p. 1527–36.
7. Hotez PJ. Hookworm infections. In: Guerrant RL, Walker DH, Weller PF, editors. Tropical Infectious Diseases: Principles, Pathogens & Practice. 2nd ed. Philadelphia: Elsevier; 2006. p. 1265–73.
8. Maguire JH. Intestinal nematodes (roundworms). In: Mandell GL, Bennett JE, Dolin R, editors. Principles and Practice of Infectious Diseases. 6th ed. Philadelphia: Elsevier; 2005. p. 3260–6.
9. Seltzer E, Barry M, Crompton DWT. Ascariasis. In: Guerrant RL, Walker DH, Weller PF, editors. Tropical Infectious Diseases: Principles, Pathogens & Practice. 2nd ed. Philadelphia: Elsevier; 2006. p. 1257–64.
10. WHO Expert Committee. Prevention and control of schistosomiasis and soil-transmitted helminthiasis. World Health Organ Tech Rep Ser. 2002;912:i–vi, 1–57, back cover.

HEPATITIS A

Umid M. Sharapov

INFECTIOUS AGENT

Hepatitis A virus (HAV) is an RNA virus classified as a picornavirus.

MODE OF TRANSMISSION

Transmission can occur through direct person-to-person contact; through exposure to contaminated water, ice, or shellfish harvested from sewage-contaminated water; or from fruits, vegetables, or other foods that are eaten uncooked and that were contaminated during harvesting or subsequent handling. HAV is shed in the feces of infected people. The virus reaches peak levels 1–2 weeks before onset of symptoms and diminishes rapidly after liver dysfunction or symptoms appear, which is concurrent with the appearance of circulating antibodies to HAV. Infants and children, however, may shed virus for up to 6 months after infection.

EPIDEMIOLOGY

Worldwide, geographic areas can be characterized by high, intermediate, low, or very low levels of endemicity (Map 3-3). The map indicates the seroprevalence of antibody to HAV (total anti-HAV) as measured in selected cross-sectional studies among each country's residents. Levels of endemicity are related to hygienic and sanitary conditions in the area. The estimates show that all high-income regions have very low HAV endemicity levels, all low-income regions have high endemicity levels, and most middle-income regions have a mix of intermediate and low endemicity levels.

HAV infection is common throughout the developing world, where infections most frequently are acquired during early childhood and usually are asymptomatic or mild, resulting in a high proportion of adults in the population that are immune to HAV and where epidemics of hepatitis A are uncommon. In developed countries, HAV infection is less common, but communitywide outbreaks may occur.

Hepatitis A is one of the most common vaccine-preventable infections acquired during travel. In 2007 in the United States, among cases for which information regarding exposures was collected, the most frequently identified risk factor for hepatitis A was international travel (reported by 18% of patients). As in previous years, most travel-related cases (85%) were associated with travel to Mexico, Central America, or South America. As HAV transmission in the United States has decreased, cases among unimmunized travelers to countries in which hepatitis is endemic have accounted for an increased proportion of all cases. The risk of HAV infection for US residents traveling abroad varies with living conditions, length of stay, and the incidence of HAV infection in the area visited. Risk is highest for those who live in or visit rural areas, trek in backcountry areas, or frequently eat or drink in settings of poor sanitation. However, cases of travel-related hepatitis A can also occur in travelers to developing countries with "standard" tourist itineraries, accommodations, and eating behaviors.

CLINICAL PRESENTATION

The incubation period for hepatitis A averages 28 days (range, 15–50 days). HAV infection may be asymptomatic, or its clinical manifestations may range in severity from a mild illness lasting 1–2 weeks to a severely disabling disease lasting several months. Clinical manifestations of hepatitis A often include the abrupt onset of fever, malaise, anorexia, nausea, and abdominal discomfort, followed within a few days by jaundice. The likelihood of having symptoms with HAV infection is related to the age of the infected person. In children aged <6 years, most (70%) infections are asymptomatic; if illness does occur, its duration is usually <2 months. Ten percent of infected people have prolonged or relapsing symptoms over a 6- to 9-month period. The overall case-fatality ratio is 0.3%; however, the ratio is 1.8% among adults aged >50 years.

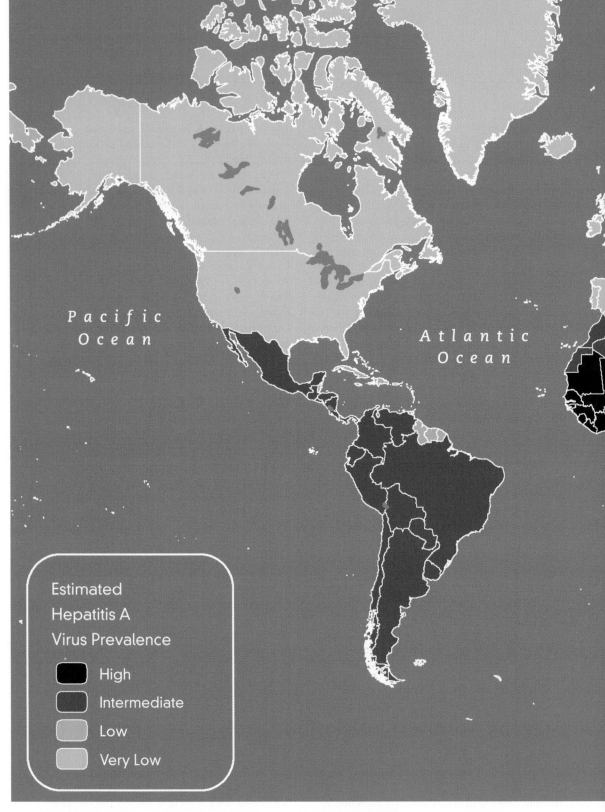

MAP 3-3. ESTIMATED PREVALENCE OF HEPATITIS A VIRUS[1,2]

Estimated
Hepatitis A
Virus Prevalence

- High
- Intermediate
- Low
- Very Low

[1] Jacobsen KH, Wiersma ST. Hepatitis A virus seroprevalence by age and world region, 1990 and 2005. Vaccine. 2010 Sep 24;28(41):6653–7. Data used with permission from Elsevier.

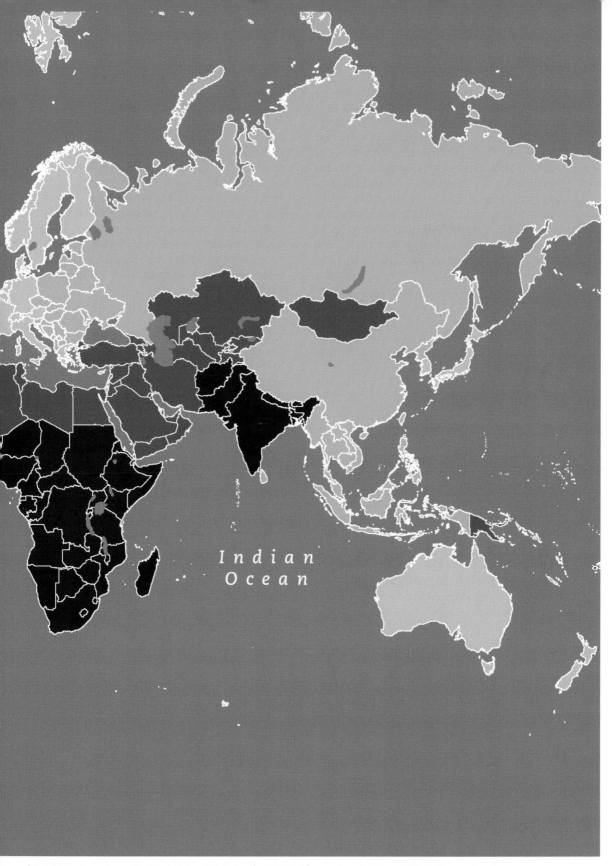

[2] Estimates of prevalence of antibody to hepatitis A virus (anti-HAV IgG), a marker of previous HAV infection, are based on systematic literature review conducted for the period of 1990–2005. In addition, anti-HAV prevalence might vary within countries by subpopulation and locality. As used on this map, the terms "high," "medium," "low" and "very low" endemicity reflect available evidence of how widespread HAV infection is within each country, rather than precise quantitative assessments.

DIAGNOSIS

Demonstration of IgM anti-HAV in the serum of acutely or recently ill patients establishes the diagnosis. IgM anti-HAV becomes detectable 5–10 days after exposure. A 4-fold or larger rise in specific antibodies in paired sera, detected by commercially available EIA, also establishes the diagnosis. If laboratory tests are not available, epidemiologic evidence may provide support for the diagnosis in a clinically compatible case. HAV RNA can be detected in blood and stools of most people during the acute phase of infection through nucleic acid amplification methods, but these generally are not used for diagnostic purposes.

TREATMENT

No specific treatment is available for people with hepatitis A; therefore, treatment is supportive.

PREVENTIVE MEASURES FOR TRAVELERS

Vaccine and Immune Globulin

Monovalent Vaccines

Two monovalent hepatitis A vaccines are licensed in the United States for people aged ≥12 months (Tables 3-2 and 3-3). Both vaccines are made of inactivated HAV adsorbed to aluminum hydroxide as an adjuvant. A full vaccination series includes 2 doses, giving the second dose 6–12 months (Havrix) or 6–18 months (Vaqta) after the first. All hepatitis A vaccines should be administered intramuscularly in the deltoid muscle.

Combination Vaccine

A combined hepatitis A and hepatitis B vaccine is licensed for people aged ≥18 years (Table 3-4). Primary immunization consists of 3 doses, given on a 0-, 1-, and 6-month schedule, the same schedule as commonly used for monovalent hepatitis B vaccine. An accelerated schedule (doses at days 0, 7, and 21–30) for travelers has been approved by the Food and Drug Administration; however, a booster dose should be given at 12 months to promote long-term immunity. The combination vaccine contains aluminum phosphate and aluminum hydroxide as adjuvants. The immunogenicity of the combination vaccine is equivalent to that of the monovalent hepatitis vaccines when tested after completion of the licensed schedule.

Indications for Use

All susceptible people traveling for any purpose, frequency, or duration to countries with high or intermediate hepatitis A endemicity should be vaccinated or receive immunoglobulin (IG) before departure. Providers also may consider its administration to travelers to any destination. The first dose of hepatitis A vaccine should be administered as soon as travel to countries with high or intermediate endemicity is considered.

People who are traveling for international adoption should be advised that hepatitis A vaccination is recommended for all previously unvaccinated household members and other people who anticipate close personal contact (such as regular babysitters) with an international adoptee from a country of high or intermediate endemicity during the first 60 days after arrival of the adoptee in the United States. The first dose of hepatitis A vaccine should be administered as soon as adoption is planned, ideally ≥2 weeks before

Table 3-2. Licensed doses and schedules for Havrix[1]

AGE GROUP (y)	DOSE (ELU)[2]	VOLUME	NUMBER OF DOSES	SCHEDULE (MONTHS)
1–18	720	0.5 mL	2	0, 6–12
≥19	1,440	1.0 mL	2	0, 6–12

[1] Hepatitis A vaccine, inactivated, GlaxoSmithKline
[2] ELU, ELISA units of inactivated hepatitis A virus

Table 3-3. Licensed doses and schedules for Vaqta[1]

AGE GROUP (y)	DOSE (U)[2]	VOLUME	NUMBER OF DOSES	SCHEDULE (MONTHS)
1–18	25	0.5 mL	2	0, 6–18
≥19	50	1.0 mL	2	0, 6–18

[1] Hepatitis A vaccine, inactivated, Merck & Co., Inc.
[2] U, units of hepatitis A virus antigen

Table 3-4. Licensed doses and schedules for Twinrix[1]

AGE GROUP (y)	VOLUME[2]	NUMBER OF DOSES	SCHEDULE
≥18 (primary immunization schedule)	1.0 mL	3	0, 1, 6 months
≥18 (accelerated schedule)	1.0 mL	4	0, 7, 21–30 days + 12 months

[1] Combined hepatitis A and hepatitis B vaccine, GlaxoSmithKline
[2] Each 1.0 mL dose contains 720 ELISA units of inactivated hepatitis A virus and 20 micrograms of hepatitis B surface antigen

the arrival of the adoptee (see Chapter 7, International Adoption).

Vaccine Administration

One dose of monovalent hepatitis A vaccine administered at any time before departure can provide adequate protection for most healthy people aged ≤40 years. Hepatitis A vaccine at the age-appropriate dose is preferred to IG. The vaccine series should be completed according to the licensed schedule for long-term protection. Many people will have detectable anti-HAV in response to the monovalent vaccine by 2 weeks after the first vaccine dose. The proportion of people who develop a detectable antibody response at 2 weeks may be lower when smaller vaccine doses are used, such as with the combination vaccine.

For optimal protection, adults aged >40 years, immunocompromised people, and people with chronic liver disease or other chronic medical conditions planning to depart to an area in <2 weeks should receive the initial dose of vaccine along with IG (0.02 mL/kg) at a separate anatomic injection site. Travelers who receive hepatitis A vaccine <2 weeks before traveling to an endemic area and who do not receive IG (either by choice or because of lack of availability) will be at lower risk for infection than those who do not receive hepatitis A vaccine or IG.

Although vaccination of an immune traveler is not contraindicated and does not increase the risk for adverse effects, screening for total anti-HAV before travel can be useful in some circumstances to determine susceptibility and eliminate unnecessary vaccination or IG prophylaxis. Such serologic screening for susceptibility might be indicated for adult travelers who are aged >40 years and those born in areas of the world with intermediate or high endemicity who are likely to have had prior HAV infection, if the cost of screening (laboratory and office visit) is less than the cost of vaccination or IG, and if testing will not delay vaccination and interfere with timely receipt of vaccine or IG before travel. Postvaccination testing for serologic response is not indicated.

Travelers who are aged <12 months, are allergic to a vaccine component, or who otherwise elect not to receive vaccine should receive a single dose of IG (0.02 mL/kg), which provides effective protection against HAV infection for up to 3 months (Table 3-5). Those who do not receive vaccination and plan to travel for >3 months should receive an IG dose of 0.06 mL/kg, which must be repeated if the duration of travel is >5 months. In addition, clinicians should be alert to opportunities to vaccinate all travelers whose plans might include future travel to an area of high or intermediate endemicity, including those whose current medical evaluation is for travel to an area where hepatitis A vaccination is not currently recommended.

Other Vaccine Considerations

Using the vaccines according to the licensed schedules is preferable. However, an interrupted series does not need to be restarted. Given their similar immunogenicity, a series that has been started with one brand of monovalent vaccine may be completed with the other brand. In adults and children who have completed the vaccine series, anti-HAV persists for ≥5–12 years after vaccination. Results of mathematical models indicate that, after completion of the vaccination series, anti-HAV will likely persist for ≥20 years. For children and adults who complete the primary series, booster doses of vaccine are not recommended.

Vaccine Safety and Adverse Reactions

Among adults, the most frequently reported side effects occurring 3–5 days after a vaccine dose are tenderness or pain at the injection site (53%–56%) or headache (14%–16%). Among children, the most common side effects reported are pain or tenderness at the injection site (15%–19%), feeding problems (8% in one study), or headache (4% in one study). No serious adverse events in children or adults have been found that could be definitively attributed to the vaccine, nor have increases in serious adverse events among vaccinated people compared with baseline rates been identified.

IG for intramuscular administration prepared in the United States has few side effects (primarily soreness at the injection site) and has never been shown to transmit infectious agents (hepatitis B virus, hepatitis C virus, or HIV). Since December 1994, all IG products commercially available in the United States have had to undergo a viral inactivation procedure or test negative for hepatitis C virus RNA before release.

Precautions and Contraindications

These vaccines should not be administered to travelers with a history of hypersensitivity to any vaccine component. Twinrix should not be administered to people with a history of hypersensitivity to yeast. Because hepatitis A vaccine consists of inactivated virus, and hepatitis B vaccine consists of a recombinant protein, no special precautions are needed for vaccination of immunocompromised travelers.

Pregnancy

The safety of hepatitis A vaccine for pregnant women has not been determined. However, because hepatitis A vaccine is produced from inactivated HAV, the theoretical risk to either the pregnant woman or the developing fetus is thought to be low. The risk of vaccination should be weighed against the risk of hepatitis A in female travelers who might be at high

Table 3-5. Recommended doses of immune globulin (IG) to protect against hepatitis A

SETTING	DURATION OF COVERAGE	DOSE (mL/kg)[1]
Preexposure	Short-term (1–2 months) Long-term (3–5 months)	0.02 0.06[2]
Postexposure	Not applicable	0.02

[1] IG should be administered by intramuscular injection into either the deltoid or gluteal muscle. For children <12 months of age, IG can be administered in the anterolateral thigh muscle.
[2] Repeat every 5 months if continued exposure to hepatitis A virus occurs.

risk for exposure to HAV. Pregnancy is not a contraindication for using IG.

Personal Protection Measures

Boiling or cooking food and beverage items for ≥1 minute to 185°F (85°C) inactivates HAV. Foods and beverages heated to this temperature and for this length of time cannot serve as vehicles for HAV infection, unless they become contaminated after heating. Adequate chlorination of water, as recommended in the United States, will inactivate HAV. Travelers should follow these recommendations, as well as those described in Chapter 2, Food and Water Precautions.

BIBLIOGRAPHY

1. Bacaner N, Stauffer B, Boulware DR, Walker PF, Keystone JS. Travel medicine considerations for North American immigrants visiting friends and relatives. JAMA. 2004 Jun 16;291(23):2856–64.
2. Bell BP, Feinstone SM. Hepatitis A vaccine. In: Plotkin SA, Orenstein WA, editors. Vaccines. 4th ed. Philadelphia: WB Saunders; 2004. p. 269–97.
3. CDC. Update: Prevention of hepatitis A after exposure to hepatitis A virus and in international travelers. Updated recommendations of the Advisory Committee on Immunization Practices (ACIP). MMWR Morb Mortal Wkly Rep. 2007 Oct 19;56(41):1080–4.
4. CDC. Updated recommendations from the Advisory Committee on Immunization Practices (ACIP) for use of hepatitis A vaccine in close contacts of newly arriving international adoptees. MMWR Morb Mortal Wkly Rep. 2009 Sep 18;58(36):1006–7.
5. Daniels D, Grytdal S, Wasley A. Surveillance for acute viral hepatitis—United States, 2007. MMWR Surveill Summ. 2009 May 22;58(3):1–27.
6. Fiore AE. Hepatitis A transmitted by food. Clin Infect Dis. 2004 Mar 1;38(5):705–15.
7. Fiore AE, Wasley A, Bell BP. Prevention of hepatitis A through active or passive immunization: recommendations of the Advisory Committee on Immunization Practices (ACIP). MMWR Recomm Rep. 2006 May 19;55(RR-7):1–23.
8. Jacobsen KH, Wiersma ST. Hepatitis A virus seroprevalence by age and world region, 1990 and 2005. Vaccine. 2010 Sep 24;28(41):6653–7.
9. Mutsch M, Spicher VM, Gut C, Steffen R. Hepatitis A virus infections in travelers, 1988–2004. Clin Infect Dis. 2006 Feb 15;42(4):490–7.
10. Van Damme P, Banatvala J, Fay O, Iwarson S, McMahon B, Van Herck K, et al. Hepatitis A booster vaccination: is there a need? Lancet. 2003 Sep 27;362(9389):1065–71.
11. Winokur PL, Stapleton JT. Immunoglobulin prophylaxis for hepatitis A. Clin Infect Dis. 1992 Feb;14(2):580–6.

HEPATITIS B

Eyasu H. Teshale

INFECTIOUS AGENT

Hepatitis B is caused by hepatitis B virus (HBV), a small, circular, partially double-stranded DNA virus in the Hepadnaviridae family.

MODE OF TRANSMISSION

HBV is transmitted by activities that involve contact with blood, blood products, and other body fluids (such as semen). Such activities include the following:

- Unprotected sexual contact
- Injection drug use with shared needles and injection paraphernalia
- Transfusions with blood or blood products that have not been screened for HBV
- Work in health care fields (medical, dental, laboratory) that entails exposure to human blood
- Dental, medical, or cosmetic (tattooing, body piercing) procedures with needles or other equipment that may be contaminated with blood
- Exposure to potentially contaminated blood through nonintact skin or mucous membranes

EPIDEMIOLOGY

Map 3-4 shows the prevalence of chronic HBV infection globally. There are no data with

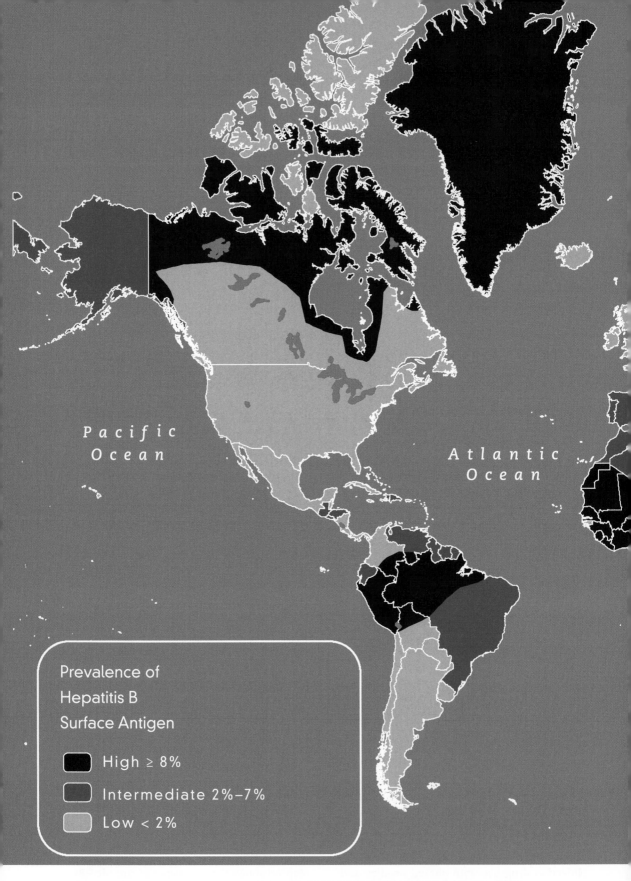

MAP 3-4. PREVALENCE OF CHRONIC INFECTION WITH HEPATITIS B VIRUS, 2006

| INFECTIOUS DISEASES RELATED TO TRAVEL

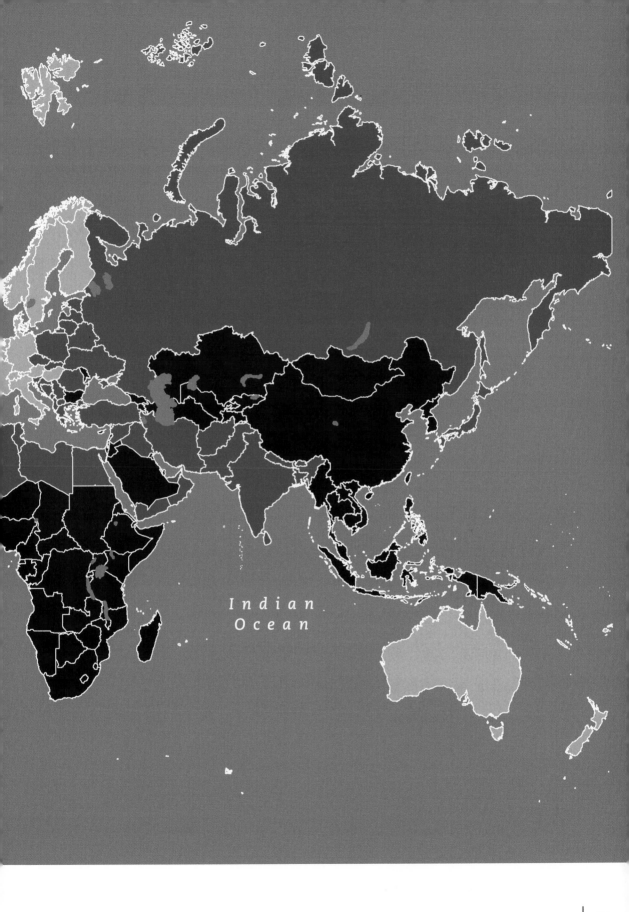

which to assess the risk for HBV infection among US travelers. Published case reports of travelers acquiring hepatitis B during travel are rare. The risk for HBV infection among international travelers is low. However, the risk of HBV infection is considered higher in countries where the prevalence of chronic HBV infection is intermediate or high. Expatriates, missionaries, and long-term aid workers may be at increased risk for HBV infection.

CLINICAL PRESENTATION

In adults and children aged ≥5 years, 30%–50% develop clinical illness typical of hepatitis B after initial exposure to the HBV. The incubation period for hepatitis B is 90 days (range, 60–150 days). Early symptoms that precede jaundice include constitutional symptoms like malaise, fatigue, and anorexia for about 1–2 weeks. The typical clinical signs and symptoms include nausea, vomiting, abdominal pain, and jaundice. In some cases, skin rashes, joint pain, and arthritis may occur. HBV infection is typically asymptomatic in children aged <5 years and immunocompromised adults. The overall case-fatality ratio of acute hepatitis B is approximately 1%.

Acute hepatitis B progresses to chronic HBV infection in 30%–90% of people infected as infants or young children and in <5% of people infected during adolescence or adulthood. Chronic infection with HBV results in chronic liver disease, including liver cirrhosis and liver cancer.

DIAGNOSIS

Serologic markers, either alone or in combination, indicate different stages of HBV infection (Table 3-6). These serologic markers are typically used to differentiate between acute, resolving, and chronic infection.

TREATMENT

No specific treatment is available for acute hepatitis B. Antiretroviral drugs are approved to treat chronic hepatitis B.

PREVENTIVE MEASURES FOR TRAVELERS
Vaccine
Indications for Use

Hepatitis B vaccination should be administered to all unvaccinated people traveling to areas with intermediate or high prevalence of chronic hepatitis B (hepatitis B surface antigen prevalence ≥2%). Hepatitis B vaccination is recommended for all US residents who work in health care settings that involve potential exposure to human blood. All unvaccinated children and adolescents (aged <19 years) should receive hepatitis B vaccine. Regardless of destination, all people who may engage in practices that place them at risk for HBV infection during travel (such as men who have sex with men, injection drug users, anyone who had a sexually transmitted disease or has had more than one sexual partner in the previous 6 months) should receive hepatitis B vaccination, if previously unvaccinated. Any adult seeking protection from HBV infection should be vaccinated; acknowledgment of a specific risk factor is not a requirement for vaccination.

Vaccine Administration

The vaccine is usually administered as a 3-dose series on a 0-, 1-, 6-month schedule. The second dose should be given 1 month after the first dose; the third dose should be given ≥2 months after the second dose and ≥4 months after the first dose. Alternatively, the vaccine Engerix-B is approved for administration on a 4-dose schedule at 0, 1, 2, and 12 months. In addition, a 2-dose schedule for Recombivax HB has been licensed for children and adolescents aged 11–15 years. According to the 2-dose schedule, the second dose is given 4–6 months after the first dose. A 3-dose series that has been started with one brand of vaccine may be completed with another brand. Twinrix is a combined hepatitis A and hepatitis B vaccine licensed for people aged ≥18 years. Primary immunization consists of 3 doses, given at 0, 1, and 6 months.

Table 3-6. Interpretation of serologic test results for hepatitis B virus infection[1]

SEROLOGIC MARKER				
HBsAG[2]	TOTAL ANTI-HBc	IgM ANTI-HBc	ANTI-HBsAG	INTERPRETATION
–	–	–	–	Never infected
+	–	–	–	Early acute infection, transient (≤18 days) after vaccination
+	+	+	–	Acute infection
–	+	+	+ or –	Acute resolving infection
–	+	–	+	Recovered from past infection and immune
+	+	–	–	Chronic infection
–	+	–	–	False-positive (susceptible), past infection, occult infection,[3] or passive transfer of anti-HBc to infant born to HBsAg-positive mother
–	–	–	+	Immune if concentration is ≥10 mIU/mL after vaccine series completion, passive transfer after hepatitis B immune globulin administration

Abbreviations: HBsAg, hepatitis B surface antigen; anti-HBc, antibody to hepatitis B core antigen.

[1] From: CDC. A comprehensive immunization strategy to eliminate transmission of hepatitis B virus infection in the United States: recommendations of the Advisory Committee on Immunization Practices (ACIP). Part II: immunization of adults. MMWR Recomm Rep. 2006 Dec 8;55(RR-16):1–33.

[2] To ensure that an HBsAg-positive test result is not a false positive, samples with reactive HBsAg results should be tested with a licensed neutralizing confirmatory test, if recommended in the manufacturer's package insert.

[3] Individuals positive only for anti-HBc are unlikely to be infectious except under unusual circumstances in which they are the source for direct percutaneous exposure of susceptible recipients to large quantities of virus (such as blood transfusion or organ transplant).

Special Situations

Ideally, vaccination should begin 6 months before travel so the full vaccine series can be completed before departure. Because some protection is provided by 1 or 2 doses, the vaccine series should be initiated, if indicated, even if it cannot be completed before departure. Optimal protection, however, is not conferred until after the final vaccine dose is received. Recently the Food and Drug Administration approved an accelerated vaccine schedule to be used for those traveling to endemic areas at short notice and facing imminent exposure or for emergency responders to disaster areas. An accelerated vaccination schedule with Twinrix (combined hepatitis A and hepatitis B vaccine) also can be used (doses at 0, 7, and 21–30 days). In this situation, a booster dose should be given at 12 months to promote long-term immunity. For children and adults with normal immune status who received the recommended vaccine series, pre-travel booster doses are not recommended (see Chapter 7, Vaccine Recommendations for Infants and Children). Serologic testing to assess antibody levels is not necessary for most fully vaccinated people.

Vaccine Safety and Adverse Reactions

Hepatitis B vaccines have been shown to be safe for people of all ages. Pain at the injection site (3%–29%) and elevated temperatures >99.9°F (37.7°C) (1%–6%) are the most frequently reported side effects among vaccine recipients. These vaccines should not be administered to people with a history of hypersensitivity to any vaccine component, including yeast. The vaccine contains a recombinant protein (hepatitis B surface antigen) that is noninfectious.

Limited data indicate no apparent risk of adverse events to the developing fetus when hepatitis B vaccine is administered to pregnant women. HBV infection in a pregnant woman can result in serious disease for the mother and chronic infection for the newborn. Neither pregnancy nor lactation should be considered a contraindication for vaccination.

Personal Protection Measures

As part of the pre-travel education process, all travelers should be given information about the risks for hepatitis B and other bloodborne pathogens from contaminated medical equipment, injection drug use, unprotected sexual activity, and other methods of transmission and be informed about prevention measures, including vaccination, to prevent transmission of HBV. When seeking medical or dental care, travelers should be alert to the use of medical, surgical, dental, and cosmetic (tattoo, piercing) equipment that has not been adequately sterilized or disinfected, reuse of contaminated equipment, and unsafe injecting practices (such as reuse of disposable needles and syringes). HBV and other bloodborne pathogens can be transmitted if tools are not sterile or if a tattoo artist or piercer does not follow proper infection control procedures. Travelers should consider the health risks when deciding to get a tattoo or body piercing in areas where adequate sterilization or disinfection procedures might not be available or practiced.

BIBLIOGRAPHY

1. Bock HL, Loscher T, Scheiermann N, Baumgarten R, Wiese M, Dutz W, et al. Accelerated schedule for hepatitis B immunization. J Travel Med. 1995 Dec 1;2(4):213–7.

2. CDC. Updated US Public Health Service guidelines for the management of occupational exposures to HBV, HCV, and HIV and recommendations for postexposure prophylaxis. MMWR Recomm Rep. 2001 Jun 29;50(RR-11):1–42.

3. Lok AS, McMahon BJ. Chronic hepatitis B: update of recommendations. Hepatology. 2004 Mar;39(3):857–61.

4. Long GE, Rickman LS. Infectious complications of tattoos. Clin Infect Dis. 1994 Apr;18(4):610–9.

5. Mariano A, Mele A, Tosti ME, Parlato A, Gallo G, Ragni P, et al. Role of beauty treatment in the spread of parenterally transmitted hepatitis viruses in Italy. J Med Virol. 2004 Oct;74(2):216–20.

6. Mast E, Goldstein S, Ward JL. Hepatitis B vaccine. In: Plotkin SA, Orenstein WA, editors. Vaccines. 5th ed. Philadelphia: WB Saunders; 2004. p. 199–337.

7. Mast EE, Margolis HS, Fiore AE, Brink EW, Goldstein ST, Wang SA, et al. A comprehensive immunization

strategy to eliminate transmission of hepatitis B virus infection in the United States: recommendations of the Advisory Committee on Immunization Practices (ACIP). Part 1: immunization of infants, children, and adolescents. MMWR Recomm Rep. 2005 Dec 23;54 (RR-16):1–31.

8. Mast EE, Weinbaum CM, Fiore AE, Alter MJ, Bell BP, Finelli L, et al. A comprehensive immunization strategy to eliminate transmission of hepatitis B virus infection in the United States: recommendations of the Advisory Committee on Immunization Practices (ACIP). Part 2: immunization of adults. MMWR Recomm Rep. 2006 Dec 8;55 (RR-16):1–33.

9. Sagliocca L, Stroffolini T, Amoroso P, Manzillo G, Ferrigno L, Converti F, et al. Risk factors for acute hepatitis B: a case-control study. J Viral Hepat. 1997 Jan;4(1):63–6.

10. Simonsen L, Kane A, Lloyd J, Zaffran M, Kane M. Unsafe injections in the developing world and transmission of bloodborne pathogens: a review. Bull World Health Organ. 1999;77(10):789–800.

HEPATITIS C

Scott Holmberg

INFECTIOUS AGENT

Hepatitis C is caused by the hepatitis C virus (HCV), a spherical, enveloped, positive-strand RNA virus, approximately 50 nm in diameter.

MODE OF TRANSMISSION

Transmission of HCV is bloodborne and occurs mainly through sharing drug-injection equipment, from transfusion of unscreened blood, or from untreated clotting factors. In developing countries, unsterile medicinal and other injection practices account for many infections. HCV is infrequently transmitted through sexual contact.

EPIDEMIOLOGY

Approximately 3% (170 million) of the world's population has been infected with HCV. For most countries, the prevalence of HCV infection is <3%. The prevalence is higher (up to 15%) in some countries in Africa and Asia and highest (>15%) in Egypt (Map 3-5). The most frequent mode of transmission in the United States is through sharing drug-injecting equipment among people who inject drugs. Travelers' risk for contracting HCV infection is generally low. For international travelers, the principal activities that can result in blood exposure are the following:

- Receiving blood transfusions that have not been screened for HCV
- Having medical or dental procedures
- Engaging in activities (such as acupuncture, tattooing, or injecting drug use) in which equipment has not been adequately sterilized or disinfected, or in which contaminated equipment is reused
- Working in health care fields (medical, dental, or laboratory) that entail direct exposure to human blood

CLINICAL PRESENTATION

Most people (80%) with acute HCV infection have no symptoms. If symptoms occur, they may include loss of appetite, abdominal pain, fatigue, nausea, dark urine, and jaundice. Approximately 75%–85% of HCV-infected people develop chronic hepatitis C. The most common symptom of chronic infection is fatigue; severe liver disease develops in 10%–20% of infected people.

DIAGNOSIS

Two major types of tests are available: IgG assays for anti-HCV and nucleic acid

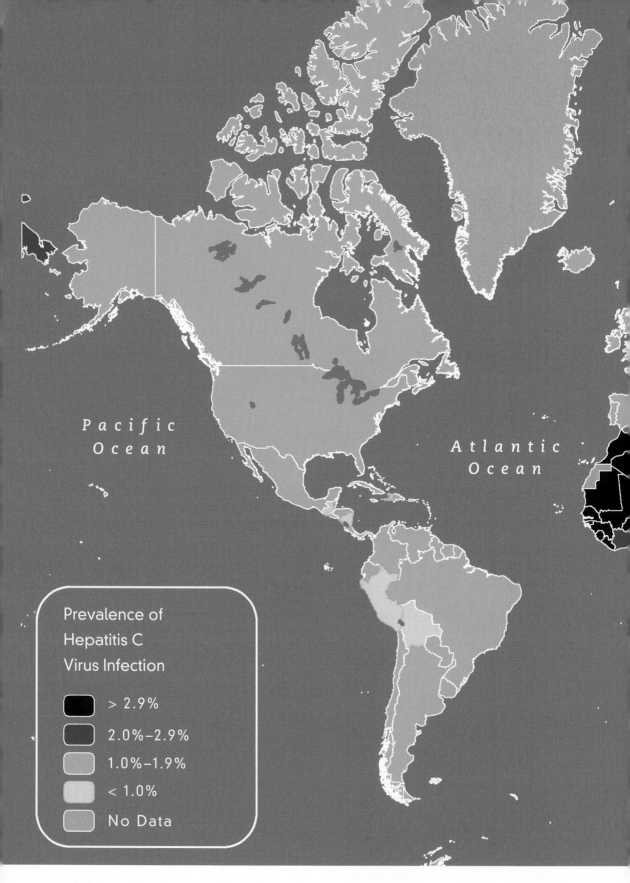

MAP 3-5. PREVALENCE OF CHRONIC HEPATITIS C INFECTION

Prevalence of Hepatitis C Virus Infection

- > 2.9%
- 2.0%–2.9%
- 1.0%–1.9%
- < 1.0%
- No Data

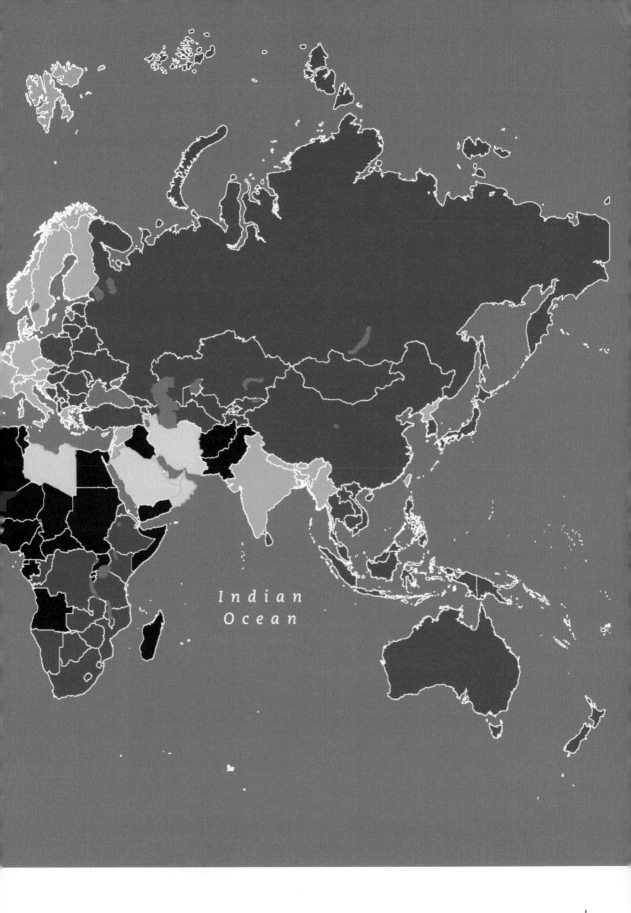

Indian Ocean

amplification testing to detect HCV RNA in blood (viremia). Assays for IgM, to detect early or acute infection, are not available. Approximately 80% of people who seroconvert to anti-HCV, indicative of acute infection, will progress to chronic infection and persistently detectable viremia. False-negative antibody test results, while rare, may occur early in the course of acute infection, usually in the first 15 weeks after exposure and infection.

TREATMENT

Treatment for hepatitis C is rapidly evolving. In general, "sustained viral response" (considered a cure) is now achieved in 50% of patients taking pegylated interferon and ribavirin for 24–48 weeks. New oral agents added to a regimen of interferon and ribavirin are increasing cure rates to 85%–90% on initial treatment attempts; these may be approved and available by the time of printing this publication.

PREVENTIVE MEASURES FOR TRAVELERS

No vaccine is available, and immune globulin does not provide protection. When seeking medical or dental care, travelers should be alert to the use of medical, surgical, and dental equipment that has not been adequately sterilized or disinfected, reuse of contaminated equipment, and unsafe injecting practices (such as reuse of disposable needles and syringes). HCV and other bloodborne pathogens can be transmitted if tools are not sterile or the clinician does not follow other proper infection-control procedures (washing hands, using latex gloves, and cleaning and disinfecting surfaces and instruments). There are still a few areas of the world, such as parts of sub-Saharan Africa, where blood donors may not be screened for HCV. Travelers should be advised to consider the health risks if they are thinking about getting a tattoo or body piercing in areas where adequate sterilization or disinfection procedures might not be available or practiced.

BIBLIOGRAPHY

1. Armstrong GL, Wasley A, Simard EP, McQuillan GM, Kuhnert WL, Alter MJ. The prevalence of hepatitis C virus infection in the United States, 1999 through 2002. Ann Intern Med. 2006 May 16;144(10):705–14.
2. Global Burden Of Hepatitis C Working Group. Global burden of disease (GBD) for hepatitis C. J Clin Pharmacol. 2004 Jan;44(1):20–9.
3. Prati D. Transmission of hepatitis C virus by blood transfusions and other medical procedures: a global review. J Hepatol. 2006 Oct;45(4):607–16.
4. Shepard CW, Finelli L, Alter MJ. Global epidemiology of hepatitis C virus infection. Lancet Infect Dis. 2005 Sep;5(9):558–67.
5. Shimakami T, Lanford RE, Lemon SM. Hepatitis C: recent successes and continuing challenges in the development of improved treatment modalities. Curr Opin Pharmacol. 2009 Oct;9(5):537–44.
6. Simonsen L, Kane A, Lloyd J, Zaffran M, Kane M. Unsafe injections in the developing world and transmission of bloodborne pathogens: a review. Bull World Health Organ. 1999;77(10):789–800.
7. Thompson ND, Perz JF, Moorman AC, Holmberg SD. Nonhospital health care–associated hepatitis B and C virus transmission: United States, 1998–2008. Ann Intern Med. 2009 Jan 6;150(1):33–9.

HEPATITIS E

Chong-Gee Teo

INFECTIOUS AGENT

Infection is caused by hepatitis E virus (HEV), a single-stranded, RNA virus belonging to the *Hepeviridae* family.

MODE OF TRANSMISSION

HEV is transmitted primarily by the fecal-oral route. Epidemics of hepatitis E are principally due to drinking fecally contaminated water. Sporadic disease in Japan and Europe is zoonotic and foodborne and is associated with eating meat and offal of deer, boars, and pigs. Sporadic disease is also observed in other temperate countries, including the United States, but its cause is unknown in most cases. Disease from blood transfusion has been reported, although rare. Perinatal HEV transmission from women infected during pregnancy is common.

EPIDEMIOLOGY

Waterborne outbreaks (often large, involving hundreds to thousands of people) have occurred in South and Central Asia, tropical East Asia, Africa, and Central America (Map 3-6). Clinical attack rates are highest in young adults aged 15–49 years. In outbreak-prone areas, interepidemic disease is sporadically encountered. In these areas, pregnant women—whether infected sporadically or during an epidemic—are at significant risk of progressing to liver failure and death.

Sporadic disease also occurs in non-outbreak-prone regions such as the Middle East, temperate East Asia (including China), North and South America, and Europe. In Europe, symptomatic disease is observed most frequently in adults aged >60 years, especially men. Primary infection acquired by people who are immunosuppressed, such as after organ transplantation, may progress to chronic infection.

People living in the United States are at risk of HEV infection when they travel to areas where epidemics have occurred. When traveling in Japan and Europe, eating raw or inadequately cooked venison, boar meat, pig liver, or food products derived from these, is a significant risk factor for infection.

CLINICAL PRESENTATION

The incubation period is 2–9 weeks (mean 6 weeks). Signs and symptoms of disease during primary infection include jaundice, fever, loss of appetite, abdominal pain, and lethargy. Acute hepatitis E is frequently self-limited. Pregnant women (particularly those infected during the second or third trimester) may present with or progress to liver failure, and their infants are at risk for spontaneous abortion and premature delivery. People with preexisting chronic liver disease may undergo further hepatic decompensation.

DIAGNOSIS

The diagnosis of acute hepatitis E is established by detecting anti-HEV IgM and IgG in serum. Detecting HEV RNA in serum or stools further confirms the serologic diagnosis but is seldom required. Longer-term, serial detection of HEV RNA in serum or stools, regardless of the HEV antibody serostatus, suggests chronic HEV infection. No diagnostic test has been approved by the Food and Drug Administration.

TREATMENT

Treatment is supportive.

PREVENTIVE MEASURES FOR TRAVELERS

No vaccine is available, nor are drugs for preventing infection. Travelers should avoid drinking unboiled or unchlorinated water and beverages that contain unboiled water or ice. Travelers should eat only thoroughly cooked food, including seafood, meat, offal, and products derived from these (see Chapter 2, Food and Water Precautions).

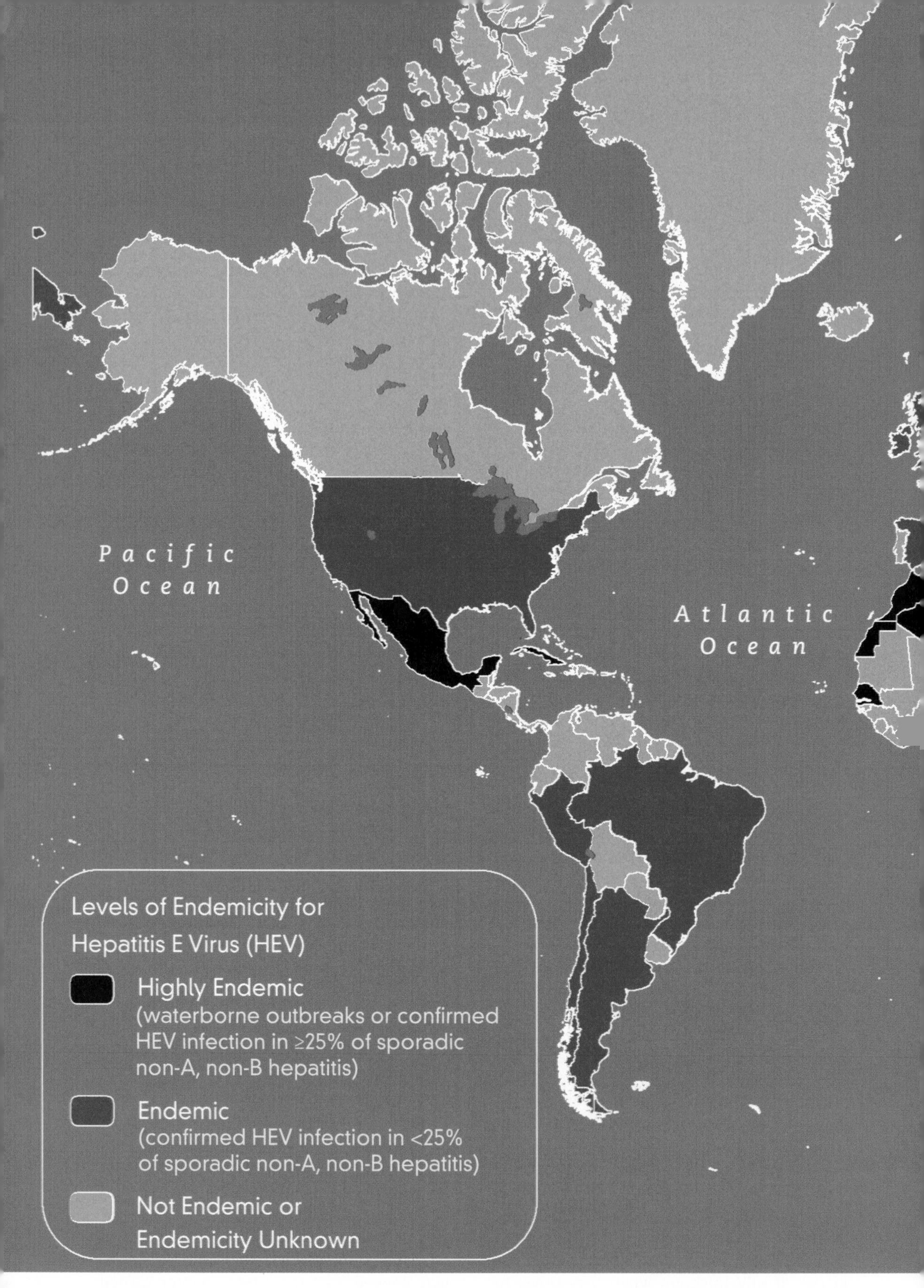

Pacific
Ocean
Atlantic
Ocean
Levels of Endemicity for
Hepatitis E Virus (HEV)
Highly Endemic
(waterborne outbreaks or confirmed
HEV infection in ≥25% of sporadic
non-A, non-B hepatitis)
Endemic
(confirmed HEV infection in <25%
of sporadic non-A, non-B hepatitis)
Not Endemic or
Endemicity Unknown

MAP 3-6. DISTRIBUTION OF HEPATITIS E INFECTION, 2010

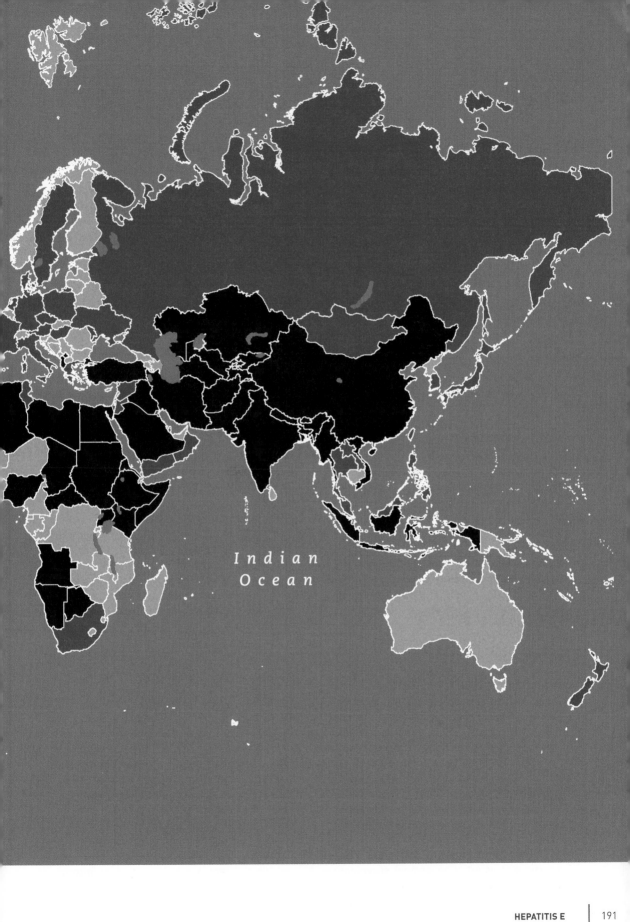

Indian Ocean

BIBLIOGRAPHY

1. Colson P, Borentain P, Queyriaux B, Kaba M, Moal V, Gallian P, et al. Pig liver sausage as a source of hepatitis E virus transmission to humans. J Infect Dis. 2010 Sep 15;202(6):825–34.

2. Labrique A, Kuniholm MH, Nelson KE. The global impact of hepatitis E—new horizons for an emerging virus. In: Grayson L, editor. Emerging Infections 9. Washington, DC: American Society for Microbiology; 2010.

3. Teo CG. Much meat, much malady: changing perceptions of the epidemiology of hepatitis E. Clin Microbiol Infect. 2010 Jan;16(1):24–32.

HISTOPLASMOSIS
Monika Roy, Tom M. Chiller

INFECTIOUS AGENT

Histoplasma capsulatum is a dimorphic fungus that grows as a mold in soil and as a yeast in animal and human hosts, as an intracellular pathogen.

MODE OF TRANSMISSION

Histoplasma is acquired via inhalation of spores (conidia) from soil contaminated with bat guano or bird droppings. Histoplasmosis is not transmitted directly from person to person.

EPIDEMIOLOGY

In the United States, *H. capsulatum* var. *capsulatum* is primarily found along the Ohio and Mississippi River Valleys, mostly in the central and southeastern states. Its occurrence has been described on every continent except Antarctica. Indigenous human cases have been reported throughout North, Central, and South America; the Caribbean; parts of the Middle East (Iran and Turkey); parts of Asia (Pakistan, India, China, Thailand, Indonesia, Vietnam, Malaysia, Philippines, Burma, and Japan); parts of Europe (northern Italy, Bulgaria, Spain, Hungary, Austria, France, Portugal, Romania, the countries of the former Soviet Union, Great Britain, Ireland, and Norway); parts of Africa; and Australia. *H. capsulatum* var. *duboisii*, also known as African *Histoplasma*, is found in central and western Africa.

Overall, histoplasmosis is rare among returning travelers. GeoSentinel surveillance data on illness in returning travelers showed that <0.5% of travelers presenting ill to clinics were diagnosed with histoplasmosis. However, exposures that lead to clusters of cases with attack rates of >50% are reported yearly.

People of all ages who visit endemic areas and are exposed to accumulations of bat guano or bird droppings are at increased risk for infection. Not all sources of exposure are obvious when visiting endemic areas; however, activities such as spelunking, mining, construction, excavation, demolition, roofing, chimney cleaning, farming, gardening, and installing heating and air-conditioning systems are associated with histoplasmosis. While in caves or mines, spending time close to the ground or kicking up dirt infested with bat guano containing *H. capsulatum* can increase the risk of infection. Other risk-prone activities may become better recognized as ecotourism and adventure tourism become more common in endemic areas of Central and South America.

CLINICAL PRESENTATION

The incubation period is typically 3–17 days. Ninety percent of infections are asymptomatic or result in a mild influenzalike illness. Some infections may cause acute pulmonary histoplasmosis, manifested by high fever, headache, nonproductive cough, chills, weakness, pleuritic chest pain, and fatigue. In general, severity of illness depends on the number of conidia inhaled, as well as the immune status of the host. Most people spontaneously recover 2–3 weeks after onset of symptoms, although fatigue may persist longer.

Dissemination, especially to the gastrointestinal tract and central nervous system, can occur in people who are immunocompromised (including patients with HIV/AIDS, hematologic malignancies, solid organ transplants, and tumor necrosis factor antagonist use). Dissemination may occur acutely or chronically as part of a clinical pattern known as progressive disseminated histoplasmosis. Other less common, chronic clinical patterns include chronic pulmonary histoplasmosis and mediastinitis. Reinfection can occur with sufficient exposure, and in these people, the incubation period can be shorter.

DIAGNOSIS

Culture of *H. capsulatum* from bone marrow, blood, sputum, and tissue specimens is the definitive method of diagnosis. Blood should be cultured by using a lysis-centrifugation method. Yield for this diagnostic is highest for patients with acute pulmonary, chronic pulmonary, and disseminated histoplasmosis.

Demonstration of the typical intracellular yeast forms by microscopic examination strongly supports the diagnosis of histoplasmosis when clinical, epidemiologic, and other laboratory studies are compatible. Yield for this method is highest for patients with acute pulmonary and disseminated histoplasmosis.

An EIA antigen detection test on urine, serum, plasma, bronchoalveolar lavage, or cerebrospinal fluid is a rapid, commercially available diagnostic test. The yield for an EIA antigen detection test is highest for severe, acute pulmonary infections and for progressive disseminated infections. It often is transiently positive early in the course of acute, self-limited pulmonary infections. A negative test does not exclude infection.

Serologic testing for antibodies is also available; however, these tests should be interpreted by an expert. Yield for serologic tests is highest for patients with subacute or chronic pulmonary infections. They are not useful for acute cases or patients with HIV.

TREATMENT

Antifungal treatment is not usually indicated for healthy, immunocompetent people with acute, localized pulmonary infection, because this form of the disease is self-limited, often resolving within 3 weeks. People with persistent symptoms beyond 1 month can be treated with itraconazole for mild to moderate illness or amphotericin B for severe infection. All people with more extensive disease, including diffuse pulmonary and disseminated histoplasmosis, should be treated with either itraconazole or amphotericin B based on illness severity. People with immunocompromising conditions and other chronic disease may require prolonged treatment. Consultation with an infectious disease specialist is advised.

PREVENTIVE MEASURES FOR TRAVELERS

No vaccine is available. People at increased risk for severe disease should be advised to avoid high-risk areas, such as bat-inhabited caves. If exposure cannot be avoided, travelers should be advised to decrease dust generation in infested areas by watering the areas and to wear masks and special protective equipment.

After engaging in high-risk activities, hosing off footwear, and placing clothing in airtight plastic bags to be laundered could also decrease the potential for exposure. Further detail about protective equipment can be obtained from www.cdc.gov/niosh/docs/2005-109. Soil, guano, and other potential fomites should not be transported.

BIBLIOGRAPHY

1. Buxton JA, Dawar M, Wheat LJ, Black WA, Ames NG, Mugford M, et al. Outbreak of histoplasmosis in a school party that visited a cave in Belize: role of antigen testing in diagnosis. J Travel Med. 2002 Jan–Feb;9(1):48–50.
2. Cano MV, Hajjeh RA. The epidemiology of histoplasmosis: a review. Semin Respir Infect. 2001 Jun;16(2):109–18.
3. CDC. Cave-associated histoplasmosis—Costa Rica. MMWR Morb Mortal Wkly Rep. 1988 May 27;37(20):312–3.
4. CDC. Outbreak of histoplasmosis among travelers returning from El Salvador—Pennsylvania and Virginia, 2008. MMWR Morb Mortal Wkly Rep. 2008 Dec 19;57(50):1349–53.

5. Freedman DO, Weld LH, Kozarsky PE, Fisk T, Robins R, von Sonnenburg F, et al. Spectrum of disease and relation to place of exposure among ill returned travelers. N Engl J Med. 2006 Jan 12;354(2):119–30.

6. Kauffman CA. Histoplasmosis. Clin Chest Med. 2009 Jun;30(2):217–25.

7. Kauffman CA. Histoplasmosis: a clinical and laboratory update. Clin Microbiol Rev. 2007 Jan;20(1):115–32.

8. Morgan J, Cano MV, Feikin DR, Phelan M, Monroy OV, Morales PK, et al. A large outbreak of histoplasmosis among American travelers associated with a hotel in Acapulco, Mexico, spring 2001. Am J Trop Med Hyg. 2003 Dec;69(6):663–9.

9. Nasta P, Donisi A, Cattane A, Chiodera A, Casari S. Acute histoplasmosis in spelunkers returning from Mato Grosso, Peru. J Travel Med. 1997 Dec 1;4(4):176–8.

10. Panackal AA, Hajjeh RA, Cetron MS, Warnock DW. Fungal infections among returning travelers. Clin Infect Dis. 2002 Nov 1;35(9):1088–95.

11. Pfaller MA, Diekema DJ. Epidemiology of invasive mycoses in North America. Crit Rev Microbiol. 2010;36(1):1–53.

12. Valdez H, Salata RA. Bat-associated histoplasmosis in returning travelers: case presentation and description of a cluster. J Travel Med. 1999 Dec;6(4):258–60.

13. Weinberg M, Weeks J, Lance-Parker S, Traeger M, Wiersma S, Phan Q, et al. Severe histoplasmosis in travelers to Nicaragua. Emerg Infect Dis. 2003 Oct;9(10):1322–5.

14. Wheat LJ. Histoplasmosis: a review for clinicians from non-endemic areas. Mycoses. 2006 Jul;49(4):274–82.

15. Wheat LJ. Improvements in diagnosis of histoplasmosis. Expert Opin Biol Ther. 2006 Nov;6(11):1207–21.

16. Wheat LJ. Laboratory diagnosis of histoplasmosis: update 2000. Semin Respir Infect. 2001 Jun;16(2):131–40.

17. Wheat LJ, Freifeld AG, Kleiman MB, Baddley JW, McKinsey DS, Loyd JE, et al. Clinical practice guidelines for the management of patients with histoplasmosis: 2007 update by the Infectious Diseases Society of America. Clin Infect Dis. 2007 Oct 1;45(7):807–25.

HIV & AIDS
John T. Brooks

INFECTIOUS AGENT

Acquired Immunodeficiency Syndrome (AIDS) is a serious disease that represents the late clinical stage of infection with human immunodeficiency virus (HIV). HIV progressively damages the immune system. Without an effective immune system, life-threatening infections and other noninfectious conditions related to failing immunity (such as certain cancers) eventually develop.

MODE OF TRANSMISSION

HIV can be transmitted through sexual contact, needle- or syringe-sharing, medical use of blood or blood components, organ or tissue transplantation, and artificial insemination; it can also be transmitted perinatally from an infected woman to her infant. HIV is not transmitted through casual contact; air, food, or water routes; contact with inanimate objects; or by mosquitoes or other arthropod vectors. The use of any public conveyance (such as airplanes, automobiles, boats, buses, or trains) by individuals with AIDS or HIV infection does not pose a risk of HIV infection for the crew members or other travelers.

EPIDEMIOLOGY

AIDS and HIV infection occur worldwide. At of the end of 2008, more than 33 million people were living with HIV/AIDS. Although sub-Saharan Africa remains the most affected part of the world (22.4 million cases), notable increases in HIV infection have occurred from 2001 to 2008 in Eastern Europe and throughout

INFECTIOUS DISEASES RELATED TO TRAVEL

Asia (Map 3-7). Ninety-seven percent of new infections come from low- and middle-income countries. Many countries lack comprehensive surveillance systems, and despite improvements, the true number of cases is likely higher than officially reported, particularly in developing countries.

The risk of HIV infection for international travelers is generally low, although the risk is determined less by geographic destination and more by behaviors such as drug use and unprotected sex. In developing countries, the blood supply might not be adequately screened, increasing the risk of HIV transmission by transfusion.

DIAGNOSIS

Any person who suspects that she or he may have been exposed to HIV should be tested. Most people develop detectable antibodies within 2–8 weeks (the average is 25 days). Ninety-seven percent of people develop antibodies in the first 3 months after infection. In very rare cases, it can take up to 6 months to develop antibodies to HIV. The time from the onset of HIV infection and a positive RNA test is about 9 days; however, these tests are costly and may not be available. Diagnosis of HIV infection and AIDS may also be made when a patient presents with an AIDS-compatible diagnosis, such as *Pneumocystis* pneumonia, and is subsequently found to be HIV-seropositive. For information on HIV testing, travelers should talk to their health care provider or identify the location of an HIV testing site near them by visiting the National HIV Testing Resources website at www.hivtest.org or call CDC-INFO at 800-CDC-INFO (800-232-4636) or 888-232-6348 (TTY), in English or Spanish. Both these resources are confidential.

TREATMENT

Prompt medical care may delay the onset of AIDS and prevent some life-threatening conditions. Detailed information on specific treatments is available from the Department of Health and Human Services AIDSinfo: www.aidsinfo.nih.gov. Information on enrolling in clinical trials is also available at AIDSinfo. Travelers may contact AIDSinfo by phone, 800-448-0440 (English or Spanish) or 888-480-3739 (TTY).

PREVENTIVE MEASURES FOR TRAVELERS

No vaccine is available to prevent infection with HIV. Travelers should be advised that they are at risk if they:

- Have sexual contact (heterosexual or homosexual) with an infected person.
- Use or allow the use of contaminated, unsterilized syringes or needles for any injections or other procedures that pierce the skin, including acupuncture, use of illicit drugs, steroid or vitamin injections, medical or dental procedures, ear or body piercing, or tattooing.
- Receive infected blood, blood components, or clotting factor concentrates. HIV infection by this route is rare in countries or cities where donated blood and plasma are screened for antibodies to HIV.

To reduce their risk of acquiring HIV, travelers should:

- Avoid sexual encounters with people who are infected with HIV, whose HIV infection status is unknown, or who are at high risk for HIV infection, such as intravenous drug users, commercial sex workers (both male and female), and other people with multiple sexual partners.
- Use condoms consistently and correctly, especially if engaging in vaginal, anal, or oral-genital sexual contact with a person who is HIV infected or whose HIV status is unknown.
- Avoid injecting drugs.
- Avoid sharing needles or other devices that can puncture skin.
- Avoid, if at all possible, blood transfusions or use of clotting factor concentrates.

Condoms

People who are sensitive to latex should use condoms made of polyurethane or other synthetic materials and should carry their own supply of condoms. When a male condom cannot be used properly, a female condom should be considered. If no condom is available, travelers should abstain from sex with people who are HIV infected or whose HIV status is unknown. Barrier methods other than condoms do not prevent HIV transmission. Spermicides alone are also not effective. The widely used spermicide nonoxynol-9 can

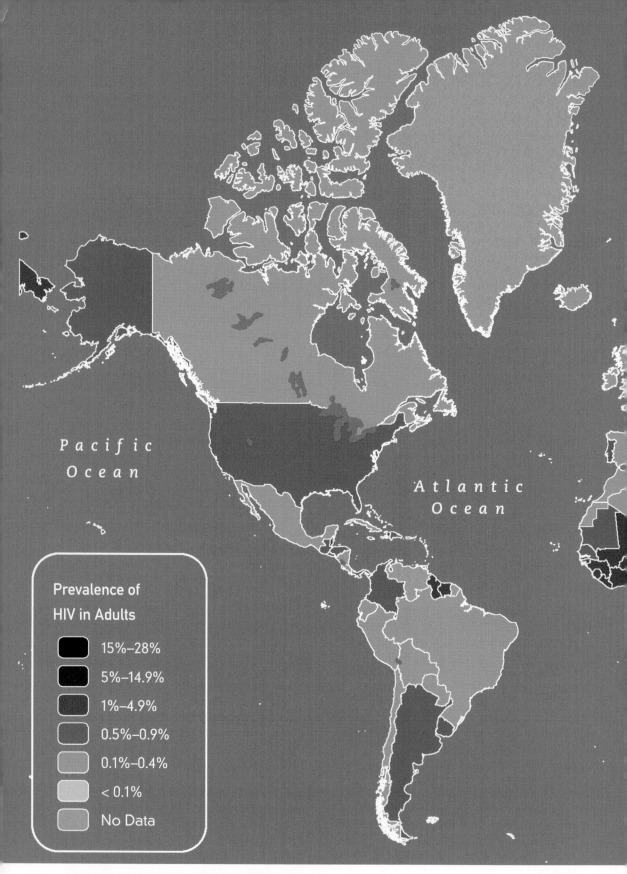

INFECTIOUS DISEASES RELATED TO TRAVEL

Prevalence of
HIV in Adults

15%–28%

5%–14.9%

1%–4.9%

0.5%–0.9%

0.1%–0.4%

< 0.1%

No Data

Pacific Ocean

Atlantic Ocean

MAP 3-7. HIV PREVALENCE IN ADULTS, 2009[1]

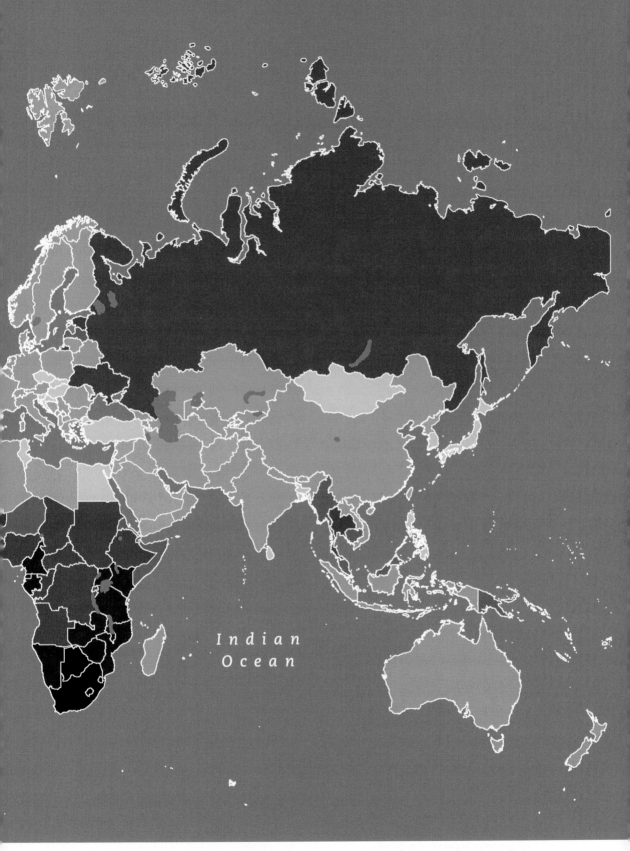

Indian
Ocean

¹ From: UNAIDS 2010 Report on the global AIDS epidemic. Available from: www.unaids.org/globalreport. Data used by kind permission of Joint United Nations Programme on HIV/AIDS (UNAIDS).

increase the risk of HIV transmission and should not be used.

Needles

Needles used to draw blood or administer injections should be sterile, single use, disposable, and prepackaged in a sealed container. If at all possible, travelers should avoid receiving medications from multidose vials, which may have become contaminated by used needles. Travelers with type 1 diabetes, hemophilia, or other conditions that necessitate routine or frequent injections should be advised to carry a supply of medication, syringes, needles, and disinfectant swabs sufficient to last their entire stay abroad. Before traveling, these travelers should consider requesting documentation of the medical necessity for traveling with these items (a doctor's letter) in case their need is questioned by inspection personnel at ports of entry (see Chapter 2, Travel Health Kits, for more information about traveling with medications).

Transfusions

In many developed countries, the risk of transfusion-associated HIV infection has been virtually eliminated through required testing of all donated blood. Developing countries may have no formal program, or inadequate technology, for testing blood or biological products for contamination with HIV. If transfusion is necessary, the blood should be tested for HIV antibody by trained laboratory technicians using a reliable test.

Postexposure Prophylaxis

People who in the course of their travel (such as a nurse volunteer drawing blood or medical missionary performing surgeries) may have contact with HIV-infected or potentially infected biological materials should ensure that they will have access to all personal protective equipment necessary (latex gloves, goggles, face shield, gowns) and that this equipment meets established international quality standards. Such travelers may also wish to consider familiarizing themselves with the principles of postexposure prophylaxis, establish a plan for seeking medical consultation, and bring a supply of antiretroviral medication of sufficient quantity to provide postexposure prophylaxis until medical care can be obtained. For more information, see Chapter 2, Occupational Exposure to HIV.

The efficacy of postexposure prophylaxis with antiretrovirals for nonoccupational exposures to HIV (such as sex or injection drug use) has not been established. It may be considered an unproven clinical intervention, after careful consideration of potential risks and benefits and with full awareness of gaps in current knowledge. Postexposure prophylaxis for potential exposure to HIV resulting from mass-casualty events is generally not warranted, except in special circumstances (for example, a blast injury in a facility that contained a large archive of HIV-infected blood specimens). Clinicians seeking advice on postexposure prophylaxis can call the US National HIV/AIDS Clinicians' Consultation Center PEPline at 888-448-4911 (www.nccc.ucsf.edu).

HIV TESTING REQUIREMENTS FOR US TRAVELERS ENTERING FOREIGN COUNTRIES

International travelers should be advised that some countries screen incoming travelers for HIV infection and may deny entry to people with AIDS or evidence of HIV infection. These countries usually screen only people planning extended visits, such as for work or study. People intending to visit a country for an extended stay should be informed of that country's policies and requirements. This information is usually available from the consular officials of the individual nations. Information about entry and exit requirements compiled by the Department of State can be found at http://travel.state.gov/travel/tips/tips_1232.html#requirement.

BIBLIOGRAPHY

1. CDC. HIV prevention bulletin: medical advice for persons who inject illicit drugs. Atlanta: CDC; 1997 [updated 2009 May 8; cited 2006 May 31]. Available from: http://www.cdc.gov/idu/pubs/hiv_prev.htm.

2. CDC. Management of possible sexual, injecting-drug-use, or other nonoccupational exposure to HIV, including considerations related to antiretroviral therapy. MMWR Recomm Rep. 1998 Sep 25; 47(RR-17):1–14.

3. Chapman LE, Sullivent EE, Grohskopf LA, Beltrami EM, Perz JF, Kretsinger K, et al. Recommendations for postexposure interventions to prevent infection with hepatitis B virus, hepatitis C virus, or human immunodeficiency virus, and tetanus in persons wounded during bombings and other mass-casualty events—United States, 2008: recommendations of the Centers for Disease Control and Prevention (CDC). MMWR Recomm Rep. 2008 Aug 1;57(RR-6):1–21.

4. Joint United Nations Programme on HIV/AIDS. 2010 report on the global AIDS epidemic. Geneva: Joint United Nations Programme on HIV/AIDS; 2010 [cited 2010 Dec 01]. Available from: www.unaids.org/globalreport.

5. Memish ZA, Osoba AO. Sexually transmitted diseases and travel. Int J Antimicrob Agents. 2003 Feb;21(2):131–4.

6. Panlilio AL, Cardo DM, Grohskopf LA, Heneine W, Ross CS. Updated US Public Health Service guidelines for the management of occupational exposures to HIV and recommendations for postexposure prophylaxis. MMWR Recomm Rep. 2005 Sep 30;54(RR-9):1–17.

7. Wright ER. Travel, tourism, and HIV risk among older adults. J Acquir Immune Defic Syndr. 2003 Jun 1;33 Suppl 2:S233–7.

HUMAN PAPILLOMAVIRUS

Eileen F. Dunne, Lauri E. Markowitz

INFECTIOUS AGENT

Human papillomavirus (HPV) is a small DNA virus.

MODE OF TRANSMISSION

There are more than 100 HPV types. More than 40 mucosal HPV types are commonly found on the genitals and are transmitted primarily by sexual contact, most commonly sexual intercourse. Sometimes transmission occurs by other routes (such as mother-to-child transmission). Infection with HPV is specific to humans.

EPIDEMIOLOGY

HPV is common worldwide. Studies in multiple countries show that the prevalence of HPV varies from 3% to 70%. There are no unique or inherent risks for travelers.

CLINICAL PRESENTATION

HPV infection is usually subclinical and asymptomatic. HPV infection is presumed when there are anogenital warts or when cervical cell changes are detected on a Papanicolaou test (Pap test). Persistent HPV infection with oncogenic types can lead to cervical cancer; >70% of cervical cancers are caused by 2 HPV types, HPV 16 or 18. HPV can also cause rare conditions and cancers, including recurrent respiratory papillomatosis; anogenital cancers such as vaginal, vulvar, anal, and penile cancers; and certain oropharyngeal and oral cancers.

DIAGNOSIS

HPV infection is most commonly asymptomatic and transient. When clinical disease occurs, diagnosis is usually made when genital warts are seen in men or women, or by results of a Pap test, HPV test, or colposcopy in women. Definitive diagnosis is made by biopsy.

TREATMENT

There is no treatment for HPV, but there are treatments for HPV-associated conditions such as genital warts and cervical cell changes.

PREVENTIVE MEASURES FOR TRAVELERS

Vaccine

Two HPV vaccines, a quadrivalent HPV vaccine (HPV4) and a bivalent HPV vaccine (HPV2), are licensed and recommended for use in adolescents and young adults (Table 3-7).

- HPV4 is approved by the Food and Drug Administration (FDA) for girls/women and

Table 3-7. Administration of human papillomavirus (HPV) vaccines

	QUADRIVALENT HPV (HPV4)[1]	BIVALENT HPV (HPV2)[2]
HPV types prevented by vaccine	6, 11, 16, 18	16, 18
Number of doses required	3	3
Schedule	0, 1–2, 6 months	0, 1–2, 6 months
Dose	0.5 mL	0.5 mL
Route of administration	Intramuscular injection	Intramuscular injection
Adjuvant	Amorphous aluminum hydroxyphosphate sulfate	50 µg 3-O-desacyl-4'-monophosphoryl lipid A and 0.5 mg aluminum hydroxide
Preservative	None	None
Storage temperature	2°C–8°C (36°F–46°F). Do not freeze.	2°C–8°C (36°F–46°F). Do not freeze.

[1] Gardasil, manufactured by Merck and Co., Inc.
[2] Cervarix, manufactured by GlaxoSmithKline

boys/men aged 9–26 years, although the Advisory Committee on Immunization Practices (ACIP) does not recommend HPV4 for routine use among boys or men.

- HPV2 is FDA approved for girls/women aged 10–25 years. HPV2 is not FDA approved for boys or men.

ACIP recommends routine vaccination of girls aged 11–12 years, although the vaccination series can be started beginning at age 9 years. Vaccination is recommended for girls/women aged 13–26 years who have

not been vaccinated previously or who have not completed the 3-dose series. If a woman reaches age 26 years before the vaccination series is complete, remaining doses can be administered after age 26 years. Ideally, vaccine should be administered before potential exposure to HPV through sexual contact.

Cervical cancer screening with a Pap test should be continued even with vaccination, because the vaccine does not prevent all types of HPV associated with cervical cancers.

BIBLIOGRAPHY

1. CDC. FDA licensure of bivalent human papillomavirus vaccine (HPV2, Cervarix) for use in females and updated HPV vaccination recommendations from the Advisory Committee on Immunization Practices (ACIP). MMWR Morb Mortal Wkly Rep. 2010 May 28;59(20):626–9.

2. CDC. FDA licensure of quadrivalent human papillomavirus vaccine (HPV4, Gardasil) for use in males and guidance from the Advisory Committee on Immunization Practices (ACIP). MMWR Morb Mortal Wkly Rep. 2010 May 28;59(20):630–2.

3. Franceschi S, Herrero R, Clifford GM, Snijders PJ, Arslan A, Anh PT, et al. Variations in the age-specific curves of human papillomavirus prevalence in women worldwide. Int J Cancer. 2006 Dec 1;119(11):2677–84.

4. Markowitz LE, Dunne EF, Saraiya M, Lawson HW, Chesson H, Unger ER. Quadrivalent human papillomavirus vaccine: recommendations of the Advisory Committee on Immunization Practices (ACIP). MMWR Recomm Rep. 2007 Mar 23;56(RR-2):1–24.

INFLUENZA (SEASONAL, ZOONOTIC, & PANDEMIC)

Margaret McCarron, David K. Shay

INFECTIOUS AGENT

Influenza in humans is caused by infection with influenza viruses; these viruses can be divided into 3 types: A, B, and C. Only types A and B cause widespread illness in humans. Influenza A viruses are further classified into subtypes on the basis of 2 surface proteins: hemagglutinin (H) and neuraminidase (N). Both influenza A and B viruses undergo continual minor antigenic change (antigenic drift), but influenza B viruses evolve more slowly and are not divided into subtypes. Only influenza A viruses demonstrate major changes (antigenic shift), in which at least the H or the H and N are replaced and a new influenza A virus with pandemic potential can result. New influenza A viruses that may emerge and spread among humans may be the result of an animal-origin influenza virus that jumps from animals to humans or the result of an influenza virus that has a new constellation of genes derived through reassortment of 2 different influenza A viruses. Influenza A (H1N1), A (H3N2), and influenza B viruses circulate globally among humans.

In April 2009, a novel A (H1N1) virus of swine origin was detected in North America. This virus is a reassortant virus, containing a combination of influenza virus gene segments not previously seen in either animal or human influenza viruses. The virus gene segments were most closely related to genes from contemporary influenza viruses circulating in North American pigs and Eurasian pigs. Contemporary North American lineage swine influenza viruses are triple reassortant viruses containing genes from human, swine, and avian influenza virus lineages, and Eurasian lineage swine influenza viruses are most closely related to Eurasian avian lineage viruses. Thus, multiple reassortant events and transmissions between animal species and humans predated the emergence of this new pandemic strain. The spread of this new virus, which was later called 2009 pandemic influenza A (H1N1) virus, resulted in a worldwide influenza pandemic.

MODE OF TRANSMISSION

Traditionally, influenza viruses have been thought to spread from person to person, primarily through large-particle respiratory droplet transmission (such as when an infected person coughs or sneezes near a susceptible person). Transmission via large-particle droplets requires close contact between the source and the recipient, because droplets generally travel only short distances (approximately ≤6 ft) through the air, but then settle out of the air. Indirect contact transmission via hand transfer of influenza virus from virus-contaminated surfaces or objects to mucosal surfaces of the face (nose, mouth) may also occur. Airborne transmission via small-particle aerosols in the vicinity of the infectious person may also occur; however, the relative contribution of the different modes of influenza transmission is unclear. All respiratory secretions and bodily fluids, including diarrheal stools, of patients with influenza should be considered infectious; however, the predominant source of infection is respiratory secretions. Viable influenza virus is rarely detected in blood or stool of infected patients. Most healthy adults who are ill with influenza may shed virus and be infectious to others from the day before symptom onset to 5–7 days after symptom onset; children, severely immunocompromised people, and more severely ill people, including those who are hospitalized, may shed influenza virus for ≥10 days after the onset of symptoms.

EPIDEMIOLOGY
Seasonal Influenza

Infection with seasonal influenza viruses is common. In temperate climates, most cases occur during the winter months. The influenza season in the Northern Hemisphere may begin as early as October and can extend until May, and the influenza season in the Southern Hemisphere may begin in April and last through September. In tropical and subtropical areas, infection with influenza virus may occur throughout the year.

CDC estimates that from 1976 through 2006, annual seasonal influenza-associated deaths in the United States ranged from a low of approximately 3,000 people to a high of approximately 49,000 people; about 90% of these deaths occur among people aged ≥65 years. Influenza virus infections can cause disease in all age groups. Infection rates are highest among infants and children, while rates of severe illness (including death) are highest among people aged ≥65 and people of any age who have underlying medical conditions that place them at increased risk for complications. Children aged <2 years have rates of influenza-related hospitalization that are as high as those in the elderly.

Zoonotic Influenza

Influenza A viruses circulate in many different animal populations. The primary reservoirs for influenza A viruses of all subtypes are wild birds. Influenza viruses found in birds are typically referred to as avian influenza viruses. Influenza A viruses are also endemic in pigs globally and in horses in many countries. Other animal species may also become infected with influenza A viruses, including domestic poultry and marine mammals. During the 2009 pandemic, infections of domesticated cat and dogs, ferrets, turkeys, a cheetah, and other animals were also reported.

Human infections with animal-origin viruses are uncommon, but they occur. Before the 2009 H1N1 pandemic, occasional swine influenza infections among humans were reported in the United States and elsewhere. In addition, more than 500 human infections with highly pathogenic avian influenza A H5N1 (HPAI-H5N1) have been reported globally since 2003. Human infections with HPAI-H5N1 are particularly concerning because of the high case-fatality ratio of approximately 60% and because this virus is widespread among poultry in some countries in Asia and the Middle East. Thus far, however, the spread of HPAI-H5N1 viruses from one ill person to another has been reported rarely and has thus far been limited, inefficient, and unsustained. Human infections with other avian influenza viruses have also included avian H7N7, H7N2, and H9N2. No sustained transmission of these other avian influenza viruses has been documented, but these viruses, along with H5N1, still have the potential to result in a pandemic.

Pandemic Influenza

A global pandemic was declared by the World Health Organization after 30,000 confirmed cases of 2009 pandemic influenza A (H1N1) virus had been reported from 74 countries. The virus spread from North America to the rest of the world. Severe illness resulting from infection with this virus was associated with risk factors such as chronic medical conditions, immunosuppression, pregnancy, young age, morbid obesity, and being a member of an indigenous population. However, in contrast to the epidemiology of seasonal influenza, CDC estimates that almost 90% of deaths from this virus occurred among people aged <65 years. The 2009 pandemic influenza A (H1N1) virus continues to circulate and was included as a component of the 2010–11 seasonal influenza vaccine.

CLINICAL PRESENTATION

Uncomplicated influenza illness is characterized by the abrupt onset of constitutional and respiratory signs and symptoms (such as fever, myalgia, headache, malaise, nonproductive cough, sore throat, vomiting, and rhinitis), typically occurring 1–4 days after exposure. However, many people will not have fever. Among children, nausea, vomiting, and diarrhea also can occur with influenza illness. Influenza illness typically resolves within 1 week for most people, although cough and malaise can persist for >2 weeks. A list of people who are at high risk of developing complications of influenza can be found on the CDC website at www.cdc.gov/flu/about/disease/high_risk.htm.

DIAGNOSIS

Respiratory illnesses caused by influenza virus infection are difficult to distinguish from illnesses caused by other respiratory pathogens on the basis of signs and symptoms alone. The predictive value of clinical definitions can vary, depending on the degree of circulation of other respiratory pathogens and the background level of influenza activity. Among studies conducted with children and adults, the positive predictive value of clinical signs and symptoms for laboratory-confirmed influenza virus infection has ranged from 30% to 88%. Laboratory testing can aid in diagnosis. Diagnostic tests available for influenza include viral culture, serology, rapid antigen testing, immunofluorescence assays, and RT-PCR. Sensitivity and specificity of any test for influenza might vary by the laboratory that performs the test, the type of test used, and the type of specimen tested. Among respiratory specimens for viral isolation or rapid detection, nasopharyngeal specimens are typically more effective than throat swab specimens.

Most patients with clinical illness consistent with uncomplicated influenza who reside in an area where influenza viruses are circulating do not require diagnostic influenza testing for clinical management. Patients who should be considered for influenza diagnostic testing include:

- Hospitalized patients with suspected influenza
- Patients for whom a diagnosis of influenza will inform decisions regarding clinical care, infection control, or management of close contacts
- Patients who died of an acute illness in which influenza was suspected

When a decision is made to use antiviral treatment for influenza, treatment should be initiated as soon as possible, without waiting for influenza test results, since antiviral treatment is most effective when administered as early as possible in the course of illness. The sensitivities of rapid influenza diagnostic tests and immunofluorescence assays are lower than those of RT-PCR tests and viral culture. Thus, a negative rapid test or immunofluorescence test result does not rule out influenza virus infection, and clinicians should not rely on a negative test to make decisions about treatment. CDC's current information on influenza diagnosis can be found on the CDC website (www.cdc.gov/flu/professionals/diagnosis).

TREATMENT

Influenza-specific antiviral drugs are adjuncts to the influenza vaccine. Empiric antiviral treatment is recommended, as early as possible, for any patient with confirmed or suspected influenza who has severe, complicated, or progressive illness, is hospitalized, or is at higher risk for influenza complications.

When indicated, antiviral treatment should be started as soon as possible after illness onset. While the most benefit is seen when antiviral treatment is started within 48 hours of illness onset, antiviral treatment may still be beneficial when started 3–4 days after illness onset, especially in people at high risk for influenza complications.

CDC recommends 2 neuraminidase inhibitors: oseltamivir and zanamivir. CDC makes revisions to antiviral recommendations periodically, in response to new data on antiviral resistance patterns among circulating strains and risk factors for influenza complications. For up-to-date antiviral recommendations, visit www.cdc.gov/flu/antivirals. People at increased risk for complications of influenza should discuss antiviral treatment and chemoprophylaxis issues with their physician before travel, if traveling to areas where influenza virus is circulating.

The effectiveness of antivirals for treating H5N1 virus infections has not been fully studied, although evidence from countries where H5N1 has caused most human cases indicates that early treatment has been associated with lower risk of death. For more information about influenza antiviral drugs, see the Avian Influenza A Virus Infections of Humans webpage at www.cdc.gov/flu/avian/gen-info/avian-flu-humans.htm.

PREVENTIVE MEASURES FOR TRAVELERS

Vaccine

Indications for Use

Annual vaccination of all people aged ≥6 months is recommended by CDC and the Advisory Committee on Immunization Practices (ACIP) as the most effective way to prevent influenza and its complications. Vaccination of pregnant women and household contacts of children aged <6 months can also reduce the risk of influenza in these children who are too young to receive influenza vaccination.

Travelers who want to reduce their risk of influenza should receive influenza vaccination ≥2 weeks before departure. Travelers who are part of large tourist groups may be exposed to influenza at any time of year through exposure to travelers from areas of the world where influenza viruses are circulating; data from cruise ships have shown that, as with other close contact environments, these settings can facilitate the transmission of influenza from person to person or through contact with contaminated environmental surfaces.

Two types of influenza vaccines are available for use in the United States: trivalent inactivated vaccine (TIV), administered by intramuscular injection, and trivalent live, attenuated influenza vaccine (LAIV), administered by nasal spray. LAIV is approved for use only in healthy people aged 2–49 years who are not pregnant.

In the United States, universal annual influenza vaccination is recommended by the ACIP for all US residents aged ≥6 months. Annual recommendations are published by CDC, including information about the season's vaccine composition, dosage and administration, and recommendations for specific populations. Current recommendations are available on the CDC website at www.cdc.gov/flu/professionals/acip/index.htm.

Vaccine Safety and Adverse Reactions

TIV

The most frequent side effects of vaccination with TIV are soreness and redness at the vaccination site that last up to 2 days. These local reactions generally are mild and rarely interfere with the ability to conduct usual daily activities. Fever, malaise, myalgia, and other systemic symptoms can occur uncommonly after vaccination and may more often affect people who have had no previous exposure to the influenza virus antigens in the vaccine (such as young children). These reactions can begin 6–12 hours after vaccination and can persist for 1–2 days. A high-dose TIV is an option for people aged ≥65 years. More information on influenza vaccine safety can be accessed on the CDC website (www.cdc.gov/mmwr/pdf/rr/rr5908.pdf).

LAIV

The most frequent side effects reported in healthy adults include runny nose or nasal congestion (28%–78%), headache (16%–44%), and sore throat (15%–27%). Some children and adolescents have reported runny nose, headache, fever, vomiting, myalgia, and wheezing. These symptoms, particularly fever, are associated more often with the first dose and are self-limited.

LAIV may result in an increase in asthma or reactive airway disease in children aged <5 years. LAIV should not be administered to any children aged <2 years or to children aged 2–4 years who have a history of wheezing in the past year or who had a diagnosis of asthma. People aged 5–49 years who have conditions that increase the risk of severe influenza, including pregnancy, should receive TIV and not LAIV.

Precautions and Contraindications

Egg allergy

Immediate reactions (such as hives, angioedema, allergic asthma, and systemic anaphylaxis) rarely occur after influenza vaccination. These reactions probably result from hypersensitivity to some vaccine component; most reactions likely are caused by residual egg protein and occur among people who have severe egg allergy. People who have developed hives, have had swelling of the lips or tongue, or have experienced acute respiratory distress or collapse after eating eggs should consult a physician for appropriate evaluation to determine if vaccine should be administered. People who have documented IgE-mediated hypersensitivity to eggs, including those who have had occupational asthma or other allergic responses due to exposure to egg protein, may also be at increased risk for reactions from influenza vaccine, and a similar consultation should be advised. Protocols have been published for safely administering influenza vaccine to people with egg allergies. There is some evidence of local hypersensitivity reactions to vaccines containing the preservative thimerosal, which is used as the preservative in multidose vials of inactivated influenza vaccine.

Personal Protection Measures

Measures that may help prevent influenza infection and other infections during travel include washing hands often with soap and water (where soap and water are not available, using an alcohol-based hand cleaner); avoiding touching one's eyes, nose, and mouth; avoiding close contact with sick people; avoiding contact with others while sick; and covering coughs and sneezes with a tissue, then disposing of the tissue.

BIBLIOGRAPHY

1. Bright RA, Shay DK, Shu B, Cox NJ, Klimov AI. Adamantane resistance among influenza A viruses isolated early during the 2005–2006 influenza season in the United States. JAMA. 2006 Feb 22;295(8):891–4.
2. CDC. Estimates of deaths associated with seasonal influenza—United States, 1976–2007. MMWR Morb Mortal Wkly Rep. 2010 Aug 27;59(33):1057–62.
3. CDC. Role of laboratory diagnosis of influenza. Atlanta: CDC; 2010 [cited 2010 Aug]. Available from: http://www.cdc.gov/flu/professionals/diagnosis/labrole.htm.
4. Dawood FS, Jain S, Finelli L, Shaw MW, Lindstrom S, Garten RJ, et al. Emergence of a novel swine-origin influenza A (H1N1) virus in humans. N Engl J Med. 2009 Jun 18;360(25):2605–15.
5. Fiore AE, Shay DK, Broder K, Iskander JK, Uyeki TM, Mootrey G, et al. Prevention and control of influenza: recommendations of the Advisory Committee on Immunization Practices (ACIP), 2008. MMWR Recomm Rep. 2008 Aug 8;57(RR-7):1–60.
6. Fiore AE, Uyeki TM, Broder K, Finelli L, Euler GL, Singleton JA, et al. Prevention and control of influenza with vaccines: recommendations of the Advisory Committee on Immunization Practices (ACIP), 2010. MMWR Recomm Rep. 2010 Aug 6;59(RR-8):1–62.
7. Jain S, Kamimoto L, Bramley AM, Schmitz AM, Benoit SR, Louie J, et al. Hospitalized patients with 2009 H1N1 influenza in the United States, April–June 2009. N Engl J Med. 2009 Nov 12;361(20):1935–44.
8. World Health Organization. Influenza A (H1N1) virus resistance to oseltamivir—2008 influenza season, Southern Hemisphere. Geneva: World Health Organization; 2008 [updated 2008 Jul 18; cited 2010 Oct 19]. Available from: http://www.paho.org/common/Display.asp?Lang=E&RecID=11596.
9. World Health Organization. New influenza A (H1N1) virus: global epidemiological situation, June 2009. Wkly Epidemiol Rec. 2009 Jun 19;84(25):249–57.

JAPANESE ENCEPHALITIS

Susan L. Hills, Randall J. Nett, Marc Fischer

INFECTIOUS AGENT

Japanese encephalitis virus (JEV) is a single-stranded RNA virus that belongs to the genus *Flavivirus* and is closely related to West Nile and Saint Louis encephalitis viruses.

MODE OF TRANSMISSION

JEV is transmitted to humans through the bite of an infected mosquito, primarily *Culex* species. The virus is maintained in an enzootic cycle between mosquitoes and amplifying vertebrate hosts, primarily pigs and wading birds. Humans are incidental or dead-end hosts, because they usually do not develop a level or duration of viremia sufficient to infect mosquitoes.

EPIDEMIOLOGY

JEV is the most common vaccine-preventable cause of encephalitis in Asia, occurring throughout most of Asia and parts of the western Pacific (Map 3-8). Local transmission of JEV has not been detected in Africa, Europe, or the Americas. Transmission principally occurs in rural agricultural areas, often associated with rice cultivation and flooding irrigation. In some areas of Asia, these ecologic conditions may occur near, or occasionally within, urban centers. In temperate areas of Asia, transmission is seasonal, and human disease usually peaks in summer and fall. In the subtropics and tropics, seasonal transmission varies with monsoon rains and irrigation practices and may be extended or even occur year-round.

In endemic countries, Japanese encephalitis (JE) is primarily a disease of children. However, travel-associated JE can occur among people of any age. The risk for JE for most travelers to Asia is extremely low but varies based on destination, duration, season, and activities.

From 1973 through 2008, there were 55 published reports of travel-associated JE among travelers from nonendemic countries. Only 4 cases among people from the United States have been reported since 1992, when a JE vaccine was first licensed in the United States.

The overall incidence of JE among people from nonendemic countries traveling to Asia is estimated to be less than 1 case per 1 million travelers. However, expatriates and travelers who stay for prolonged periods in rural areas with active JEV transmission are likely at similar risk as the susceptible resident population (5–50 cases per 100,000 children per year). Travelers on even brief trips might be at increased risk if they have extensive outdoor or nighttime exposure in rural areas during periods of active transmission. Short-term (<1 month) travelers whose visits are restricted to major urban areas are at minimal risk for JE. In endemic areas there are few human cases among residents because of vaccination or natural immunity. JEV is often still maintained in an enzootic cycle between animal and mosquitoes. Therefore, susceptible visitors may be at risk for infection.

CLINICAL PRESENTATION

Most human infections with JEV are asymptomatic; <1% of people infected with JEV develop clinical disease. Acute encephalitis is the most commonly recognized clinical manifestation of JEV infection. Milder forms of disease, such as aseptic meningitis or undifferentiated febrile illness, can also occur. The incubation period is 5–15 days. Illness usually begins with sudden onset of fever, headache,

and vomiting. Mental status changes, focal neurologic deficits, generalized weakness, and movement disorders may develop over the next few days.

- The classical description of JE includes a parkinsonian syndrome with masklike facies, tremor, cogwheel rigidity, and choreoathetoid movements.
- Acute flaccid paralysis, with clinical and pathological features similar to those of poliomyelitis, has also been associated with JEV infection.
- Seizures are common, especially among children.
- Clinical laboratory findings might include a moderate leukocytosis, mild anemia, and hyponatremia. Cerebrospinal fluid (CSF) typically has a mild to moderate pleocytosis with a lymphocytic predominance, slightly elevated protein, and normal ratio of CSF to plasma glucose.

The case-fatality ratio is approximately 20%–30%. Among survivors, 30%–50% have significant neurologic, cognitive, or psychiatric sequelae.

DIAGNOSIS

JE should be suspected in a patient with evidence of a neurologic infection (such as encephalitis, meningitis, or acute flaccid paralysis) who has recently traveled to or resided in an endemic country in Asia or the western Pacific. Laboratory diagnosis of JEV infection should be performed by using a JEV-specific IgM-capture ELISA on CSF or serum. JEV-specific IgM can be measured in the CSF of most patients by 4 days after onset of symptoms and in serum by 7 days after onset. A ≥4-fold rise in JEV-specific neutralizing antibodies between acute- and convalescent-phase serum specimens may be used to confirm the diagnosis. Vaccination history, date of onset of symptoms, and information regarding other flaviviruses known to circulate in the geographic area that may cross-react in serologic assays need to be considered when interpreting results.

Humans have low levels of transient viremia and usually have neutralizing antibodies by the time distinctive clinical symptoms are recognized. Virus isolation and nucleic-acid amplification tests are insensitive in

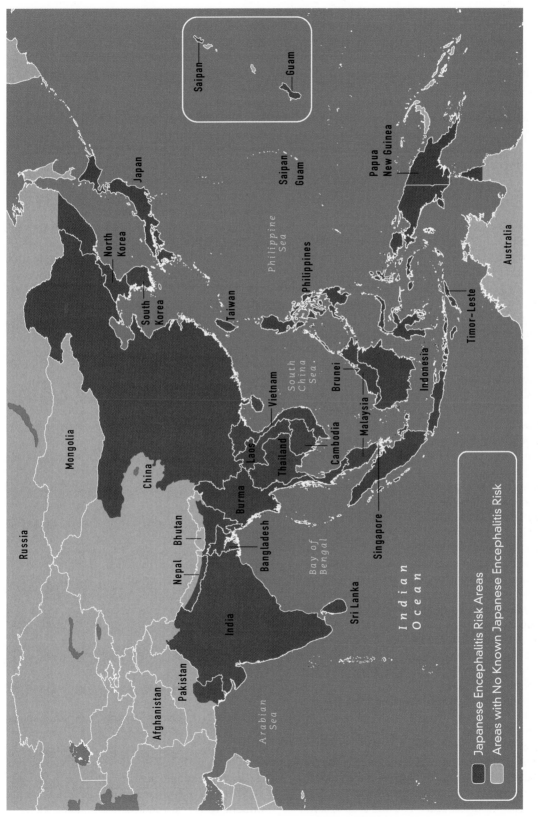

MAP 3-8. GEOGRAPHIC DISTRIBUTION OF JAPANESE ENCEPHALITIS

Japanese Encephalitis Risk Areas

Areas with No Known Japanese Encephalitis Risk

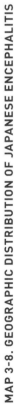

detecting JEV or JE viral RNA in blood or CSF and should not be used for ruling out a diagnosis of JE. Clinicians should contact their state or local health department or CDC's Division of Vector-Borne Diseases at 970-221-6400 for assistance with diagnostic testing.

TREATMENT

There is no specific antiviral treatment for JE; therapy consists of supportive care and management of complications.

PREVENTIVE MEASURES FOR TRAVELERS
Vaccine

Two JE vaccines are licensed in the United States: an inactivated mouse brain–derived vaccine (JE-Vax) and an inactivated Vero cell culture–derived vaccine (Ixiaro).

- JE-Vax, manufactured by Biken and distributed by Sanofi Pasteur, has been licensed in the United States since 1992 for use in travelers aged ≥1 year. In 2006, production of JE-Vax was discontinued, and all remaining doses expired in May 2011.
- Ixiaro, manufactured by Intercell and distributed by Novartis Vaccines, was approved in March 2009 for use in people aged ≥17 years. Pediatric clinical trials are being conducted to enable licensure of Ixiaro for use in children.

Other inactivated and live attenuated JE vaccines are manufactured and used in Asia but are not licensed for use in the United States.

Ixiaro
Efficacy and immunogenicity

There are no efficacy data for Ixiaro. The vaccine was licensed in the United States on the basis of its ability to induce JEV neutralizing antibodies as a surrogate for protection, as well as safety evaluations in almost 5,000 adults. In the pivotal noninferiority immunogenicity study, 96% of adults developed protective neutralizing antibodies after receiving a primary immunization series of 2 doses administered 28 days apart.

Dosage and administration

The primary immunization schedule for Ixiaro is 2 doses administered intramuscularly on days 0 and 28. The dose is 0.5 mL for people aged ≥17 years, and the 2-dose series should be completed ≥1 week before travel.

Booster doses

The full duration of protection after primary immunization with Ixiaro is unknown. In one study, 83% of people who received two doses of Ixiaro maintained protective levels of antibodies at 12 months after the first vaccine dose, and in a second study, 58% and 48% of people had protective antibodies at 12 and 24 months, respectively.

If the primary series of Ixiaro was administered ≥1 year previously, a booster dose should be given prior to potential reexposure or if there is a continued risk for JEV infection. Data on the response to a booster dose administered ≥2 years after the primary series are not available. Data on the need for and timing of additional booster doses are also not available.

Vaccine safety and adverse reactions

Pain and tenderness were the most commonly reported symptoms in a safety study with 1,993 participants who received 2 doses of Ixiaro. Systemic side effects, including headache, myalgia, fatigue, and an influenzalike illness, were each reported at a rate of >10%. Because Ixiaro was licensed after study in <5,000 recipients, the possibility of rare serious adverse events cannot be excluded. Postlicensure studies and surveillance are further evaluating the safety of Ixiaro in a larger population.

JE-Vax
Efficacy and immunogenicity

A randomized controlled trial among 65,000 children in Thailand showed an efficacy of 91% (95% confidence interval, 70%–97%) after 2 doses. From 87% to 100% of adults from nonendemic settings developed neutralizing antibodies after receiving 3 doses of vaccine.

Dosage and administration

The recommended primary immunization series for JE-Vax is 3 doses administered subcutaneously on days 0, 7, and 30. For travelers aged ≥3 years, each dose is 1.0 mL, and for children aged 1–2 years, each dose is 0.5 mL. An abbreviated schedule (days 0, 7, and 14) provides similar rates of seroconversion but lower neutralizing antibody titers at 2 and 6 months. The last dose should be administered ≥10 days before travel begins to ensure an adequate immune response and access to medical care in the event of a delayed adverse reaction.

Booster doses

The duration of protection after primary immunization is unknown, but circulating neutralizing antibodies appear to last for at least 2–3 years. A booster dose may be administered 2 years after the primary series. There are no data on interchangeability of JE vaccines or the use of Ixiaro as a booster dose after a primary series with JE-Vax. If JE-Vax is unavailable, people who have received JE-Vax previously and require further vaccination against JEV should receive a 2-dose primary series of Ixiaro.

Vaccine safety and adverse reactions

Local side effects including erythema, tenderness, and swelling at the injection site occur in about 20% of recipients. Systemic side effects, including fever, chills, headache, rash, myalgia, and gastrointestinal symptoms, have been reported in approximately 10% of vaccinees. Serious allergic hypersensitivity reactions, including generalized urticaria and angioedema of the extremities, face, and oropharynx, have been reported. Accompanying bronchospasm, respiratory distress, and hypotension have been observed in some of these patients, although there have been no deaths among vaccine recipients with these symptoms. Estimates of the frequency of these reactions range from 10 to 260 cases per 100,000 vaccinees and vary by country, year, case definition, surveillance method, and vaccine lot.

Although most hypersensitivity reactions occur within 24–48 hours after the first dose, when they occur after a subsequent dose the onset of symptoms is often delayed (median, 3 days; range, 1–14 days). Most reactions can be treated with antihistamines or corticosteroids on an outpatient basis; however, up to 10% of vaccinees with hypersensitivity reactions are hospitalized. At least 4 deaths attributed to anaphylactic shock have been associated temporally with receipt of this vaccine. None of these patients had evidence of urticaria or angioedema, and 2 had received other vaccines simultaneously. Moderate to severe neurologic symptoms, including encephalitis, seizures, gait disturbances, and parkinsonian syndrome, have been reported at a rate of 0.1–2 cases per 100,000 vaccinees. In addition, there have been case reports of children in Japan and Korea with severe or fatal acute disseminated encephalomyelitis temporally associated with JE vaccination.

Indications for Use of JE Vaccine for Travelers

When making recommendations regarding the use of JE vaccine for travelers, clinicians must weigh the overall low risk of travel-associated JEV disease, the high rate of death and disability when JE occurs, the low probability of serious adverse events after immunization, and the cost of the vaccine. Evaluation of an individual traveler's risk should take into account the planned itinerary, including travel location, duration, activities, and seasonal patterns of disease in the areas to be visited (see Table 3-8). The data in the table should be interpreted cautiously, because JEV transmission activity varies within countries and from year to year.

The Advisory Committee on Immunization Practices recommends JE vaccine for travelers who plan to spend ≥1 month in endemic areas during the JEV transmission season. This includes long-term travelers, recurrent travelers, or expatriates who will be based in urban areas but are likely to visit endemic rural or agricultural areas during a high-risk period of JEV transmission. Vaccine should also be considered for the following:

- Short-term (<1 month) travelers to endemic areas during the JEV transmission season, if they plan to travel outside an urban area and their activities will increase the risk of JEV exposure. Examples of higher-risk activities or itineraries include: 1) spending substantial time outdoors in rural or agricultural areas, especially during the evening or night; 2) participating in extensive outdoor activities (such as camping, hiking, trekking, biking, fishing, hunting, or farming); and 3) staying in accommodations without air conditioning, screens, or bed nets.
- Travelers to an area with an ongoing JE outbreak.
- Travelers to endemic areas who are uncertain of specific destinations, activities, or duration of travel.

JE vaccine is not recommended for short-term travelers whose visits will be restricted to urban areas or times outside a well-defined JEV transmission season.

Table 3-8. Risk for Japanese encephalitis, by country[1]

COUNTRY	AFFECTED AREAS	TRANSMISSION SEASON	COMMENTS
Australia	Outer Torres Strait islands	December–May; all human cases reported February–April	1 human case reported from north Queensland mainland
Bangladesh	Limited data, probably widespread	Unknown; most human cases reported May–October	1 outbreak of human disease reported from Tangail District in 1977; sentinel surveillance has recently identified human cases in Chittagong, Dhaka, Khulna, Rajshahi, and Sylhet Divisions; highest incidence reported from Rajshahi Division
Bhutan	No data	No data	
Brunei	No data; presumed to be endemic countrywide	Unknown; presumed year-round transmission	
Burma (Myanmar)	Limited data; presumed to be endemic countrywide	Unknown; most human cases reported from May–October	Outbreaks of human disease documented in Shan State; antibodies documented in animals and humans in other areas
Cambodia	Presumed to be endemic countrywide	Year round with peaks reported May–October	Sentinel surveillance has identified human cases in at least 14 provinces, including Phnom Penh, Takeo, Kampong Cham, Battambang, Svay Rieng, and Siem Reap
China	Human cases reported from all provinces except Xizang (Tibet), Xinjiang, and Qinghai; not considered endemic in Hong Kong and Macau, but rare cases reported from the New Territories	Most human cases reported June–October	Highest rates reported from Chongqing, Guizhou, Shaanxi, Sichuan, and Yunnan provinces; vaccine not routinely recommended for travel limited to Beijing or other major cities
India	Human cases reported from all states except Dadra, Daman, Diu, Gujarat, Himachal Pradesh, Jammu, Kashmir, Lakshadweep, Meghalaya, Nagar Haveli, Punjab, Rajasthan, and Sikkim	Most human cases reported May–October, especially in northern India; the season may be extended or year-round in some areas, especially in southern India	Highest rates of human disease reported from the states of Andhra Pradesh, Assam, Bihar, Goa, Haryana, Karnataka, Kerala, Tamil Nadu, Uttar Pradesh, and West Bengal

continued

TABLE 3-8. RISK FOR JAPANESE ENCEPHALITIS, BY COUNTRY[1] (continued)

COUNTRY	AFFECTED AREAS	TRANSMISSION SEASON	COMMENTS
Indonesia	Presumed to be endemic countrywide	Human cases reported year-round; peak season varies by island	Sentinel surveillance has identified human cases in Bali, Kalimantan, Java, Nusa Tenggara, Papua, and Sumatra
Japan[2]	Rare sporadic human cases on all islands except Hokkaido; enzootic activity ongoing	Most human cases reported July–October	Large number of human cases reported until JE vaccination program introduced in late 1960s; most recent small outbreak reported from Chugoku district in 2002; enzootic transmission without human cases observed on Hokkaido; vaccine not routinely recommended for travel limited to Tokyo or other major cities
Korea, North	No data	No data	
Korea, South[2]	Rare sporadic human cases countrywide; enzootic activity ongoing	Most human cases reported May–October	Large number of human cases reported until routine JE vaccination program introduced in mid-1980s; highest rates of disease were reported from the southern provinces; last major outbreak reported in 1982; vaccine not routinely recommended for travel limited to Seoul or other major cities
Laos	Limited data; presumed to be endemic countrywide	Year round, with peak June–September	Sentinel surveillance has identified human cases in north, central, and southern Laos
Malaysia	Endemic in Sarawak; sporadic cases reported from all other states; occasional outbreaks reported	Year-round transmission; peak October–December in Sarawak	Most human cases reported from Sarawak; vaccine not routinely recommended for travel limited to Kuala Lumpur or other major cities
Mongolia	Not considered endemic		

continued

TABLE 3-8. RISK FOR JAPANESE ENCEPHALITIS, BY COUNTRY[1] (continued)

COUNTRY	AFFECTED AREAS	TRANSMISSION SEASON	COMMENTS
Nepal	Endemic in southern lowlands (Terai); cases also reported from hill and mountain districts, including the Kathmandu valley	Most human cases reported June–October	Highest rates of human disease reported from western Terai districts, including Banke, Bardiya, Dang, and Kailali; vaccine not routinely recommended for those trekking in high-altitude areas or spending short periods in Kathmandu or Pokhara en route to such trekking routes
Pakistan	Limited data; human cases reported from around Karachi	Unknown	
Papua New Guinea	Limited data; probably widespread	Unknown	Sporadic human cases reported from Western Province; serologic evidence of disease from Gulf and Southern Highland Provinces; a case of JE was reported from near Port Moresby in 2004
Philippines	Limited data; presumed to be endemic on all islands	Unknown; probably year-round	Outbreaks reported in Nueva Ecija and Manila; sporadic human cases reported from other areas of Luzon and the Visayas
Russia	Rare human cases reported from the Far Eastern maritime areas south of Khabarovsk	Most human cases reported July–September	
Singapore	Rare sporadic human cases reported	Year-round transmission	Vaccine not routinely recommended
Sri Lanka	Endemic countrywide except in mountainous areas	Year-round with variable peaks based on monsoon rains	Highest rates of human disease reported from Anuradhapura, Gampaha, Kurunegala, Polonnaruwa, and Puttalam districts
Taiwan[2]	Rare sporadic human cases islandwide	Most human cases reported May–October	Large number of human cases reported until routine JE vaccination introduced in 1968; vaccine not routinely recommended for travel limited to Taipei or other major cities

continued

TABLE 3-8. RISK FOR JAPANESE ENCEPHALITIS, BY COUNTRY[1] (continued)

COUNTRY	AFFECTED AREAS	TRANSMISSION SEASON	COMMENTS
Thailand	Endemic countrywide; seasonal epidemics in the northern provinces	Year-round with seasonal peaks May–October, especially in the north	Highest rates of human disease reported from the Chiang Mai Valley; sporadic human cases reported from Bangkok suburbs
Timor-Leste	Limited data; sporadic human cases reported	No data	
Vietnam	Endemic countrywide; seasonal epidemics in the northern provinces	Year-round with seasonal peaks May–October, especially in the north	Highest rates of disease in the northern provinces around Hanoi and northwestern and northeastern provinces bordering China
Western Pacific Islands	Outbreaks of human disease reported in Guam in 1947–1948 and Saipan in 1990	Unknown; most human cases reported October–March	Enzootic cycle might not be sustainable; outbreaks may follow introductions of virus

[1] Data are based on published reports and personal correspondence. Risk assessments should be performed cautiously, because risk can vary within areas and from year to year, and surveillance data regarding human cases and JEV transmission are incomplete.

[2] In some endemic areas, human cases among residents are limited because of vaccination or natural immunity. However, because JEV is maintained in an enzootic cycle between animals and mosquitoes, susceptible visitors to these areas still may be at risk for infection.

Precautions and Contraindications

Ixiaro

A severe allergic reaction after a previous dose of Ixiaro is a contraindication to administration of further doses. Ixiaro contains protamine sulfate, a compound known to cause hypersensitivity reactions in some people. The safety and effectiveness of Ixiaro among children aged ≤16 years have not yet been determined. Limited data on the use of Ixiaro in people aged ≥65 years suggest safety and immunogenicity are similar to that among younger people, but further data are needed. No studies of Ixiaro in pregnant women have been conducted. Therefore, administration of Ixiaro to pregnant women usually should be deferred. However, pregnant women who must travel to an area where risk for JEV infection is high should be vaccinated when the theoretical risk of immunization is outweighed by the risk of infection.

JE-Vax

A history of an allergic or hypersensitivity reaction to a previous dose of mouse brain–derived JE vaccine is a contraindication to receiving additional doses. Proven or suspected hypersensitivity to thimerosal or proteins of rodent or neural origin is a contraindication to vaccination. People with a previous history of urticaria attributed to any cause are more likely to develop a hypersensitivity reaction after receipt of JE vaccine. No data are available on the safety and efficacy of JE-Vax in infants aged <1 year, and vaccination of infants should be deferred until they are ≥1 year of age.

Personal Protection Measures

The best way to prevent mosquitoborne diseases, including JE, is to avoid mosquito bites (see Chapter 2, Protection against Mosquitoes, Ticks, and Other Insects and Arthropods).

BIBLIOGRAPHY

1. CDC. Japanese encephalitis among three US travelers returning from Asia, 2003–2008. MMWR Morb Mortal Wkly Rep. 2009 Jul 17;58(27):737–40.

2. Defraites RF, Gambel JM, Hoke CH, Jr., Sanchez JL, Withers BG, Karabatsos N, et al. Japanese encephalitis vaccine (inactivated, BIKEN) in US soldiers: immunogenicity and safety of vaccine administered in two dosing regimens. Am J Trop Med Hyg. 1999 Aug;61(2):288–93.

3. Fischer M, Lindsey N, Staples JE, Hills S. Japanese encephalitis vaccines: recommendations of the Advisory Committee on Immunization Practices (ACIP). MMWR Recomm Rep. 2010 Mar 12;59(RR-1):1–27.

4. Halstead SB, Jacobson J. Japanese encephalitis vaccines. In: Plotkin SA, Orenstein WA, Offit PA, editors. Vaccines. 5th ed. Philadelphia: Saunders; 2008. p. 311–52.

5. Hills SL, Griggs AC, Fischer M. Japanese encephalitis in travelers from non-endemic countries, 1973–2008. Am J Trop Med Hyg. 2010 May;82(5):930–6.

6. Hoke CH, Nisalak A, Sangawhipa N, Jatanasen S, Laorakapongse T, Innis BL, et al. Protection against Japanese encephalitis by inactivated vaccines. N Engl J Med. 1988 Sep 8;319(10):608–14.

7. Marfin AA, Eidex RS, Kozarsky PE, Cetron MS. Yellow fever and Japanese encephalitis vaccines: indications and complications. Infect Dis Clin North Am. 2005 Mar;19(1):151–68, ix.

8. Plesner AM. Allergic reactions to Japanese encephalitis vaccine. Immunol Allergy Clin North Am. 2003 Nov;23(4):665–97.

9. Shlim DR, Solomon T. Japanese encephalitis vaccine for travelers: exploring the limits of risk. Clin Infect Dis. 2002 Jul 15;35(2):183–8.

10. Solomon T. Flavivirus encephalitis. N Engl J Med. 2004 Jul 22;351(4):370–8.

11. Takahashi H, Pool V, Tsai TF, Chen RT. Adverse events after Japanese encephalitis vaccination: review of post-marketing surveillance data from Japan and the United States. The VAERS Working Group. Vaccine. 2000 Jul 1;18(26):2963–9.

12. Tauber E, Kollaritsch H, Korinek M, Rendi-Wagner P, Jilma B, Firbas C, et al. Safety and immunogenicity of a Vero-cell-derived, inactivated Japanese encephalitis vaccine: a non-inferiority, phase III, randomised controlled trial. Lancet. 2007 Dec 1;370(9602):1847–53.

13. Tauber E, Kollaritsch H, von Sonnenburg F, Lademann M, Jilma B, Firbas C, et al. Randomized, double-blind, placebo-controlled phase 3 trial of the safety and tolerability of IC51, an inactivated Japanese encephalitis vaccine. J Infect Dis. 2008 Aug 15;198(4):493–9.

14. World Health Organization. Japanese encephalitis vaccines. Wkly Epidemiol Rec. 2006 Aug 25;81(34/35):331–40.

LEGIONELLOSIS (LEGIONNAIRES' DISEASE & PONTIAC FEVER)

Lauri A. Hicks, Laurel E. Garrison

INFECTIOUS AGENT

Legionellosis is caused by gram-negative bacteria of the genus *Legionella*.

MODE OF TRANSMISSION

Transmission occurs by inhalation of a water aerosol containing the bacteria. The bacterium grows in warm freshwater environments. Person-to-person transmission does not occur with either Legionnaires' disease or Pontiac fever.

EPIDEMIOLOGY

Legionellae are ubiquitous worldwide. Most cases of legionellosis are caused by *Legionella pneumophila*. Disease occurs after exposure to aquatic settings that promote bacterial growth—the aquatic environment is somewhat stagnant, the water is warm (77°F–108°F [25°C–42°C]), and the water must be aerosolized so that the bacteria can be inhaled into the lungs. These 3 conditions are met almost exclusively in developed or industrialized settings. Disease does not occur in association with natural settings such as waterfalls, lakes, or streams.

Outbreaks of legionellosis have been described in numerous countries throughout the world. In Australia and the United States, rare cases of legionellosis caused by *L. longbeachae* have been associated with exposure to potting soil. The largest outbreak (449 cases) ever reported was traced to a cooling tower on the roof of a city hospital in Murcia, Spain, in 2001.

Despite the presence of *Legionella* bacteria in many aquatic environments, the risk of developing legionellosis for most people is low. Travelers who are exposed to aerosolized, warm water are at risk for infection. Elderly and immunocompromised travelers, such as those being treated for cancer, are at higher risk. Many outbreaks have been associated with exposure to cruise ships, hotels, and resorts. Exposures can occur during recreation in or near a whirlpool spa, while showering in a hotel, or touring in cities with buildings that have cooling towers. Patients often do not recall specific water exposures, as they frequently occur during activities of daily living.

CLINICAL PRESENTATION
Legionnaires' disease typically presents with pneumonia, which usually requires hospitalization and can be fatal in 10%–15% of cases. Symptom onset occurs 2–14 days after exposure. In outbreak settings, <5% of people exposed to the source of the outbreak develop Legionnaires' disease.

Pontiac fever is milder than Legionnaires' disease and presents as an influenzalike illness, with fever, headache, and myalgias, but no signs of pneumonia. Pontiac fever can affect healthy people, as well as those with underlying illnesses, and symptoms occur within 72 hours of exposure. Most patients fully recover. Up to 95% of people exposed in outbreak settings can develop symptoms of Pontiac fever.

DIAGNOSIS
Isolation of *Legionella* from respiratory secretions, lung tissue, pleural fluid, or a normally sterile site is an important method for diagnosis of Legionnaires' disease. Clinical isolates are often necessary to interpret the findings of an environmental investigation. Because of differences in mechanism of disease, *Legionella* cannot be isolated in people who have Pontiac fever.

The most used diagnostic method is the *Legionella* urinary antigen assay. However, the assay can only detect *L. pneumophila* serogroup 1, the most common cause of legionellosis. Paired serology showing a 4-fold rise in antibody titer between acute- and convalescent-phase specimens confirms the diagnosis. A single antibody titer of any level is not diagnostic of legionellosis. Additional information can be found at CDC's Legionellosis Resource Site (www.cdc.gov/legionella/index.htm).

TREATMENT
For travelers with suspected Legionnaires' disease, specific antibiotic treatment is necessary and should be administered promptly while diagnostic tests are being processed. Appropriate antibiotics include fluoroquinolones and macrolides. Treatment may be necessary for up to 3 weeks. In severe cases, patients may have prolonged stays in intensive care units. Consultation with an infectious diseases specialist is advised. Pontiac fever is a self-limited illness that requires supportive care only; antibiotics have no benefit.

PREVENTIVE MEASURES FOR TRAVELERS
There is no vaccine for legionellosis, and antibiotic prophylaxis is not effective. Travelers at increased risk for infection, such as the elderly or those with immunocompromising conditions such as cancer or diabetes, may choose to avoid high-risk areas, such as whirlpool spas. If exposure cannot be avoided, travelers should be advised to seek medical attention promptly if they develop symptoms of Legionnaires' disease or Pontiac fever.

BIBLIOGRAPHY
1. Burnsed LJ, Hicks LA, Smithee LM, Fields BS, Bradley KK, Pascoe N, et al. A large, travel-associated outbreak of legionellosis among hotel guests: utility of the urine antigen assay in confirming Pontiac fever. Clin Infect Dis. 2007 Jan 15;44(2):222–8.

2. CDC. Cruise ship-associated Legionnaires disease, November 2003–May 2004. MMWR Morb Mortal Wkly Rep. 2005 Nov 18;54(45):1153–5.

3. CDC. Legionnaires' disease associated with potting soil—California, Oregon, and Washington, May–June

2000. MMWR Morb Mortal Wkly Rep. 2000 Sep 1;49(34):777–8.

4. CDC. Surveillance for travel-associated legionnaires disease—United States, 2005–2006. MMWR Morb Mortal Wkly Rep. 2007 Dec 7;56(48):1261–3.

5. Fields BS, Benson RF, Besser RE. *Legionella* and legionnaires' disease: 25 years of investigation. Clin Microbiol Rev. 2002 Jul;15(3):506–26.

6. Garcia-Fulgueiras A, Navarro C, Fenoll D, Garcia J, Gonzalez-Diego P, Jimenez-Bunuales T, et al.

Legionnaires' disease outbreak in Murcia, Spain. Emerg Infect Dis. 2003 Aug;9(8):915–21.

7. Jernigan DB, Hofmann J, Cetron MS, Genese CA, Nuorti JP, Fields BS, et al. Outbreak of legionnaires' disease among cruise ship passengers exposed to a contaminated whirlpool spa. Lancet. 1996 Feb 24;347(9000):494–9.

8. Ricketts K, Joseph CA, Yadav R. Travel-associated legionnaires disease in Europe in 2008. Euro Surveill. 2010 May 27;15(21):19578.

LEISHMANIASIS, CUTANEOUS

Barbara L. Herwaldt, Alan J. Magill

Leishmaniasis is a parasitic disease found in parts of the tropics, subtropics, and southern Europe. Leishmaniasis has several different forms. This section focuses on cutaneous leishmaniasis (CL), the most common form, both in general and in travelers.

INFECTIOUS AGENT

Leishmaniasis is caused by obligate intracellular protozoan parasites; approximately 20 *Leishmania* species cause CL.

MODE OF TRANSMISSION

CL is transmitted through the bite of infected female phlebotomine sand flies. CL also can occur after accidental occupational (laboratory) exposures to *Leishmania* parasites.

EPIDEMIOLOGY

In the Old World (Eastern Hemisphere), CL is found in parts of the Middle East, Asia (particularly southwest and central Asia), Africa (particularly the tropical region and North Africa), and southern Europe. In the New World (Western Hemisphere), CL is found in parts of Mexico, Central America, and South America. Occasional cases have been reported in Texas and Oklahoma. CL is not found in Chile, Uruguay, or Canada. Overall, CL is found in focal areas of about 90 countries. Most (>90%) of the world's cases of CL occur in 10 countries: Afghanistan, Algeria, Iran, Iraq, Saudi Arabia, and Syria in the Old

World; and Bolivia, Brazil, Colombia, and Peru in the New World.

The geographic distribution of cases of CL evaluated in countries such as the United States reflects travel and immigration patterns. More than 75% of the cases diagnosed in US civilians have been acquired in Latin America, including popular tourist destinations such as Costa Rica. Cases in US service personnel reflect military activities (in Iraq, for example). CL is usually more common in rural than urban areas, but it is found in some periurban and urban areas (such as in Baghdad, Iraq, and Kabul, Afghanistan). The ecologic settings range from rainforests to arid regions.

The risk is highest from dusk to dawn because sand flies typically feed (bite) at night and during twilight hours. Although sand flies are less active during the hottest time of the day, they may bite if they are disturbed (for example, if hikers brush up against tree trunks or other sites where sand flies are resting). Vector activity can easily be overlooked: sand flies do not make noise, they are small (approximately one-third the size of mosquitoes), and their bites might not be noticed.

Examples of types of travelers who might have an increased risk for CL include ecotourists, adventure travelers, bird watchers, Peace Corps volunteers, missionaries, soldiers, construction workers, and people who do research outdoors at night or twilight. However, even short-term travelers in endemic areas have developed CL.

CLINICAL PRESENTATION

CL is characterized by skin lesions (open or closed sores), which typically develop within several weeks or months after exposure. In some people, the sores first appear months or years later, in the context of trauma (such as skin wounds or surgery). The sores can change in size and appearance over time. They typically progress from small papules to nodular plaques, and eventually lead to open sores with a raised border and central crater (ulcer), which can be covered with scales or crust. The lesions usually are painless but can be painful, particularly if open sores become infected with bacteria. Satellite lesions, regional lymphadenopathy (swollen glands), and nodular lymphangitis can be noted. The sores usually heal eventually, even without treatment. However, they can last for months or years and typically result in scarring.

Another potential concern applies to some of the *Leishmania* species in South and Central America—occasionally, these parasites spread from the skin to the mucosal surfaces of the nose or mouth and cause sores there. This form of leishmaniasis, mucosal leishmaniasis (ML), might not be noticed until years after the original skin sores appear to have healed. Although ML is uncommon, it has occurred in travelers and expatriates whose cases of CL were not treated or were inadequately treated. The initial clinical manifestations typically involve the nose (chronic stuffiness, bleeding, and inflamed mucosa or sores) and less often the mouth; in advanced cases, ulcerative destruction of the nose, mouth, and pharynx can be noted (such as perforation of the nasal septum).

DIAGNOSIS

Clinicians should consider CL in people with chronic (nonhealing) skin lesions who have been in areas where leishmaniasis is found. Laboratory confirmation of the diagnosis is achieved by detecting *Leishmania* parasites (or DNA) in infected tissue, through light-microscopic examination of stained specimens, culture techniques, or molecular methods.

CDC can assist in all aspects of the diagnostic evaluation. Identification of the *Leishmania* species can be important,

particularly if more than one species is found where the patient traveled and if the species can have different clinical and prognostic implications. Serologic testing generally is not useful for CL but can provide supportive evidence for the diagnosis of ML.

For consultative services, contact CDC Public Inquiries (770-488-7775; parasites@cdc.gov). Additional information can be found on the CDC website at www.cdc.gov/parasites/leishmaniasis.

TREATMENT

Decisions about whether and how to treat CL should be individualized. All cases of ML should be treated. Clinicians may consult with CDC staff about the relative merits of various approaches (see the Diagnosis section above for contact information).

The pentavalent antimonial compound sodium stibogluconate (Pentostam) is available to US-licensed physicians through the CDC Drug Service (404-639-3670) for intravenous or intramuscular administration under an investigational new drug protocol (see www.cdc.gov/laboratory/drugservice/index.html).

PREVENTIVE MEASURES FOR TRAVELERS

No vaccines or drugs to prevent infection are available. Preventive measures are aimed at reducing contact with sand flies by using personal protective measures (see Chapter 2, Protection against Mosquitoes, Ticks, and Other Insects and Arthropods). Travelers should be advised to:

- Avoid outdoor activities, especially from dusk to dawn, when sand flies generally are the most active.
- Wear protective clothing and apply insect repellent to exposed skin and under the edges of clothing, such as sleeves and pant legs, according to the manufacturer's instructions.
- Sleep in air-conditioned or well-screened areas. Spraying the quarters with insecticide might provide some protection. Fans or ventilators might inhibit the movement of sand flies, which are weak fliers.

Sand flies are so small (approximately 2–3 mm, less than one-eighth of an inch) that they can pass through the holes in ordinary bed nets. Although closely woven nets are available, they may be uncomfortable in hot climates. The effectiveness of bed nets can be enhanced by treatment with a pyrethroid-containing insecticide (permethrin or delta-methrin). The same treatment can be applied to window screens, curtains, bed sheets, and clothing.

BIBLIOGRAPHY

1. Ahluwalia S, Lawn SD, Kanagalingam J, Grant H, Lockwood DN. Mucocutaneous leishmaniasis: an imported infection among travellers to central and South America. BMJ. 2004 Oct 9;329(7470):842–4.
2. Blum J, Desjeux P, Schwartz E, Beck B, Hatz C. Treatment of cutaneous leishmaniasis among travellers. J Antimicrob Chemother. 2004 Feb;53(2):158–66.
3. Herwaldt BL. Leishmaniasis. Lancet. 1999 Oct 2;354(9185):1191–9.
4. Herwaldt BL, Stokes SL, Juranek DD. American cutaneous leishmaniasis in US travelers. Ann Intern Med. 1993 May 15;118(10):779–84.
5. Magill AJ. Cutaneous leishmaniasis in the returning traveler. Infect Dis Clin North Am. 2005 Mar;19(1):241–66, x–xi.
6. Murray HW, Berman JD, Davies CR, Saravia NG. Advances in leishmaniasis. Lancet. 2005 Oct 29–Nov 4;366(9496):1561–77.
7. Schwartz E, Hatz C, Blum J. New world cutaneous leishmaniasis in travellers. Lancet Infect Dis. 2006 Jun;6(6):342–9.

LEISHMANIASIS, VISCERAL
Barbara L. Herwaldt, Alan J. Magill

Leishmaniasis is a parasitic disease found in parts of the tropics, subtropics, and southern Europe. Leishmaniasis has several different forms. This section focuses on visceral leishmaniasis (VL), which affects some of the internal organs of the body (such as spleen, liver, and bone marrow).

INFECTIOUS AGENT
VL is caused by obligate intracellular protozoan parasites, particularly by the species *Leishmania donovani* and *L. infantum/ L. chagasi*.

MODE OF TRANSMISSION
VL is predominantly transmitted through the bite of infected female phlebotomine sand flies, although congenital and parenteral transmission (through blood transfusions and needle sharing) have been reported.

EPIDEMIOLOGY
VL is usually more common in rural than urban areas, but it is found in some periurban areas (such as in northeastern Brazil).

In the Old World (Eastern Hemisphere), VL is found in parts of Asia (particularly the Indian subcontinent and southwest and central Asia), the Middle East, Africa (particularly East Africa), and southern Europe. In the New World (Western Hemisphere), most cases occur in Brazil; some cases occur in scattered foci elsewhere in Latin America. Overall, VL is found in focal areas of approximately 65 countries. Most (>90%) of the world's cases of VL occur in the Indian subcontinent (India, Bangladesh, and Nepal), Sudan, Ethiopia, and Brazil; none of the affected areas in these 6 countries are common tourist destinations.

The geographic distribution of cases of VL evaluated in countries such as the United States reflects travel and immigration patterns. VL is uncommon in US travelers and expatriates. Occasional cases have been diagnosed in short-term travelers (tourists) to southern Europe and also in longer-term travelers (such as expatriates and deployed soldiers) to the Mediterranean region and other areas where VL is found.

CLINICAL PRESENTATION

Among symptomatic people, the incubation period typically ranges from weeks to months. The onset of illness can be abrupt or gradual. Stereotypical manifestations of VL include fever, weight loss, hepatosplenomegaly (especially splenomegaly), and pancytopenia (anemia, leukopenia, and thrombocytopenia). If untreated, severe (advanced) cases of VL typically are fatal. Latent infection can become clinically manifest years to decades after exposure in people who become immunocompromised for other medical reasons.

DIAGNOSIS

Clinicians should consider VL in people with a relevant travel history (even in the distant past) and a persistent, unexplained febrile illness, especially if accompanied by other suggestive manifestations (such as splenomegaly and pancytopenia). Laboratory confirmation of the diagnosis is achieved by detecting *Leishmania* parasites or DNA in infected tissue (such as in bone marrow, liver, lymph node, or blood), through light-microscopic examination of stained specimens, culture techniques, or molecular methods. Serologic testing can provide supportive evidence for the diagnosis.

CDC can assist in all aspects of the diagnostic evaluation, including species identification. For consultative services, contact CDC Public Inquiries (770-488-7775; parasites@cdc.gov). Additional information can be found on the CDC website (www.cdc.gov/parasites/leishmaniasis).

TREATMENT

Infected travelers should be advised to consult an infectious disease or tropical medicine specialist. Therapy for VL should be individualized with expert consultation. The relative merits of various approaches can be discussed with CDC staff (see the Diagnosis section above for contact information).

Liposomal amphotericin B (AmBisome) is approved by the Food and Drug Administration to treat VL. The pentavalent antimonial compound sodium stibogluconate (Pentostam) is available to US-licensed physicians through the CDC Drug Service (404-639-3670) under an investigational new drug protocol (see www.cdc.gov/laboratory/drugservice/index.html).

PREVENTIVE MEASURES FOR TRAVELERS

No vaccines or drugs to prevent infection are available. Preventive measures are aimed at reducing contact with sand flies (see the Protection against Mosquitoes, Ticks, and Other Insects and Arthropods section in Chapter 2 and Preventive Measures for Travelers in the previous section, Cutaneous Leishmaniasis). In particular, travelers should be advised to avoid outdoor activities, especially from dusk to dawn, when sand flies generally are the most active, and to sleep in air-conditioned or well-screened quarters. Preventive measures also include wearing protective clothing, applying insect repellent to exposed skin, using bed nets treated with a pyrethroid-containing insecticide, and spraying dwellings with residual-action insecticides.

BIBLIOGRAPHY

1. Herwaldt BL. Leishmaniasis. Lancet. 1999 Oct 2;354(9185):1191–9.
2. Malik AN, John L, Bruceson AD, Lockwood DN. Changing pattern of visceral leishmaniasis, United Kingdom, 1985–2004. Emerg Infect Dis. 2006 Aug;12(8):1257–9.
3. Murray HW, Berman JD, Davies CR, Saravia NG. Advances in leishmaniasis. Lancet. 2005 Oct 29–Nov 4;366(9496):1561–77.
4. Myles O, Wortmann GW, Cummings JF, Barthel RV, Patel S, Crum-Cianflone NF, et al. Visceral leishmaniasis: clinical observations in 4 US army soldiers deployed to Afghanistan or Iraq, 2002–2004. Arch Intern Med. 2007 Sep 24;167(17):1899–901.
5. Weisser M, Khanlari B, Terracciano L, Arber C, Gratwohl A, Bassetti S, et al. Visceral leishmaniasis: a threat to immunocompromised patients in non-endemic areas? Clin Microbiol Infect. 2007 Aug;13(8):751–3.

LEPTOSPIROSIS

Robyn Stoddard, Sean V. Shadomy

INFECTIOUS AGENT

Leptospirosis is caused by obligate aerobic spirochete bacteria in the genus *Leptospira*, which grow optimally at 28°C–30°C.

MODE OF TRANSMISSION

Infection occurs through abrasions or cuts in the skin or through the conjunctiva and mucous membranes. Humans may be infected by direct contact with urine or reproductive fluids from infected animals or with water or soil contaminated with those fluids. Prolonged immersion in contaminated water increases the risk for infection. Infection rarely occurs through animal bites or human-to-human contact.

EPIDEMIOLOGY

Leptospirosis has worldwide distribution, with a higher incidence in tropical climates. Domestic, peridomestic, and wild animals are maintenance hosts of the bacteria and excrete the bacteria in their urine, amniotic fluid, or placental tissue, which can contaminate the soil and water. Most *Leptospira* species can persist 2–3 weeks in fresh water, damp soil, or mud. Flooding after hurricanes or heavy rainfall facilitates the spread of the organism, contributing to outbreaks. This is especially true in regions with high endemic rates of infection. Leptospirosis is associated with animal husbandry.

Rodentborne leptospirosis may be a risk to people exposed to rat urine in infested urban areas. Travelers participating in recreational water activities, such as whitewater rafting, adventure racing, kayaking, or triathlon events may be at increased risk for leptospirosis, particularly after heavy rainfall or flooding. Outbreaks of leptospirosis have occurred in the United States after flooding in Hawaii and Puerto Rico. Leptospirosis has also been reported in international travelers to regions experiencing epidemics after heavy rainfall or flooding.

CLINICAL PRESENTATION

The incubation period is 2 days to 3 weeks. The symptoms of leptospirosis are varied and often biphasic. The acute or bacteremic phase lasts a week, followed by the immune phase that is characterized by antibody production and the presence of leptospires in the urine. The acute, generalized illness mimics other acute febrile illnesses, such as dengue fever, malaria, or typhus. Common symptoms include headache, fever, chills, myalgia, nausea, diarrhea, abdominal pain, uveitis, adenopathy, conjunctival suffusion without purulent discharge, and occasionally, a skin rash. The headache is often severe and includes retroorbital pain and photophobia. Aseptic meningitis occurs in up to 25% of cases.

The icteric or severe form of the disease (Weil disease) occurs in 5%–10% of patients with leptospirosis. Symptoms include jaundice, renal failure, hemorrhage, cardiac arrhythmias, pneumonitis, and hemodynamic collapse. The death rate in patients with severe leptospirosis is 5%–15%.

DIAGNOSIS

Diagnosis of leptospirosis is usually based on serology. Antibodies may be detected in the blood within 5–7 days of symptom onset. Culture and demonstration of the organism under darkfield microscopy are both relatively insensitive. No PCR assay has been validated with clinical specimens. Confirmation of leptospirosis requires seroconversion between acute- and convalescent-phase serum specimens, as demonstrated by the microscopic agglutination test (MAT), culture of the organism from clinical specimens, or demonstration of *Leptospira* in a clinical specimen by immunofluorescence.

MAT, the recognized standard reference test for serologic diagnosis of leptospirosis, is performed only in reference laboratories. Although MAT is not specific for diagnosis of acute cases, a single elevated MAT titer in a patient with a compatible febrile illness and suspected exposure suggests acute leptospirosis. Seroconversion with a 4-fold or larger rise in titer between acute- and convalescent-phase serum specimens obtained 2 weeks or more apart confirms the diagnosis.

Several rapid, reliable serologic assays are commercially available for diagnostic screening for an acute infection. A recent evaluation of 4 of these assays concluded that both a microplate IgM ELISA and an IgM dot-ELISA dipstick test exhibited high sensitivity and specificity on acute-phase samples.

TREATMENT

Missed or delayed diagnosis of leptospirosis is common because of its nonspecific clinical presentation and a low index of suspicion among clinicians seeing returned travelers. Antimicrobial therapy should be initiated early in the course of the disease if leptospirosis is suspected. Intravenous penicillin is a drug of choice for patients with severe leptospirosis. As with other spirochete infections, a Jarisch-Herxheimer reaction (an acute febrile reaction that can range from rash to anaphylaxis) can develop after initiation of penicillin therapy. Various methods have been described to prevent or control Jarisch-Herxheimer reactions, and management should follow the appropriate standards for patient care. Doxycycline is effective in decreasing the severity and duration of leptospirosis and the occurrence of leptospiruria. Parenteral third-generation cephalosporins and azithromycin may also be used for treatment. Because of the risk for potential complications, including cardiac arrhythmia, renal failure, pulmonary involvement and respiratory distress, or myocarditis, patients with leptospirosis may require hospitalization, supportive therapy, and close monitoring.

PREVENTIVE MEASURES FOR TRAVELERS

No vaccine is available in the United States. Travelers who might be at an increased risk for infection because of recreational water activities or exposure to contaminated surface waters and soil should be advised to consider preventive measures such as wearing protective clothing, especially footwear, and covering cuts and abrasions with occlusive dressings. They should avoid contact with, submersion in, or swallowing potentially contaminated water.

Travelers at risk because of destination or activities during travel may benefit from chemoprophylaxis. Until further data become available, CDC recommends that adult travelers who might be at increased risk for leptospirosis be advised to consider chemoprophylaxis with doxycycline (200 mg orally, weekly), begun 1–2 days before and continuing through the period of exposure. Indications for prophylactic doxycycline use for children have not been established. Travelers at increased risk for leptospirosis and in need of malaria chemoprophylaxis should consider using doxycycline for both indications.

BIBLIOGRAPHY

1. Bajani MD, Ashford DA, Bragg SL, Woods CW, Aye T, Spiegel RA, et al. Evaluation of four commercially available rapid serologic tests for diagnosis of leptospirosis. J Clin Microbiol. 2003 Feb;41(2):803–9.
2. Gaynor K, Katz AR, Park SY, Nakata M, Clark TA, Effler PV. Leptospirosis on Oahu: an outbreak associated with flooding of a university campus. Am J Trop Med Hyg. 2007 May;76(5):882–5.
3. Griffith ME, Hospenthal DR, Murray CK. Antimicrobial therapy of leptospirosis. Curr Opin Infect Dis. 2006 Dec;19(6):533–7.
4. Guidugli F, Castro AA, Atallah AN. Antibiotics for preventing leptospirosis. Cochrane Database Syst Rev. 2000(4):CD001305.
5. Haake DA, Dundoo M, Cader R, Kubak BM, Hartskeerl RA, Sejvar JJ, et al. Leptospirosis, water sports, and chemoprophylaxis. Clin Infect Dis. 2002 May 1;34(9):e40–3.
6. Levett PN. Leptospirosis. Clin Microbiol Rev. 2001 Apr;14(2):296–326.
7. Morgan J, Bornstein SL, Karpati AM, Bruce M, Bolin CA, Austin CC, et al. Outbreak of leptospirosis among triathlon participants and community residents in Springfield, Illinois, 1998. Clin Infect Dis. 2002 Jun 15;34(12):1593–9.
8. Pappas G, Cascio A. Optimal treatment of leptospirosis: queries and projections. Int J Antimicrob Agents. 2006 Dec;28(6):491–6.
9. Phimda K, Hoontrakul S, Suttinont C, Chareonwat S, Losuwanaluk K, Chueasuwanchai S, et al. Doxycycline versus azithromycin for treatment of leptospirosis and scrub typhus. Antimicrob Agents Chemother. 2007 Sep;51(9):3259–63.
10. Sanders EJ, Rigau-Perez JG, Smits HL, Deseda CC, Vorndam VA, Aye T, et al. Increase of leptospirosis in dengue-negative patients after a hurricane in Puerto Rico in 1966. Am J Trop Med Hyg. 1999 Sep;61(3):399–404.
11. Vinetz JM, Glass GE, Flexner CE, Mueller P, Kaslow DC. Sporadic urban leptospirosis. Ann Intern Med. 1996 Nov 15;125(10):794–8.

LYME DISEASE

Jeffrey R. Miller, Paul S. Mead

INFECTIOUS AGENT

Lyme borreliosis (Lyme disease) is caused by spirochetes belonging to the *Borrelia burgdorferi* sensu lato complex, including *B. afzelii*, *B. burgdorferi* sensu stricto, and *B. garinii*.

MODE OF TRANSMISSION

Lyme disease is transmitted through the bite of nymph and adult *Ixodes* ticks, which are found in temperate forested and woodland areas of North America and Eurasia. Adult and nymphal *Ixodes* ticks are tiny, roughly the size of sesame seed and poppy seed, respectively; infected people are often unaware that they have been bitten.

EPIDEMIOLOGY

In Europe, Lyme disease occurs from southern Scandinavia into the northern Mediterranean countries of Italy, Spain, and Greece. Incidence is highest in central and Eastern European countries, such as Slovenia, where the annual reported incidence is 155 cases per 100,000 population. In North America, highly endemic areas are the northeastern and north-central United States. Transmission has not been documented in the tropics.

Lyme disease is rarely reported in returning travelers. All ages are at risk for infection during travel to endemic areas. Infection is associated with exposure to tick habitats (such as wooded, brushy, or grassy areas).

CLINICAL PRESENTATION

Incubation period is 3–32 days. Approximately 80% of people infected with *B. burgdorferi* develop a characteristic rash, erythema migrans (EM), within 30 days of exposure. EM is a red, expanding rash, with or without central clearing, that is often accompanied by symptoms of fatigue, fever, headache, mild stiff neck, arthralgia, or myalgia. A rash <5 cm in diameter that develops while the tick is still attached or within 48 hours of tick bite is likely caused by a hypersensitivity reaction and is not an indication of infection.

Within days or weeks, infection can spread to other parts of the body, causing more serious neurologic conditions (meningitis, radiculopathy, and facial palsy) or cardiac abnormalities (myocarditis with atrioventricular heart block). Untreated, infection can progress over a period of months to cause monoarticular or oligoarticular arthritis, peripheral neuropathy, or encephalopathy. Long-term sequelae can be typically observed over a number of months, ranging from 1 week to a few years.

The clinical presentation of Lyme disease in Eurasia is generally similar to the presentation of infection in North America. Multiple EM rashes have been described more often in patients infected in North America than in Europe. Patients infected in Europe may be more likely to develop neuroborreliosis or the rare skin manifestations, acrodermatitis chronic atrophicans and borrelial lymphocytoma.

DIAGNOSIS

Observation of an EM rash with a history of recent travel to an endemic area (with or without history of tick bite) is sufficient to make a diagnosis of Lyme disease. Serologic testing is often negative in the first few weeks of illness and should not delay treatment in patients with a recent onset (2–3 weeks) of a characteristic EM rash. For patients with evidence of disseminated infection (musculoskeletal, neurologic, or cardiac manifestations) 2-tiered serologic testing, consisting of an ELISA/IFA and confirmatory Western blot, is recommended. Patients suspected of acquiring Lyme disease overseas should be tested by using a C6-based ELISA, as other serologic tests may not detect infection with European species of *Borrelia*.

TREATMENT

Guidelines for treatment of Lyme disease have been published by the Infectious Diseases Society of America and are available at http://cid.oxfordjournals.org/content/43/9/1089.full. Depending on the stage of disease, most patients can be treated with either oral doxycycline or intravenous ceftriaxone. Physicians unfamiliar with Lyme disease may wish to consult an infectious disease specialist for further guidance. Additional information about Lyme disease can be found on the CDC website (www.cdc.gov/ncidod/dvbid/lyme/index.htm).

PREVENTIVE MEASURES FOR TRAVELERS

No vaccine is available. Measures to prevent Lyme disease and other tickborne infections include avoiding tick habitats, using insect repellent on exposed skin and clothing, and carefully checking every day for attached ticks (see Chapter 2, Protection against Mosquitoes, Ticks, and Other Insects and Arthropods). Remove ticks by grasping them firmly with tweezers as close to the skin as possible and lifting gently. Avoid crushing the tick's body. Do not use petroleum jelly, a hot match, nail polish, or other products to remove a tick. Postexposure prophylaxis is generally not recommended unless the traveler sustained a tick bite in a highly endemic area. Prophylactic antibiotics are not recommended for travelers.

BIBLIOGRAPHY

1. Gern L, Humair P. Ecology of Borrelia burgdorferi sensu lato in Europe. In: Gray JS KO, Lane RS, Stanek G, editors. Lyme Borreliosis: Biology, Epidemiology and Control. New York: CABI Publishing; 2002. p. 149–74.
2. Korenberg E, Gorelova N, Kovalevskii Y. Ecology of Borrelia burgdorferi sensu lato in Russia. In: Gray JS, Kahl O, Lane RS, Stanek G, editors. Lyme Borreliosis: Biology, Epidemiology and Control. New York: CABI Publishing; 2002. p. 175–200.
3. Miyamoto K, Masuzawa T. Ecology of Borrelia burgdorferi sensu lato in Japan and East Asia. In: Gray JS KO, Lane RS, Stanek G, editors. Lyme Borreliosis: Biology, Epidemiology and Control. New York: CABI Publishing; 2002. p. 201–22.
4. O'Connell S. Lyme borreliosis: current issues in diagnosis and management. Curr Opin Infect Dis. 2010 Jun;23(3):231–5.
5. Stanek G, Strle F. Lyme disease: European perspective. Infect Dis Clin North Am. 2008 Jun;22(2):327–39.
6. Steere AC. Lyme disease. N Engl J Med. 2001 Jul 12;345(2):115–25.
7. Weber K. Aspects of Lyme borreliosis in Europe. Eur J Clin Microbiol Infect Dis. 2001 Jan;20(1):6–13.
8. Wormser GP, Dattwyler RJ, Shapiro ED, Halperin JJ, Steere AC, Klempner MS, et al. The clinical assessment, treatment, and prevention of Lyme disease, human granulocytic anaplasmosis, and babesiosis: clinical practice guidelines by the Infectious Diseases Society of America. Clin Infect Dis. 2006 Nov 1;43(9):1089–134.

MALARIA

Paul M. Arguin, Sonja Mali

INFECTIOUS AGENT

Malaria in humans is caused by 1 of 4 protozoan species of the genus Plasmodium: Plasmodium falciparum, P. vivax, P. ovale, or P. malariae. In addition, P. knowlesi, a parasite of Old World (Eastern Hemisphere) monkeys, has been documented as a cause of human infections and some deaths in Southeast Asia.

MODE OF TRANSMISSION

All species are transmitted by the bite of an infective female Anopheles mosquito.

Occasionally, transmission occurs by blood transfusion, organ transplantation, needle sharing, or congenitally from mother to fetus.

EPIDEMIOLOGY

Malaria is a major international public health problem, causing 350–500 million infections worldwide and approximately 1 million deaths annually. Information about malaria transmission in specific countries (see the Yellow Fever and Malaria Information, by Country section later in this chapter) is derived from various sources, including the World Health Organization. The information presented herein was accurate at the time of publication; however, factors that can change rapidly and from year to year (such as local weather conditions, mosquito vector density, and prevalence of infection) can markedly affect local malaria transmission patterns. Updated information may be found on the CDC website at www.cdc.gov/malaria. Tools such as the malaria map application can assist in locating more unusual destinations and determining if malaria transmission occurs there (www.cdc.gov/malaria/map).

Malaria transmission occurs in large areas of Africa, Central and South America, parts of the Caribbean, Asia (including South Asia, Southeast Asia, and the Middle East), Eastern Europe, and the South Pacific (Maps 3-9 and 3-10).

The risk for acquiring malaria differs substantially from region to region and from traveler to traveler, even within a single country. This variability is a function of the intensity of transmission within the various regions and the itinerary, duration, season and type of travel. From 1999 through 2008, 8,117 cases of travel-associated malaria among US residents were reported to CDC. Of these, 5,372 (66%) were acquired in sub-Saharan Africa, 1,170 (14%) in Asia, 940 (12%) in the Caribbean and Central and South America, 220 (3%) in Oceania, and 60 (1%) in North America (all from Mexico). During this period, 43 fatal malaria infections occurred among US residents; 35 (81%) were caused by *P. falciparum*, of which 32 (91%) were acquired in sub-Saharan Africa.

These absolute numbers of cases should be considered in the context of the volume of travel to these locations. Travelers with the highest estimated relative risk for infection are those going to West Africa and Oceania. Travelers going to other parts of Africa, South Asia, and South America have a moderate estimated relative risk for infection. Travelers with lower estimated relative risk are those going to Central America and other parts of Asia.

CLINICAL PRESENTATION

Malaria is characterized by fever and influenzalike symptoms, including chills, headache, myalgias, and malaise; these symptoms can occur at intervals. Uncomplicated disease may be associated with anemia and jaundice. In severe disease, seizures, mental confusion, kidney failure, acute respiratory disease syndrome (ARDS), coma, and death may occur. Malaria symptoms can develop as early as 7 days (usually ≥14 days) after initial exposure in a malaria-endemic area and as late as several months or more after departure. Suspected or confirmed malaria, especially *P. falciparum*, is a medical emergency, requiring urgent intervention as clinical deterioration can occur rapidly and unpredictably.

DIAGNOSIS

Travelers who have symptoms of malaria should seek medical evaluation **as soon as possible**. Physicians should consider malaria in any patient with a febrile illness who has recently returned from a malaria-endemic country.

Smear microscopy remains the gold standard for malaria diagnosis. Microscopy can also be used to determine the species of malaria parasite and quantify the parasitemia—both of which are necessary pieces of information for providing the most appropriate treatment. Microscopy results should be available within a few hours. It is an unacceptable practice to send these tests to an offsite laboratory or batch them with results provided days later.

Various test kits are available to detect antigens derived from malaria parasites. Such immunologic (immunochromatographic) tests most often use a dipstick or cassette format and provide results in 2–15 minutes. These rapid diagnostic tests (RDTs) offer a useful alternative to microscopy in situations where reliable microscopic diagnosis is not available. Although RDTs can detect malaria parasites within minutes, they cannot determine the species or

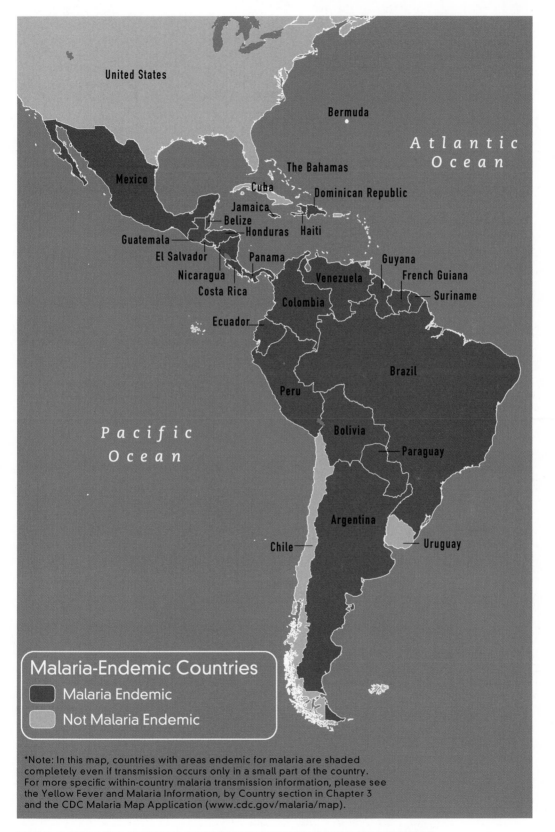

MAP 3-9. MALARIA-ENDEMIC COUNTRIES IN THE WESTERN HEMISPHERE

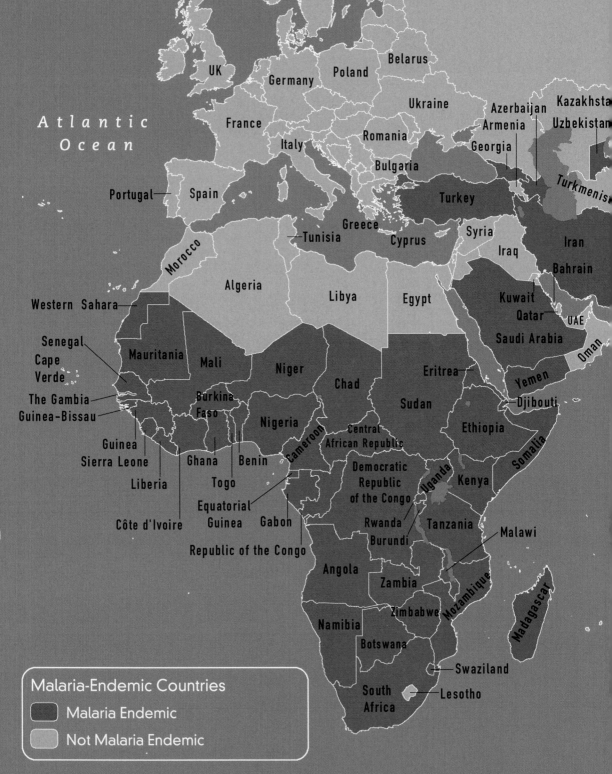

Malaria-Endemic Countries

| Malaria Endemic |
| Not Malaria Endemic |

*Note: In this map, countries with areas endemic for malaria are shaded completely even if transmission occurs only in a small part of the country. For more specific within-country malaria transmission information, please see the Yellow Fever and Malaria Information, by Country section in Chapter 3 and the CDC Malaria Map Application (www.cdc.gov/malaria/map).

MAP 3-10. MALARIA-ENDEMIC COUNTRIES IN THE EASTERN HEMISPHERE

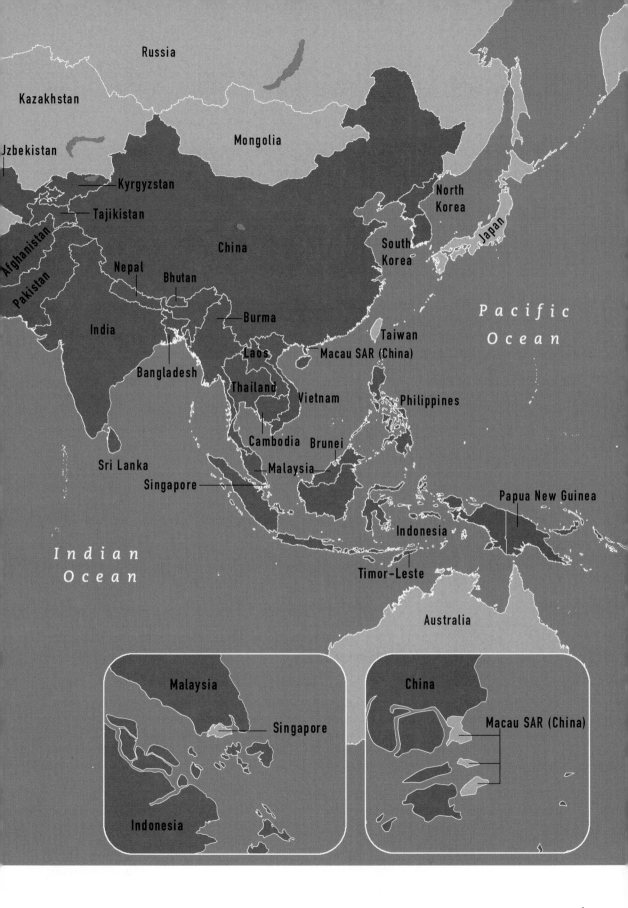

quantify parasitemia. In addition, positive and negative results must always be confirmed by microscopy. The Food and Drug Administration (FDA) has approved one RDT for use in the United States by hospital and commercial laboratories, not by individual clinicians or by patients themselves. This RDT, called BinaxNOW Malaria test, is produced by Inverness Medical Professional Diagnostics, located in Scarborough, Maine.

PCR tests are also available for detecting malaria parasites; however, none are FDA-approved. Although these tests are slightly more sensitive than routine microscopy, results are not usually available as quickly as microscopy results should be, thus limiting the utility of this test for acute diagnosis. PCR testing is most useful for definitively identifying the species of malaria parasite and detecting mixed infections. Species confirmation by PCR is available at the CDC malaria laboratory.

In sub-Saharan Africa, clinical overdiagnosis and the rate of false-positive tests for malaria may be high. Travelers to this region should be warned they may be diagnosed with malaria incorrectly, even though they are taking a reliable antimalarial regimen. In such cases, acutely ill travelers should be advised to seek the best available medical services and follow the treatment offered locally (except the use of halofantrine, which is not recommended; see below) but **not** to stop their chemoprophylaxis regimen.

TREATMENT

Malaria can be treated effectively early in the course of the disease, but delay of appropriate therapy can have serious or even fatal consequences. Travelers who have symptoms of malaria should be advised to seek medical evaluation **as soon as possible**. Specific treatment options depend on the species of malaria, the likelihood of drug resistance (based on where the infection was acquired), the age of the patient, pregnancy status, and the severity of infection.

Detailed CDC recommendations for malaria treatment can be found at www.cdc.gov/malaria/diagnosis_treatment/treatment.html. Clinicians who require assistance with the diagnosis or treatment of malaria should call the CDC Malaria Hotline (770-488-7788)

from 8:00 AM to 4:30 PM Eastern Time. After hours or on weekends and holidays, clinicians requiring assistance should call the CDC Emergency Operations Center at 770-488-7100 and ask the operator to page the person on call for the Malaria Branch. In addition, it is advisable to consult with a clinician who has specialized travel or tropical medicine expertise or with an infectious disease physician.

Medications that are not used in the United States for the treatment of malaria, such as halofantrine, are widely available overseas. CDC does not recommend halofantrine for treatment because of cardiac adverse events, including deaths, which have been documented after treatment. These adverse events have occurred in people with and without preexisting cardiac problems and both in the presence and absence of other antimalarial drugs (such as mefloquine).

Travelers who reject the advice to take prophylaxis, who choose a suboptimal drug regimen (such as chloroquine in an area with chloroquine-resistant *P. falciparum*), or who require a less-than-optimal drug regimen for medical reasons are at increased risk for acquiring malaria and needing prompt treatment while overseas. In addition, some travelers who are taking effective prophylaxis but who will be in remote areas may decide, in consultation with their travel health provider, to take along a reliable supply of a full course of an approved malaria treatment regimen. In the event that they are diagnosed with malaria, they will have immediate access to this treatment regimen, which if acquired in their home country is unlikely to be counterfeit and will not deplete local resources. In rare instances when access to medical care is not available and the traveler develops a febrile illness consistent with malaria, the reliable supply medication can be self-administered presumptively. **Travelers should be advised that this self-treatment of a possible malarial infection is only a temporary measure and that prompt medical evaluation is imperative.**

Two malaria treatment regimens can be prescribed as stand-by emergency treatment (SBET): atovaquone-proguanil and artemether-lumefantrine. The use of the same or related drugs that have been taken

Table 3-9. Stand-by emergency treatment regimens for the treatment of malaria

DRUG[1]	ADULT DOSE	PEDIATRIC DOSE	COMMENTS
Atovaquone-proguanil The adult tablet contains 250 mg atovaquone and 100 mg proguanil. The pediatric tablet contains 62.5 mg atovaquone and 25 mg proguanil.	4 adult tablets, orally as a single daily dose for 3 consecutive days	Daily dose to be taken for 3 consecutive days: 5–8 kg: 2 pediatric tablets 9–10 kg: 3 pediatric tablets 11–20 kg: 1 adult tablet 21–30 kg: 2 adult tablets 31–40 kg: 3 adult tablets >41 kg: 4 adult tablets	Contraindicated in people with severe renal impairment (creatinine clearance <30 mL/min) Not recommended for people on atovaquone-proguanil prophylaxis Not recommended for children weighing <5 kg, pregnant women, and women breastfeeding infants weighing <5 kg
Artemether-lumefantrine One tablet contains 20 mg artemether and 120 mg lumefantrine.	A 3-day treatment schedule with a total of 6 oral doses is recommended for both adult and pediatric patients based on weight. The patient should receive the initial dose, followed by the second dose 8 hours later, then 1 dose twice per day for the following 2 days. 5–<15 kg: 1 tablet per dose 15–<25 kg: 2 tablets per dose 25–<35 kg: 3 tablets per dose ≥35 kg: 4 tablets per dose	Not for people on mefloquine prophylaxis Not recommended for children weighing <5 kg, pregnant women, and women breastfeeding infants weighing <5 kg

[1] If used for presumptive self-treatment, medical care should be sought as soon as possible.

for prophylaxis is not recommended to treat malaria. For example, atovaquone-proguanil may be used as SBET by travelers not taking atovaquone-proguanil for prophylaxis. See Table 3-9 for the dosing recommendation.

PREVENTIVE MEASURES FOR TRAVELERS

Malaria prevention consists of a combination of mosquito avoidance measures and chemoprophylaxis. Although efficacious, the recommended interventions are not 100% effective. For details about how CDC determines malaria prevention recommendations for travelers, see Box 3-1.

Preventing malaria involves striking a balance between ensuring that all people at risk for infection use the appropriate prevention measures, while preventing rare occurrences of adverse effects of these interventions among people using them unnecessarily. An individual risk assessment should be conducted for every traveler, taking into account not only the destination country but also the detailed itinerary, including specific cities, types of accommodation, season,

BOX 3-1. HOW CDC ARRIVES AT RECOMMENDATIONS FOR PREVENTING MALARIA AMONG TRAVELERS

Countries are not required to submit malaria surveillance data to CDC. On an ongoing basis, we actively solicit data from multiple sources, including WHO (main and regional offices); national malaria control programs; international organizations, such as the International Society of Travel Medicine; CDC overseas staff; US Military; academic, research, and aid organizations; and published records from the medical literature. We also make judgments about the reliability and accuracy of those data. When possible, we assess trends and consider the data in the context of what we know about the malaria control activities within that country or other mitigating factors, such as natural disasters, wars, and other events that may be affecting the ability to control malaria or accurately count and report it. We consider factors such as the volume of travel to that country and the number of acquired cases reported in the US surveillance system. Based on all those considerations, we then try to accurately describe areas of that country where transmission occurs, significant occurrences of antimalarial drug resistance, the proportions of species present, and the recommended chemoprophylaxis options.

BOX 3-2. CLINICAL HIGHLIGHTS FOR MALARIA

- Overdose of antimalarial drugs, particularly chloroquine, can be fatal. Medication should be stored in childproof containers out of the reach of infants and children.
- Chemoprophylaxis can be started earlier if there are particular concerns about tolerating one of the medications. For example, mefloquine can be started 3–4 weeks in advance to allow potential adverse events to occur before travel. If unacceptable side effects develop, there would be time to change the medication before the traveler's departure.
- The drugs used for antimalarial chemoprophylaxis are generally well tolerated. However, side effects can occur. Minor side effects usually do not require stopping the drug. Travelers who have serious side effects should see a clinician who can determine if their symptoms are related to the medicine and make an appropriate medication change.
- In comparison with drugs with short half-lives, which are taken daily, drugs with longer half-lives, which are taken weekly, offer the advantage of a wider margin of error if the traveler is late with a dose. For example, if a traveler is 1–2 days late with a weekly drug, prophylactic blood levels can remain adequate; if the traveler is 1–2 days late with a daily drug, protective blood levels are less likely to be maintained.
- In those who are G6PD deficient, primaquine can cause hemolysis, which can be fatal. Be sure to document a normal G6PD level before prescribing primaquine.
- Travelers should be informed that malaria can be fatal if treatment is delayed. Medical help should be sought promptly if malaria is suspected, and a blood sample should be taken and examined for malaria parasites on one or more occasions.
- Malaria smear results or a rapid diagnostic test must be available immediately (within a few hours). Sending specimens to offsite laboratories where results are not available for extended periods of time (days) is not acceptable. If a patient has an illness suggestive of severe malaria and a compatible travel history in an area where malaria transmission occurs, it is advisable to start treatment as soon as possible, even before the diagnosis is established. CDC recommendations for malaria treatment can be found at www.cdc.gov/malaria/diagnosis_treatment/index.html.

and style of travel. In addition, conditions such as pregnancy or antimalarial drug resistance at the destination may modify the risk assessment.

Depending on level of risk, it may be appropriate to recommend no specific interventions, mosquito avoidance measures only, or mosquito avoidance measures plus chemoprophylaxis. For areas of intense transmission, such as West Africa, exposure for even short periods of time can result in transmission, so travelers to this area should be considered high risk. Malaria transmission is not distributed homogeneously throughout all countries. Some destinations have malaria transmission occurring throughout the whole country, while in others it occurs in defined areas. If travelers are going to the high-transmission areas during peak transmission times, even though the country as a whole may have lower amounts of malaria transmission, they may be at high risk for infection while there.

Geography is just one part of determining a traveler's risk for infection. Risk can differ substantially for different travelers if their behaviors and circumstances differ. For example, travelers staying in air-conditioned hotels may be at lower risk than backpackers or adventure travelers. Similarly, long-term residents living in screened and air-conditioned housing are less likely to be exposed than are people living without such amenities. The highest risk is associated with first- and second-generation immigrants living in nonendemic countries who return to their countries of origin to visit friends and relatives (VFRs). VFR travelers often consider themselves to be at no risk, because they grew up in a malarious country and consider themselves immune. However, acquired immunity is lost quickly, and VFRs should be considered to have the same risk as otherwise nonimmune travelers. Travelers should also be reminded that even if one has had malaria before, one can get it again, and preventive measures are still necessary.

Mosquito Avoidance Measures

Because of the nocturnal feeding habits of *Anopheles* mosquitoes, malaria transmission occurs primarily between dusk and dawn. Contact with mosquitoes can be reduced by remaining in well-screened areas, using mosquito bed nets (preferably insecticide-treated nets), using a pyrethroid-containing insect spray in living and sleeping areas during evening and nighttime hours, and wearing clothes that cover most of the body.

All travelers should use an effective mosquito repellent (see Chapter 2, Protection against Mosquitoes, Ticks, and Other Insects and Arthropods). Repellents should be applied to exposed parts of the skin when mosquitoes are likely to be present. If travelers are also wearing sunscreen, sunscreen should be applied first and insect repellent second. In addition to using a topical insect repellent, a permethrin-containing product may be applied to bed nets and clothing for additional protection against mosquitoes.

Chemoprophylaxis

All recommended primary chemoprophylaxis regimens involve taking a medicine before, during, and after travel to an area with malaria. Beginning the drug before travel allows the antimalarial agent to be in the blood before the traveler is exposed to malaria parasites. In choosing an appropriate chemoprophylactic regimen before travel, the traveler and the travel health provider should consider several factors. The travel itinerary should be reviewed in detail and compared with the information on where malaria transmission occurs within a given country, to determine whether the traveler will be traveling in a part of the country where malaria occurs and if significant antimalarial drug resistance has been reported in that location (see the Yellow Fever and Malaria Information, by Country section later in this chapter). Additional factors to consider are the patient's other medical conditions, medications being taken (to assess potential drug interactions), the cost of the medicines, and the potential side effects. Table 3-10 lists some of the benefits and limitations of medicines used for malaria chemoprophylaxis; additional information about choosing a malaria chemoprophylaxis regimen can be found at www.cdc.gov/malaria/travelers/drugs.html.

Table 3-10. Considerations when choosing a drug for malaria prophylaxis

DRUG	REASONS TO CONSIDER USE OF THIS DRUG	REASONS TO CONSIDER AVOIDING USE OF THIS DRUG
Atovaquone-proguanil	• Good for last-minute travelers because the drug is started 1–2 days before travel • Some people prefer to take a daily medicine • Good choice for shorter trips because you have to take the medicine for only 7 days after traveling rather than 4 weeks • Well tolerated—side effects uncommon • Pediatric tablets are available and may be more convenient	• Cannot be used by women who are pregnant or breastfeeding a child that weighs <5 kg • Cannot be taken by people with severe renal impairment • Tends to be more expensive than some of the other options (especially for long trips) • Some people (including children) would rather not take a medicine every day
Chloroquine	• Some people would rather take medicine weekly • Good choice for long trips because it is taken only weekly • Some people are already taking hydroxychloroquine chronically for rheumatologic conditions; in those instances, they may not have to take an additional medicine • Can be used in all trimesters of pregnancy	• Cannot be used in areas with chloroquine or mefloquine resistance • May exacerbate psoriasis • Some people would rather not take a weekly medication • For short trips, some people would rather not take medication for 4 weeks after travel • Not a good choice for last-minute travelers, because drug needs to be started 1–2 weeks before travel
Doxycycline	• Some people prefer to take a daily medicine • Good for last-minute travelers because the drug is started 1–2 days before travel • Tends to be the least expensive antimalarial • People who are already taking doxycycline chronically to prevent acne do not have to take an additional medicine • Doxycycline also can prevent some additional infections (such as rickettsial infections and leptospirosis), so it may be preferred by people planning to hike, camp, and swim in fresh water	• Cannot be used by pregnant women and children aged <8 years • Some people would rather not take a medicine every day • For short trips, some people would rather not take medication for 4 weeks after travel • Women prone to getting vaginal yeast infections when taking antibiotics may prefer taking a different medicine • People may want to avoid the increased risk of sun sensitivity • Some people are concerned about the potential of getting an upset stomach from doxycycline
Mefloquine	• Some people would rather take medicine weekly • Good choice for long trips because it is taken only weekly • Can be used in second and third trimester of pregnancy and in first trimester if there is no other option	• Cannot be used in areas with mefloquine resistance • Cannot be used in patients with certain psychiatric conditions • Cannot be used in patients with a seizure disorder • Not recommended for people with cardiac conduction abnormalities

continued

TABLE 3-10. CONSIDERATIONS WHEN CHOOSING A DRUG FOR MALARIA PROPHYLAXIS (continued)

DRUG	REASONS TO CONSIDER USE OF THIS DRUG	REASONS TO CONSIDER AVOIDING USE OF THIS DRUG
		• Not a good choice for last-minute travelers because drug needs to be started at least 2 weeks before travel • Some people would rather not take a weekly medication • For short trips, some people would rather not take medication for 4 weeks after travel
Primaquine	• It is the most effective medicine for preventing *P. vivax*, so it is a good choice for travel to places with more than 90% *P. vivax* • Good choice for shorter trips because you only have to take the medicine for 7 days after traveling rather than 4 weeks • Good for last-minute travelers because the drug is started 1–2 days before travel • Some people prefer to take a daily medicine	• Cannot be used in patients with glucose-6-phosphate dehydrogenase (G6PD) deficiency • Cannot be used in patients who have not been tested for G6PD deficiency • There are costs and delays associated with getting a G6PD test; however, it only has to be done once. Once a normal G6PD level is verified and documented, the test does not have to be repeated the next time primaquine is considered • Cannot be used by pregnant women • Cannot be used by women who are breastfeeding, unless the infant has also been tested for G6PD deficiency • Some people (including children) would rather not take a medicine every day • Some people are concerned about the potential of getting an upset stomach from primaquine

The resistance of *P. falciparum* to chloroquine has been confirmed in all areas with *P. falciparum* malaria except the Caribbean, Central America west of the Panama Canal, and some countries in the Middle East. In addition, resistance to sulfadoxine-pyrimethamine is widespread in the Amazon River Basin area of South America, much of Southeast Asia, other parts of Asia, and in large parts of Africa. Resistance to mefloquine has been confirmed on the borders of Thailand with Burma (Myanmar) and Cambodia, in the western provinces of Cambodia, in the eastern states of Burma on the border between Burma and China, along the borders of Laos and Burma, the adjacent parts of the Thailand-Cambodia border, and in southern Vietnam (Map 3-11).

In addition to primary prophylaxis, presumptive antirelapse therapy (also known as terminal prophylaxis) uses a medication toward the end of the exposure period (or immediately thereafter) to prevent relapses or delayed-onset clinical presentations of

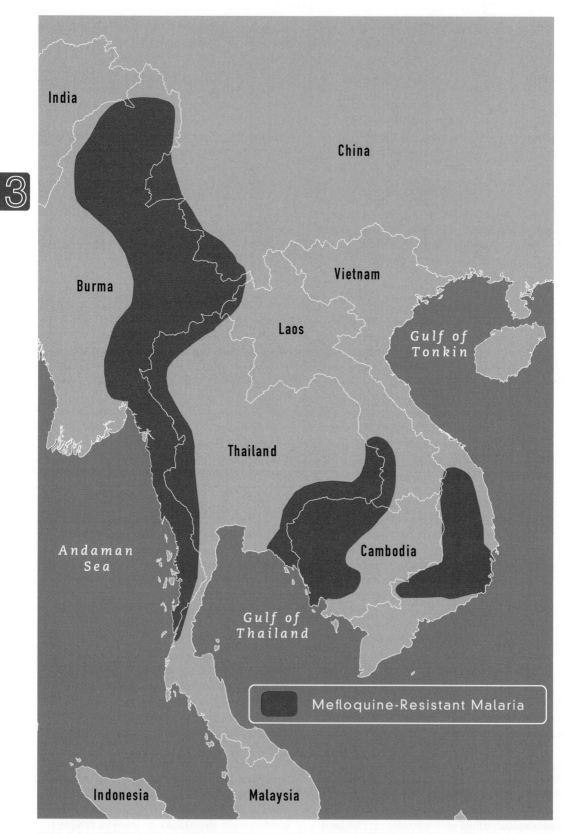

MAP 3-11. GEOGRAPHIC DISTRIBUTION OF MEFLOQUINE-RESISTANT MALARIA

malaria caused by hypnozoites (dormant liver stages) of *P. vivax* or *P. ovale*. Because most malarious areas of the world (except the Caribbean) have at least one species of relapsing malaria, travelers to these areas have some risk for acquiring either *P. vivax* or *P. ovale*, although the actual risk for an individual traveler is difficult to define. Presumptive antirelapse therapy is generally indicated only for people who have had prolonged exposure in malaria-endemic areas (such as missionaries or volunteers).

The medications recommended for chemoprophylaxis of malaria may also be available at overseas destinations. However, combinations of these medications and additional drugs that are not recommended may be commonly prescribed and used in other countries. Travelers should be strongly discouraged from obtaining chemoprophylactic medications while abroad. The quality of these products is not known; they may not be protective and could be dangerous. These medications may have been produced by substandard manufacturing practices, may be counterfeit, or may contain contaminants. Additional information on this topic can be found in Chapter 2, Perspectives: Counterfeit Drugs, and on the FDA website (www.fda.gov/Drugs/ResourcesForYou/ Consumers/BuyingUsingMedicineSafely/ BuyingMedicinefromOutsidetheUnitedStates/ default.htm).

Medications Used for Chemoprophylaxis
Atovaquone-Proguanil
Atovaquone-proguanil is a fixed combination of the drugs atovaquone and proguanil.

Prophylaxis should begin 1–2 days before travel to malarious areas and should be taken daily, at the same time each day, while in the malarious areas, and daily for 7 days after leaving the areas (see Table 3-11 for recommended dosages). Atovaquone-proguanil is well tolerated, and side effects are rare. The most common adverse effects reported in people using atovaquone-proguanil for prophylaxis or treatment are abdominal pain, nausea, vomiting, and headache. Atovaquone-proguanil is not recommended for prophylaxis in children weighing <5 kg (11 lb), pregnant women, or patients with severe renal impairment

(creatinine clearance <30 mL/min). There is a theoretical interaction between proguanil and warfarin that can increase the effect of warfarin; however, adverse events related to this theoretical interaction have not been reported.

Chloroquine and Hydroxychloroquine
Chloroquine phosphate or hydroxychloroquine sulfate can be used for prevention of malaria only in destinations where chloroquine resistance is not present (see Maps 3-9 and 3-10 and the Yellow Fever and Malaria Information, by Country section later in this chapter). Prophylaxis should begin 1–2 weeks before travel to malarious areas. It should be continued by taking the drug once a week, on the same day of the week, during travel in malarious areas and for 4 weeks after a traveler leaves these areas (see Table 3-11 for recommended dosages). Reported side effects include gastrointestinal disturbance, headache, dizziness, blurred vision, insomnia, and pruritus, but generally these effects do not require that the drug be discontinued. High doses of chloroquine, such as those used to treat rheumatoid arthritis, have been associated with retinopathy; this serious side effect appears to be extremely unlikely when chloroquine is used for routine weekly malaria prophylaxis. Chloroquine and related compounds have been reported to exacerbate psoriasis. People who experience uncomfortable side effects after taking chloroquine may tolerate the drug better by taking it with meals. As an alternative, the related compound hydroxychloroquine sulfate may be better tolerated.

Doxycycline
Doxycycline prophylaxis should begin 1–2 days before travel to malarious areas. It should be continued once a day, at the same time each day, during travel in malarious areas and daily for 4 weeks after the traveler leaves such areas. Insufficient data exist on the antimalarial prophylactic efficacy of related compounds such as minocycline (commonly prescribed for the treatment of acne). People on a long-term regimen of minocycline who need malaria prophylaxis should stop taking minocycline 1–2 days before travel and start doxycycline instead. Minocycline can

Table 3-11. Drugs used in the prophylaxis of malaria

DRUG	USAGE	ADULT DOSE	PEDIATRIC DOSE	COMMENTS
Atovaquone-proguanil	Prophylaxis in all areas	Adult tablets contain 250 mg atovaquone and 100 mg proguanil hydrochloride. 1 adult tablet orally, daily	Pediatric tablets contain 62.5 mg atovaquone and 25 mg proguanil hydrochloride. 5–8 kg: 1/2 pediatric tablet daily >8–10 kg: 3/4 pediatric tablet daily >10–20 kg: 1 pediatric tablet daily >20–30 kg: 2 pediatric tablets daily >30–40 kg: 3 pediatric tablets daily >40 kg: 1 adult tablet daily	Begin 1–2 days before travel to malarious areas. Take daily at the same time each day while in the malarious area and for 7 days after leaving such areas. Contraindicated in people with severe renal impairment (creatinine clearance <30 mL/min). Atovaquone-proguanil should be taken with food or a milky drink. Not recommended for prophylaxis for children weighing <5 kg, pregnant women, and women breastfeeding infants weighing <5 kg. Partial tablet doses may need to be prepared by a pharmacist and dispensed in individual capsules, as described in the text.
Chloroquine phosphate	Prophylaxis only in areas with chloroquine-sensitive malaria	300 mg base (500 mg salt) orally, once/week	5 mg/kg base (8.3 mg/kg salt) orally, once/week, up to a maximum adult dose of 300 mg base	Begin 1–2 weeks before travel to malarious areas. Take weekly on the same day of the week while in the malarious area and for 4 weeks after leaving such areas. May exacerbate psoriasis.
Doxycycline	Prophylaxis in all areas	100 mg orally, daily	≥8 years of age: 2.2 mg/kg up to adult dose of 100 mg/day	Begin 1–2 days before travel to malarious areas. Take daily at the same time each day while in the malarious area and for 4 weeks after leaving such areas. Contraindicated in children <8 years of age and pregnant women.
Hydroxychloroquine sulfate	An alternative to chloroquine for prophylaxis only in areas with chloroquine-sensitive malaria	310 mg base (400 mg salt) orally, once/week	5 mg/kg base (6.5 mg/kg salt) orally, once/week, up to a maximum adult dose of 310 mg base	Begin 1–2 weeks before travel to malarious areas. Take weekly on the same day of the week while in the malarious area and for 4 weeks after leaving such areas.

Drug	Use	Adult dose	Pediatric dose	Comments
Mefloquine	Prophylaxis in areas with mefloquine-sensitive malaria	228 mg base (250 mg salt) orally, once/week	≤9 kg: 4.6 mg/kg base (5 mg/kg salt) orally, once/week >9–19 kg: 1/4 tablet once/week >19–30 kg: 1/2 tablet once/week >30–45 kg: 3/4 tablet once/week >45 kg: 1 tablet once/week	Begin ≥2 weeks before travel to malarious areas. Take weekly on the same day of the week while in the malarious area and for 4 weeks after leaving such areas. Contraindicated in people allergic to mefloquine or related compounds (quinine, quinidine) and in people with active depression, a recent history of depression, generalized anxiety disorder, psychosis, schizophrenia, other major psychiatric disorders, or seizures. Use with caution in people with psychiatric disturbances or a previous history of depression. Not recommended for people with cardiac conduction abnormalities.
Primaquine[1]	Prophylaxis for short-duration travel to areas with principally P. vivax	30 mg base (52.6 mg salt) orally, daily	0.5 mg/kg base (0.8 mg/kg salt) up to adult dose orally, daily	Begin 1–2 days before travel to malarious areas. Take daily at the same time each day while in the malarious area and for 7 days after leaving such areas. Contraindicated in people with G6PD deficiency. Also contraindicated during pregnancy and lactation, unless the infant being breastfed has a documented normal G6PD level.
	Used for presumptive antirelapse therapy (terminal prophylaxis) to decrease the risk for relapses of P. vivax and P. ovale	30 mg base (52.6 mg salt) orally, daily for 14 days after departure from the malarious area	0.5 mg/kg base (0.8 mg/kg salt) up to adult dose orally, daily for 14 days after departure from the malarious area	Indicated for people who have had prolonged exposure to P. vivax, P. ovale, or both. Contraindicated in people with G6PD deficiency. Also contraindicated during pregnancy and lactation, unless the infant being breastfed has a documented normal G6PD level.

Abbreviation: G6PD, glucose-6-phosphate dehydrogenase.

[1] All people who take primaquine should have a documented normal G6PD level before starting the medication.

be restarted after the full course of doxycycline is completed (see Table 3-11 for recommended dosages).

Doxycycline can cause photosensitivity, usually manifested as an exaggerated sunburn reaction. The risk for such a reaction can be minimized by avoiding prolonged, direct exposure to the sun and by using sunscreen. In addition, doxycycline use is associated with an increased frequency of vaginal yeast infections. Gastrointestinal side effects (nausea or vomiting) may be minimized by taking the drug with a meal or by specifically prescribing doxycycline monohydrate or the enteric-coated doxycycline hyclate, rather than the generic doxycycline hyclate, which is often less expensive. To reduce the risk for esophagitis, travelers should be advised not to take doxycycline before going to bed. Doxycycline is contraindicated in people with an allergy to tetracyclines, during pregnancy, and in infants and children aged <8 years. Vaccination with the oral typhoid vaccine Ty21a should be delayed for ≥24 hours after taking a dose of doxycycline.

Mefloquine

Mefloquine prophylaxis should begin ≥2 weeks before travel to malarious areas. It should be continued once a week, on the same day of the week, during travel in malarious areas and for 4 weeks after a traveler leaves such areas (see Table 3-11 for recommended dosages). Mefloquine has been associated with rare but serious adverse reactions (such as psychoses or seizures) at prophylactic doses; these reactions are more frequent with the higher doses used for treatment. Other side effects that have occurred in chemoprophylaxis studies include gastrointestinal disturbance, headache, insomnia, abnormal dreams, visual disturbances, depression, anxiety disorder, and dizziness. Other more severe neuropsychiatric disorders occasionally reported during postmarketing surveillance include sensory and motor neuropathies (including paresthesia, tremor, and ataxia), agitation or restlessness, mood changes, panic attacks, forgetfulness, confusion, hallucinations, aggression, paranoia, and encephalopathy. On occasion, psychiatric symptoms have been reported to continue long after mefloquine has been stopped. Mefloquine is contraindicated for use by travelers with a known hypersensitivity to mefloquine or related compounds (such as quinine or quinidine) and in people with active depression, a recent history of depression, generalized anxiety disorder, psychosis, schizophrenia, other major psychiatric disorders, or seizures. It should be used with caution in people with psychiatric disturbances or a history of depression. A review of available data suggests that mefloquine may be used in people concurrently on β-blockers, if they have no underlying arrhythmia. However, mefloquine is not recommended for people with cardiac conduction abnormalities. Any traveler receiving a prescription for mefloquine must also receive a copy of the FDA medication guide, which can be found at www.fda.gov/down loads/Drugs/DrugSafety/ucm088616.pdf.

Primaquine

Primaquine phosphate has 2 distinct uses for malaria prevention: primary prophylaxis in areas with primarily P. vivax and presumptive antirelapse therapy (terminal prophylaxis).

When taken for primary prophylaxis, primaquine should be taken 1–2 days before travel to malarious areas, daily, at the same time each day, while in the malarious areas, and daily for 7 days after leaving the areas (see Table 3-11 for recommended dosages). Primary prophylaxis with primaquine obviates the need for presumptive antirelapse therapy.

When used for presumptive antirelapse therapy, primaquine is administered for 14 days after the traveler has left a malarious area. When chloroquine, doxycycline, or mefloquine is used for primary prophylaxis, primaquine is usually taken during the last 2 weeks of postexposure prophylaxis. When atovaquone-proguanil is used for prophylaxis, primaquine may be taken during the final 7 days of atovaquone-proguanil, and then for an additional 7 days. Primaquine should be given concurrently with the primary prophylaxis medication. However, if that is not feasible, the primaquine course should still be administered after the primary prophylaxis medication has been completed.

The most common adverse event in people with normal glucose-6-phosphate dehydrogenase (G6PD) levels is gastrointestinal upset if primaquine is taken on an empty stomach. This problem is minimized or eliminated if primaquine is taken with food. In G6PD-deficient people, primaquine can cause hemolysis that can be fatal. **Before primaquine is used, G6PD deficiency MUST be ruled out by appropriate laboratory testing.**

Travel to Areas with Limited Malaria Transmission

For destinations where malaria cases occur sporadically and risk for infection to travelers is assessed as being low, CDC recommends that travelers use mosquito avoidance measures only, and no chemoprophylaxis should be prescribed (see the Yellow Fever and Malaria Information, by Country section later in this chapter).

Travel to Areas with Mainly *P. vivax* Malaria

For destinations where the main species of malaria present is *P. vivax*, in addition to mosquito avoidance measures, primaquine is a good choice for primary prophylaxis for travelers who are not G6PD deficient. Its use for this indication is considered off-label in the United States. The predominant species of malaria and the recommended chemoprophylaxis medicines are listed in the Yellow Fever and Malaria Information, by Country section later in this chapter. For people unable to take primaquine, other drugs can be used as described below, depending on the presence of antimalarial drug resistance.

Travel to Areas with Chloroquine-Sensitive Malaria

For destinations where chloroquine-sensitive malaria is present, in addition to mosquito avoidance measures, the many effective chemoprophylaxis options include chloroquine, atovaquone-proguanil, doxycycline, mefloquine, and in some instances, primaquine for travelers who are not G6PD-deficient. Longer-term travelers may prefer the convenience of weekly chloroquine, while shorter-term travelers may prefer the shorter course of atovaquone-proguanil or primaquine.

Travel to Areas with Chloroquine-Resistant Malaria

For destinations where chloroquine-resistant malaria is present, in addition to mosquito avoidance measures, chemoprophylaxis options are atovaquone-proguanil, doxycycline, and mefloquine.

Travel to Areas with Mefloquine-Resistant Malaria

For destinations where mefloquine-resistant malaria is present, in addition to mosquito avoidance measures, chemoprophylaxis options are either atovaquone-proguanil or doxycycline.

Chemoprophylaxis for Infants, Children, and Adolescents

Infants of any age or weight or children and adolescents of any age can contract malaria. Therefore, all children traveling to malaria-endemic areas should use the recommended prevention measures, which often include taking an antimalarial drug. In the United States, antimalarial drugs are available only in oral formulations and may taste bitter. Pediatric doses should be carefully calculated according to body weight but should never exceed adult dose. Pharmacists can pulverize tablets and prepare gelatin capsules for each measured dose. If the child is unable to swallow the capsules or tablets, parents should prepare the child's dose of medication by breaking open the gelatin capsule and mixing the drug with a small amount of something sweet, such as applesauce, chocolate syrup, or jelly, to ensure the entire dose is delivered to the child. Giving the dose on a full stomach may minimize stomach upset and vomiting.

Chloroquine and mefloquine are options for use in infants and children of all ages and weights, depending on drug resistance at their destination. Primaquine can be used for children who are not G6PD-deficient traveling to areas with principally *P. vivax*. Doxycycline may be used for children who are aged ≥8 years. Atovaquone-proguanil may be used for prophylaxis for infants and children weighing ≥5 kg (11 lb). Prophylactic dosing for children weighing <11 kg (24 lb) constitutes off-label use in the United States. Pediatric dosing regimens are contained in Table 3-11.

Chemoprophylaxis during Pregnancy and Breastfeeding

Malaria infection in pregnant women can be more severe than in nonpregnant women. Malaria can increase the risk for adverse pregnancy outcomes, including prematurity, spontaneous abortion, and stillbirth. For these reasons, and because no chemoprophylactic regimen is completely effective, women who are pregnant or likely to become pregnant should be advised to avoid travel to areas with malaria transmission if possible (see Chapter 8, Pregnant Travelers). If travel to a malarious area cannot be deferred, use of an effective chemoprophylaxis regimen is essential.

Pregnant women traveling to areas where chloroquine-resistant *P. falciparum* has not been reported may take chloroquine prophylaxis. Chloroquine has not been found to have any harmful effects on the fetus when used in the recommended doses for malaria prophylaxis; therefore, pregnancy is not a contraindication for malaria prophylaxis with chloroquine phosphate or hydroxychloroquine sulfate. For travel to areas where chloroquine resistance is present, mefloquine is the only medication recommended for malaria chemoprophylaxis during pregnancy. A review of mefloquine use in pregnancy, from clinical trials and reports of inadvertent use of mefloquine during pregnancy, suggests that its use at prophylactic doses during the second and third trimesters of pregnancy is not associated with adverse fetal or pregnancy outcomes. More limited data suggest it is also safe to use during the first trimester. Because of insufficient data regarding the use during pregnancy, atovaquone-proguanil is not recommended to prevent malaria in pregnant women.

Doxycycline is contraindicated for malaria prophylaxis during pregnancy because of the risk for adverse effects seen with tetracycline, a related drug, on the fetus, which include discoloration and dysplasia of the teeth and inhibition of bone growth. Primaquine should not be used during pregnancy because the drug may be passed transplacentally to a G6PD-deficient fetus and cause hemolytic anemia in utero.

Very small amounts of antimalarial drugs are excreted in the breast milk of lactating women. Because the quantity of antimalarial drugs transferred in breast milk is insufficient to provide adequate protection against malaria, infants who require chemoprophylaxis must receive the recommended dosages of antimalarial drugs listed in Table 3-11. Because chloroquine and mefloquine may be safely prescribed to infants, it is also safe for infants to be exposed to the small amounts excreted in breast milk. Although data are very limited about the use of doxycycline in lactating women, most experts consider the theoretical possibility of adverse events to the infant to be remote.

Although no information is available on the amount of primaquine that enters human breast milk, the mother and infant should be tested for G6PD deficiency before primaquine is given to a woman who is breastfeeding. Because data are not yet available on the safety of atovaquone-proguanil prophylaxis in infants weighing <5 kg (11 lb), CDC does not recommend it to prevent malaria in women breastfeeding infants weighing <5 kg. However, it can be used to treat women who are breastfeeding infants of any weight when the potential benefit outweighs the potential risk to the infant (such as treating a breastfeeding woman who has acquired *P. falciparum* malaria in an area of multidrug-resistant strains and who cannot tolerate other treatment options).

Choosing a Drug to Prevent Malaria

Recommendations for drugs to prevent malaria differ by country of travel and can be found in the Yellow Fever and Malaria Information, by Country section later in this chapter. Recommended drugs for each country are listed in alphabetical order and have comparable efficacy in that country. No antimalarial drug is 100% protective and must be combined with the use of personal protective measures (such as insect repellent, long sleeves, long pants, sleeping in a mosquito-free setting or using an insecticide-treated bed net). When several different drugs are recommended for an area, Table 3-10 may help in the decision-making process.

Changing Medications as a Result of Side Effects during Chemoprophylaxis

Medications recommended for prophylaxis against malaria have different modes of action that affect the parasites at different stages of the life cycle. Thus, if the medication needs to be changed because of side effects before a full course has been completed, there are some special considerations (see Table 3-12).

BLOOD DONATION AFTER TRAVEL TO MALARIOUS AREAS

People who have been in an area where malaria transmission occurs, either during daytime or nighttime hours, are not permitted to donate blood in the United States

Table 3-12. Changing medications as a result of side effects during chemoprophylaxis

DRUG BEING STOPPED	DRUG BEING STARTED	COMMENTS
Mefloquine	Doxycycline	Begin doxycycline, continue daily while in malaria-endemic area, and continue for 4 weeks after leaving malaria-endemic area.
	Atovaquone-proguanil	• If the switch occurs ≥3 weeks before departure from the endemic area, atovaquone-proguanil should be taken daily for the remainder of the stay in the endemic area and for 1 week thereafter. • If the switch occurs <3 weeks before departure from the endemic area, atovaquone-proguanil should be taken daily for 4 weeks after the switch. • If the switch occurs after departure from the risk area, atovaquone-proguanil should be taken daily until 4 weeks after the date of departure from the endemic area.
	Chloroquine	Not recommended
	Primaquine	Not recommended
Doxycycline	Mefloquine	Not recommended
	Atovaquone-proguanil	If the switch occurs ≥3 weeks before departure from the endemic area, atovaquone-proguanil should be taken daily for the remainder of the stay in the endemic area and for 1 week thereafter. If the switch occurs <3 weeks before departure from the endemic area, atovaquone-proguanil should be taken daily for 4 weeks after the switch. If the switch occurs after departure from the risk area, atovaquone-proguanil should be taken daily until 4 weeks after the date of departure from the endemic area.
	Chloroquine	Not recommended
	Primaquine	Not recommended

continued

TABLE 3-12. CHANGING MEDICATIONS AS A RESULT OF SIDE EFFECTS DURING CHEMOPROPHYLAXIS (continued)

DRUG BEING STOPPED	DRUG BEING STARTED	COMMENTS
Atovaquone-proguanil	Doxycycline	Begin doxycycline, continue daily while in malaria-endemic area, and continue for 4 weeks after leaving malaria-endemic area.
	Mefloquine	Not recommended
	Chloroquine	Not recommended
	Primaquine	This switch would be unlikely as primaquine is only recommended for primary prophylaxis in areas with mainly *P. vivax* for people with normal G6PD activity. Should that be the case, begin primaquine, continue daily while in malaria-endemic area, and continue for 7 days after leaving malaria-endemic area.
Chloroquine	Doxycycline	Begin doxycycline, continue daily while in malaria-endemic area, and continue for 4 weeks after leaving malaria-endemic area.
	Atovaquone-proguanil	If the switch occurs ≥3 weeks before departure from the endemic area, atovaquone-proguanil should be taken daily for the remainder of the stay in the endemic area and for 1 week thereafter. If the switch occurs <3 weeks before departure from the endemic area, atovaquone-proguanil should be taken daily for 4 weeks after the switch. If the switch occurs following departure from the risk area, atovaquone-proguanil should be taken daily until 4 weeks after the date of departure from the endemic area.
	Mefloquine	Not recommended
	Primaquine	Not recommended
Primaquine	Doxycycline	Begin doxycycline, continue daily while in malaria-endemic area, and continue for 4 weeks after leaving malaria-endemic area.
	Atovaquone-proguanil	Begin atovaquone-proguanil, continue daily while in malaria-endemic area, and continue for 7 days after leaving malaria-endemic area.
	Chloroquine	Not recommended
	Mefloquine	Not recommended

for a period of time after returning from the malarious area. People who are residents of nonmalarious countries are not permitted to donate blood for 1 year after they have returned from a malarious area. People who are residents of malarious countries are not permitted to donate blood for 3 years after leaving a malarious area. People who have had malaria are not allowed to donate blood for 3 years after treatment for malaria. Risk assessments may differ between travel health providers and blood banks. A travel health provider advising a traveler going to a country with a relatively low amount of malaria transmission for a short period of time and engaging in low-risk behaviors may choose insect avoidance only and no chemoprophylaxis for the traveler. However, upon the traveler's return, a blood bank may still choose to defer that traveler for 1 year because of the travel to an area where transmission occurs.

BIBLIOGRAPHY

1. Baird JK, Fryauff DJ, Hoffman SL. Primaquine for prevention of malaria in travelers. Clin Infect Dis. 2003 Dec 15;37(12):1659–67.
2. Boggild AK, Parise ME, Lewis LS, Kain KC. Atovaquone-proguanil: report from the CDC expert meeting on malaria chemoprophylaxis (II). Am J Trop Med Hyg. 2007 Feb;76(2):208–23.
3. CDC. CDC malaria map application. Atlanta: CDC; 2010 [updated 2010 Feb 8; cited 2010 Oct 22]. Available from: http://www.cdc.gov/malaria/map/index.html.
4. CDC. Malaria. Atlanta: CDC; 2010 [updated 2010 Feb 8; cited 2010 Oct 22]. Available from: http://www.cdc.gov/malaria.
5. Cox-Singh J, Davis TM, Lee KS, Shamsul SS, Matusop A, Ratnam S, et al. *Plasmodium knowlesi* malaria in humans is widely distributed and potentially life threatening. Clin Infect Dis. 2008 Jan 15;46(2):165–71.
6. Fradin MS, Day JF. Comparative efficacy of insect repellents against mosquito bites. N Engl J Med. 2002 Jul 4;347(1):13–8.
7. Hill DR, Baird JK, Parise ME, Lewis LS, Ryan ET, Magill AJ. Primaquine: report from CDC expert meeting on malaria chemoprophylaxis I. Am J Trop Med Hyg. 2006 Sep;75(3):402–15.
8. Kitchen AD, Chiodini PL. Malaria and blood transfusion. Vox Sang. 2006 Feb;90(2):77–84.
9. Kochar DK, Saxena V, Singh N, Kochar SK, Kumar SV, Das A. *Plasmodium vivax* malaria. Emerg Infect Dis. 2005 Jan;11(1):132–4.
10. Leder K, Black J, O'Brien D, Greenwood Z, Kain KC, Schwartz E, et al. Malaria in travelers: a review of the GeoSentinel surveillance network. Clin Infect Dis. 2004 Oct 15;39(8):1104–12.
11. Leder K, Tong S, Weld L, Kain KC, Wilder-Smith A, von Sonnenburg F, et al. Illness in travelers visiting friends and relatives: a review of the GeoSentinel Surveillance Network. Clin Infect Dis. 2006 Nov 1;43(9):1185–93.
12. Mali S, Steele S, Slutsker L, Arguin PM. Malaria surveillance—United States, 2007. MMWR Surveill Summ 2009;58(SS-2):1–16.
13. Newman RD, Parise ME, Barber AM, Steketee RW. Malaria-related deaths among US travelers, 1963–2001. Ann Intern Med. 2004 Oct 5;141(7):547–55.
14. Reyburn H, Mbatia R, Drakeley C, Carneiro I, Mwakasungula E, Mwerinde O, et al. Overdiagnosis of malaria in patients with severe febrile illness in Tanzania: a prospective study. BMJ. 2004 Nov 20;329(7476):1212.
15. Schwartz E, Parise M, Kozarsky P, Cetron M. Delayed onset of malaria—implications for chemoprophylaxis in travelers. N Engl J Med. 2003 Oct 16;349(16):1510–6.
16. Whitty CJ, Edmonds S, Mutabingwa TK. Malaria in pregnancy. BJOG. 2005 Sep;112(9):1189–95.
17. World Health Organization. World malaria report 2009. Geneva: World Health Organization; 2009. Available from: http://whqlibdoc.who.int/publications/2009/9789241563901_eng.pdf.

MEASLES (RUBEOLA)

Amy Parker Fiebelkorn, Amra Uzicanin

INFECTIOUS AGENT

Measles virus is a member of the genus *Morbillivirus* of the family Paramyxoviridae. Humans are the only known natural host for the measles virus. Measles is one of the most highly communicable infectious diseases.

MODE OF TRANSMISSION

Measles virus spreads by airborne droplets or by direct contact with nasal or throat secretions of infected people. It is less commonly spread by articles freshly soiled with nose and throat secretions. Infected people are usually contagious from 4 days before until 4 days after the onset of signs or symptoms.

EPIDEMIOLOGY

The number of reported measles cases in the United States has declined from nearly 900,000 per year in the early 1940s to fewer than 150 cases annually since 1997. As a result of high vaccination coverage, in 2000 measles was declared eliminated in the United States. Indigenous measles virus circulation was interrupted in 2002 in the rest of the Western Hemisphere. However, measles virus continues to be imported into the United States from other parts of the world. Globally, an estimated 20 million measles cases occur each year. Given the large global incidence and high communicability of the disease, travelers may be exposed to the virus in almost any country they visit, but the risks are higher in countries where measles is endemic or where large outbreaks are occurring. Of the 67 reported measles cases in the United States in 2009, 13 occurred among US residents who were traveling abroad (4 people became infected in the United Kingdom, 4 in India, 2 in China, and 1 each in Cape Verde, the Philippines, and Vietnam), and 5 cases occurred among foreign visitors to the United States (from the United Kingdom, France, Italy, South Africa, and India).

People who do not have evidence of measles immunity should be considered at risk for measles during international travel.

Acceptable presumptive evidence of immunity to measles for international travelers includes meeting one or more of the following criteria:

- For infants aged 6–11 months, documented administration of 1 dose of live measles-containing vaccine (MCV) and for people aged ≥12 months, 2 doses of MCV ≥28 days apart, on or after the first birthday
- Laboratory evidence of immunity
- Birth before 1957
- Documented physician-diagnosed measles

CLINICAL PRESENTATION

The incubation period is about 10 days (range, 7–18 days) from exposure to onset of fever, usually 14 days before appearance of rash. Symptoms include prodromal fever, conjunctivitis, coryza (runny nose), cough, and small spots with white or bluish-white centers on an erythematous base on the buccal mucosa (Koplik spots). Characteristic red, blotchy (maculopapular) rash appears on the third to seventh day; it begins on the face, becomes generalized, and lasts 4–7 days. Common complications include diarrhea (8%), middle ear infection (7%–9%), and pneumonia (1%–6%). Encephalitis, frequently resulting in permanent brain damage, occurs in approximately 1 per 1,000–2,000 cases of measles. Subacute sclerosing panencephalitis (SSPE), a rare but serious degenerative central nervous system disease, is thought to occur in 1 per 100,000 cases, although a rate of 22 SSPE cases per 100,000 measles cases was found during the 1989–1991 measles resurgence in the United States. SSPE, which is caused by a persistent infection with a defective measles virus, is manifested by mental and motor deterioration that starts an average of 7 years after measles virus infection (most frequently in children who were infected at age <2 years), progressing to coma and death. The risk of serious complications and death is highest for children aged ≤5 years and adults aged ≥20 years. It is also higher in populations with poor nutritional status.

DIAGNOSIS

A clinical case of measles illness is characterized by all of the following:

- Generalized maculopapular rash lasting ≥3 days
- Temperature of ≥101°F (38.3°C)
- Cough, coryza, or conjunctivitis

Laboratory criteria for diagnosis include any of the following: a positive serologic test for measles IgM, seroconversion, a significant rise in measles IgG level by any standard serologic assay, isolation of measles virus, or identification by PCR of measles virus RNA from a clinical specimen. A confirmed case is one that is either laboratory-confirmed or that meets the clinical case definition and is epidemiologically linked to a confirmed case. A laboratory-confirmed case does not need to meet the clinical case definition.

TREATMENT

Treatment is supportive. The World Health Organization recommends vitamin A for all children with acute measles, regardless of their country of residence, to reduce the risk of complications. Vitamin A is administered once a day for 2 days at the following doses:

- 50,000 IU for infants aged <6 months
- 100,000 IU for infants aged 6–11 months
- 200,000 IU for children aged ≥12 months

A third, age-specific dose of vitamin A is to be given 2–4 weeks later to patients with clinical signs and symptoms of vitamin A deficiency. Parenteral and oral formulations of vitamin A are available in the United States.

PREVENTIVE MEASURES FOR TRAVELERS
Vaccine

People traveling abroad, including people traveling to industrialized countries, who do not have evidence of measles immunity should be up to date on their MCV vaccination before departure. Measles vaccine contains live, attenuated measles virus. In the United States, it is available only in combination formulations, such as measles-mumps-rubella (MMR) and measles-mumps-rubella-varicella (MMRV). MMRV vaccine is licensed for children aged 12 months to 12 years and may be used in place of MMR vaccine if vaccination for measles, mumps, rubella, and varicella is needed. However, compared with use of separate MMR and varicella vaccines at the same visit, use of MMRV vaccine is associated with a higher risk for fever and febrile seizures.

Most international travelers should receive 1 or 2 doses before travel:

- Infants aged 6–11 months should have at least 1 MCV dose. Infants vaccinated before age 12 months must be revaccinated on or after the first birthday with 2 doses of MCV separated by ≥28 days. MMRV is not licensed for children aged <12 months.
- Preschool children aged ≥12 months should have 2 MCV doses separated by ≥28 days.
- School-age children should have 2 MCV doses separated by ≥28 days.
- Adults born in or after 1957 should have 2 MCV doses separated by ≥28 days.

If administered at ≥12 months of age, 1 dose of MCV or MMR is 95% effective in preventing measles disease, and 2 doses are 99% effective. One dose of MCV or MMR is approximately 85% effective if administered at 9 months of age.

MCV and immune globulin (IG) are effective as postexposure prophylaxis. MCV, if administered within 72 hours after initial exposure, may provide some protection. If the exposure does not result in infection, the vaccine should induce protection against subsequent measles virus infection. IG can be used to prevent or mitigate measles in a susceptible person when administered within 6 days of exposure. However, any immunity conferred is temporary unless modified or typical measles occurs, and the person should receive MCV 5–6 months after IG administration.

Vaccine Safety and Adverse Reactions

In rare circumstances, MMR vaccination has been associated with the following adverse events:

- Anaphylaxis (approximately 1–3.5 occurrences per million doses administered)
- Thrombocytopenia (a rate of 1 case in every 25,000 doses during the 6 weeks after immunization)
- Febrile seizures (The risk of febrile seizures increases approximately 3-fold 8–14 days after receipt of MMR vaccine, but overall, the rate of febrile seizure after MCV is much lower than the rate after measles disease.)

- Acute arthritis (Arthralgia develops among approximately 25% of susceptible postpubertal females after MMR vaccination, and approximately 10% have acute arthritislike signs and symptoms.)
- Joint symptoms (If they occur, they generally persist for 1 day to 3 weeks and rarely recur. Chronic joint symptoms attributable to the rubella component of the MMR vaccine are rare, if they occur at all.)

Evidence does not support a link between MMR vaccination and any of the following: hearing loss, retinopathy, optic neuritis, ocular palsies, Guillain-Barré syndrome, cerebellar ataxia, Crohn's disease, or autism. A published report on MMR vaccination and inflammatory bowel disease and pervasive developmental disorders (such as autism) has never been replicated by other studies and has subsequently been retracted by the journal.

Compared with use of MMR and varicella vaccines at the same visit, use of MMRV vaccine is associated with a higher risk for fever and febrile seizures 5–12 days after the first dose among children aged 12–23 months (about 1 extra febrile seizure for every 2,300–2,600 MMRV vaccine doses). Use of separate MMR and varicella vaccines avoids this increased risk for fever and febrile seizures.

Precautions and Contraindications
Allergy
People with severe allergy (hives, swelling of the mouth or throat, difficulty breathing, hypotension, and shock) to gelatin or neomycin, or who have had a severe allergic reaction to a prior dose of MMR or MMRV, should not be revaccinated, except with extreme caution. MMR or MMRV vaccines may be administered to people who are allergic to eggs without prior routine skin testing or the use of special protocols.

Immunosuppression
Enhanced replication of vaccine viruses can occur in people who have immune deficiency disorders. Death related to vaccine-associated measles virus infection has been reported among severely immunocompromised people. Therefore, severely immunosuppressed people should not be vaccinated with MMR or MMRV vaccines (see Chapter 8 for a thorough discussion of recommendations for immunocompromised travelers):

- People who have received high-dose corticosteroid therapy (in general considered to be >20 mg prednisone or equivalent) daily or on alternate days for an interval of ≥14 days should avoid vaccination with MMR or MMRV for ≥1 month after cessation of steroid therapy.
- People who have received high-dose corticosteroid therapy daily or on alternate days for an interval of <14 days generally can be vaccinated with MMR or MMRV immediately after cessation of treatment, although some experts prefer waiting until 2 weeks after completion of therapy.
- Other immunosuppressive therapy: in general, MMR or MMRV vaccines should be withheld for ≥3 months after cessation of the immunosuppressive therapy and remission of the underlying disease. This interval is based on the assumptions that the immune response will have been restored in 3 months and the underlying disease for which the therapy was given remains in remission.

Thrombocytopenia
The benefits of primary immunization are usually greater than the potential risks of thrombocytopenia. However, avoiding a subsequent dose of MMR or MMRV vaccine may be prudent if an episode of thrombocytopenia occurred within approximately 6 weeks after a previous dose of vaccine.

BIBLIOGRAPHY

1. American Academy of Pediatrics. Measles. In: Pickering LK, Baker CJ, Kimberlin DW, Long SS, editors. Red Book: 2009 Report of the Committee on Infectious Diseases. 28th ed. Elk Grove Village, IL: American Academy of Pediatrics; 2009. p. 444–55.
2. Bellini WJ, Rota JS, Lowe LE, Katz RS, Dyken PR, Zaki SR, et al. Subacute sclerosing panencephalitis: more cases of this fatal disease are prevented by measles immunization than was previously recognized. J Infect Dis. 2005 Nov 15;192(10):1686–93.
3. CDC. Measles (rubeola): 2009 case definition. Atlanta: CDC; 2009 [cited 2010 February 24]. Available from: http://www.cdc.gov/ncphi/disss/nndss/casedef/measles_2009.htm.
4. CDC. Progress toward measles elimination—region of the Americas, 2002–2003. MMWR Morb Mortal Wkly Rep. 2004 Apr 16;53(14):304–6.

5. CDC. Recommended Childhood and Adolescent Immunization Schedule—United States, 2006. MMWR Morb Mortal Wkly Rep. 2006;54(52):Q1–4.

6. CDC. Update: recommendations from the Advisory Committee on Immunization Practices (ACIP) regarding administration of combination MMRV vaccine. MMWR Morb Mortal Wkly Rep. 2008 Mar 14;57(10):258–60.

7. Editors of the Lancet. Retraction—Ileal-lymphoid-nodular hyperplasia, non-specific colitis, and pervasive development disorder in children. Lancet [serial on the Internet]. 2010 [cited 2010 February 2]. Available from: http://press.thelancet.com/wakefieldretraction.pdf.

8. Katz SL, Hinman AR. Summary and conclusions: measles elimination meeting, 16–17 March 2000. J Infect Dis. 2004 May 1;189 Suppl 1:S43–7.

9. Marin M, Broder KR, Temte JL, Snider DE, Seward JF. Use of combination measles, mumps, rubella, and varicella vaccine: recommendations of the Advisory Committee on Immunization Practices (ACIP). MMWR Recomm Rep. 2010 May 7;59(RR-3):1–12.

10. Murch SH, Anthony A, Casson DH, Malik M, Berelowitz M, Dhillon AP, et al. Retraction of an interpretation. Lancet. 2004 Mar 6;363(9411):750.

11. Perry RT, Halsey NA. The clinical significance of measles: a review. J Infect Dis. 2004 May 1;189 Suppl 1:S4–16.

12. Strebel PM, Papania MJ, Dayan GH. Measles vaccine. In: Plotkin SA, Orenstein WA, Offit PA, editors. Vaccines. 5th ed. Philadelphia: Saunders Elsevier; 2008. p. 353–98.

13. Wakefield AJ, Murch SH, Anthony A, Linnell J, Casson DM, Malik M, et al. Ileal-lymphoid-nodular hyperplasia, non-specific colitis, and pervasive developmental disorder in children. Lancet. 1998 Feb 28;351(9103):637–41.

14. Watson JC, Hadler SC, Dykewicz CA, Reef S, Phillips L. Measles, mumps, and rubella—vaccine use and strategies for elimination of measles, rubella, and congenital rubella syndrome and control of mumps: recommendations of the Advisory Committee on Immunization Practices (ACIP). MMWR Recomm Rep. 1998 May 22;47(RR-8):1–57.

15. WHO. Measles fact sheet. Geneva: World Health Organization; 2009 [updated 2009 Dec; cited 2010 Oct 19]. Available from: http://www.who.int/mediacentre/factsheets/fs286/en/index.html.

MELIOIDOSIS

David D. Blaney, Jay E. Gee, Theresa L. Smith

INFECTIOUS AGENT

Burkholderia pseudomallei is a saprophytic, gram-negative bacillus widely distributed in tropical soil and water.

MODE OF TRANSMISSION

Human infection with *B. pseudomallei* usually occurs by inhalation or subcutaneous inoculation, or occasionally by ingestion; person-to-person transmission is rare via contact with the blood and body fluids of an infected person.

EPIDEMIOLOGY

Melioidosis is an infectious disease endemic in Southeast Asia, northern Australia, Papua New Guinea, much of the Indian subcontinent, southern China, Hong Kong, and Taiwan. It is considered highly endemic in northeast Thailand, Malaysia, Singapore, and northern Australia (Map 3-12). In northern Australia and northeast Thailand, melioidosis accounts for 20% of all community-acquired septicemias. Melioidosis is the most common cause of severe community-acquired pneumonia in northern Australia.

Melioidosis has been reported in Puerto Rico, suspected in El Salvador, and may be underdiagnosed in India, Africa, the Caribbean, and Central and South America. In 2009, an imported case from Aruba was identified in the United States. In northern Brazil, clusters of melioidosis have recently been recognized and are associated with periods of heavy rainfall.

Travelers of all ages are at risk for infection when visiting areas endemic for melioidosis. The highest risk for melioidosis exists for military personnel, adventure travelers, ecotourists, construction and resource extraction workers, and other people whose contact with contaminated soil or water may expose them to the bacteria. *B. pseudomallei* has been isolated from ill troops of all nationalities who served in areas with endemic disease, with a latency of as long as 62 years.

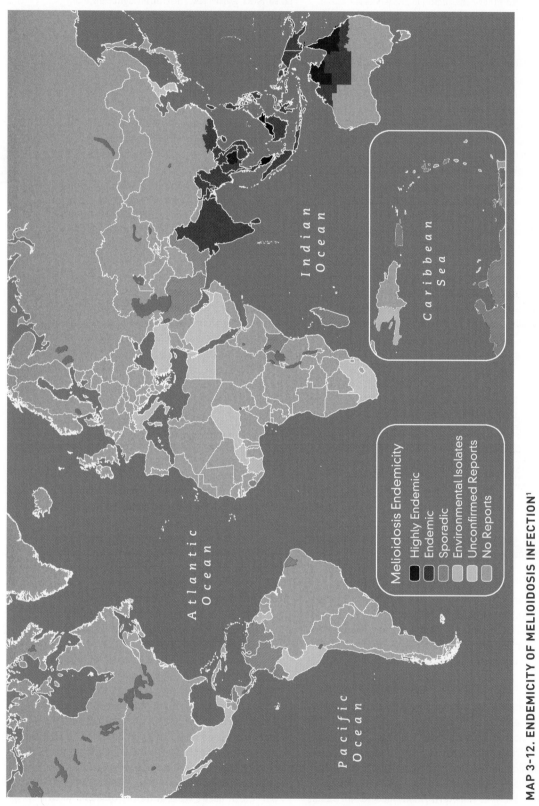

MAP 3-12. ENDEMICITY OF MELIOIDOSIS INFECTION[1]

Melioidosis Endemicity
- Highly Endemic
- Endemic
- Sporadic
- Environmental Isolates
- Unconfirmed Reports
- No Reports

[1] Cheng AC, Currie BJ. Melioidosis: epidemiology, pathophysiology, and management. Clin Microbiol Rev. 2005;18:383–416. Modified with permission from the American Society of Microbiology.

As much as 85% of cases occur during the rainy season, when exposure to the organism is believed to be highest. Melioidosis has been diagnosed among travelers who contracted the disease while staying in endemic areas during the rainy season. After the 2004 Southeast Asian tsunami, an increase in the number of melioidosis cases was observed among repatriated tourists. Risk factors for systemic melioidosis include diabetes, excessive alcohol use, chronic renal disease, chronic lung disease (such as associated with cystic fibrosis and chronic obstructive pulmonary disease), thalassemia, and malignancy or other non-HIV-related immune suppression.

CLINICAL PRESENTATION

Melioidosis may occur as a subclinical infection, localized infection (such as cutaneous), pneumonia, meningoencephalitis, sepsis, or chronic suppurative infection. The latter may mimic tuberculosis, with fever, weight loss, productive cough, and upper lobe infiltrate, with or without cavitation. The incubation period is generally 1–21 days, although it may extend for months or years. With a high inoculum, symptoms can develop in a few hours. More than 50% of cases present with pneumonia. Without appropriate treatment, case-fatality ratio may reach 90% within 48 hours of developing symptoms. Morbidity and mortality of melioidosis are higher in people with underlying diseases such as diabetes mellitus, renal dysfunction, chronic pulmonary disease,

or compromised immune system. However, HIV infection does not appear to be a major risk factor for developing melioidosis.

DIAGNOSIS

Culture of the organism may be done from blood, sputum, pus, urine, synovial fluid, peritoneal fluid, and pericardial fluid. The most widely used serologic test for melioidosis is the indirect hemagglutination assay (IHA). Diagnostic assistance, including IHA serology and molecular, biochemical, and genetic characterization of isolates, is available through the CDC Zoonoses and Select Agent Laboratory (http://www.cdc.gov/nczved/divisions/dfbmd/bzb/lab_submission.html#zsal).

TREATMENT

Melioidosis often requires long courses of antimicrobial therapy. Some of the more common antibiotics used are ceftazidime, imipenem, meropenem, trimethoprim-sulfamethoxazole, and doxycycline. Relapse may be seen in patients, especially those who do not complete a full course of recommended eradication-phase therapy.

PREVENTIVE MEASURES FOR TRAVELERS

No vaccine is available to protect against melioidosis. In areas of endemic disease, skin lacerations, abrasions, or burns that have been contaminated with soil or surface water should be immediately and thoroughly cleaned.

BIBLIOGRAPHY

1. Cheng AC, Currie BJ. Melioidosis: epidemiology, pathophysiology, and management. Clin Microbiol Rev. 2005 Apr;18(2):383–416.
2. Currie BJ. Advances and remaining uncertainties in the epidemiology of Burkholderia pseudomallei and melioidosis. Trans R Soc Trop Med Hyg. 2008 Mar;102(3):225–7.
3. Currie BJ, Dance DA, Cheng AC. The global distribution of Burkholderia pseudomallei and melioidosis: an update. Trans R Soc Trop Med Hyg. 2008 Dec;102 Suppl 1:S1–4.
4. Currie BJ, Fisher DA, Howard DM, Burrow JN, Lo D, Selva-Nayagam S, et al. Endemic melioidosis in tropical northern Australia: a 10-year prospective study and review of the literature. Clin Infect Dis. 2000 Oct;31(4):981–6.
5. Dance DA. Ecology of Burkholderia pseudomallei and the interactions between environmental Burkholderia

spp. and human-animal hosts. Acta Trop. 2000 Feb 5;74(2–3):159–68.
6. Inglis TJ, Rolim DB, Sousa Ade Q. Melioidosis in the Americas. Am J Trop Med Hyg. 2006 Nov;75(5):947–54.
7. Inglis TJ, Sagripanti JL. Environmental factors that affect the survival and persistence of Burkholderia pseudomallei. Appl Environ Microbiol. 2006 Nov;72(11):6865–75.
8. Ko WC, Cheung BM, Tang HJ, Shih HI, Lau YJ, Wang LR, et al. Melioidosis outbreak after typhoon, southern Taiwan. Emerg Infect Dis. 2007 Jun;13(6):896–8.
9. Ngauy V, Lemeshev Y, Sadkowski L, Crawford G. Cutaneous melioidosis in a man who was taken as a prisoner of war by the Japanese during World War II. J Clin Microbiol. 2005 Feb;43(2):970–2.

10. Peacock SJ. Melioidosis. Curr Opin Infect Dis. 2006 Oct;19(5):421–8.

11. Suputtamongkol Y, Chaowagul W, Chetchotisakd P, Lertpatanasuwun N, Intaranongpai S, Ruchutrakool T, et al. Risk factors for melioidosis and bacteremic melioidosis. Clin Infect Dis. 1999 Aug;29(2): 408–13.

12. White NJ. Melioidosis. Lancet. 2003 May 17;361(9370):1715–22.

MENINGOCOCCAL DISEASE

Amanda Cohn, Michael L. Jackson

INFECTIOUS AGENT

The infectious agent is a gram-negative diplococci, *Neisseria meningitidis*. Meningococci are classified into serogroups on the basis of the composition of the capsular polysaccharide. The 5 major meningococcal serogroups associated with disease are A, B, C, Y, and W-135.

MODE OF TRANSMISSION

Person-to-person transmission occurs by close contact with respiratory secretions or saliva.

EPIDEMIOLOGY

N. meningitidis is found worldwide. At any time, 5%–10% of the population may be carriers of *N. meningitidis*. Invasive disease is rare in nonepidemic areas, occurring at a rate of 0.5–10 cases per 100,000 population per year, but can occur at a rate of up to 1,000 cases per 100,000 population per year in epidemic regions.

The incidence of meningococcal disease is highest in the "meningitis belt" of sub-Saharan Africa (Map 3-13). The incidence of meningococcal disease is several times higher in the meningitis belt than in the United States, with periodic epidemics during the dry season (December–June). During nonepidemic periods, the rate of meningococcal disease is roughly 5–10 cases per 100,000 population per year. During epidemics, the rate can be as high as 1,000 cases per 100,000 population. Although most common in the African meningitis belt, meningococcal outbreaks can occur anywhere in the world. Serogroup A predominates in the meningitis belt, although serogroups C, X, and W-135 are also found.

Young children have the highest risk for meningococcal disease, but 60% of cases occur in adolescents and adults. Risk is highest in travelers who have prolonged contact with local populations in the meningitis belt during an epidemic. The Hajj pilgrimage to Saudi Arabia has been associated with outbreaks of meningococcal disease in returning pilgrims and their contacts.

CLINICAL PRESENTATION

Meningococcal disease generally occurs 1–14 days after exposure. Meningococcal disease presents as meningitis in ≥50% of cases. Meningococcal meningitis is characterized by sudden onset of headache, fever, and stiffness of the neck, sometimes accompanied by nausea, vomiting, photophobia, or altered mental status. Up to 20% of people with meningococcal disease present with meningococcal sepsis, known as meningococcemia. Meningococcemia is characterized by an abrupt onset of fever and a petechial or purpuric rash. The rash may progress to purpura fulminans. Meningococcemia may often involve hypotension, acute adrenal hemorrhage, and multiorgan failure. Among infants and children aged <2 years, meningococcal disease may have nonspecific symptoms. Neck stiffness, usually seen in people with meningitis, may be absent.

DIAGNOSIS

Early diagnosis and treatment are critical. If possible, a lumbar puncture should be done before starting antibiotic therapy to ensure that bacteria, if any, can be cultured from cerebrospinal fluid (CSF). Diagnosis is generally made by isolating *N. meningitidis* from blood or CSF, by detecting meningococcal antigen in CSF by latex agglutination, or by evidence of *N. meningitidis* DNA by PCR.

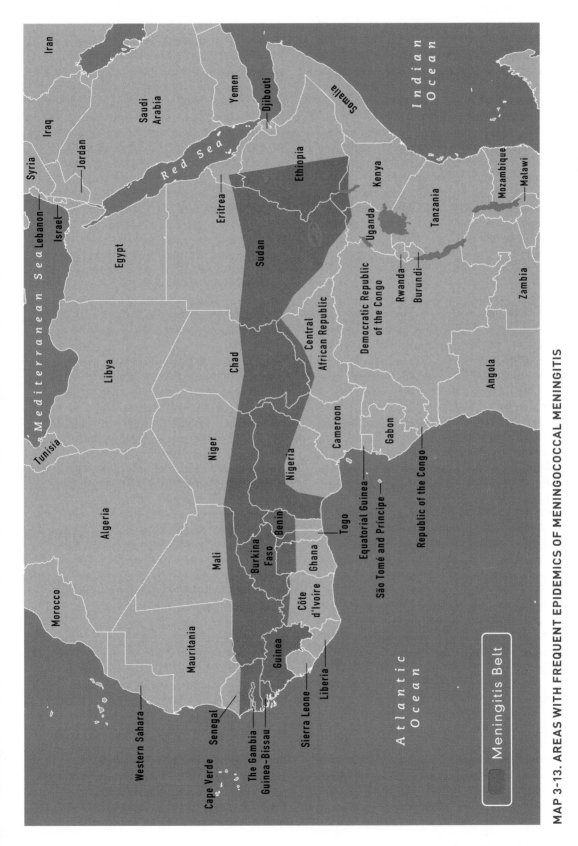

MAP 3-13. AREAS WITH FREQUENT EPIDEMICS OF MENINGOCOCCAL MENINGITIS

Meningitis Belt

The signs and symptoms of meningococcal meningitis are similar to those of other causes of bacterial meningitis, such as *Haemophilus influenzae* and *Streptococcus pneumoniae*. The causative organism should be identified so that the correct antibiotics can be used for treatment and prophylaxis.

TREATMENT

Meningococcal disease is potentially fatal and should always be viewed as a medical emergency. Antibiotic treatment must be started early in the course of the disease. Several antibiotic choices are available, including ceftriaxone, chloramphenicol, cefotaxime, and benzylpenicillin.

PREVENTIVE MEASURES FOR TRAVELERS
Vaccine
Indications for Use

The Advisory Committee for Immunization Practices (ACIP) recommends vaccination against meningococcal disease to people who travel to or reside in countries where *N. meningitidis* is hyperendemic or epidemic, particularly if contact with the local population will be prolonged. Hyperendemic regions include the meningitis belt of Africa during the dry season (December–June). Advisories for travelers to other countries are issued when epidemics of meningococcal disease caused by vaccine-preventable serogroups are recognized (see the CDC Travelers' Health website at www.cdc.gov/travel). Note that proof of receipt of quadrivalent vaccination against meningococcal disease is required for people traveling to Mecca during the annual Hajj and Umrah pilgrimages.

Vaccine Administration

Two quadrivalent meningococcal polysaccharide–protein conjugate vaccines (MenACWY) (Menactra, Menveo) are licensed for use in the United States and are differentiated by their protein conjugate. Both vaccines are licensed for people aged 2–55 years. Quadrivalent meningococcal polysaccharide vaccine (MPVS4) (Menomune) is licensed for use among people aged ≥2 years. These vaccines protect against meningococcal disease caused by serogroups A, C, Y, and W-135. Approximately 7–10 days are required after vaccination for development of protective antibody levels.

MenACWY is the preferred vaccine for people aged 2–55 years; MPSV4 should be used for people >55 years. In the United States, there is no licensed vaccine for people <2 years. For travelers to Mecca for the Hajj pilgrimage, CDC recommends giving MPSV4 to children <2 years if they require vaccination. Limited experience in this age group suggests that MPSV4 may be less immunogenic, but there are no safety concerns.

CDC recommends routine vaccination of people with MenACWY at age 11 or 12 years, with a booster dose at age 16 years. For adolescents who receive the first dose at age 13–15 years, a one-time booster dose should be administered, preferably at age 16–18 years. People who receive their first dose of MenACWY at or after age 16 years do not need a booster dose, unless they remain at continued risk for meningococcal disease.

Travelers who were vaccinated previously and are living in or returning to the meningitis belt may need to be revaccinated. ACIP recommends that children previously vaccinated with MenACWY or MPVS4 at ages 2–6 years with a single dose who remain at an increased risk for meningococcal disease should receive an additional dose of MenACWY 3 years after their previous meningococcal vaccine and every 5 years thereafter, if at continued risk. Likewise, individuals who were previously vaccinated with MenACWY or MPVS4 at ages 7–55 years and who remain at an increased risk for meningococcal disease should receive an additional dose of MenACWY 5 years after their previous dose and every 5 years thereafter, if at continued risk. Travelers aged >55 years should be vaccinated or revaccinated with MPSV4 if it has been >5 years since their last meningococcal vaccine. Travelers to the Hajj must show proof of vaccination in the previous 3 years. Previously unvaccinated travelers who have a history of complement component deficiency (C3, properdin, factor D, or late component), functional or anatomic asplenia, or HIV should receive a two-dose primary series of meningococcal conjugate vaccine, 2 months apart, prior to travel if possible.

Vaccine Safety and Adverse Reactions

For MPSV4, the incidence of local reactions (such as pain and redness at the injection site) has ranged from 4% to 56% across studies. Severe reactions are rare, with an incidence of <0.1

per 100,000 vaccinees. In comparison trials, the incidence of severe reactions after MenACWY was similar to the incidence after MPSV4 vaccination; however, local reactions (including pain that limited movement of the arm of injection) were more common after MenACWY.

Precautions and Contraindications

People with moderate or severe acute illness should defer vaccination until their condition improves. MenACWY and MPSV4 are contraindicated for people who have severe allergic reaction to any component of the vaccines. People with dry natural rubber latex allergy should not receive Menactra.

MPSV4 is an acceptable alternative for protection against meningococcal disease. Both MenACWY and MPSV4 are inactivated vaccines and may be given to immunosuppressed people.

Antibiotic Chemoprophylaxis

In the United States and most industrialized countries, antibiotic chemoprophylaxis among close contacts of a patient with invasive meningococcal disease is recommended to prevent secondary cases. Antibiotic regimens for prophylaxis include rifampin, ciprofloxacin, and ceftriaxone. Ceftriaxone is recommended for pregnant women.

BIBLIOGRAPHY

1. American Academy of Pediatrics. Meningococcal infections. In: Pickering LK, editor. Red Book: 2003 Report of the Committee on Infectious Disease. 26th ed. Elk Grove Village, IL: American Academy of Pediatrics; 2003. p. 430–6.
2. Bilukha OO, Rosenstein N. Prevention and control of meningococcal disease. Recommendations of the Advisory Committee on Immunization Practices (ACIP). MMWR Recomm Rep. 2005 May 27;54(RR-7):1–21.
3. CDC. Updated recommendation from the Advisory Committee on Immunization Practices (ACIP) for revaccination of persons at prolonged increased risk for meningococcal disease. MMWR Morb Mortal Wkly Rep. 2009 Sep 25;58(37):1042–3.
4. CDC. Updated recommendations for use of meningococcal conjugate vaccines—Advisory Committee on Immunization Practices (ACIP), 2010. MMWR Morb Mortal Wkly Rep. 2011 Jan 28;60(3):72–6.
5. Greenwood B. Manson Lecture. Meningococcal meningitis in Africa. Trans R Soc Trop Med Hyg. 1999 Jul–Aug;93(4):341–53.
6. Koch S, Steffen R. Meningococcal disease in travelers: vaccination recommendations. J Travel Med. 1994 Mar 1;1(1):4–7.
7. Raghunathan PL, Bernhardt SA, Rosenstein NE. Opportunities for control of meningococcal disease in the United States. Annu Rev Med. 2004;55:333–53.
8. Rosenstein NE, Perkins BA, Stephens DS, Popovic T, Hughes JM. Meningococcal disease. N Engl J Med. 2001 May 3;344(18):1378–88.
9. Stephens DS, Greenwood B, Brandtzaeg P. Epidemic meningitis, meningococcaemia, and *Neisseria meningitidis*. Lancet. 2007 Jun 30;369(9580):2196–210.
10. Wilder-Smith A. Meningococcal disease: risk for international travellers and vaccine strategies. Travel Med Infect Dis. 2008 Jul;6(4):182–6.

MUMPS

Preeta K. Kutty, Albert E. Barskey IV, Kathleen M. Gallagher

INFECTIOUS AGENT

Mumps virus is an enveloped, negative-strand RNA virus, a member of the genus *Rubulavirus*. Humans are the only known natural host for mumps virus.

MODE OF TRANSMISSION

Transmission is by respiratory droplets, saliva, or contact with contaminated fomites. Patients are usually contagious from approximately 5 days before until 5 days after symptom onset.

EPIDEMIOLOGY

Because of a successful immunization program in the United States, mumps disease rates declined >99% since a vaccine was licensed in 1967. However, large outbreaks occurred in highly vaccinated populations in 2006 (more than 6,500 cases) and 2009–2010 (approximately 3,000 cases). Mumps virus remains endemic in many countries throughout the world, because mumps vaccine is used in only 61% of the World Health Organization member countries. The risk of exposure to mumps among travelers is variable but remains high in many countries of the world, including industrialized countries, such as the United Kingdom, which has had several outbreaks since 2004, and Japan, which does not routinely vaccinate against mumps. Risk is especially high for travelers aged >12 months who do not have evidence of mumps immunity.

CLINICAL PRESENTATION

The incubation period from exposure to onset of symptoms is generally 16–18 days (range, 12–25 days). Mumps is most often characterized by parotitis (swelling of the parotid salivary glands), either unilateral or bilateral. Onset of illness is usually nonspecific, with symptoms of fever, headache, malaise, myalgia, and anorexia. Approximately 30% of mumps cases are asymptomatic.

Mumps is generally a mild and self-limited disease, but complications do occur. Orchitis (inflammation of the testicles) is the most common complication, occurring in up to one-third of postpubertal males. Other complications include oophoritis or mastitis (inflammation of the ovaries or breasts, respectively), pancreatitis, meningitis, and encephalitis. With the exception of deafness, these complications are more frequent in adults than in children.

DIAGNOSIS

Mumps may occur in epidemics; mumps virus is the only known cause of epidemic parotitis. Diagnosis is usually clinical, based on the presence of parotitis and associated signs, symptoms, or complications. The clinical case definition is an illness with acute onset of unilateral or bilateral tender, self-limited swelling of the parotid glands, other salivary glands, or both, lasting ≥2 days, and without other apparent cause. Laboratory criteria include the following:

- Isolation of mumps virus from clinical specimen
- Detection of mumps nucleic acid (standard or real-time RT-PCR assays)
- Detection of mumps IgM
- Demonstration of specific mumps antibody response, in the absence of recent vaccination, either by a 4-fold increase in IgG titer as measured by quantitative assays or by seroconversion from negative to positive by using a standard serologic assay of paired acute- and convalescent-phase serum specimens

Laboratory specimens that can be collected are serum for serology (IgM, IgG) and a buccal swab (or a throat swab) for viral detection or isolation. For more information, see the CDC Laboratory Testing for Mumps Infection website (www.cdc.gov/mumps/lab/index.html). Laboratory confirmation is more challenging in highly vaccinated populations. Serologic tests should be interpreted with caution. A negative laboratory test should not rule out a clinically compatible case, especially in a 2-dose vaccine recipient.

TREATMENT

There is no specific antiviral therapy for mumps, and the basic treatment consists of supportive care.

PREVENTIVE MEASURES FOR TRAVELERS
Vaccine

Although vaccination against mumps is not a requirement for entry into any country (including the United States), travelers leaving the United States or living abroad should ensure they are immune to mumps. Acceptable presumptive evidence of immunity to mumps for international travelers includes the following:

- Documented administration of 2 doses of live mumps virus vaccine ≥28 days apart, on or after the first birthday
- Laboratory evidence of immunity
- Birth before 1957
- Documentation of physician-diagnosed mumps

Mumps vaccine contains live attenuated mumps virus. It is available as a combination

3

formulation, such as measles, mumps, and rubella (MMR). Combined MMR vaccine is recommended whenever one or more of the individual components are indicated to provide optimal protection against all 3 viruses. Mumps vaccine is effective in preventing mumps but is not 100% effective. One dose of mumps vaccine is approximately 80% (range, 62%–91%) effective in preventing clinical mumps with parotitis, and 2 doses are approximately 90% (range, 79%–95%) effective.

Mumps vaccine has not been demonstrated to be effective in preventing infection when administered after exposure; however, it can be administered after exposure to protect against subsequent exposures. Immune globulin is not effective in preventing mumps infection after an exposure and is not recommended.

Vaccine Safety, Adverse Reactions, Precautions, and Contraindications to Mumps Vaccine

Refer to the Measles (Rubeola) section earlier in this chapter for information on reactions after MMR vaccine and additional precautions and contraindications. For routine vaccine recommendations, pediatric and catch-up schedules, and recommendations for special populations, refer to Chapters 7 and 8.

BIBLIOGRAPHY

1. American Academy of Pediatrics. Mumps. In: Pickering LK, Baker CJ, Kimberlin DW, Long SS, editors. Red Book: 2009 Report of the Committee on Infectious Diseases. 28th ed. Elk Grove Village, IL: American Academy of Pediatrics; 2009. p. 468–72.

2. CDC. Measles prevention: recommendations of the Immunization Practices Advisory Committee on Infectious Diseases (ACIP). MMWR Morb Mortal Wkly Rep. 1989 Dec 29;38 Suppl 9:1–18.

3. CDC. Notice to readers: updated recommendations of the Advisory Committee on Immunization Practices (ACIP) for the control and elimination of mumps. MMWR Morb Mortal Wkly Rep. 2006 Jun 9;55(22):629–30.

4. CDC. Update: mumps outbreak—New York and New Jersey, June 2009–January 2010. MMWR Morb Mortal Wkly Rep. 2010 Feb 12;59(5):125–9.

5. CDC. Updated recommendations for isolation of persons with mumps. MMWR Morb Mortal Wkly Rep. 2008 Oct 10;57(40):1103–5.

6. Dayan GH, Quinlisk MP, Parker AA, Barskey AE, Harris ML, Schwartz JM, et al. Recent resurgence of mumps in the United States. N Engl J Med. 2008 Apr 10;358(15):1580–9.

7. Harling R, White JM, Ramsay ME, Macsween KF, van den Bosch C. The effectiveness of the mumps component of the MMR vaccine: a case control study. Vaccine. 2005 Jul 1;23(31):4070–4.

8. Kutty PK, Kyaw MH, Dayan GH, Brady MT, Bocchini JA, Reef SE, et al. Guidance for isolation precautions for mumps in the United States: a review of the scientific basis for policy change. Clin Infect Dis. 2010 Jun 15;50(12):1619–28.

9. Plotkin SA, Rubin S. Mumps vaccine. In: Plotkin SA, Orenstein WA, Offit PA, editors. Vaccines. 5th ed. Philadelphia: Elsevier Saunders; 2008. p. 436–65.

10. Quinlisk P. Revision of the surveillance case definition for mumps. Council of State and Territorial Epidemiologists. Infectious Disease Committee; 2007. Available from: http://www.cste.org/ PS/2007ps/2007psfinal/ID/07-ID-02.pdf.

11. Watson JC, Hadler SC, Dykewicz CA, Reef S, Phillips L. Measles, mumps, and rubella—vaccine use and strategies for elimination of measles, rubella, and congenital rubella syndrome and control of mumps: recommendations of the Advisory Committee on Immunization Practices (ACIP). MMWR Recomm Rep. 1998 May 22;47(RR-8):1–57.

12. World Health Organization. Immunization schedules by antigen, selection centre [database on the Internet]. World Health Organization Vaccine Preventable Diseases Monitoring System. 2010 [cited Apr 29 2010]. Available from: http://apps.who.int/ immunization_monitoring/en/globalsummary/ ScheduleSelect.cfm.

NOROVIRUS

Aron J. Hall, Ben Lopman

INFECTIOUS AGENT

Norovirus infection is caused by nonenveloped, single-stranded RNA viruses of the genus *Norovirus*, which have also been referred to as "Norwalk-like viruses," Norwalk viruses, human caliciviruses, and small round-structured viruses.

MODE OF TRANSMISSION

Transmission occurs primarily through the fecal-oral route, either through direct person-to-person contact or indirectly via contaminated food or water. Norovirus is also indirectly spread through aerosols of vomitus and contaminated environmental surfaces and objects.

EPIDEMIOLOGY

Seroprevalence studies in the Amazon, southern Africa, Mexico, Chile, and Canada have shown that norovirus infections are common throughout the world, and most children will have experienced at least 1 infection by the age of 5 years. Norovirus infections can occur year round; in temperate climates, norovirus activity peaks during the winter. In the United States, norovirus is the leading cause of sporadic cases and outbreaks of gastroenteritis, estimated to cause 23 million illnesses a year and up to 50% of all foodborne outbreaks. In both developing and developed countries, noroviruses are estimated to cause 12% of all severe diarrheal disease.

Norovirus appears to be increasing as a cause of travelers' diarrhea; rates range from 3% to 17% of returning travelers. However, coinfection and asymptomatic infection with norovirus is common, so focused studies are needed to determine exactly how frequently norovirus is the cause of disease. Risk for infection is present anywhere food is prepared in an unsanitary manner and may become contaminated, or where drinking water is inadequately treated. Of particular risk are "ready-to-eat" cold foods, such as sandwiches and salads. Raw shellfish, especially oysters, are also a frequent source of infection, because virus from contaminated water concentrates in the gut of these filter feeders. Contaminated ice has also been previously implicated in outbreaks.

Large norovirus outbreaks are associated with settings where people live in close quarters and can easily infect each other, such as hotels, cruise ships, and camps. Viral contamination of inanimate objects may persist during outbreaks and be a source of infection. On cruise ships, for instance, such environmental contamination has caused recurrent norovirus outbreaks on successive cruises with newly boarded passengers. Transmission of norovirus on airplanes has been reported during both domestic and international flights, and likely results from contamination of lavatories or from symptomatic passengers in the cabin.

CLINICAL PRESENTATION

Infected people usually have an acute onset of violent vomiting with nonbloody diarrhea. The incubation period is 24–48 hours. Other symptoms include abdominal cramps, nausea, and occasionally a low-grade fever. Illness is generally self-limited, and full recovery can be expected in 1–4 days. In some cases, dehydration, especially in patients who are very young or elderly, may require medical attention.

DIAGNOSIS

Norovirus infection is generally diagnosed by symptoms. No laboratory tests have been approved by the Food and Drug Administration to guide clinical management, but laboratory testing is used during outbreak investigations by public health agencies. Norovirus diagnostic testing is usually not available in developing countries.

The most common diagnostic test used at state public health laboratories and CDC is RT-PCR, which rapidly and reliably detects the virus in stool specimens. Several commercial EIAs are available to detect the virus in stool specimens. The specificity and sensitivity of these assays are poor compared with RT-PCR.

These tests have been used occasionally by cruise lines during outbreaks on ships.

TREATMENT

The mainstay of management is supportive care, such as rest and oral or intravenous rehydration.

PREVENTIVE MEASURES FOR TRAVELERS

No vaccines are available. Noroviruses are common and highly contagious, but the risk for infection can be minimized by frequent and proper handwashing and avoiding possibly contaminated food and water.

In addition to handwashing, measures to prevent transmission of noroviruses between people traveling together include carefully cleaning up fecal material or vomit and disinfecting contaminated surfaces and toilet areas. Products should be approved by the Environmental Protection Agency for norovirus disinfection; alternatively, a high concentration of domestic bleach (at least a 1:50 solution of bleach and water) may be used. Soiled articles of clothing should be washed and machine-dried at high heat.

To help prevent the spread of noroviruses, ill people have been confined on cruise ships and in institutional settings.

BIBLIOGRAPHY

1. Glass RI, Parashar UD, Estes MK. Norovirus gastroenteritis. N Engl J Med. 2009 Oct 29;361(18):1776–85.
2. Kirking HL, Cortes J, Burrer S, Hall AJ, Cohen NJ, Lipman H, et al. Likely transmission of norovirus on an airplane, October 2008. Clin Infect Dis. 2010 May 1;50(9):1216–21.
3. Koo HL, Ajami NJ, Jiang ZD, Neill FH, Atmar RL, Ericsson CD, et al. Noroviruses as a cause of diarrhea in travelers to Guatemala, India, and Mexico. J Clin Microbiol. 2010 May;48(5):1673–6.
4. Kornylo K, Kim DK, Widdowson MA, Turabelidze G, Averhoff FM. Risk of norovirus transmission during air travel. J Travel Med. 2009 Sep–Oct;16(5):349–51.
5. Mead PS, Slutsker L, Dietz V, McCaig LF, Bresee JS, Shapiro C, et al. Food-related illness and death in the United States. Emerg Infect Dis. 1999 Sep–Oct;5(5):607–25.
6. Parashar U, Quiroz ES, Mounts AW, Monroe SS, Fankhauser RL, Ando T, et al. "Norwalk-like viruses." Public health consequences and outbreak management. MMWR Recomm Rep. 2001 Jun 1;50 (RR-9):1–17.
7. Patel MM, Widdowson MA, Glass RI, Akazawa K, Vinje J, Parashar UD. Systematic literature review of role of noroviruses in sporadic gastroenteritis. Emerg Infect Dis. 2008 Aug;14(8):1224–31.
8. Widdowson MA, Cramer EH, Hadley L, Bresee JS, Beard RS, Bulens SN, et al. Outbreaks of acute gastroenteritis on cruise ships and on land: identification of a predominant circulating strain of norovirus—United States, 2002. J Infect Dis. 2004 Jul 1;190(1):27–36.

ONCHOCERCIASIS (RIVER BLINDNESS)
LeAnne M. Fox

INFECTIOUS AGENT

Onchocerciasis, also known as river blindness, is caused by the filarial nematode, *Onchocerca volvulus*.

MODE OF TRANSMISSION

Infection occurs through the bite of female blackflies of the genus *Simulium*, which bite during the day and are found near rapidly flowing rivers and streams.

EPIDEMIOLOGY

Onchocerciasis is endemic in more than 25 nations located in a broad band across the central part of Africa. Small endemic foci are also present in the Arabian Peninsula (Yemen) and in the Americas (Brazil, Colombia, Ecuador, Guatemala, southern Mexico, and Venezuela). An estimated 17 million people are infected worldwide.

Short-term travelers to endemic areas are at low risk for this infection. Travelers who visit endemic areas for extended periods of time (generally >3 months) and live or work near blackfly habitats are at higher risk for infection. Most infections seen in the United States occur in expatriate groups, such as missionaries, field scientists, and Peace Corps volunteers.

A recent report from the GeoSentinel Surveillance Network showed only 0.6% (271 of 43,722) of medical conditions reported from 1995 through 2004 were caused by any filarial infection, and only 101 (37% of the total) were caused by O. volvulus. Most (95%) of those who acquired onchocerciasis did so in sub-Saharan Africa; 3 infections were acquired elsewhere. As expected, most cases (62%) were seen in immigrants or refugees. Nevertheless, in this study, 7 travelers from nonendemic regions who acquired onchocerciasis did so during trips of ≤31 days.

CLINICAL PRESENTATION

Infection with O. volvulus can result in a highly pruritic, papular dermatitis; subcutaneous nodules; lymphadenitis; and ocular lesions, which can progress to visual loss and blindness. Symptoms in travelers are primarily dermatologic and may occur months to years after departure from endemic areas. Immigrants from endemic areas may present with skin or ocular disease.

DIAGNOSIS

Onchocerciasis is diagnosed by finding the microfilariae in superficial skin shavings or punch biopsy, adult worms in histologic sections of excised nodules, or characteristic eye lesions. Serologic testing is most useful for detecting infection in specific groups, such as expatriates with a brief exposure history, when microfilariae are not identifiable. Determination of serum antifilarial IgG is available through the National Institutes of Health (301-496-5398) or the CDC's Division of Parasitic Diseases and Malaria (770-488-7775; parasites@cdc.gov).

TREATMENT

Ivermectin (150–200 µg/kg orally, once or twice per year) is the drug of choice for onchocerciasis. Repeated annual or semiannual doses may be required, because the drug kills the microfilariae but not the adult worms, which can live for many years. Antibiotic trials with doxycycline (100 mg orally per day) directed against Wolbachia, an endosymbiont of O. volvulus, have demonstrated a decrease in onchocercal microfiladermia with 6 weeks of therapy. Therefore, some experts recommend treating patients with 1 dose of ivermectin followed by 6 weeks of doxycycline.

Diethylcarbamazine (DEC) is contraindicated in onchocerciasis, because it has been associated with severe and fatal posttreatment reactions. Any subcutaneous nodules should be excised if their anatomic location allows it to be done safely. To ensure correct diagnosis and treatment, travelers should be advised to consult with an infectious diseases or tropical medicine specialist.

PREVENTIVE MEASURES FOR TRAVELERS

No vaccine or drug to prevent infection is available. Protective measures include avoiding blackfly habitats and the use of personal protection measures against biting insects (see Chapter 2, Protection against Mosquitoes, Ticks, and Other Insects and Arthropods).

BIBLIOGRAPHY

1. Abiose A. Onchocercal eye disease and the impact of Mectizan treatment. Ann Trop Med Parasitol. 1998 Apr;92 Suppl 1:S11–22.
2. Abramowicz M. Drugs for Parasitic Infections. New Rochelle (NY): The Medical Letter, Inc; 2007.
3. Albiez EJ, Buttner DW, Duke BO. Diagnosis and extirpation of nodules in human onchocerciasis. Trop Med Parasitol. 1988 Dec;39 Suppl 4:331–46.
4. Brieger WR, Awedoba AK, Eneanya CI, Hagan M, Ogbuagu KF, Okello DO, et al. The effects of ivermectin on onchocercal skin disease and severe itching: results of a multicentre trial. Trop Med Int Health. 1998 Dec;3(12):951–61.
5. Burnham G. Onchocerciasis. Lancet. 1998 May 2;351(9112):1341–6.
6. Hoerauf A. Filariasis: new drugs and new opportunities for lymphatic filariasis and onchocerciasis. Curr Opin Infect Dis. 2008 Dec;21(6):673–81.
7. Hoerauf A, Mand S, Adjei O, Fleischer B, Buttner DW. Depletion of Wolbachia endobacteria in Onchocerca volvulus by doxycycline and microfilaridermia after ivermectin treatment. Lancet. 2001 May 5;357(9266):1415–6.
8. Lipner EM, Law MA, Barnett E, Keystone JS, von Sonnenburg F, Loutan L, et al. Filariasis in travelers

presenting to the GeoSentinel Surveillance Network. PLoS Negl Trop Dis. 2007;1(3):e88.

9. Murdoch ME, Asuzu MC, Hagan M, Makunde WH, Ngoumou P, Ogbuagu KF, et al. Onchocerciasis: the clinical and epidemiological burden of skin disease in Africa. Ann Trop Med Parasitol. 2002 Apr;96(3):283–96.

10. Tielsch JM, Beeche A. Impact of ivermectin on illness and disability associated with onchocerciasis. Trop Med Int Health. 2004 Apr;9(4):A45–56.

11. WHO Expert Committee. Onchocerciasis and its control. Report of a WHO Expert Committee on Onchocerciasis Control. World Health Organ Tech Rep Ser. 1995;852:1–104.

PERTUSSIS
Tami H. Skoff, Cynthia G. Thomas

INFECTIOUS AGENT
Pertussis is caused by a fastidious gram-negative coccobacillus, *Bordetella pertussis*.

MODE OF TRANSMISSION
Pertussis is spread by person-to-person transmission via aerosolized respiratory droplets or by direct contact with respiratory secretions.

EPIDEMIOLOGY
Pertussis is endemic worldwide, even in areas with high vaccination rates. From 2004 through 2008, the annual number of reported pertussis cases in the United States ranged from approximately 4,000 to 25,000. Disease rates are highest among young children in countries where vaccination coverage is low, which is primarily in the developing world. In developed countries, the incidence of pertussis is highest among unvaccinated infants and increases again among adolescents.

Immunity from childhood vaccination and natural disease wanes with time; therefore, adolescents and adults who have not received a Tdap booster vaccination can become infected or reinfected. US travelers are not at increased risk for disease specifically because of international travel, but they are at risk if they come in close contact with infected people. Infants too young to be protected by a complete vaccination series are at highest risk for severe pertussis that requires hospitalization.

CLINICAL PRESENTATION
In classic disease, mild upper respiratory tract symptoms begin 7–10 days (range, 6–21 days) after exposure, followed by a cough that becomes paroxysmal. Coughing paroxysms may be frequent or relatively infrequent and are often followed by vomiting. Fever is absent or minimal. The clinical case definition for pertussis includes cough for ≥2 weeks with paroxysms, whoop, or posttussive vomiting.

Disease in infants aged <6 months can be atypical, with a short catarrhal stage, gagging, gasping, or apnea as early manifestations; among infants aged <2 months, the case-fatality ratio is approximately 1%. Recently immunized children who develop disease may have mild cough illness; older children and adults may have prolonged cough with or without paroxysms. The cough gradually wanes over several weeks to months.

DIAGNOSIS
Factors such as prior vaccination status, stage of disease, antibiotic use, specimen collection and transport conditions, and nonstandardized tests may affect the sensitivity, specificity, and interpretation of available diagnostic tests for *B. pertussis*. CDC guidelines for the laboratory confirmation of pertussis cases include culture and PCR (when the above clinical case definition is met); serology and direct fluorescent antibody (DFA) tests are not confirmatory tests included in the case definition.

TREATMENT
Macrolide antibiotics (azithromycin, clarithromycin, and erythromycin) are recommended for the treatment of pertussis in people aged ≥1 month; for infants aged <1 month, azithromycin

is the preferred antibiotic. Antimicrobial therapy with a macrolide antibiotic administered <3 weeks after cough onset can limit transmission to others. Postexposure prophylaxis is recommended for close contacts of cases and for people at high risk of developing severe disease. The recommended agents and dosing regimens for prophylaxis are the same as for the treatment of pertussis.

PREVENTIVE MEASURES FOR TRAVELERS
Vaccine

Travelers should be up to date with pertussis vaccinations before departure. Multiple pertussis vaccines are available in the United States for infants and children, and 2 vaccines are available for adolescents and adults. A complete listing of licensed vaccines can be found at www.fda.gov/BiologicsBloodVaccines/Vaccines/ApprovedProducts/ucm093833.htm.

Complete vaccination of children aged <7 years with 5 doses of acellular pertussis vaccine in combination with diphtheria and tetanus toxoids (DTaP) is recommended; an accelerated schedule of doses may be used to complete the DTaP series. Children aged 7–10 years who are not fully vaccinated against pertussis and for whom no contraindication to pertussis vaccine exists should receive a single dose of Tdap to provide protection against pertussis. If additional doses of tetanus and diphtheria toxoid-containing vaccines are needed, then children aged 7–10 years should be vaccinated according to catch-up guidance, with Tdap preferred as the first dose. Adolescents aged 11–18 years who have completed the recommended childhood DTwP/DTaP vaccination series should receive a single dose of Tdap instead of Td for booster immunization against tetanus, diphtheria, and pertussis. Tdap vaccine, when indicated, should be administered to adolescents regardless of interval since the last dose of Td vaccine.

Adults aged 19–64 years who have not previously received Tdap should receive a single dose of Tdap to replace a single dose of Td for booster immunization against tetanus, diphtheria, and pertussis regardless of interval since their last tetanus toxoid-containing vaccine (such as Td). Adults aged ≥65 years who have or who anticipate having close contact with an infant aged <12 months and who have not previously received Tdap should receive a single dose of Tdap to protect against pertussis and reduce the likelihood of transmission; all other adults ≥65 years who have not previously received Tdap may be given a single dose of Tdap instead of Td.

Tdap can be given regardless of interval from the last Td to provide pertussis protection before travel, except to people for whom vaccination is contraindicated or for people who have been previously received Tdap. Adolescents and adults who have never been immunized against pertussis, tetanus, or diphtheria, who have incomplete immunization, or whose immunity is uncertain should follow the catch-up schedule established for Td/Tdap. Tdap can be substituted for any one of the Td doses in the series.

BIBLIOGRAPHY

1. American Academy of Pediatrics. Pertussis. In: Pickering LK, Baker CJ, Long SS, McMillan JA, editors. Red Book: 2006 report of the Committee on Infectious Diseases. 27th ed. Elk Grove Village, IL: American Academy of Pediatrics; 2006. p. 498–520.
2. Broder KR, Cortese MM, Iskander JK, Kretsinger K, Slade BA, Brown KH, et al. Preventing tetanus, diphtheria, and pertussis among adolescents: use of tetanus toxoid, reduced diphtheria toxoid and acellular pertussis vaccines. Recommendations of the Advisory Committee on Immunization Practices (ACIP). MMWR Recomm Rep. 2006 Dec 15;55(RR-17):1–33.
3. CDC. Pertussis vaccination: use of acellular pertussis vaccines among infants and young children. Recommendations of the Advisory Committee on Immunization Practices (ACIP). MMWR Recomm Rep. 1997 Mar 28;46(RR-7):1–25.
4. CDC. Updated recommendations for use of tetanus toxoid, reduced diphtheria toxoid and acellular pertussis (Tdap) vaccine from the Advisory Committee on Immunization Practices, 2010. MMWR Morb Mortal Wkly Rep. 2011 Jan 14;60(1):13–5.
5. Edwards KM, Decker MD. Pertussis vaccines. In: Plotkin SA, Orenstein WA, editors. Vaccines. 4th ed. Philadelphia: WB Saunders; 2004. p. 471–528.
6. Tiwari T, Murphy TV, Moran J. Recommended antimicrobial agents for the treatment and postexposure prophylaxis of pertussis: 2005 CDC Guidelines. MMWR Recomm Rep. 2005 Dec 9;54 (RR-14):1–16

PINWORM (ENTEROBIASIS, OXYURIASIS, THREADWORM)

Els Mathieu

INFECTIOUS AGENT

The intestinal nematode (roundworm) *Enterobius vermicularis* causes pinworm infection. Other helminth infections are discussed in the Helminths, Intestinal section earlier in this chapter.

MODE OF TRANSMISSION

Fecal-oral ingestion of the egg, direct person-to-person contact, or indirect contact via contaminated hands, dust, food, or objects (such as bedding, clothing, toys, bathwater, toilet seats) are modes of transmission. The incubation period from when the egg is ingested to when the adult worm migrates to the anus is 1–2 months, but may be longer. Eggs can remain infective indoors for 2–3 weeks. Humans are the only known natural host; animal pinworms do not infect humans.

EPIDEMIOLOGY

Pinworm infection is found worldwide and is the most frequent worm infection in the United States. Infections cluster in households; are common in school-age and preschool-age children and their household members, caregivers, and playmates; and are common in child care and institutional care settings. Crowded living conditions facilitate transmission. People of all ages are at risk. Risk factors include the following:

* Poor hygiene (including failure to follow proper handwashing practices and poor toilet hygiene)
* Unsanitary or inadequate toilet facilities
* Crowded living conditions or living in same household as infected person
* Close day-to-day contact (living and working) with people, particularly institutionalized people or preschool- and school-age children

CLINICAL PRESENTATION

Although infections can be asymptomatic, common symptoms include nocturnal perianal and perineal pruritus and restless sleep. Urethritis, vaginitis, salpingitis, hepatitis, or peritonitis may occur if adult worms migrate from the perineum to other sites. Secondary bacterial infection of skin may occur from scratching.

DIAGNOSIS

Diagnosis is made by identifying the worm or its eggs by:

* Direct visualization of female adult worms near anus or on sheets or underclothing or pajamas at night, about 2–3 hours after patient falls asleep.
* Microscopic identification of worm eggs by using the "scotch tape test" on 3 consecutive mornings. The adhesive side of clear transparent—not translucent—cellophane tape is pressed to the skin around the anus when patient first awakens, before washing or bathing. The tape is then directly affixed to a microscope slide and examined under low power for eggs.
* Eosinophilia is unusual (because of absence of tissue invasion); serologic testing is not useful or widely available.
* Eggs and worms are rarely found in routine stool samples.

TREATMENT

Administer an antihelminthic as a single oral dose; repeat in 2 weeks. Drugs of choice are mebendazole, albendazole, or pyrantel pamoate. Treat all household contacts and caretakers at the same time as the patient. Daily morning bathing removes a large proportion of eggs; change underclothing and bedding frequently and launder in hot water. Reinfection occurs easily; instruction about prevention is mandatory to eliminate continued infection and spread.

PREVENTIVE MEASURES FOR TRAVELERS

Strict observance of good hand hygiene is essential (proper handwashing; maintaining clean, short fingernails; avoiding or preventing nail biting and scratching the perianal and perineal region). Daily morning bathing, as well as careful handling and frequent changing and laundering of underclothing and bedding with hot water, can help reduce infection and prevent reinfection and environmental contamination with eggs.

BIBLIOGRAPHY

1. American Academy of Pediatrics. Pinworm infection (*Enterobius vermicularis*). In: Pickering LK, Baker CJ, Long SS, McMillan JA, editors. Red Book: 2006 Report of the Committee on Infectious Diseases. 27th ed. Elk Grove Village, IL: American Academy of Pediatrics; 2006. p. 520–2.
2. American Public Health Association. Enterobiasis. In: Heyman DL, editor. Control of Communicable Diseases Manual. 18th ed. Washington, DC: American Public Health Association; 2004. p. 194–6.
3. Kucik CJ, Martin GL, Sortor BV. Common intestinal parasites. Am Fam Physician. 2004 Mar 1;69(5): 1161–8.
4. Meinking TL, Burkhart CN, Burkhart CG. Changing paradigms in parasitic infections: common dermatological helminthic infections and cutaneous myiasis. Clin Dermatol. 2003 Sep–Oct;21(5):407–16.
5. St Georgiev V. Chemotherapy of enterobiasis (oxyuriasis). Expert Opin Pharmacother. 2001 Feb;2(2):267–75.

PLAGUE (BUBONIC, PNEUMONIC, SEPTICEMIC)

Kevin S. Griffith, Paul S. Mead

INFECTIOUS AGENT
Plague is caused by the gram-negative bacterium *Yersinia pestis*.

MODE OF TRANSMISSION
Zoonotic disease is usually transmitted to humans by the bites of infected rodent fleas. Less common exposures include handling infected animal tissues (hunters, wildlife personnel), inhalation of infectious droplets from cats or dogs with plague, and rarely, contact with a pneumonic plague patient.

EPIDEMIOLOGY
Each year, 1,000–2,500 cases occur globally. Plague is endemic in rural areas in central and southern Africa, central Asia and the Indian subcontinent, the northeastern part of South America, and parts of the southwestern United States. Although rare, urban outbreaks of plague have been reported in Mahajanga, Madagascar. All ages are at risk for infection; however, risk to travelers is largely restricted to rural endemic areas. Only 1 case associated with international travel has been reported in the United States in the past 2 decades.

CLINICAL PRESENTATION
The incubation period is typically 1–6 days. History is suggestive of exposure to rodents, rodent fleas, wild rabbits, sick or dead carnivores, or patients with pneumonic plague. Symptoms and signs of the 3 clinical presentations of plague illness are as follows:

- Bubonic (more than 80%)—rapid onset of fever; painful, swollen, and tender lymph nodes, usually inguinal, axillary, or cervical
- Pneumonic—high fever, overwhelming pneumonia, cough, bloody sputum, chills
- Septicemic—fever, prostration, hemorrhagic or thrombotic phenomena, progressing to acral gangrene

DIAGNOSIS
Y. pestis can be isolated from bubo aspirates, blood cultures, or sputum culture if pneumonic. Diagnosis can be confirmed through culture rapid assays, available through public

health laboratories, or serologic tests that show a 4-fold change in antibody titer to F1 antigen between acute- and convalescent-phase sera.

TREATMENT

Physicians should report all suspected plague cases to state or local health departments and consult with CDC to obtain information and access diagnostic services. Parenteral antibiotic therapy with streptomycin is the recommended first-line therapy; alternatively, gentamicin or, where treatment is limited to oral therapy, doxycycline can be used. Additional information can be found on the Division of Vector-Borne Diseases website at www.cdc.gov/ncidod/dvbid/plague/index.htm.

PREVENTIVE MEASURES FOR TRAVELERS

No vaccine is currently available in the United States. Preventive measures are aimed at reducing contact with fleas and potentially infected rodents and other wild-life. Prophylactic antibiotic treatment is given only in the event of exposure to bites of wild rodent fleas during an outbreak, exposure to tissues of a plague-infected animal, or close exposure to another person or animal with suspected plague pneumonia. People working in health care settings should follow droplet precautions while working with suspected plague patients, especially if patient is coughing.

BIBLIOGRAPHY

1. Boisier P, Rahalison L, Rasolomaharo M, Ratsitorahina M, Mahafaly M, Razafimahefa M, et al. Epidemiologic features of four successive annual outbreaks of bubonic plague in Mahajanga, Madagascar. Emerg Infect Dis. 2002 Mar;8(3):311–6.
2. Boulanger LL, Ettestad P, Fogarty JD, Dennis DT, Romig D, Mertz G. Gentamicin and tetracyclines for the treatment of human plague: review of 75 cases in new Mexico, 1985–1999. Clin Infect Dis. 2004 Mar 1;38(5):663–9.
3. CDC. Human plague—India, 1994. MMWR Morb Mortal Wkly Rep. 1994 Sep 30;43(38):689–91.
4. CDC. Prevention of plague: recommendations of the Advisory Committee on Immunization Practices (ACIP). MMWR Recomm Rep. 1996 Dec 13;45(RR-14):1–15.
5. Dennis DT, Mead P. *Yersinia* species, including plague. In: Mandell GS, Bennett JE, Dolin R, editors. Principles and Practice of Infectious Diseases. 7th ed. Philadelphia: Churchill Livingstone Elsevier; 2010. p. 2943–53.
6. Gage KL. Plague. In: Collier L, editor. Microbiology and Microbial Infections. 9th ed. New York: Arnold; 1998.
7. Inglesby TV, Dennis DT, Henderson DA, Bartlett JG, Ascher MS, Eitzen E, et al. Plague as a biological weapon: medical and public health management. Working Group on Civilian Biodefense. JAMA. 2000 May 3;283(17):2281–90.
8. Kool JL. Risk of person-to-person transmission of pneumonic plague. Clin Infect Dis. 2005 Apr 15;40(8):1166–72.
9. Neerinckx S, Bertherat E, Leirs H. Human plague occurrences in Africa: an overview from 1877 to 2008. Trans R Soc Trop Med Hyg. 2010 Feb;104(2):97–103.
10. Perry RD, Fetherston JD. *Yersinia pestis*—etiologic agent of plague. Clin Microbiol Rev. 1997 Jan;10(1):35–66.
11. World Health Organization. Human plague: review of regional morbidity and mortality, 2004–2009. Wkly Epidemiol Rec. 2009 Feb 5;85(6):40–5.

PNEUMOCOCCAL DISEASE (*STREPTOCOCCUS PNEUMONIAE*)

J. Pekka Nuorti

INFECTIOUS AGENT

Pneumococcal disease is caused by the bacterium *Streptococcus pneumoniae* (pneumococcus), which has more than 91 known serotypes.

The major clinical syndromes include life-threatening infections such as meningitis, bacteremia, and pneumonia. Pneumococcus is the most commonly identified cause of community-acquired pneumonia. It is also a major cause of milder but more common illnesses, such as sinusitis and otitis media.

MODE OF TRANSMISSION

S. pneumoniae is transmitted directly from person to person through close contact via respiratory droplets. The organism frequently colonizes the nasopharynx of healthy people, particularly young children, without causing illness. Transmission is thought to be common, but clinical illness occurs infrequently among casual contacts.

EPIDEMIOLOGY

Pneumococcal disease occurs worldwide. The reported rates are higher in developing than in industrialized countries. Pneumococcal disease is more common during winter and early spring, when respiratory viruses are circulating. Most illnesses are sporadic. Outbreaks of pneumococcal disease are uncommon but may occur in closed populations, such as nursing homes, childcare centers, or other institutions. In the United States, most deaths from pneumococcal disease occur in older adults, although in developing countries, many children die of pneumococcal pneumonia.

Routine use of the 7-valent pneumococcal conjugate vaccine (PCV7) in the United States since 2000 has dramatically reduced the incidence of pneumococcal disease in both children and adults. Because the vaccine interrupts transmission of vaccine-type pneumococci, rates of pneumococcal disease in unvaccinated older children and adults have also decreased. Many other industrialized countries are also using pneumococcal conjugate vaccines.

The risk for pneumococcal disease is generally highest among young children, the elderly, and people of any age who have chronic medical conditions, such as heart disease, lung disease, diabetes, or asplenia or conditions that suppress the immune system, such as HIV. Cigarette smokers are also at increased risk. While most travelers are not in the high-risk categories, healthy travelers of any age can develop pneumococcal pneumonia while traveling.

CLINICAL PRESENTATION

Sudden onset of fever and malaise are typical symptoms for all forms of pneumococcal infections and may be the only symptoms in young children with bacteremia. In pneumococcal pneumonia, fever may precede the usual symptoms of cough, pleuritic chest pain, and production of purulent or blood-tinged sputum by 12–24 hours. In elderly people, the onset of pneumococcal pneumonia may be less abrupt, with fever, shortness of breath, or altered mental status as the initial symptoms; sputum production may be absent. Pneumococcal meningitis may present with a stiff neck, headache, lethargy, or seizures.

DIAGNOSIS

A definitive diagnosis of pneumococcal infection can be made by isolating the bacterium from blood or other normally sterile body sites, such as cerebrospinal fluid. Most patients with pneumococcal pneumonia, however, do not have detectable bacteremia. The diagnosis of pneumococcal pneumonia can be suspected if, on microscopy, a sputum specimen contains many gram-positive diplococci and polymorphonuclear leukocytes and few epithelial cells. Detection of pneumococcal antigen in urine is a useful diagnostic test for adults.

In pneumococcal pneumonia, typical chest radiography may show lobar, segmental, or multilobar consolidation. Pneumococcal pneumonia is usually, but not always, associated with a high white blood cell count. High white blood cell counts should raise suspicion for this diagnosis, since other serious travel-related diseases causing fever, such as hepatitis, typhoid fever, malaria, dengue fever, or typhus, are all associated with normal or low white blood cell counts.

TREATMENT

All types of pneumococcal infections are usually treated with antibiotics. Empiric therapy for suspected pneumococcal infection depends on the syndrome but usually includes a penicillin or cephalosporin. Worldwide, many strains are increasingly resistant to penicillin, cephalosporins, and macrolides, and some are resistant to multiple classes of drugs, complicating treatment choices. Antimicrobial susceptibility of strains isolated from blood and cerebrospinal fluid should be determined, and definitive treatment should be targeted on the basis of susceptibility results.

In 2008, the Clinical and Laboratory Standards Institute adopted new susceptibility breakpoints for penicillin treatment of nonmeningitis cases of pneumococcal disease. However, empiric antibiotic therapy should not be delayed and should begin before microbiologic confirmation. In the United States and other countries where β-lactam resistance among pneumococcal isolates is common, the initial regimen for suspected pneumococcal meningitis should include vancomycin or a fluoroquinolone along with a third-generation cephalosporin, until the antimicrobial susceptibility pattern of the organism is available.

PREVENTIVE MEASURES FOR TRAVELERS
Vaccine

As of 2010, 3 vaccines are available to prevent pneumococcal disease in the United States. These vaccines induce antibodies to the specific types of pneumococcal capsule. No specific recommendations for the use of pneumococcal vaccines in travelers have been formulated.

Pneumococcal Conjugate Vaccines

The 7-valent pneumococcal conjugate vaccine (PCV7) has been part of the routine infant immunization schedule in the United States since 2000. It is recommended for all children aged <5 years. In 2010, a 13-valent pneumococcal conjugate vaccine (PCV13) was approved by the Food and Drug Administration and is replacing PCV7. PCV13 is recommended for routine vaccination of all children aged 2–59 months and for children aged 60–71 months with underlying medical conditions that increase their risk for pneumococcal disease or complications. Children with HIV, sickle cell anemia, asplenia, cerebrospinal fluid leak, or cochlear implant can receive PCV13 through age 18 years. The PCV7 and PCV13 vaccines are recommended as a 4-dose series at ages 2, 4, 6, and 12–15 months. Fewer doses are required for children who begin the series after age 7 months.

Pneumococcal Polysaccharide Vaccine

A 23-valent pneumococcal polysaccharide vaccine (PPSV23) is recommended for all adults aged ≥65 years and for people aged 2–64 years with underlying medical conditions. People with underlying conditions should be vaccinated as soon as possible after the condition is diagnosed. Children with underlying medical conditions that are vaccine indications should also receive PPSV23, after receiving the conjugate vaccine series. Routine revaccination with PPSV23 is not recommended for most people. A second dose is recommended 5 years after the first dose for people with functional or anatomic asplenia and for people with immunocompromising conditions. People ≥65 years who received PPSV23 before age 65 for an underlying medical condition should be administered another dose of PPSV23, if ≥5 years have passed since their previous dose.

The World Health Organization recommends that inclusion of pneumococcal conjugate vaccines in all national immunization programs should be a priority. As of 2008, 26 industrialized countries were routinely using pneumococcal conjugate vaccines, including the United States, Canada, Australia, the United Kingdom, and other Western European and Middle Eastern countries. A 10-valent pneumococcal conjugate vaccine formulation is available in many countries, including Europe, Canada, and Australia.

Vaccine Safety and Adverse Reactions

After receipt of PCV7, mild local reactions such as redness, swelling, or tenderness occur in 10%–23% of infants. Larger areas of redness or swelling or limitations in arm movement may occur in 1%–9% of infants. Low-grade fever can occur in up to 24%, and fever higher than 102.2°F (39°C) may occur in up to 2.5% of vaccinees. The safety profiles of PCV13 and PCV7 are comparable: the most commonly reported (more than 20% of recipients) adverse reactions after PCV13 were injection-site reactions, fever, decreased appetite, irritability, and increased or decreased sleep.

After receipt of PPV23, self-limiting local side effects occur in approximately half of vaccine recipients and are more common after revaccination than after the first dose. These reactions usually resolve within 48 hours. More severe local reactions and systemic symptoms, including myalgias and fever, are rare.

Precautions and Contraindications

PCV7 is contraindicated for children known to have hypersensitivity to any component of the vaccine. PCV13 is contraindicated among people known to have a severe allergic reaction (anaphylaxis) to any component of PCV13 or PCV7 or to any diphtheria toxoid–containing vaccine. Clinicians may delay vaccination of children with moderate or severe illness until the child has recovered, although minor illnesses, such as mild upper respiratory tract infection with or without low-grade fever, are not contraindications to vaccination. Revaccination with PPV23 is contraindicated for people who had a severe reaction (anaphylactic reaction or localized Arthus-type reaction) to the initial dose.

Other Preventive Measures

Chemoprophylaxis is not routinely recommended for travelers or for close contacts of people with pneumococcal meningitis or other cases of invasive disease unless otherwise recommended by the clinician supervising their care.

BIBLIOGRAPHY

1. American Academy of Pediatrics. Pneumococcal infections. In: Pickering LK, Baker CJ, Kimberlin DW, Long SS, editors. Red Book: 2009 Report of the Committee on Infectious Diseases. 28th ed. Elk Grove Village, IL: American Academy of Pediatrics; 2009. p. 524–35.
2. CDC. Licensure of a 13-valent pneumococcal conjugate vaccine (PCV13) and recommendations for use among children—Advisory Committee on Immunization Practices (ACIP), 2010. MMWR Morb Mortal Wkly Rep. 2010 Mar 12;59(9):258–61.
3. CDC. Preventing pneumococcal disease among infants and young children. Recommendations of the Advisory Committee on Immunization Practices (ACIP). MMWR Recomm Rep. 2000 Oct 6;49(RR-9):1–38.
4. CDC. Prevention of pneumococcal disease: recommendations of the Advisory Committee on Immunization Practices (ACIP). MMWR Recomm Rep. 1997 Apr 4;46(RR-8):1–24.
5. Fedson DS, Scott JA. The burden of pneumococcal disease among adults in developed and developing countries: what is and is not known. Vaccine. 1999 Jul 30;17 Suppl 1:S11–8.
6. Greenwood B. The epidemiology of pneumococcal infection in children in the developing world. Philos Trans R Soc Lond B Biol Sci. 1999 Apr 29;354(1384):777–85.
7. Tunkel AR, Hartman BJ, Kaplan SL, Kaufman BA, Roos KL, Scheld WM, et al. Practice guidelines for the management of bacterial meningitis. Clin Infect Dis. 2004 Nov 1;39(9):1267–84.
8. Wikler MA. Performance Standards for Antimicrobial Susceptibility Testing, Eighteenth Informational Supplement. Wayne, PA: Clinical and Laboratory Standards Institute; 2008.
9. World Health Organization. Pneumococcal conjugate vaccine for childhood immunisation—WHO position paper. Wkly Epidemiol Rec. 2007;82(12):93–104.

POLIOMYELITIS
James P. Alexander, Gregory S. Wallace, Steven G. F. Wassilak

INFECTIOUS AGENT

The infectious agent is poliovirus (genus *Enterovirus*) types 1, 2, and 3. Polioviruses are small (27–30 nm), nonenveloped viruses with capsids enclosing a single-stranded, positive-sense RNA genome about 7,500 nucleotides long. Most of the properties of polioviruses are shared with the other enteroviruses.

MODE OF TRANSMISSION

Polioviruses are spread through fecal-oral or oral transmission. Acute infection involves the oropharynx, gastrointestinal tract, and occasionally the central nervous system.

EPIDEMIOLOGY

In the prevaccine era, infection with poliovirus was common worldwide, with seasonal peaks and epidemics in the summer and fall in temperate areas. The incidence of poliomyelitis in the United States declined rapidly after the licensure of inactivated polio vaccine (IPV) in 1955 and live oral polio vaccine (OPV) in the 1960s. The last cases of indigenously acquired polio in the United States occurred in 1979. The Global Polio Eradication Initiative (GPEI) subsequently eliminated polio in the Americas, where the last wild poliovirus (WPV)-associated polio case was detected in 1991.

In 1999, a change in vaccination policy in the United States from use of OPV to exclusive use of IPV eliminated the 8–10 vaccine-associated paralytic poliomyelitis (VAPP) cases that had occurred annually since the introduction of OPV in the 1960s. In the United States, 2 events in 2005 highlighted the continuing but low risk for poliovirus infection for unvaccinated people, whether residing in the United States or traveling:

- A case of imported VAPP occurred in an unvaccinated US adult who had traveled abroad, likely from contact with an infant recently vaccinated with OPV.
- An unvaccinated, immunocompromised infant and 4 children in 2 other families in the same small rural community were found to be asymptomatically infected with a vaccine-derived poliovirus, presumably originating outside the United States in a country that uses OPV.

GPEI has built upon the success in the Americas and made great progress in eradicating WPVs, reducing the number of reported polio cases worldwide by more than 99% since the mid-1980s. Wild poliovirus circulation has never been interrupted in only 4 countries: Afghanistan, India, Nigeria, and Pakistan. In spite of progress made in eradicating WPVs globally, countries are still at risk for imported cases, primarily from these 4 countries. From 2008 through 2010, WPV outbreaks from importations have occurred in 28 countries in Africa, Eastern Europe and North Asia, and South Asia. In 4 of these countries (Angola, Chad, Democratic Republic of the Congo, and southern Sudan), WPV transmission has been reestablished.

Because of polio eradication efforts, the number of countries where travelers are at risk for polio has decreased dramatically. The last documented case of WPV-associated paralysis in a US resident travelling abroad occurred in 1986 in a 29-year-old vaccinated adult who had been traveling in South and Southeast Asia. As noted above, in 2005 an unvaccinated US adult traveling abroad acquired VAPP after contact with an infant recently vaccinated with OPV.

At the time of publication, most of the world's population resides in areas considered free of WPV circulation, including the Western Hemisphere, the Western Pacific region (which encompasses China), and most of Europe. Vaccination is recommended for all travelers to polio-endemic or epidemic areas, including countries with recent proven WPV circulation and neighboring countries. As of October 2010, these areas include some but not all countries in East, Central and West Africa, Eastern Europe and Northern Asia, and South Asia. For current information on the status of polio eradication efforts and vaccine recommendations, consult the travel notices on the CDC Travelers' Health website (www.cdc.gov/travel) or the GPEI website (www.polioeradication.org).

CLINICAL PRESENTATION

Clinical manifestations of poliovirus infection range from asymptomatic (most infections) to symptomatic, including acute flaccid paralysis of a single limb to quadriplegia, respiratory failure, and rarely, death.

DIAGNOSIS

The diagnosis is made by identifying poliovirus in clinical specimens (usually stool) obtained from an acutely ill patient. Poliovirus may be detected by culture on appropriate cell lines followed by identification by neutralization tests or by PCR. Poliovirus may also be identified by direct amplification from stool specimens followed by partial genomic sequencing to establish identity and possible source of the virus. Shedding in fecal specimens can be intermittent, but usually poliovirus can be detected for up to 4 weeks after onset of illness. During the first 3–10 days of the illness, poliovirus can also be detected from oropharyngeal specimens. Poliovirus is rarely detected in the blood or cerebrospinal fluid.

TREATMENT

Only treatment for symptoms is available, ranging from pain and fever relief to intubation and mechanical ventilation for patients with respiratory insufficiency.

PREVENTIVE MEASURES FOR TRAVELERS

Vaccine

In the United States, infants and children should be vaccinated against polio as part of a routine immunization series (see Infants and Children below). Before traveling to areas where poliomyelitis cases are still occurring, travelers should ensure that they have completed the recommended age-appropriate polio vaccine series and have received a booster dose, if necessary (see Infants and Children and Adults below). To eliminate the risk for VAPP, since 2000, IPV has been the only polio vaccine available in the United States; however, OPV continues to be used in many countries and for global polio eradication activities.

Infants and Children

In the United States, all infants and children should receive 4 doses of IPV at ages 2, 4, and 6–18 months and 4–6 years. The final dose should be administered at age ≥4 years, regardless of the number of previous doses, and should be given ≥6 months after the previous dose. A fourth dose in the routine IPV series is not necessary if the third dose was administered at age ≥4 years and ≥6 months after the previous dose. If both OPV and IPV were administered as part of the routine series, a combined total of 4 doses should be administered, regardless of the child's age. If the routine series cannot be administered within the recommended intervals before protection is needed, the following alternatives are recommended:

- The first dose should be given to infants ≥6 weeks old.
- The second and third doses should be administered ≥4 weeks after the previous doses.
- The minimum interval between the third and fourth doses is 6 months.

If the age-appropriate series is not completed before departure, the remaining IPV doses to complete a full series should be administered when feasible, at the intervals recommended above, if the child remains at increased risk for poliovirus exposure.

Adults

Adults who are traveling to areas where poliomyelitis cases are still occurring and who are unvaccinated, incompletely vaccinated, or whose vaccination status is unknown should receive 2 doses of IPV administered at an interval of 4–8 weeks; a third dose should be administered 6–12 months after the second. If 3 doses of IPV cannot be administered within the recommended intervals before protection is needed, the following alternatives are recommended:

- If >8 weeks is available before protection is needed, 3 doses of IPV should be administered ≥4 weeks apart.
- If <8 weeks but >4 weeks is available before protection is needed, 2 doses of IPV should be administered ≥4 weeks apart.
- If <4 weeks is available before protection is needed, a single dose of IPV is recommended.

If <3 doses are administered, the remaining IPV doses to complete a 3-dose series should be administered when feasible, at the intervals recommended above, if the person remains at increased risk for poliovirus exposure. Adults who have completed a routine series of polio vaccine are considered to have lifelong immunity to poliomyelitis, but data are lacking. As a precaution, adults (≥18 years of age) who are traveling to areas where poliomyelitis cases are occurring and who have received a routine series with either IPV or OPV in childhood should receive another dose of IPV before departure. For adults, available data do not indicate the need for more than a single lifetime booster dose with IPV.

Vaccine Safety and Adverse Reactions

Minor local reactions (pain and redness) can occur with IPV. No serious adverse reactions to IPV have been documented. IPV should not be administered to people who have experienced a severe allergic reaction (anaphylaxis) after a previous dose of IPV or after receiving streptomycin, polymyxin B, or neomycin, which IPV contains in trace amounts; hypersensitivity reactions can occur after IPV administration among people sensitive to these 3 antibiotics.

Pregnancy and Breastfeeding

If a pregnant woman is unvaccinated or incompletely vaccinated and requires immediate protection against polio because of planned travel to a country or area where polio cases are occurring, IPV can be administered as recommended for adults. Breastfeeding is not a contraindication to vaccination of an infant or mother against polio.

Precautions and Contraindications

IPV may be administered to people with diarrhea. Minor upper respiratory illnesses with or without fever, mild to moderate local reactions to a previous dose of IPV, current antimicrobial therapy, and the convalescent phase of acute illness are not contraindications for vaccination.

Immunosuppression

IPV may be administered safely to immunodeficient travelers and their household contacts. Although a protective immune response cannot be ensured, IPV might confer some protection to the immunodeficient person. People with certain primary immunodeficiency diseases should not be given OPV and should avoid contact with excreted OPV virus (such as exposure to a child vaccinated with OPV in the previous 6 weeks); however, this situation no longer occurs in the United States unless a child receives OPV overseas.

BIBLIOGRAPHY

1. Alexander JP, Ehresmann K, Seward J, Wax G, Harriman K, Fuller S, et al. Transmission of imported vaccine-derived poliovirus in an undervaccinated community in Minnesota. J Infect Dis. 2009 Feb 1;199(3):391–7.
2. Alexander LN, Seward JF, Santibanez TA, Pallansch MA, Kew OM, Prevots DR, et al. Vaccine policy changes and epidemiology of poliomyelitis in the United States. JAMA. 2004 Oct 13;292(14):1696–701.
3. CDC. Certification of poliomyelitis eradication—the Americas, 1994. MMWR Morb Mortal Wkly Rep. 1994 Oct 7;43(39):720–2.
4. CDC. Immunization schedules. Atlanta: CDC; 2010 [cited 2010 Apr 6]. Available from: http://www.cdc.gov/vaccines/recs/schedules/default.htm.
5. CDC. Imported vaccine-associated paralytic poliomyelitis—United States, 2005. MMWR Morb Mortal Wkly Rep. 2006 Feb 3;55(4):97–9.
6. CDC. Laboratory surveillance for wild and vaccine-derived polioviruses—worldwide, January 2008–June 2009. MMWR Morb Mortal Wkly Rep. 2009 Sep 4;58(34):950–4.
7. CDC. Poliomyelitis. In: Atkinson W, Hamborsky J, McIntyre L, Wolfe S, editors. Epidemiology and Prevention of Vaccine-Preventable Diseases. 9th ed. Washington, DC: Public Health Foundation; 2006. p. 97–110.
8. CDC. Poliomyelitis—United States, 1975–1984. MMWR Morb Mortal Wkly Rep. 1986 Mar 21;35(11):180–2.
9. CDC. Progress toward interruption of wild poliovirus transmission—worldwide, 2009. MMWR Morb Mortal Wkly Rep. 2010 May 14;59(18):545–50.
10. CDC. Update on vaccine-derived polioviruses—worldwide, January 2008–June 2009. MMWR Morb Mortal Wkly Rep. 2009 Sep 18;58(36):1002–6.
11. CDC. Updated recommendations of the Advisory Committee on Immunization Practices (ACIP) regarding routine poliovirus vaccination. MMWR Morb Mortal Wkly Rep. 2009 Aug 7;58(30):829–30.
12. CDC. Wild poliovirus type 1 and type 3 importations—15 countries, Africa, 2008–2009. MMWR Morb Mortal Wkly Rep. 2009 Apr 17;58(14):357–62.
13. Plotkin SA, Vidor E. Vaccine-inactivated. In: Plotkin SA, Orenstein WA, Offit PA, editors. Vaccines. 5th ed. Philadelphia: Saunders Elsevier; 2008. p. 605–30.
14. Prevots DR, Burr RK, Sutter RW, Murphy TV. Poliomyelitis prevention in the United States. Updated recommendations of the Advisory Committee on Immunization Practices (ACIP). MMWR Recomm Rep. 2000 May 9;49(RR-5):1–22.
15. Sutter RW, Kew OM, Cochi SL. Poliovirus vaccine-live. In: Plotkin SA, Orenstein WA, Offit PA, editors. Vaccines. Philadelphia: Saunders Elsevier; 2008. p. 631–86.
16. World Health Organization. Wild poliovirus weekly update. World Health Organization; 2010 [updated 2010 Mar 6; cited 2010 Apr 6]. Available from: http://www.polioeradication.org/casecount.asp.
17. WHO Advisory Committee. Conclusions and recommendations of the Advisory Committee on Poliomyelitis Eradication, Geneva, 27–28 November 2007. Wkly Epidemiol Rec. 2008 Jan 18;83(3):25–35.

Q FEVER

Alicia Anderson, Jennifer McQuiston

INFECTIOUS AGENT

Q fever is caused by the organism *Coxiella burnetii*, which is an obligate intracellular bacterium.

MODE OF TRANSMISSION

Q fever is a zoonotic disease that is often associated with exposure to cattle, sheep, and goats. The most common mode of transmission to humans is inhalation of aerosols or dust contaminated with dried birth fluids or excreta from infected animals. Direct animal contact is not required for transmission to occur. Infections via ingestion of contaminated dairy products and human-to-human transmission via sexual contact or during parturition have been rarely reported.

EPIDEMIOLOGY

Q fever is found worldwide. Human cases of Q fever have been reported from across the United States and are most commonly reported in those who are occupationally exposed to livestock. The average annual reported incidence of Q fever in the United States is 0.28 cases per million population per year, with an estimated national seroprevalence of 3.1%. The incidence in the United Kingdom also appears to be low (2 cases per million), whereas the reported incidence in France (500 cases per million) and Australia (38 cases per million) is much higher. Q fever is believed to be underdiagnosed and underreported throughout the world, so the number of reported cases likely does not reflect the true incidence of disease.

The largest outbreak of Q fever ever reported is ongoing in the Netherlands. From 2007 through 2009, more than 3,500 cases were reported: most in the southern region, although cases have been confirmed throughout the country. Cases have continued throughout 2010.

Travelers who visit rural areas or farms with cattle, sheep, goats, or other livestock may be exposed to Q fever. Transmission is also possible by drinking unpasteurized milk. Occupational exposure to infected animals (such as in farmers, veterinarians, butchers, meat packers, and seasonal or migrant farm workers), particularly during parturition, poses a high risk for disease transmission. Recent cases of Q fever in military personnel returning from deployments to Iraq and Afghanistan should alert clinicians to consider this diagnosis among people presenting with compatible symptoms.

CLINICAL PRESENTATION

Approximately half of infected people are asymptomatic. Symptomatic illness typically occurs within 2–3 weeks after exposure. Variable incubation periods may be dose-dependent, with shorter incubation periods after exposure to high organism numbers. The most common presentation is a mild and self-limiting influenza-like illness. Other potential manifestations include pneumonia, hepatitis, myocarditis, encephalitis, osteomyelitis, and miscarriage in pregnant women. Chronic Q fever is uncommon (<1% of acutely infected patients). Most chronic cases (60%–70%) present as culture-negative endocarditis in patients with a preexistent valvulopathy. Pregnant women and immunosuppressed people are also considered at high risk for developing chronic Q fever.

DIAGNOSIS

Serologic evidence of a 4-fold rise in phase II IgG by indirect immunofluorescent assay (IFA) between paired sera taken 2–4 weeks apart is the gold standard for diagnosis of acute infection. A single high serum phase II IgG titer (higher than 1:128) by IFA may be considered evidence of probable infection.

C. burnetii may be detected in infected tissues by using immunohistochemical staining, DNA detection methods, or by direct isolation of the agent via culture. PCR assays may be used on whole blood samples in the early stages of illness and before initiation of antibiotic therapy.

Chronic Q fever may occur months or years after an acute infection and is typically diagnosed based on the presence of a rising phase I IgG titer (typically 1:800 or higher) that is most often higher than phase II IgG and an identifiable nidus of infection (such as endocarditis, vascular infection, osteomyelitis, chronic hepatitis). Treatment for chronic Q fever should not be given on the basis of elevated serologic titers alone without clinical manifestation of persistent infection.

TREATMENT

Doxycycline is the treatment of choice for acute Q fever. Pregnant women, children aged <8 years with mild illness, and patients allergic to doxycycline may be treated with other antibiotics. Treatment should not be delayed while awaiting laboratory results, and consultation with an infectious diseases physician is recommended. Treatment for acute Q fever is not recommended for asymptomatic people or for those whose symptoms have resolved. Chronic Q fever endocarditis is more difficult to treat effectively and typically requires long-term combination therapy.

Prophylactic treatment for chronic Q fever endocarditis should be considered on the basis of a rising phase I IgG titer (typically 1:800 or higher) that is most often higher than phase II IgG and preexisting valvular heart disease (such as a history of a valvular graft, prosthetic heart valve, or congenital heart defect). Additional information can be found on the CDC website at www.bt.cdc.gov/agent/qfever.

PREVENTIVE MEASURES FOR TRAVELERS

A human vaccine for Q fever has been developed and used successfully in Australia. No vaccine is commercially available in the United States. No drugs for preventing infection are available, and doxycycline is not recommended as prophylaxis after a known Q fever exposure, because it will not prevent infection. Preventive measures are aimed at restricting access to areas where potentially infected animals are kept and at properly disposing birth products from livestock. People at highest risk for developing chronic Q fever (pregnant women, people with preexisting valvulopathy, and immunosuppressed people) should be educated on the risks and sources of infection. Travelers should also avoid consumption of unpasteurized dairy products.

BIBLIOGRAPHY

1. Anderson AD, Kruszon-Moran D, Loftis AD, McQuillan G, Nicholson WL, Priestley RA, et al. Seroprevalence of Q fever in the United States, 2003–2004. Am J Trop Med Hyg. 2009 Oct;81(4):691–4.
2. Gikas A, Kofteridis DP, Manios A, Pediaditis J, Tselentis Y. Newer macrolides as empiric treatment for acute Q fever infection. Antimicrob Agents Chemother. 2001 Dec;45(12):3644–6.
3. Gleeson TD, Decker CF, Johnson MD, Hartzell JD, Mascola JR. Q fever in US military returning from Iraq. Am J Med. 2007 Sep;120(9):e11–2.
4. Karakousis PC, Trucksis M, Dumler JS. Chronic Q fever in the United States. J Clin Microbiol. 2006 Jun;44(6):2283–7.
5. Leung-Shea C, Danaher PJ. Q fever in members of the United States armed forces returning from Iraq. Clin Infect Dis. 2006 Oct 15;43(8): e77–82.
6. Maurin M, Raoult D. Q fever. Clin Microbiol Rev. 1999 Oct;12(4):518–53.
7. McQuiston JH, Childs JE, Thompson HA. Q fever. J Am Vet Med Assoc. 2002 Sep 15;221(6):796–9.
8. McQuiston JH, Holman RC, McCall CL, Childs JE, Swerdlow DL, Thompson HA. National surveillance and the epidemiology of human Q fever in the United States, 1978–2004. Am J Trop Med Hyg. 2006 Jul;75(1):36–40.
9. Schimmer B, Morroy G, Dijkstra F, Schneeberger PM, Weers-Pothoff G, Timen A, et al. Large ongoing Q fever outbreak in the south of The Netherlands, 2008. Euro Surveill. 2008 Jul 31;13(31).

RABIES

Charles E. Rupprecht, David R. Shlim

INFECTIOUS AGENTS

Rabies is an acute, progressive, fatal encephalomyelitis caused by neurotropic viruses in the family Rhabdoviridae, genus *Lyssavirus*. Regardless of the viral variants found throughout the world, all lyssaviruses cause rabies, resulting in tens of millions of exposures and tens of thousands of human deaths each year.

MODE OF TRANSMISSION

Virus is present in the saliva of the biting rabid mammal. Transmission almost always occurs by an animal bite that inoculates virus into wounds. Virus inoculated into a wound does not enter the bloodstream but is taken up at a nerve synapse to travel to the brain, where it causes encephalitis. Virus may enter the nervous system fairly rapidly or may remain at the bite site for an extended period before gaining access to the nervous system. The approximate density of nerve endings in the region of the bite may increase the risk of developing encephalitis more rapidly. The hands and face, because of the relative density of nerve endings, are considered higher-risk exposures. Rarely, virus has been transmitted by exposures other than bites that introduce the agent into open wounds or mucous membranes.

All mammals are believed to be susceptible to infection, but major reservoirs are carnivores and bats. Although dogs are the main reservoir in developing countries, the epidemiology of the disease from one region or country to another differs enough to warrant the medical evaluation of all mammal bites. Bat bites anywhere in the world are a cause of concern and an indication for prophylaxis.

EPIDEMIOLOGY

Rabies is found on all continents, except Antarctica. Regionally, different viral variants are adapted to various mammalian hosts and perpetuate in dogs and wildlife, such as bats and some carnivores, including foxes, jackals, mongooses, raccoons, and skunks. In certain areas of the world, canine rabies remains highly enzootic, including but not limited to, parts of Africa, Asia, and Central and South America. Table 3-13 lists countries that have reported no cases of rabies during the most recent period for which information is available (formerly referred to as "rabies-free" countries).

Additional information about the global occurrence of rabies can be obtained from the following sources:

- World Health Organization (www.who.int/rabies/rabnet/en/)
- Rabies Bulletin—Europe (www.rbe.fli.bund.de)
- World Organization for Animal Health (www.oie.int/eng/en_index.htm)
- Local health authorities of the country, the embassy, or the local consulate's office in the United States

These lists are provided only as a guide, because up-to-date information may not be available, surveillance standards vary, and reporting status can change suddenly as a result of disease reintroduction or emergence. The actual rate of possible rabies exposure in travelers has not been calculated with accuracy. However, studies have found a range of roughly 16–200 per 100,000 travelers based on differing criteria.

CLINICAL PRESENTATION

Most patients will present after a documented, highly suspected, or likely exposure from a rabid animal. Clinical illness is compatible with acute, progressive encephalitis. After infection, the incubation period is highly variable, but it lasts approximately 1–3 months. The disease progresses acutely from a nonspecific, prodromal phase with fever and vague symptoms, to a neurologic phase, characterized by anxiety, paresis, paralysis, and other signs of encephalitis; spasms of swallowing muscles can be stimulated by the sight, sound, or perception of water (hydrophobia); and delirium and convulsions can develop, followed rapidly by coma and death.

Table 3-13. Countries and political units that reported no indigenous cases of rabies during 2009[1]

REGION	COUNTRIES
Africa	Cape Verde, Libya, Mauritius, Réunion, São Tomé and Príncipe, and Seychelles
Americas	North: Bermuda, Saint Pierre and Miquelon Caribbean: Antigua and Barbuda, Aruba, The Bahamas, Barbados, Cayman Islands, Dominica, Guadeloupe, Jamaica, Martinique, Montserrat, Netherlands Antilles, Saint Kitts (Saint Christopher) and Nevis, Saint Lucia, Saint Martin, Saint Vincent and Grenadines, Turks and Caicos, and Virgin Islands (UK and US)
Asia and the Middle East	Hong Kong, Japan, Kuwait, Lebanon, Malaysia (Sabah), Qatar, Singapore, United Arab Emirates
Europe	Austria, Belgium, Cyprus, Czech Republic,[2] Denmark,[2] Finland, Gibraltar, Greece, Iceland, Ireland, Isle of Man, Luxembourg, Netherlands,[2] Norway, Portugal, Spain[2] (except Ceuta and Melilla), Sweden, Switzerland, and United Kingdom[2]
Oceania[3]	Australia,[2] Cook Islands, Fiji, French Polynesia, Guam, Hawaii, Kiribati, Micronesia, New Caledonia, New Zealand, Northern Mariana Islands, Palau, Papua New Guinea, Samoa, and Vanuatu

[1] Bat rabies may exist in some areas that are reportedly free of rabies in other mammals.
[2] Bat lyssaviruses are known to exist in these areas that are reportedly free of rabies in other mammals.
[3] Most of Pacific Oceania is reportedly "rabies-free."

Once clinical signs manifest, most patients die in 7–14 days.

DIAGNOSIS

Diagnosis is straightforward in an encephalitic patient recently exposed to a rabid animal. However, in lieu of a history of a documented exposure and the potential for long incubation periods of weeks to months after initial viral transmission, clinical diagnosis may be complicated by the variety of symptoms and the differential exclusion of other etiologic agents associated with encephalitis.

Definitive diagnosis can be made by demonstrating virus in neuronal tissue, corneal impressions, or nuchal biopsy, either by detecting viral antigens or amplicons. Additional detailed information on diagnostic testing may be obtained from CDC (www.cdc.gov/rabies). A specific serologic response to virus can also support the diagnosis in an encephalitic patient.

TREATMENT

No treatment is effective after the development of clinical signs, but the extremely rare case of recovery after extensive medical interventions offers hope that future experimental therapeutics may be developed.

PREVENTIVE MEASURES FOR TRAVELERS
Avoiding Animal Bites

Travelers to rabies-enzootic countries should be warned about the risk of acquiring rabies and educated in animal bite-prevention strategies. Travelers should avoid stray animals, be aware of their surroundings so that they do not accidentally surprise a stray dog, avoid contact with bats and other wildlife, and not carry or eat food while nonhuman primates are near. Casual exposure to cave air is not a concern, but visitors should be educated not to handle bats or other wildlife. Noncavers can occasionally encounter a bat, particularly during ecotourism events. Many bats have tiny teeth, and not all wounds may be apparent, compared with the lesions caused by carnivores. Any suspected or documented bite or scratch from a bat should be grounds for seeking postexposure prophylaxis.

Children are at higher risk for rabies exposures because of their smaller stature, which makes extensive bites more likely; their curiosity and attraction to animals; and the possibility that they may not report a possible exposure. Although licks to fresh wounds or mucus membranes are a theoretical risk of acquiring rabies and postexposure prophylaxis should be considered, there are no reported examples of rabies in travelers who were exposed in this manner.

Preexposure Vaccination

For certain international travelers, preexposure rabies vaccine may be recommended, based on the prevalence of rabies in the country to be visited, the availability of appropriate antirabies biologics, intended activities, and duration of stay. A decision to receive preexposure rabies immunization may also be based on the likelihood of repeat travel to at-risk destinations or taking up residence in a high-risk destination. Preexposure vaccination may be recommended for veterinarians, animal handlers, field biologists, cavers, missionaries, and certain laboratory workers. Table 3-14 provides criteria for preexposure vaccination. Serology for rabies virus neutralizing antibodies is used as one gauge for revaccination considerations. Lists of US laboratories performing rabies serology may be found on the CDC website (www.cdc.gov/rabies). Regardless of whether or not preexposure vaccine is administered, travelers going to areas with a high risk for rabies should be encouraged to purchase medical evacuation insurance (see Chapter 2, Travel Health Insurance and Evacuation Insurance).

In the United States, preexposure vaccination consists of a series of 3 injections with human diploid cell rabies vaccine (HDCV) or purified chick embryo cell (PCEC) vaccine. The schedule for this series is given in Table 3-15.

Travelers should receive all 3 preexposure immunizations before travel. If 3 doses of rabies vaccine cannot be completed before travel, the traveler should not start the series, as it would be problematic to plan postexposure prophylaxis after a partial immunization series. Preexposure vaccination does not eliminate the need for additional medical attention after a rabies exposure, but it simplifies postexposure prophylaxis. Preexposure vaccination may also provide some degree of protection when there is an unapparent or unrecognized exposure to rabies virus and when postexposure prophylaxis might be delayed.

Travelers who have completed a 3-dose preexposure rabies immunization series or have received the full postexposure prophylaxis are considered preimmunized and do not require routine boosters, except after a likely rabies exposure. Periodic serum testing for rabies virus neutralizing antibody is not necessary in routine international travelers.

From 2007 through 2009, the supply of rabies vaccine in the United States was limited, and preexposure vaccination was not available to international travelers, except under special circumstances; supplies of vaccine were reserved for postexposure prophylaxis. This supply limitation has been resolved, and preexposure vaccination is now available to travelers.

Wound Management

Any animal bite or scratch should be thoroughly cleaned with copious amounts of soap and water and povidone iodine, if available. This local care will substantially reduce the risk for rabies. Wounds that might require suturing should have the suturing delayed for a few days. If suturing is necessary to control bleeding, or for functional or cosmetic reasons, rabies immune globulin (RIG), if indicated, should be administered into the wound before closing. The use of local anesthetic is not contraindicated in wound management.

Postexposure Prophylaxis
In Travelers Who Received Preexposure Vaccination

In the event of a possible rabies exposure in someone who received preexposure rabies vaccination, 2 boosters of an acceptable rabies vaccine are given on days 0 and 3 after the exposure. The booster doses should be modern

Table 3-14. Criteria for preexposure immunization for rabies

RISK CATEGORY	NATURE OF RISK	TYPICAL POPULATIONS	PREEXPOSURE REGIMEN
Continuous	Virus present continuously, often in high concentrations Specific exposures likely to go unrecognized Bite, nonbite, or aerosol exposure	Rabies research laboratory workers,[1] rabies biologics production workers	Primary course; serologic testing every 6 months; booster vaccination if antibody titer is below acceptable level[2]
Frequent	Exposure usually episodic with source recognized, but exposure might also be unrecognized Bite, nonbite, or aerosol exposure possible	Rabies diagnostic laboratory workers,[1] cavers, veterinarians and staff, and animal control and wildlife workers in rabies-epizootic areas	Primary course; serologic testing every 2 years; booster vaccination if antibody titer is below acceptable level[2]
Infrequent (more than general population)	Exposure nearly always episodic with source recognized Bite or nonbite exposure	Veterinarians, animal control, and wildlife workers in areas with low rabies rates; veterinary students; and travelers visiting areas where rabies is enzootic and immediate access to appropriate medical care, including biologics, is limited	Primary course; no serologic testing or booster vaccination
Rare (general population)	Exposure always episodic, with source recognized	US population at large, including people in rabies-epizootic areas	No preexposure immunization necessary

[1] Judgment of relative risk and extra monitoring of vaccination status of laboratory workers is the responsibility of the laboratory supervisor (see www.cdc.gov/biosafety/publications/bmbl5 for more information).

[2] Preexposure booster immunization consists of 1 dose of human diploid cell (rabies) vaccine or purified chick embryo cell vaccine, 1.0-mL dose, intramuscular (deltoid area). Minimum acceptable antibody level is complete virus neutralization at a 1:5 serum dilution by the rapid fluorescent focus inhibition test. A booster dose should be administered if titer falls below this level.

cell culture vaccines, but they do not have to be the same brand as the vaccine given in the original preexposure immunization series.

In Travelers Who Did Not Receive Preexposure Vaccination

If preexposure rabies vaccination has not been given, postexposure prophylaxis consists of injections of RIG (20 IU/kg) and a series of 4 injections of rabies vaccine over 14 days (or 5 doses over a 1-month period in immunosuppressed patients). After wound cleansing, as much of the calculated amount of RIG (Table 3-16) as is anatomically feasible should be infiltrated around the wound. The dose injected around the wound may be as small as

Table 3-15. Preexposure immunization for rabies[1]

VACCINE	DOSE (mL)	NUMBER OF DOSES	SCHEDULE (DAYS)	ROUTE
HDCV	1.0	3	0, 7, and 21 or 28	Intramuscular
PCEC	1.0	3	0, 7, and 21 or 28	Intramuscular

Abbreviations: HDCV, human diploid cell vaccine; PCEC, purified chick embryo cell.

[1] Patients who are immunosuppressed by disease or medications should postpone preexposure vaccinations and consider avoiding activities for which rabies preexposure prophylaxis is indicated. When this course is not possible, immunosuppressed people who are at risk for rabies should have their antibody titers checked after vaccination.

Table 3-16. Postexposure immunization for rabies[1]

IMMUNIZATION STATUS	VACCINE/ PRODUCT	DOSE	NUMBER OF DOSES	SCHEDULE (DAYS)	ROUTE
Not previously immunized	RIG plus	20 IU/kg body weight	1	0	Infiltrated at bite site (if possible); remainder intramuscular
	HDCV or PCEC	1.0 mL	4[2]	0, 3, 7, 14	Intramuscular
Previously immunized[3,4]	HDCV or PCEC	1.0 mL	2	0, 3	Intramuscular

Abbreviations: RIG, rabies immune globulin; HDCV, human diploid cell vaccine; PCEC, purified chick embryo cell.

[1] All postexposure prophylaxis should begin with immediate, thorough cleansing of all wounds with soap and water.
[2] Five vaccine doses for the immunosuppressed patient.
[3] Preexposure immunization with HDCV or PCEC, prior postexposure prophylaxis with HDCV or PCEC, or people previously immunized with any other type of rabies vaccine and a documented history of positive rabies virus neutralizing antibody response to the prior vaccination.
[4] RIG should not be administered.

0.5 mL if the wound is small or on a finger. If the wounds are extensive, the calculated dose of RIG must not be exceeded. If the calculated dose is inadequate to inject all the wounds, the RIG should be diluted with normal saline to extend the number of wounds that can be injected. This is a particular issue in children, whose body weight may be small in relation to the size and number of wounds.

The remainder of the RIG dose, if any, should be injected intramuscularly. Care should be taken to guarantee that this remaining amount of RIG is deposited in a muscle and not injected subcutaneously, which may decrease its effectiveness. The remaining RIG can be given in the deltoid muscle, on the opposite side of the initial vaccine dose. The anterior thigh is an alternative site.

RIG should not be given >7 days after the start of the postexposure vaccine series. This 7-day period does not relate to the time of the bite exposure itself. Postexposure prophylaxis, including RIG, should be initiated after a possible bite exposure even if there has been a considerable delay between the exposure and the traveler presenting for evaluation.

Human RIG is manufactured by plasmapheresis of blood from hyperimmunized volunteers. The manufactured quantity of human RIG falls short of worldwide requirements, and it is not available in many developing countries. Equine RIG or purified fractions of equine RIG have been used effectively in some developing countries where human RIG might not be available. If necessary, such heterologous products are preferable to no RIG.

The incidence of adverse reactions after the use of equine-derived RIG is low (0.8%–6.0%), and most reactions are minor. However, such products are not evaluated by US standards or regulated by the Food and Drug Administration, and their use cannot be unequivocally recommended. In addition, unpurified antirabies serum of equine origin might still be used in some countries where neither human nor equine RIG is available. The use of this antirabies serum is associated with higher rates of serious adverse reactions, including anaphylaxis.

Different postexposure vaccine schedules, alternative routes of administration, and other rabies vaccines besides HDCV and PCEC may be used abroad. Although not approved for sale in the United States, purified Vero cell rabies vaccine and purified chick embryo cell vaccine (manufactured abroad) are acceptable alternatives if available in a destination country. Assistance in managing complicated postexposure scenarios may be obtained from experienced travel medicine professionals, health departments, and CDC.

Rabies vaccine was once manufactured from viruses grown in animal brains, and some of these vaccines are still in use in developing countries. Typically, the brain-derived vaccines can be identified if the traveler is offered a large injection (5 mL) daily for 14–21 days. The traveler should not accept these vaccines, but rather travel to where acceptable vaccines and immune globulin are available.

Rabies Vaccine
Vaccine Safety and Adverse Reactions
Travelers should be advised that they may experience local reactions after vaccination, such as pain, erythema, swelling, or itching at the injection site, or mild systemic reactions, such as headache, nausea, abdominal pain, muscle aches, and dizziness. Approximately 6% of people receiving booster vaccinations with HDCV may experience an immune complex–like reaction characterized by urticaria, pruritus, and malaise. The likelihood of these reactions is less with PCEC. Once initiated, rabies postexposure prophylaxis should not be interrupted or discontinued because of local or mild systemic reactions to rabies vaccine.

Precautions and Contraindications
Pregnancy is not a contraindication to postexposure prophylaxis. In infants and children, the dose of HDCV or PCEC for preexposure or postexposure prophylaxis is the same as that recommended for adults. The dose of RIG for postexposure prophylaxis is based on body weight (Table 3-16).

BIBLIOGRAPHY

1. Gautret P, Adehossi E, Soula G, Soavi MJ, Delmont J, Rotivel Y, et al. Rabies exposure in international travelers: do we miss the target? Int J Infect Dis. 2010 Mar;14(3):e243–6.
2. Rupprecht CE, Briggs D, Brown CM, Franka R, Katz SL, Kerr HD, et al. Use of a reduced (4-dose) vaccine schedule for postexposure prophylaxis to prevent human rabies: recommendations of the advisory committee on immunization practices. MMWR Recomm Rep. 2010 Mar 19;59(RR-2):1–9.
3. Rupprecht CE, Gibbons RV. Clinical practice. Prophylaxis against rabies. N Engl J Med. 2004 Dec 16;351(25):2626–35.
4. Shaw MT, O'Brien B, Leggat PA. Rabies postexposure management of travelers presenting to travel health clinics in Auckland and Hamilton, New Zealand. J Travel Med. 2009 Jan–Feb;16(1):13–7.
5. Smith A, Petrovic M, Solomon T, Fooks A. Death from rabies in a UK traveller returning from India. Euro Surveill. 2005 Jul;10(7):E050728 5.
6. Strauss R, Granz A, Wassermann-Neuhold M, Krause R, Bago Z, Revilla-Fernandez S, et al. A human case of travel-related rabies in Austria, September 2004. Euro Surveill. 2005 Nov;10(11):225–6.
7. van Thiel PP, de Bie RM, Eftimov F, Tepaske R, Zaaijer HL, van Doornum GJ, et al. Fatal human rabies due to Duvenhage virus from a bat in Kenya: failure of treatment with coma-induction, ketamine, and antiviral drugs. PLoS Negl Trop Dis. 2009;3(7):e428.

8. Warrell MJ, Warrell DA. Rabies and other lyssavirus diseases. Lancet. 2004 Mar 20;363(9413):959–69.

9. Yamamoto S, Iwasaki C, Oono H, Ninomiya K, Matsumura T. The first imported case of rabies into Japan in 36 years: a forgotten life-threatening disease. J Travel Med. 2008 Sep–Oct;15(5):372–4.

10. WHO Expert Committee. WHO expert consultation on rabies. World Health Organ Tech Rep Ser. 2005;931:1–88.

RICKETTSIAL (SPOTTED & TYPHUS FEVERS) & RELATED INFECTIONS (ANAPLASMOSIS & EHRLICHIOSIS)

Marina E. Eremeeva, Gregory A. Dasch

INFECTIOUS AGENT

Rickettsial infections are caused by a variety of obligate intracellular, gram-negative bacteria from the genera *Rickettsia*, *Orientia*, *Ehrlichia*, *Neorickettsia*, and *Anaplasma* (Table 3-17). *Rickettsia* are further classified into the typhus group and spotted fever group (SFG), and *Orientia* makes up the classic scrub typhus group.

MODE OF TRANSMISSION

Most rickettsial pathogens are transmitted by ectoparasites such as fleas, lice, mites, and ticks during feeding or by scratching infectious feces into the skin. Inhaling dust contaminated with dried infected lice or flea feces may also cause infections. The specific vectors that transmit each form of rickettsiae are listed in Table 3-17. Transmission of infection after blood transfusion is rare but has been reported during the asymptomatic incubation period of some diseases.

EPIDEMIOLOGY

All age groups are at risk for rickettsial infections during travel to endemic areas. Transmission is increased during outdoor activities in the spring and summer months when ticks and fleas are most active. However, infection can occur throughout the year. Because of the 5- to 14-day incubation period for most rickettsial diseases, tourists may not necessarily experience symptoms during their trip, and onset may coincide with their return home or develop within a week after returning.

SFG rickettsial infections among travelers include Mediterranean (or Boutonneuse) spotted fever from southern Europe and Africa, Indian tick typhus from India, Astrakhan fever from southeastern Europe and central Africa, Israeli tick typhus from Mediterranean countries, Thai tick typhus from Asia and Australia, Queensland tick typhus and Australian spotted fever from eastern Australia, tickborne lymphadenopathy from European countries, north Asian tick typhus from China and Russia, Rocky Mountain spotted fever and *Rickettsia parkeri* from the Americas, and African tick-bite fever from Africa and the Caribbean islands. Game hunting and traveling to southern Africa from November through April are risk factors for African tick-bite fever in travelers. Contact with tick-infested dogs in areas endemic for certain SFG rickettsiae may increase the risk of disease. One study estimated that the risk of a traveler contracting a rickettsiosis in southern Africa is 4–5 times higher than that of acquiring malaria.

Rickettsialpox, transmitted by house-mouse mites, circulates in urban centers in Ukraine, South Africa, Korea, Balkan states, and the United States. Outbreaks of rickettsialpox most often occur after contact with infected rodents and their mites, especially during natural die-offs or extermination of infected rodents that causes the mites to seek

Table 3-17. Classification, primary vector, and reservoir occurrence of rickettsiae known to cause disease in humans

ANTIGENIC GROUP	DISEASE	SPECIES	VECTOR	ANIMAL RESERVOIR(S)	GEOGRAPHIC DISTRIBUTION
Anaplasma	Human granulocytic anaplasmosis	*Anaplasma phagocytophilum*	Tick	Deer, elk, small mammals, and rodents	Worldwide
Ehrlichia	Human monocytic ehrlichiosis	*Ehrlichia chaffeensis*	Tick	Deer, wild and domestic dogs, domestic ruminants, and rodents	Worldwide
	Ehrlichiosis	*E. muris*	Tick	Deer and rodents	Western United States, Russia, Japan
	Ehrlichiosis	*E. ewingii*	Tick	Deer, wild and domestic dogs, and rodents	North America
Neorickettsia	Sennetsu fever	*Neorickettsia sennetsu*	Trematode	Fish	Japan, Malaysia, possibly other parts of Asia
Scrub typhus	Scrub typhus	*Orientia tsutsugamushi*	Larval mite (chigger)	Rodents	Asia–Pacific region from maritime Russia and China to Indonesia and North Australia to Afghanistan
Spotted fever	Rickettsiosis	*Rickettsia aeschlimannii*	Tick	Unknown	South Africa, Morocco, Mediterranean littoral
	African tick-bite fever	*R. africae*	Tick	Ruminants	Sub-Saharan Africa, West Indies

continued

3

TABLE 3-17. CLASSIFICATION, PRIMARY VECTOR, AND RESERVOIR OCCURRENCE OF RICKETTSIAE KNOWN TO CAUSE DISEASE IN HUMANS (continued)

ANTIGENIC GROUP	DISEASE	SPECIES	VECTOR	ANIMAL RESERVOIR(S)	GEOGRAPHIC DISTRIBUTION
	Rickettsialpox	R. akari	Mite	House mice, wild rodents	Countries of the former Soviet Union, South Africa, Korea, Turkey, Balkan countries, North and South America
	Queensland tick typhus	R. australis	Tick	Rodents	Australia, Tasmania
	Mediterranean spotted fever or Boutonneuse fever	R. conorii[1]	Tick	Dogs, rodents	Southern Europe, southern and western Asia, Africa, India
	Cat flea rickettsiosis	R. felis	Flea	Domestic cats, rodents, opossums	Europe, North and South America, Africa, Asia
	Far Eastern spotted fever	R. heilongjiangensis	Tick	Rodents	Far East of Russia, Northern China, eastern Asia
	Aneruptive fever	R. helvetica	Tick	Rodents	Central and northern Europe, Asia
	Flinders Island spotted fever; Thai tick typhus	R. honei	Tick	Unknown	Australia, Thailand
	Japanese spotted fever	R. japonica	Tick	Rodents	Japan
	Australian spotted fever	R. marmionii	Tick	Rodents, reptiles	Australia

Disease	Species	Vector	Reservoir	Distribution
Mediterranean spotted fever-like disease	*R. massiliae*	Tick	Unknown	France, Greece, Spain, Portugal, Switzerland, Sicily, central Africa, and Mali
Maculatum infection	*R. parkeri*	Tick	Rodents	North and South America
Rocky Mountain spotted fever, febre maculosa, São Paulo exanthematic typhus, Minas Gerais exanthematic typhus, Brazilian spotted fever	*R. rickettsii*	Tick	Rodents	North, Central, and South America
North Asian tick typhus, Siberian tick typhus	*R. sibirica*	Tick	Rodents	Russia, China, Mongolia
Lymphangitis-associated rickettsiosis	*R. sibirica mongolotimonae*	Tick	Rodents	Southern France, Portugal, China, sub-Saharan Africa
Tickborne lymphadenopathy (TIBOLA), *Dermacentor*-borne necrosis and lymphadenopathy (DEBONEL)	*R. slovaca*	Tick	Lagomorphs, rodents	Southern and eastern Europe, Asia
Typhus fever Epidemic typhus, sylvatic typhus	*R. prowazekii*	Human body louse, flying squirrel ectoparasites, *Amblyomma* ticks	Humans, flying squirrels	Central Africa, Asia, Central, North, and South America
Murine typhus	*R. typhi*	Flea	Rodents	Tropical and subtropical areas worldwide

[1] Includes 4 different subspecies that can be distinguished serologically and by PCR assay and respectively are the etiologic agents of Boutonneuse fever and Mediterranean tick fever in southern Europe and Africa (*R. conorii* subsp. *conorii*), Indian tick typhus in south Asia (*R. conorii* subsp. *indica*), Israeli tick typhus in southern Europe and Middle East (*R. conorii* subsp. *israelensis*), and Astrakhan spotted fever in the North Caspian region of Russia (*R. conorii* subsp. *caspiae*).

out new hosts, including humans. The agent may spill over and occasionally be found in other wild rodent populations.

Scrub typhus is endemic in northern Japan, Southeast Asia, the western Pacific Islands, eastern Australia, China, maritime areas and several parts of south-central Russia, India, and Sri Lanka. More than 1 million cases occur annually. Unusual travel-associated cases of scrub typhus have been diagnosed in people returning from Ghana to Japan and from Dubai to Australia. Most travel-acquired cases of scrub typhus occur during visits to rural areas in endemic countries for activities such as camping, hiking, or rafting, but urban cases have also been described.

Fleaborne rickettsioses caused by R. typhi and R. felis are widely distributed, especially throughout the tropics and subtropics and in port cities and coastal regions with rodents. Humans exposed to flea-infested cats, dogs, and peridomestic animals while traveling in endemic regions or entering areas infested with rats are at most risk for flea-borne rickettsioses. Murine typhus has been reported among travelers returning from Asia, Africa, and southern Europe and has also been reported from Hawaii, California, and Texas in the United States.

Epidemic typhus occurs in communities and refugee populations where body lice are prevalent. Outbreaks often occur during the colder months when infested clothing is not laundered. Travelers at most risk for epidemic typhus include those who may work with or visit areas with large homeless populations, impoverished areas, refugee camps, and regions that have recently experienced war or natural disasters. Sylvatic epidemic typhus cases occur only from direct contact with flying squirrels or their nesting materials. Active foci of endemic typhus are known in the Andes regions of South America and in Burundi and Ethiopia. Sylvatic epidemic typhus is also endemic among flying squirrels in the eastern United States. Sylvatic typhus cases occur only from direct contact with flying squirrel ectoparasites or their nest materials. Tick-associated reservoirs of R. prowazekii have been described in Ethiopia, Mexico, and Brazil.

Ehrlichiosis is most commonly reported in the southeastern and south-central United States where the lonestar tick, Amblyomma americanum, and white-tailed deer are commonplace. In Europe and Asia, transmission of monocytic ehrlichiosis may be due to Ehrlichia chaffeensis or related organisms such as E. muris that are associated with ticks of the Ixodes persulcatus complex, found on small rodents and passerine birds. Recent publications indicate that E. chaffeensis or similar agents also circulate in Brazil, Panama, and Africa, and E. muris circulates in the United States.

Anaplasmosis occurs worldwide, corresponding with the ranges of I. persulcatus–group ticks. Known endemic regions include the United States, Europe, China, Russia, and Korea.

Sennetsu fever occurs in Japan, Malaysia, and possibly other parts of Asia. Sennetsu fever can be contracted from eating raw infected fish.

CLINICAL PRESENTATION

Although the clinical presentations vary with the causative agent, some common symptoms that typically develop within 1–2 weeks of infection include fever, headache, malaise, and sometimes nausea and vomiting. Most symptoms associated with acute rickettsial infections are nonspecific and require further tests to make an accurate diagnosis. Most tick-transmitted rickettsioses are accompanied by a maculopapular, vesicular, or petechial rash or an eschar at the site of the tick bite. While many rickettsial diseases cause mild or moderate illness, epidemic typhus and Rocky Mountain spotted fever can be severe and may be fatal in 20%–60% of untreated cases.

DIAGNOSIS

If clinical symptoms and the epidemiologic history are compatible with rickettsial infections, the following diagnostic tests should be used during the acute stage of illness and at the time antibiotic treatment is initiated:

- PCR test on skin biopsy of rash or eschar or EDTA whole blood
- Specific immunohistologic detection of rickettsiae in skin biopsy of rash or eschar
The diagnosis can be confirmed at a later time by testing acute- and convalescent-phase serum from the patient or by isolation of a

rickettsial agent by culture from samples collected at initial suspicion of disease. In patients suspected of having rickettsial disease, an acute-phase serum should be drawn and held in case serology is warranted at a later time. Most serum specimens collected during the acute stage of rickettsial diseases do not contain significant titers of antirickettsial antibodies, although immune responses to scrub typhus rickettsiae can be rapid. Detection of IgM class antibody alone should not be interpreted as recent exposure to the rickettsial agents and should be confirmed by detection of IgG or, preferably, IgG seroconversion by parallel evaluation with a convalescent-phase serum collected 4–6 weeks after onset of the illness. Contact the CDC Rickettsial Zoonoses Branch at 404-639-1075 for further information about testing and patient management.

TREATMENT

Diagnosing a rickettsial infection can be difficult, but early treatment with appropriate antibiotic therapy is critical for rapid recovery. Treatment must be based on clinical suspicion and not be delayed pending results of laboratory tests. The standard treatment regimen consists of 200 mg of doxycycline daily for 3–14 days or 2.2 mg/kg body weight per dose administered twice a day (orally or intravenously) for children weighing <45.4 kg (100 lb). However, the specific type and duration of antibiotic administered may vary, depending on the disease and kinetics of defervescence.

Antibiotics of the tetracycline class (doxycycline in particular) have a high degree of efficacy and low toxicity in treating rickettsial infections, even in children and pregnant women. Depending on the specific pathogen, chloramphenicol, azithromycin, fluoroquinolones, and rifampin may also be considered, but these are not universally effective for all rickettsial agents, nor have they been evaluated by controlled clinical trials.

PREVENTIVE MEASURES FOR TRAVELERS

No vaccines or drugs are available for preventing rickettsial infections. Antibiotics are not recommended for prophylaxis of rickettsial diseases and should not be prescribed to asymptomatic people exposed to ticks.

The best prevention is to minimize exposure to infectious arthropods (particularly lice, fleas, ticks, mites) and animal reservoirs, particularly dogs and cats, when traveling in endemic areas. The proper use of insect repellents, self-examination after visits to vector-infested areas, and wearing protective clothing are ways to reduce risk. These precautions are especially important for people with underlying conditions that may compromise their immune systems, as these people may be more susceptible to severe disease. For more detailed information, see Chapter 2, Protection against Mosquitoes, Ticks, and Other Insects and Arthropods.

BIBLIOGRAPHY

1. Dumler JS, Madigan JE, Pusterla N, Bakken JS. Ehrlichioses in humans: epidemiology, clinical presentation, diagnosis, and treatment. Clin Infect Dis. 2007 Jul 15;45 Suppl 1:S45–51.

2. Jensenius M, Davis X, von Sonnenburg F, Schwartz E, Keystone JS, Leder K, et al. Multicenter GeoSentinel analysis of rickettsial diseases in international travelers, 1996–2008. Emerg Infect Dis. 2009 Nov;15(11):1791–8.

3. Jensenius M, Fournier PE, Raoult D. Rickettsioses and the international traveler. Clin Infect Dis. 2004 Nov 15;39(10):1493–9.

4. Jensenius M, Fournier PE, Raoult D. Tick-borne rickettsioses in international travellers. Int J Infect Dis. 2004 May;8(3):139–46.

5. Nachega JB, Bottieau E, Zech F, Van Gompel A. Travel-acquired scrub typhus: emphasis on the differential diagnosis, treatment, and prevention strategies. J Travel Med. 2007 Sep–Oct;14(5):352–5.

6. Paddock CD, Eremeeva ME. Rickettsialpox. In: Raoult D, Parola P, editors. Rickettsial Diseases. New York: Informa Healthcare USA, Inc; 2007. p. 63–86.

7. Parola P, Paddock CD, Raoult D. Tick-borne rickettsioses around the world: emerging diseases challenging old concepts. Clin Microbiol Rev. 2005 Oct;18(4):719–56.

8. Raoult D, Parola P, editors. Rickettsial Diseases. New York: Informa Healthcare USA, Inc; 2007.

9. Roch N, Epaulard O, Pelloux I, Pavese P, Brion JP, Raoult D, et al. African tick bite fever in elderly patients: 8 cases in French tourists returning from South Africa. Clin Infect Dis. 2008 Aug 1;47(3):e28–35.

10. Walker DH. Rickettsial diseases in travelers. Travel Med Infect Dis. 2003 Feb;1(1):35–40.

RUBELLA

Huong Q. McLean, Susan E. Reef

INFECTIOUS AGENT

Rubella virus is a member of the *Togaviridae* family and the only member of the genus *Rubivirus*. Humans are the only known natural host for the rubella virus.

MODE OF TRANSMISSION

Rubella virus is transmitted through person-to-person contact or droplets shed from the respiratory secretions of infected people. If a woman is infected with rubella virus during pregnancy, the virus can cross the placenta and infect the fetus.

EPIDEMIOLOGY

Rubella used to occur worldwide. However, in September 2010, the Pan American Health Organization announced that the region of the Americas had achieved the rubella elimination goals, based on surveillance data; documentation of elimination is in progress. In the United States, endemic rubella virus transmission has been eliminated. However, from 2005 through 2009, an average of 11 cases (range, 4–16) were reported each year, of which approximately 30% were imported or linked to an imported case. Of the imported cases, 32% occurred in US residents returning from foreign countries. All susceptible people are at risk for infection during travel outside the United States. Because asymptomatic rubella virus infections are common, travelers may be unaware that they have been in contact with an infected person.

CLINICAL PRESENTATION

The average incubation period is 14 days, with a range of 12–23 days. Rubella usually presents as a nonspecific, maculopapular, generalized rash that lasts ≤3 days (hence the term "3-day measles") with generalized lymphadenopathy, particularly of the posterior auricular, suboccipital and posterior cervical lymph nodes. Asymptomatic rubella virus infections are common; 20%–50% of infections occur without rash or are asymptomatic. In adults and adolescents, the rash may be preceded by a 1- to 5-day prodrome of low-grade fever, malaise, anorexia, mild conjunctivitis, runny nose, sore throat, and lymphadenopathy. When rubella virus infection occurs during early pregnancy, consequences may include miscarriage, fetal death, or an infant born with the constellation of severe birth defects known as congenital rubella syndrome. The most common congenital defects are cataracts, heart defects, and hearing impairment.

DIAGNOSIS

A clinical case of rubella is characterized by the following characteristics:

- Acute onset of generalized maculopapular rash
- Temperature >99°F (37.2°C)
- Arthralgia or arthritis, lymphadenopathy, or conjunctivitis

Many illnesses can mimic rubella, and rubella virus infections can occur without a rash or be asymptomatic. Therefore, the only reliable evidence of acute rubella virus infection is laboratory diagnosis. Serologic testing for rubella-specific IgM is most commonly used to diagnose rubella. Diagnosis can also be made by demonstrating seroconversion of rubella-specific IgG titers and by detecting virus either through virus culture or PCR. A confirmed case of rubella is either laboratory confirmed or meets the clinical case definition and is epidemiologically linked to a laboratory-confirmed case.

TREATMENT

There is no specific antiviral therapy for rubella; basic treatment consists of supportive care.

PREVENTIVE MEASURES FOR TRAVELERS

Vaccine

Before international travel, travelers should be immune to rubella. This is the most important prevention message, because many imported cases result from US residents returning from countries where rubella vaccination is not widespread. Acceptable presumptive evidence of immunity to rubella for international travelers includes the following:

- Documentation of receipt of ≥1 dose of rubella-containing vaccine on or after the first birthday
- Laboratory evidence of rubella immunity (a positive serologic test for rubella-specific IgG)
- Born before 1957 (except women of childbearing age who could become pregnant)

Travelers who do not meet the above criteria for rubella immunity should be vaccinated before departure.

Vaccine Safety, Adverse Reactions, Precautions, and Contraindications to Rubella Vaccine

Refer to the Measles (Rubeola) section earlier in this chapter for information on reactions after MMR vaccine and additional precautions and contraindications.

BIBLIOGRAPHY

1. CDC. Measles, mumps, and rubella—vaccine use and strategies for elimination of measles, rubella, and congenital rubella syndrome and control of mumps: recommendations of the Advisory Committee on Immunization Practices (ACIP). MMWR Recomm Rep. 1998;47(RR-8):1–57.
2. CDC. Progress toward control of rubella and prevention of congenital rubella syndrome—worldwide, 2009. MMWR Morb Mortal Wkly Rep. 2010 Oct 15;59(40):1307–10.
3. CDC. Rubella. In: Atkinson W, Hamborsky J, McIntyre L, Wolfe S, editors. Epidemiology and Prevention of Vaccine-Preventable Diseases. 11th ed. Washington, DC: Public Health Foundation; 2009. p. 257–71.
4. Kroger AT, Atkinson WL, Marcuse EK, Pickering LK. General recommendations on immunization: recommendations of the Advisory Committee on Immunization Practices (ACIP). MMWR Recomm Rep. 2006 Dec 1;55(RR-15):1–48.
5. Meissner HC, Reef SE, Cochi S. Elimination of rubella from the United States: a milestone on the road to global elimination. Pediatrics. 2006 Mar;117(3):933–5.
6. Plotinsky RN, Talbot EA, Kellenberg JE, Reef SE, Buseman SK, Wright KD, et al. Congenital rubella syndrome in a child born to Liberian refugees: clinical and public health perspectives. Clin Pediatr (Phila). 2007 May;46(4):349–55.
7. Plotkin SA, Reef SE. Rubella vaccine. In: Plotkin SA, Orenstein WA, Offit PA, editors. Vaccines. 5th ed. Philadelphia: Saunders Elsevier; 2008. p. 735–71.
8. Reef S, Redd SB, Abernathy E, Kutty PK, Icenogle J. Evidence used to support the achievement and maintenance of elimination of rubella and congenital rubella syndrome in the United States. J Infect Dis. 2011. In Press.
9. Reef SE, Cochi SL. The evidence for the elimination of rubella and congenital rubella syndrome in the United States: a public health achievement. Clin Infect Dis. 2006 Nov 1;43 Suppl 3:S123–5.
10. Reef SE, Redd SB, Abernathy E, Zimmerman L, Icenogle JP. The epidemiological profile of rubella and congenital rubella syndrome in the United States, 1998–2004: the evidence for absence of endemic transmission. Clin Infect Dis. 2006 Nov 1;43 Suppl 3:S126–32.
11. Strebel P, Gacic-Dobo M, Reef S, Cochi S. Global use of rubella vaccines, 1980–2009. J Infect Dis. 2011. In Press.

SCABIES (SARCOPTIC ITCH, SARCOPTIC ACARIASIS)

Els Mathieu

INFECTIOUS AGENT

Scabies is caused by the microscopic human itch mite (*Sarcoptes scabiei* var. *hominis*).

MODE OF TRANSMISSION

Transmission occurs directly via prolonged skin-to-skin contact with a person with conventional scabies or via brief skin-to-skin contact with a person with crusted (Norwegian) scabies. Indirect transmission occurs via contact with objects (such as bedding, clothing, or furniture) contaminated by a person with crusted (Norwegian) scabies, but rarely via contact with fomites used by a person with conventional scabies. Human scabies is not spread by pets or other animals.

EPIDEMIOLOGY

Scabies occurs worldwide; it is epidemic in much of the developing world and common in the tropics. Outbreaks are reported most commonly in nursing-care facilities, prisons, and schools. Infection occurs in all races and social classes, and all ages are at risk. Household members and sexual partners of infested people are at high risk.

Exposure to crusted (Norwegian) scabies is more likely in institutions that care for elderly, immunocompromised, or mentally or physically disabled people. Crowded living conditions and settings where close body and skin contact are common (such as refugee settings, schools, and childcare facilities) increase the risk of scabies, as does close day-to-day contact with local populations in areas where the prevalence is high.

CLINICAL PRESENTATION

Symptom onset occurs 2–8 weeks after first exposure and 1–4 days after subsequent exposures. A patient is contagious from the time of exposure, even while asymptomatic, until successfully treated and all mites and eggs are killed. Head, neck, palms, and soles are usually not affected in older children and adults in temperate climates.

Conventional scabies is characterized by intense pruritus, particularly at night, and papular or papulovesicular, pruritic (itchy), erythematous rash; common sites are wrists, elbows, axillae, groin/genitals, breasts/nipples, beltline, buttocks, between fingers/shoulder blades; itching can be generalized; papules are often excoriated; secondary bacterial infection can occur. Tiny, raised, grayish or skin-colored, serpiginous lines on skin surface represent mite burrows; they are most commonly seen on the wrist, penis, and between fingers. Burrows are often few and difficult to find. Crusted (Norwegian) scabies is characterized by often mild or absent pruritus and exfoliating hyperkeratotic scales or crusts that contain large numbers of mites.

DIAGNOSIS

Scabies is generally diagnosed by identifying burrows in a patient with pruritus and characteristic rash. Diagnosis can be confirmed by microscopically identifying mites, mite eggs, or scybala (mite feces) in skin scrapings of fresh lesions (intact papules/burrows). Placing a drop of mineral oil on the skin can facilitate scraping and subsequent microscopic examination. Excoriated lesions rarely contain mites.

TREATMENT

Permethrin (5%) cream is considered by many to be the drug of choice; it is not Food and Drug Administration (FDA)-approved for use in children aged <2 months. Ivermectin, an oral antiparasitic agent, is reported safe and effective to treat scabies, including crusted (Norwegian) scabies. Two or more doses may be necessary to eliminate infestation. It is not FDA-approved but should be considered for patients in whom treatment has failed or who cannot tolerate other approved medications.

Crotamiton (10%) lotion or cream is associated with frequent treatment failure and is not FDA-approved for use in children. Lindane (1%) lotion is not recommended as first-line therapy because of neurotoxicity. Its use is restricted to patients in whom treatment has failed or who cannot tolerate other medications that pose less risk. It should not be used to treat premature infants, people with a seizure disorder, women who are pregnant or breastfeeding, people who have very irritated skin or sores where lindane will be applied, infants, children, the elderly, and people who weigh <110 pounds (50 kg). Other medications that are used in some areas include topical precipitated sulfur in petrolatum and benzyl benzoate solution or emulsion.

All household members and intimate contacts should be treated at the same time. To prevent reinfestation, exposed clothing and bed linen should be washed in hot water (≥122°F [50°C]) or be dry-cleaned at the same time as treatment.

PREVENTIVE MEASURES FOR TRAVELERS

No vaccine is available. Preventive measures are aimed at reducing skin-to-skin contact with affected people and with items such as clothing and bed linen used by an affected person.

BIBLIOGRAPHY

1. American Academy of Pediatrics. Scabies. In: Pickering LK, Baker CJ, Long SS, McMillan JA, editors. Red Book: 2006 Report of the Committee on Infectious Diseases. 27th ed. Elk Grove Village, IL: American Academy of Pediatrics; 2006. p. 584–7.
2. Ansart S, Perez L, Jaureguiberry S, Danis M, Bricaire F, Caumes E. Spectrum of dermatoses in 165 travelers returning from the tropics with skin diseases. Am J Trop Med Hyg. 2007 Jan;76(1):184–6.
3. Chosidow O. Clinical practices. Scabies. N Engl J Med. 2006 Apr 20;354(16):1718–27.
4. Hengge UR, Currie BJ, Jager G, Lupi O, Schwartz RA. Scabies: a ubiquitous neglected skin disease. Lancet Infect Dis. 2006 Dec;6(12):769–79.
5. Heukelbach J, Feldmeier H. Scabies. Lancet. 2006 May 27;367(9524):1767–74.
6. Meinking TL. Infestations. Curr Probl Dermatol. 1999;11(3):73–118.
7. Strong M, Johnstone PW. Interventions for treating scabies. Cochrane Database Syst Rev. 2007(3):CD000320.
8. Strother MS, Colven R. Ectoparasites, cutaneous parasites, and cnidarian envenomation. In: Jong EC, McMullen WR, editors. The Travel and Tropical Medicine Manual. 3rd ed. Philadelphia: Saunders; 2003. p. 459–70.
9. Wilson ME, Chen LH. Dermatologic infectious diseases in international travelers. Curr Infect Dis Rep. 2004 Feb;6(1):54–62.

SCHISTOSOMIASIS
Susan Montgomery

INFECTIOUS AGENT

Schistosomiasis is caused by helminth parasites of the genus *Schistosoma*. Other helminth infections are discussed in the Helminths, Intestinal section earlier in this chapter.

MODE OF TRANSMISSION

Waterborne transmission occurs via penetration of larval cercariae in contaminated bodies of freshwater.

EPIDEMIOLOGY

An estimated 85% of the world's cases of schistosomiasis are in Africa, where prevalence rates can exceed 50% in local populations. *Schistosoma mansoni* and *S. haematobium* are distributed throughout Africa; only *S. haematobium* is found in areas of the Middle East, and *S. japonicum* is found in Indonesia and parts of China and Southeast Asia (Map 3-14). Two other species can infect humans: *S. mekongi*, found in Cambodia and Laos, and *S. intercalatum*, found in parts of Central and West Africa. These 2 species are rarely reported causes of infection.

All ages are at risk for infection with travel to endemic areas and freshwater exposure. Swimming, bathing, and wading in contaminated freshwater can result in infection. Human schistosomiasis cannot be acquired by contact with saltwater (oceans or seas). The distribution of schistosomiasis is very focal and determined by the presence of competent snail vectors, inadequate sanitation, and infected humans. The geographic distribution of cases of schistosomiasis acquired by travelers reflects travel and immigration patterns. Most travel-associated cases of schistosomiasis are acquired in sub-Saharan Africa. Sites in Africa frequently visited by travelers are commonly reported sites of infection. These sites include rivers and water sources in the Banfora region (Burkina Faso) and areas populated by the Dogon people (Mali); Lake Malawi; Lake Tanganyika; Lake Victoria; the Omo River (Ethiopia); the Zambezi River; and the Nile River. However, as visitors travel to more uncommon sites, it is important to remember that most freshwater surface water sources in Africa are potentially contaminated and can be sources of infection.

The specific snail vectors can be difficult to identify, and snail infection with human schistosome species must be determined in the laboratory. The types of travelers and expatriates potentially at increased risk for

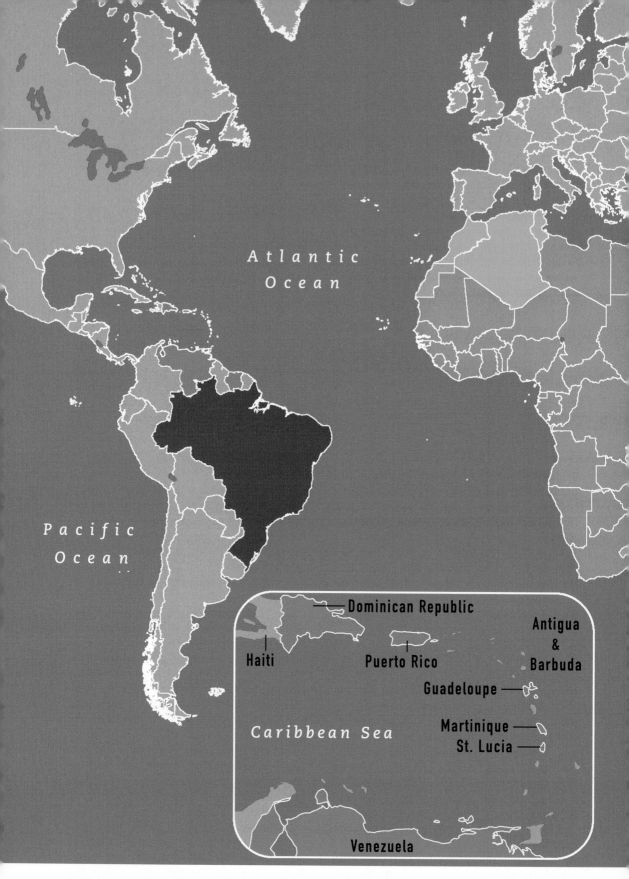

MAP 3-14. GEOGRAPHIC DISTRIBUTION OF SCHISTOSOMIASIS

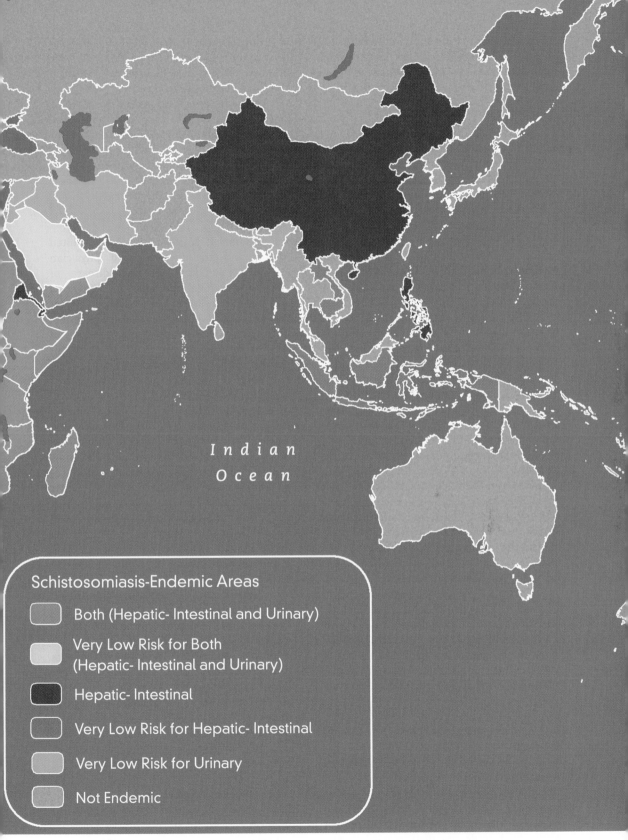

Schistosomiasis-Endemic Areas

Both (Hepatic- Intestinal and Urinary)

Very Low Risk for Both
(Hepatic- Intestinal and Urinary)

Hepatic- Intestinal

Very Low Risk for Hepatic- Intestinal

Very Low Risk for Urinary

Not Endemic

Indian Ocean

infection include adventure travelers, Peace Corps volunteers, missionaries, soldiers, and ecotourists. Outbreaks of schistosomiasis have occurred among adventure travelers on river trips in Africa.

CLINICAL PRESENTATION

Incubation period is typically 14–84 days for acute schistosomiasis (Katayama syndrome), but chronic infection can remain asymptomatic for years. Penetration of cercariae can be associated with a rash that develops within hours or up to a week after contaminated water exposures. Acute schistosomiasis is characterized by fever, headache, myalgia, diarrhea, and respiratory symptoms. Eosinophilia is present, as well as often painful hepatomegaly or splenomegaly.

The clinical manifestations of chronic schistosomiasis are the result of host immune responses to schistosome eggs. Eggs secreted by adult worm pairs enter the circulation and lodge in organs and cause granulomatous reactions. Eosinophilia may be present. S. mansoni and S. japonicum eggs most commonly lodge in the blood vessels of the liver or intestine and can cause diarrhea, constipation, and blood in the stool. Chronic inflammation can lead to bowel wall ulceration, hyperplasia, and polyposis and, with heavy infections, to periportal liver fibrosis. S. haematobium eggs typically lodge in the urinary tract and can cause dysuria and hematuria. Calcifications in the bladder may appear late in the disease. S. haematobium infection has been associated with increased risk of bladder cancer.

Rarely, central nervous system schistosomiasis may develop; this form is thought to result from aberrant migration of adult worms or eggs depositing in the spinal cord or brain. Signs and symptoms are related to the site of the granulomas in the central nervous system and can present as transverse myelitis.

DIAGNOSIS

Diagnosis is made by microscopic identification of parasite eggs in stool (S. mansoni or S. japonicum) or urine (S. haematobium). Serologic tests are useful to diagnose light infections where egg shedding may not be consistent and in travelers and others who have not had schistosomiasis previously. Antibody tests do not distinguish between past and current infection. Available test sensitivity and specificity vary, depending on the antigen preparation used and how the test is performed.

It is important to consider screening asymptomatic people who may have been exposed during travel. These people may benefit from treatment. Additional information and assistance with diagnosis may be obtained through CDC's Division of Parasitic Diseases and Malaria (www.dpd.cdc.gov/dpdx).

TREATMENT

Schistosomiasis is uncommon in the United States, and the inexperienced physician should consult an infectious disease or tropical medicine specialist for diagnosis and treatment. Praziquantel is used to treat schistosomiasis. Praziquantel is most effective against adult forms of the parasite and requires an immune response to the adult worm to be fully effective.

PREVENTIVE MEASURES FOR TRAVELERS

No vaccine is available. No drugs for preventing infection are available. Preventive measures are primarily avoiding wading, swimming, or other contact with freshwater in disease-endemic countries. Untreated piped water coming directly from freshwater sources may contain cercariae, but filtering with fine-mesh filters, heating bathing water to 50°C (122°F) for 5 minutes, or allowing water to stand for ≥24 hours before exposure can eliminate risk for infection.

Swimming in adequately chlorinated swimming pools is virtually always safe, even in disease-endemic countries. Vigorous towel-drying after accidental exposure to water has been suggested as a way to remove cercariae before they can penetrate, but this may only prevent some infections and should not be recommended as a preventive measure. Topical applications of the insect repellent DEET can block penetrating cercariae, but the effect depends on the repellent formulation, may be short-lived and cannot reliably prevent infection. Repellents with active ingredients other than DEET have not been evaluated, so there is no evidence of their effectiveness of preventing cercarial penetration.

BIBLIOGRAPHY

1. Bierman WF, Wetsteyn JC, van Gool T. Presentation and diagnosis of imported schistosomiasis: relevance of eosinophilia, microscopy for ova, and serology. J Travel Med. 2005 Jan–Feb;12(1): 9–13.
2. Corachan M. Schistosomiasis and international travel. Clin Infect Dis. 2002 Aug 15;35(4):446–50.
3. Doenhoff MJ, Cioli D, Utzinger J. Praziquantel: mechanisms of action, resistance and new derivatives for schistosomiasis. Curr Opin Infect Dis. 2008 Dec;21(6):659–67.
4. Grobusch MP, Muhlberger N, Jelinek T, Bisoffi Z, Corachan M, Harms G, et al. Imported schistosomiasis in Europe: sentinel surveillance data from TropNetEurop. J Travel Med. 2003 May–Jun;10(3): 164–9.
5. King CH, Sturrock RF, Kariuki HC, Hamburger J. Transmission control for schistosomiasis—why it matters now. Trends Parasitol. 2006 Dec;22(12): 575–82.
6. Meltzer E, Artom G, Marva E, Assous MV, Rahav G, Schwartzt E. Schistosomiasis among travelers: new aspects of an old disease. Emerg Infect Dis. 2006 Nov;12(11):1696–700.
7. Morgan OW, Brunette G, Kapella BK, McAuliffe I, Katongole-Mbidde E, Li W, et al. Schistosomiasis among recreational users of Upper Nile River, Uganda, 2007. Emerg Infect Dis. 2010 May;16(5): 866–8.
8. Nicolls DJ, Weld LH, Schwartz E, Reed C, von Sonnenburg F, Freedman DO, et al. Characteristics of schistosomiasis in travelers reported to the GeoSentinel Surveillance Network 1997–2008. Am J Trop Med Hyg. 2008 Nov;79(5):729–34.
9. Ross AG, Bartley PB, Sleigh AC, Olds GR, Li Y, Williams GM, et al. Schistosomiasis. N Engl J Med. 2002 Apr 18;346(16):1212–20.
10. Ross AG, Vickers D, Olds GR, Shah SM, McManus DP. Katayama syndrome. Lancet Infect Dis. 2007 Mar;7(3):218–24.
11. WHO Expert Committee. Prevention and control of schistosomiasis and soil-transmitted helminthiasis. World Health Organ Tech Rep Ser. 2002;912:1–57.

SEXUALLY TRANSMITTED DISEASES
Kimberly Workowski

INFECTIOUS AGENT

Sexually transmitted diseases (STDs) are the infections and resulting clinical syndromes caused by more than 25 infectious organisms.

MODE OF TRANSMISSION

Sexual activity is the predominant mode of transmission, through genital, anal, or oral mucosal contact.

EPIDEMIOLOGY

STDs are among the most common infections. Annually, an estimated 448 million infections occur worldwide, and 19 million infections occur in the United States. Some STDs can be more prevalent in developing countries (chancroid, lymphogranuloma venereum, granuloma inguinale) and may be more likely to be imported into developed countries by travelers returning from such locales. International travelers are at risk for contracting STDs, including HIV, if they have sexual contact with partners in locales where the prevalence of STDs is high.

Increased sexual promiscuity and casual sexual relationships tend to occur during travel to foreign countries and are frequently detected in long-term overseas travelers. Commercial sex in various destinations, such as Southeast Asia, attracts many foreign travelers. Travelers who have sex with commercial sex workers in endemic areas may have high rates of STDs, such as gonorrhea.

Knowledge of the clinical presentation, frequency of infection, and antimicrobial resistance patterns is needed to manage STDs that occur in travelers to specific destinations. Assessing risk for men who have sex with men is important because of the recent increased rates of infectious syphilis, quinolone-resistant gonorrhea, and lymphogranuloma venereum in various geographic locations.

CLINICAL PRESENTATION

Many infections may be asymptomatic (chlamydia, gonorrhea), so screening for such infections at anatomic sites of contact and serologic testing for syphilis should be encouraged among travelers who might have been exposed to an STD. Any traveler who might have been exposed and who develops vaginal, urethral, or rectal discharge, an unexplained rash or genital lesion, or genital or pelvic pain should be advised to cease sexual activity and promptly seek medical evaluation.

DIAGNOSIS

Genital ulcer evaluation should include a serologic test for syphilis, a culture or antigen test for genital herpes, and a culture for chancroid (if exposure occurred in areas where chancroid can occur, such as Africa, Asia, and Latin America). Lymphadenopathy can accompany genital ulceration with these infections, as well as with lymphogranuloma venereum and donovanosis. Lymphogranuloma venereum should be suspected in a traveler with tender unilateral inguinal or femoral lymphadenopathy or proctocolitis. Genital and lymph node specimens should be tested for *Chlamydia trachomatis* by culture, direct immunofluorescence, or nucleic acid testing. Donovanosis is endemic in some areas, including India, Papua New Guinea, central Australia, and southern Africa, and is diagnosed with a crush tissue preparation from the lesion.

Chlamydia and gonorrhea testing at the anatomic site of exposure with nucleic acid amplification testing or culture is available to detect *C. trachomatis* and *Neisseria gonorrhoeae*. Culture and antibiotic susceptibility testing should be done when gonorrhea is suspected, because of geographic differences in antimicrobial susceptibility. Various diagnostic methods are available to identify the origin of an abnormal vaginal discharge, including microscopic evaluation and pH testing of vaginal secretions, DNA probe-based testing, and culture. Anyone who seeks evaluation and treatment for STDs should be screened for HIV infection.

TREATMENT

Etiologic treatment directed toward the specific pathogen is the historical norm for most STDs in industrialized countries. Syndromic management, of interest in developing countries, requires broad clinical manifestations with risk assessment, followed by treatment of the main causes of the syndrome without identification of a specific pathogen. Evaluation and management of STDs should be based on standard guidelines (CDC and the World Health Organization), and the frequency of antimicrobial resistance in different geographic areas should be considered. Early detection and treatment are important. STDs can often result in serious and long-term complications, including pelvic inflammatory disease, infertility, stillbirths and neonatal infections, genital cancers, and an increased risk for HIV acquisition and transmission.

PREVENTIVE MEASURES FOR TRAVELERS

The prevention and control of STDs are based on education and counseling. Specific messages to avoid acquiring or transmitting STDs should be part of the health advice given to travelers. Abstinence or mutual monogamy is the most reliable way to avoid acquiring and transmitting STDs.

For people whose sexual behaviors place them at risk for STDs, correct and consistent use of the male latex condom can reduce the risk of HIV infection and some STDs, including chlamydia, gonorrhea, and trichomoniasis, and by limiting lower genital tract infections might reduce the risk of pelvic inflammatory disease in women. Condoms might protect against herpes simplex virus-2 and syphilis, although data are limited. Only water-based lubricants (such as K-Y Jelly or glycerin) should be used with latex condoms because oil-based lubricants (such as petroleum jelly, shortening, mineral oil, or massage oil) can weaken latex condoms. Vaginal spermicides containing nonoxynol-9 are not recommended for STD/HIV prevention, as nonoxynol-9 can increase the risk of HIV transmission. Contraceptive methods that are not mechanical barriers offer no protection against HIV or other STDs.

Prompt evaluation of sexual partners is necessary to prevent reinfection and disrupt transmission of many STDs. Preexposure vaccination is among the most effective methods for preventing some STDs. Two human papillomavirus (HPV) vaccines are available and licensed for girls and women aged 9–26 years to prevent cervical precancers and cancers: the quadrivalent HPV and the bivalent HPV vaccine. The quadrivalent vaccine also prevents genital warts. Preexposure vaccination against hepatitis A and B is recommended, as these infections can be sexually transmissible. Hepatitis A vaccine is recommended for all unvaccinated sexually active men who have sex with men or injection drug users. Hepatitis B vaccine is recommended for all unvaccinated men who have sex with men, people with a history of an STD, people who have had more than 1 sexual partner in the previous 6 months, and people who use or who have a sex partner who uses injection drugs.

BIBLIOGRAPHY

1. Abdullah AS, Ebrahim SH, Fielding R, Morisky DE. Sexually transmitted infections in travelers: implications for prevention and control. Clin Infect Dis. 2004 Aug 15;39(4):533–8.

2. Ansart S, Hochedez P, Perez L, Bricaire F, Caumes E. Sexually transmitted diseases diagnosed among travelers returning from the tropics. J Travel Med. 2009 Mar–Apr;16(2):79–83.

3. Holmes KK, Levine R, Weaver M. Effectiveness of condoms in preventing sexually transmitted infections. Bull World Health Organ. 2004 Jun;82(6):454–61.

4. Leder K, Tong S, Weld L, Kain KC, Wilder-Smith A, von Sonnenburg F, et al. Illness in travelers visiting friends and relatives: a review of the GeoSentinel Surveillance Network. Clin Infect Dis. 2006 Nov 1;43(9):1185–93.

5. Martin ET, Krantz E, Gottlieb SL, Magaret AS, Langenberg A, Stanberry L, et al. A pooled analysis of the effect of condoms in preventing HSV-2 acquisition. Arch Intern Med. 2009 Jul 13;169(13):1233–40.

6. Matteelli A, Carosi G. Sexually transmitted diseases in travelers. Clin Infect Dis. 2001 Apr 1;32(7):1063–7.

7. Memish ZA, Osoba AO. Sexually transmitted diseases and travel. Int J Antimicrob Agents. 2003 Feb;21(2):131–4.

8. Peterman TA, Heffelfinger JD, Swint EB, Groseclose SL. The changing epidemiology of syphilis. Sex Transm Dis. 2005 Oct;32(10 Suppl):S4–10.

9. Schmid G, Steen R, N'Dowa F. Control of bacterial sexually transmitted diseases in the developing world is possible. Clin Infect Dis. 2005 Nov 1;41(9):1313–5.

10. Tietz A, Davies SC, Moran JS. Guide to sexually transmitted disease resources on the Internet. Clin Infect Dis. 2004 May 1;38(9):1304–10.

11. US Preventive Services Task Force. Behavioral counseling to prevent sexually transmitted infections: US Preventive Services Task Force recommendation statement. Ann Intern Med. 2008 Oct 7;149(7):491–6, W95.

12. Ward BJ, Plourde P. Travel and sexually transmitted infections. J Travel Med. 2006 Sep–Oct;13(5):300–17.

13. Ward H, Martin I, Macdonald N, Alexander S, Simms I, Fenton K, et al. Lymphogranuloma venereum in the United kingdom. Clin Infect Dis. 2007 Jan 1;44(1):26–32.

14. Weinstock H, Berman S, Cates W Jr. Sexually transmitted diseases among American youth: incidence and prevalence estimates, 2000. Perspect Sex Reprod Health. 2004 Jan–Feb;36(1):6–10.

15. Workowski KA, Berman S. Sexually transmitted diseases treatment guidelines, 2010. MMWR Recomm Rep. 2010 Dec 17;59(RR-12):1–110.

16. Workowski KA, Berman SM, Douglas JM, Jr. Emerging antimicrobial resistance in *Neisseria gonorrhoeae*: urgent need to strengthen prevention strategies. Ann Intern Med. 2008 Apr 15;148(8):606–13.

SEX TOURISM

Emilia H. Koumans

SEX DURING INTERNATIONAL TRAVEL

Two studies in sexually transmitted disease (STD) clinics found that 20%–42% of international travelers had sex with a new partner during travel. STDs, including HIV, are a risk worldwide, not only in local people but also in fellow travelers. However, official data on the prevalence of STDs are often unknown, and many travelers may be unaware of the risks.

SEX TOURISM

"Sex tourism" has been defined as travel specifically planned to procure sex. However, travelers may solicit or engage in sex during travel whether or not this was the intended purpose of the trip. In certain destinations, travelers may find that sex workers are readily available and culturally acceptable, lowering the threshold for purchasing sexual encounters. Alcohol, drugs, and the encouragement of friends may lead to encounters that the traveler may later regret.

SEXUAL EXPLOITATION

While commercial sex work is legal in some countries, child prostitution is universally illegal. The International Labor Organization works globally with governmental and nongovernmental partners to reduce child exploitation. Sex with a minor may be prosecuted in the United States, even if the behavior occurred while abroad.

PRE-TRAVEL INFORMATION

Regardless of whether or not sex is purchased, sex with a new partner during travel places the traveler at risk for an STD, including HIV. All travelers should be counseled before travel on risks and prevention of STDs and be given information on the illegality of child prostitution. Travelers may also benefit from the following information about child prostitution:

- Report suspected commercial child sexual exploitation in tourist destinations to the authorities abroad or to the Department of Homeland Security's Immigration and Customs Enforcement. If travelers have information regarding a person who has sexually exploited a child or suspect someone of child sex tourism, they can e-mail the Immigration and Customs Enforcement (ICE) Operation Predator (operation.predator@DHS.gov) or call the ICE hotline: 866-347-2423.
- Federal law prohibits adult US residents and citizens from engaging in sexual acts with people aged <18 outside the United States (18 USC 2423). Travelers should be aware that any US citizen or permanent legal resident arrested in a foreign country for sexually abusing minors may be subject to return to the United States and, if convicted, can face up to 30 years in prison.

- Governmental and nongovernmental organizations are working to protect children from commercial sexual exploitation.
- If immediate assistance is needed, contact the regional security officer at the local American embassy or consulate or foreign law enforcement officials.

BIBLIOGRAPHY

1. Carter S, Horn K, Hart G, Dunbar M, Scoular A, MacIntyre S. The sexual behaviour of international travellers at two Glasgow GUM clinics. Glasgow genitourinary medicine. Int J STD AIDS. 1997 May;8(5):336–8.
2. Hamlyn E, Peer A, Easterbrook P. Sexual health and HIV in travellers and expatriates. Occup Med (Lond). 2007 Aug;57(5):313–21.
3. Hawkes S, Hart GJ, Bletsoe E, Shergold C, Johnson AM. Risk behaviour and STD acquisition in genitourinary clinic attenders who have travelled. Genitourin Med. 1995 Dec;71(6):351–4.
4. International Labour Organization, International Programme on the Elimination of Child Labour. Commercial sexual exploitation of children. Geneva: International Labour Organization; 2010 [cited 2008 Nov 20]. Available from: http://www.ilo.org/ipec/areas/CSEC/lang--en/index.htm.
5. Marrazzo JM. Sexual tourism: implications for travelers and the destination culture. Infect Dis Clin North Am. 2005 Mar;19(1):103–20.
6. Pan American Health Organization. Trafficking of Women and Children for Sexual Exploitation in the Americas. Washington DC: Women, Health and Development Program. Pan American Health Organization; 2001 [cited 2008 Nov 30]. Available from: http://www.paho.org/English/AD/GE/TraffickingPaper.pdf.
7. US Department of Justice. Child sex tourism. Washington, DC: US Department of Justice. Available from: http://www.usdoj.gov/criminal/ceos/sextour.html.
8. US Department of State. Office to monitor and combat trafficking in persons. Washington, DC: US Department of State. Available from: http://www.state.gov/g/tip/.

SHIGELLOSIS
Anna Bowen, Katharine A. Schilling, Eric Mintz

INFECTIOUS AGENT

Shigellosis is an acute infection of the intestine caused by bacteria in the genus *Shigella*. There are 4 species of *Shigella*: *Shigella dysenteriae*, *S. flexneri*, *S. boydii*, and *S. sonnei* (also referred to as group A, B, C, and D, respectively). Several distinct serotypes are recognized within the first 3 species. Disease severity varies according to species and serotype. *S. dysenteriae* serotype 1 (Sd1) is the agent of epidemic dysentery, while *S. sonnei* is a common cause of mild diarrheal illness.

MODE OF TRANSMISSION

Transmission occurs via the fecal-oral route, either indirectly through contaminated food, water, or fomites, or via direct person-to-person contact. As few as 10 organisms are sufficient to cause infection. Only humans and higher primates carry *Shigella*. Outbreaks have been traced to contaminated produce and other foods, contaminated drinking water, swimming in contaminated water, and sexual contact between men. In the United States, outbreaks of *S. sonnei* infection among young children in daycare settings are common.

EPIDEMIOLOGY

Worldwide, *Shigella* is estimated to cause 80–165 million cases and 600,000 deaths annually. *Shigella* spp. are endemic in temperate and tropical climates. *Shigella sonnei* is found most frequently in industrialized countries, while *S. flexneri* more commonly affects people in the developing world. *Shigella* spp. are an uncommon cause of travelers' diarrhea among travelers to Mexico but are common among travelers to Asia. *Shigella* spp. are found in the stools of 5%–18% of patients with travelers' diarrhea. A FoodNet study found that approximately 26% of US residents with sporadic shigellosis reported international travel in the week before symptom onset.

CLINICAL PRESENTATION

Disease onset occurs 12–96 hours after exposure. The symptoms of shigellosis range from mild to severe and typically last 4–7 days. The disease is characterized by watery, bloody or mucoid diarrhea, fever, stomach cramps, and nausea. On rare occasions, patients experience toxemia, vomiting, tenesmus, postinfectious arthritis, hemolytic uremic syndrome (after infection with Shiga toxin–producing strains), or seizures (young children).

DIAGNOSIS

Shigellosis is confirmed through culture of a stool specimen or rectal swab. To effectively isolate *Shigella*, samples must be processed rapidly, because *Shigella* cannot survive outside the body for long periods of time. *Shigella* isolates may then be speciated and serotyped and their antimicrobial susceptibilities determined.

TREATMENT

In healthy people, shigellosis will typically resolve within 4–7 days, even without treatment. Antimicrobial treatment, when given early in the course of illness, can shorten the duration of symptoms and of carriage. Because multidrug resistance among *Shigella* strains is common, empiric treatment should begin with a fluoroquinolone (for adults and, if infection is acquired in regions with high rates of multidrug resistance, children) or ceftriaxone (for children) until information about antimicrobial susceptibility is available. Resistance to fluoroquinolones has been reported, more often among *Shigella* isolates acquired in south and east Asia.

PREVENTIVE MEASURES FOR TRAVELERS

No vaccines are available for *Shigella*. The best defense against shigellosis is thorough, frequent handwashing and strict adherence to standard food and water safety recommendations, as described in Chapter 2, Food and Water Precautions.

BIBLIOGRAPHY

1. American Academy of Pediatrics. Shigella infections. In: Pickering L, Baker CJ, Long SS, McMillan JA, editors. Red Book: 2009 report of the Committee on Infectious Diseases. 28th ed. Elk Grove Village, IL: American Academy of Pediatrics; 2009. p. 593–96.
2. American Public Health Association. Shigellosis. In: Heymann DL, editor. Control of communicable diseases manual. 19 ed. Washington, DC: American Public Health Association; 2008. p. 556–60.
3. CDC. *Shigella* surveillance: annual summary, 2006. Atlanta: CDC; 2008. Available from: http://www.cdc.gov/ncidod/DBMD/phlisdata/shigtab/2006/ShigellaAnnualSummary2006.pdf.
4. Dutta S, Dutta P, Matsushita S, Bhattacharya SK, Yoshida S. *Shigella dysenteriae* serotype 1, Kolkata, India. Emerg Infect Dis. 2003 Nov;9(11):1471–4.
5. Gaynor K, Park SY, Kanenaka R, Colindres R, Mintz E, Ram PK, et al. International foodborne outbreak of *Shigella sonnei* infection in airline passengers. Epidemiol Infect. 2009 Mar;137(3):335–41.
6. Haley CC, Ong KL, Hedberg K, Cieslak PR, Scallan E, Marcus R, et al. Risk factors for sporadic shigellosis, FoodNet 2005. Foodborne Pathog Dis. 2010 Jul;7(7):741–7.
7. Kotloff KL, Winickoff JP, Ivanoff B, Clemens JD, Swerdlow DL, Sansonetti PJ, et al. Global burden of *Shigella* infections: implications for vaccine development and implementation of control strategies. Bull World Health Organ. 1999;77(8):651–66.
8. Ram PK, Crump JA, Gupta SK, Miller MA, Mintz ED. Part II. Analysis of data gaps pertaining to *Shigella* infections in low and medium human development index countries, 1984–2005. Epidemiol Infect. 2008 May;136(5):577–603.
9. von Seidlein L, Kim DR, Ali M, Lee H, Wang X, Thiem VD, et al. A multicentre study of *Shigella* diarrhoea in six Asian countries: disease burden, clinical manifestations, and microbiology. PLoS Med. 2006 Sep;3(9):e353.

SMALLPOX & OTHER ORTHOPOXVIRUS-ASSOCIATED INFECTIONS

Mary G. Reynolds

INFECTIOUS AGENT

Smallpox is caused by variola virus, a member of the *Poxvirus* family, genus *Orthopoxvirus*. Other members of this genus known to cause infection in humans are vaccinia virus, monkeypox virus, and cowpox virus. In 1980, the World Health Organization declared that smallpox had been eradicated globally. As a result, smallpox is not considered a risk for international travelers. International travelers may, however, be at risk for contracting other orthopoxvirus infections, including vaccinia, monkeypox, and cowpox.

MODE OF TRANSMISSION
Smallpox

During the smallpox era, disease transmission from person to person occurred principally through face-to-face contact, via respiratory routes. Respiratory droplets produced during the first 3–7 days of illness in a person suffering from smallpox are heavily laden with virus and can efficiently establish infection in a susceptible person who is exposed. Less commonly, new infections were the result of a person's inhaling or having mucus membrane exposure to virus-containing material shed from skin lesions or scabs.

Monkeypox

Monkeypox virus infection can occur after contact with infected animals or from people who are ill with monkeypox. Person-to-person transmission is thought to occur by way of large respiratory droplets and, less commonly, through contact with lesions or objects contaminated with lesion material (fluid, scab). Multiple species of African rodents and primates have been observed to harbor the virus, and could transmit infection to humans, but the precise reservoir host for monkeypox virus remains unknown.

Vaccinia

Vaccinia virus causes a localized infection of the skin that is typically confined to the portal of entry, often a freshly abraded (scratched) area. Vaccinia virus is the live virus component of contemporary smallpox vaccines. Rarely, social contacts of people recently vaccinated for smallpox develop infections with vaccinia virus. These infections occur either when a susceptible person's skin comes into direct contact with fluid from the inoculation lesion of a recent smallpox vaccinee, or when a person is exposed to objects (towels, clothing) contaminated with lesion material. Zoonotic infections with vaccinialike viruses have been reported in Brazil and India.

Cowpox

Cowpox virus also causes localized infections of the skin that occur at the portal of entry, typically a freshly abraded (scratched) area. Human infections with cowpox virus stem from contact with infected animals; transmission of the virus between humans has not been observed. Rodents, predators of rodents (cats), and occasionally exotic animal species in zoos can become infected with cowpox virus. Infected animals typically demonstrate signs of illness, including skin lesions.

EPIDEMIOLOGY
Smallpox

The last reported case of endemic smallpox occurred in Somalia in 1977, and the last reported case of laboratory-acquired smallpox occurred in the United Kingdom in 1978.

Monkeypox

Monkeypox virus is endemic in tropical forested regions of West and Central Africa, notably the Congo Basin. Hundreds of monkeypox virus infections are reported to health authorities annually in the Democratic Republic of the Congo. Rodents imported from

West Africa were the source of an outbreak of human monkeypox that occurred in the United States in 2003. Travelers should avoid contact with forest-dwelling animals that appear sick or that have been found dead.

Vaccinia

Infections with wild vaccinialike viruses have been reported among cattle and buffalo herders in India and among dairy workers in southern Brazil.

Cowpox

Human infections with cowpox virus have been reported in Europe.

CLINICAL PRESENTATION
Monkeypox

Monkeypox virus infection causes an illness clinically identical to smallpox, with fever and widespread vesiculopustular rash involving the palms and soles. One feature distinctive to monkeypox is marked lymphadenopathy. The case-fatality ratio for monkeypox is estimated to be 10%.

Vaccinia and Cowpox

Human infections with vaccinia, wild vaccinialike viruses, and cowpox virus are most often self-limited, characterized by localized pustular (occasionally ulcerative) lesions. Fever and other constitutional symptoms may occur briefly after lesions first appear. Lesions can be painful and can persist for weeks. Orthopoxvirus infections in humans are rare. People who are immunocompromised or who have exfoliative skin conditions (such as eczema or atopic dermatitis) are at substantially higher risk of severe illness or fatal outcomes.

DIAGNOSIS

Orthopoxvirus infection is confirmed by PCR or virus isolation. Physicians can refer to CDC smallpox website (www.bt.cdc.gov/agent/smallpox/diagnosis) for guidance in the application of a clinical algorithm designed to aid in distinguishing smallpox from other disseminated rash illnesses, namely chickenpox.

TREATMENT

Treatment of human orthopoxvirus infection is mainly supportive, to include hydration, nutritional supplementation, and prevention of secondary infections. Vaccinia lesions should remain covered by bandage, gauze, or clothing until the scab detaches, in order to diminish chances of inadvertent inoculation of the virus to other parts of the body or transmission to another person. To prevent person-to-person transmission of smallpox and monkeypox, patients should be isolated and cared for by someone who has received the smallpox vaccine. Physicians managing orthopoxvirus infection in a patient who is at high risk for severe outcome (such as a patient who is immunocompromised or has an underlying skin condition) should consult with CDC to explore investigational treatment options; contact the CDC Emergency Operations Center at 770-488-7100.

PREVENTIVE MEASURES FOR TRAVELERS

Smallpox vaccine is not recommended for international travelers. Live vaccinia virus is the main component of the smallpox vaccine. Because of the elimination of smallpox, routine smallpox vaccination ceased worldwide in 1980. Smallpox vaccination is recommended only for laboratory workers who handle variola virus (the agent of smallpox) or viruses closely related to variola virus and health care and public health officials who would be designated first responders in the event of an intentional release of variola virus. In addition, members of the US military may be required to receive the vaccine.

There are no preventive vaccines for other orthopoxvirus infections. No drugs for preventing or treating orthopoxvirus infection are licensed. Travelers are advised to avoid contact with rodents and sick or dead animals, including pets and domestic ruminants (cattle, buffalo). For more information about monkeypox and other orthopoxviruses, contact the CDC Poxvirus Inquiry Line (404-639-4129).

BIBLIOGRAPHY

1. Baxby D, Bennett M, Getty B. Human cowpox 1969–93: a review based on 54 cases. Br J Dermatol. 1994 Nov;131(5):598–607.

2. Campe H, Zimmermann P, Glos K, Bayer M, Bergemann H, Dreweck C, et al. Cowpox virus transmission from pet rats to humans, Germany. Emerg Infect Dis. 2009 May;15(5):777–80.

3. CDC. Human monkeypox—Kasai Oriental, Democratic Republic of Congo, February 1996–October 1997. MMWR Morb Mortal Wkly Rep. 1997 Dec 12;46(49):1168–71.

4. Damon IK, Roth CE, Chowdhary V. Discovery of monkeypox in Sudan. N Engl J Med. 2006 Aug 31;355(9):962–3.

5. de Souza Trindade G, Drumond BP, Guedes MI, Leite JA, Mota BE, Campos MA, et al. Zoonotic vaccinia virus infection in Brazil: clinical description and implications for health professionals. J Clin Microbiol. 2007 Apr;45(4):1370–2.

6. Learned LA, Reynolds MG, Wassa DW, Li Y, Olson VA, Karem K, et al. Extended interhuman transmission of monkeypox in a hospital community in the Republic of the Congo, 2003. Am J Trop Med Hyg. 2005 Aug;73(2):428–34.

7. Levine RS, Peterson AT, Yorita KL, Carroll D, Damon IK, Reynolds MG. Ecological niche and geographic distribution of human monkeypox in Africa. PLoS One. 2007;2(1):e176.

8. Reynolds MG, Davidson WB, Curns AT, Conover CS, Huhn G, Davis JP, et al. Spectrum of infection and risk factors for human monkeypox, United States, 2003. Emerg Infect Dis. 2007 Sep;13(9):1332–9.

9. Rotz LD, Dotson DA, Damon IK, Becher JA. Vaccinia (smallpox) vaccine: recommendations of the Advisory Committee on Immunization Practices (ACIP), 2001. MMWR Recomm Rep. 2001 Jun 22;50 (RR-10):1–25.

10. Trindade GS, Guedes MI, Drumond BP, Mota BE, Abrahao JS, Lobato ZI, et al. Zoonotic vaccinia virus: clinical and immunological characteristics in a naturally infected patient. Clin Infect Dis. 2009 Feb 1; 48(3):e37–40.

STRONGYLOIDIASIS
LeAnne M. Fox

INFECTIOUS AGENT
Strongyloidiasis is caused by an intestinal nematode, *Strongyloides stercoralis*.

MODE OF TRANSMISSION
Infection occurs when filariform larvae found in infected soil penetrate human skin. Person-to-person transmission is rare but has been documented.

EPIDEMIOLOGY
Strongyloides is endemic in the tropics and subtropics, and in limited foci in the southeastern United States, Europe, Australia, and Japan. Estimates of global prevalence vary between 3 million and 100 million. Most infections seen in the United States occur in immigrants, refugees, and military veterans who have lived in endemic areas for long periods of time. Risk for short-term travelers is very low, but infections can occur.

CLINICAL PRESENTATION
Most infections are asymptomatic. With acute infections, a localized, pruritic, erythematous papular rash can develop at the site of skin penetration, followed by pulmonary symptoms (a Löffler-like pneumonitis), diarrhea, abdominal pain, and eosinophilia. Migrating larvae in the skin can cause larva currens, a serpiginous urticarial rash.

Immunocompromised people, especially those receiving systemic corticosteroids or patients with human T-cell lymphotropic virus type 1 infection, are at risk for hyperinfection or disseminated disease, characterized by abdominal pain, diffuse pulmonary infiltrates, and septicemia or meningitis from enteric gram-negative bacilli. The death rate from untreated disseminated strongyloidiasis is high. Unexplained eosinophilia may be a presenting sign of strongyloidiasis.

DIAGNOSIS
Diagnosis is made by finding rhabditiform larvae on microscopic examination of the stool, either directly or by culture on agar plates. Repeated stool examinations or examination of duodenal contents may be necessary, given the low sensitivity of a single stool examination. Hyperinfection and disseminated strongyloidiasis are readily diagnosed by examining stool, sputum, cerebrospinal fluid, and other body fluids and tissues, which typically contain high numbers of larvae. Serologic testing using an immunoassay is useful and available through the National Institutes of Health and CDC's Division of Parasitic Diseases and Malaria (www.dpd.cdc.gov/dpdx).

TREATMENT
Ivermectin (200 µg/kg orally for 2 days) is the treatment of choice for both chronic infection and disseminated disease with hyperinfection. Albendazole is an alternative agent, although associated with slightly lower cure rates. Prolonged or repeated treatment may be necessary in patients with hyperinfection and disseminated strongyloidiasis, and relapse can occur.

PREVENTIVE MEASURES FOR TRAVELERS
No vaccine is available. No drugs for preventing infection are available. Protective measures include wearing shoes when walking in areas where humans may have defecated.

BIBLIOGRAPHY
1. Abramowicz M. Drugs for Parasitic Infections. New Rochelle (NY): The Medical Letter, Inc; 2007.
2. Adedayo O, Grell G, Bellot P. Hyperinfective strongyloidiasis in the medical ward: review of 27 cases in 5 years. South Med J. 2002 Jul;95(7):711–6.
3. Arthur RP, Shelley WB. Larva currens; a distinctive variant of cutaneous larva migrans due to Strongyloides stercoralis. AMA Arch Derm. 1958 Aug;78(2):186–90.
4. Cappello M, Hotez PJ. Disseminated strongyloidiasis. Semin Neurol. 1993 Jun;13(2):169–74.
5. Genta RM, Weesner R, Douce RW, Huitger-O'Connor T, Walzer PD. Strongyloidiasis in US veterans of the Vietnam and other wars. JAMA. 1987 Jul 3;258(1):49–52.
6. Grove DI. Human strongyloidiasis. Adv Parasitol. 1996;38:251–309.
7. Gyorkos TW, Genta RM, Viens P, MacLean JD. Seroepidemiology of Strongyloides infection in the Southeast Asian refugee population in Canada. Am J Epidemiol. 1990 Aug;132(2):257–64.
8. Keiser PB, Nutman TB. Strongyloides stercoralis in the immunocompromised population. Clin Microbiol Rev. 2004 Jan;17(1):208–17.
9. Siddiqui AA, Berk SL. Diagnosis of Strongyloides stercoralis infection. Clin Infect Dis. 2001 Oct 1;33(7):1040–7.
10. Zaha O, Hirata T, Kinjo F, Saito A. Strongyloidiasis—progress in diagnosis and treatment. Intern Med. 2000 Sep;39(9):695–700.

TAENIASIS
Jeffrey L. Jones

INFECTIOUS AGENT
Taeniasis is caused by intestinal infection with the adult stage of tapeworms Taenia solium (pork tapeworm) and T. saginata (beef tapeworm).

MODE OF TRANSMISSION
Humans acquire T. solium when they eat raw or undercooked contaminated pork; the adult worm then develops in the intestine. Eggs passed by humans in the stool are infectious

to pigs; the larval stage lives in the flesh of pigs (pig cysticercosis). Eggs passed by humans in the stool are also infectious to humans and can be transferred by the fecal-oral route. Eggs are infectious when shed. When humans ingest *T. solium* eggs, the larvae penetrate the intestinal wall and spread to the tissues via the blood and lymphatics (human cysticercosis, see the Cysticercosis section earlier in this chapter).

T. saginata eggs passed in the stool of an infected person are infectious only to cattle; the larval stage lives in the flesh of cattle (cysticercosis bovis) and infects humans when they eat raw or undercooked contaminated beef. *T. asiatica* is a third species, similar to *T. saginata*.

EPIDEMIOLOGY

Taeniasis is distributed worldwide but is more common where pigs and cattle can eat human feces. The highest prevalences are in Latin America, Africa, and South and Southeast Asia. The disease has been reported, but at lower rates, from Eastern Europe, Spain, and Portugal. Transmission of *T. solium* is rare in the United States, Canada, Western Europe, and many areas of Asia and the Pacific. The risk is higher in developing countries where inadequate sanitation leads to pork and beef contamination with larvae, as well as food and water contamination with *Taenia* eggs. Immigrants from endemic areas may have taeniasis or cysticercosis.

CLINICAL PRESENTATION

Taeniasis (intestinal tape worm) may be asymptomatic or associated with abdominal discomfort, weight loss, anorexia, nausea, insomnia, weakness, perianal pruritus, and nervousness. Proglottids may be passed from the rectum. Rarely, these infections result in intestinal, biliary, or pancreatic obstruction. Tapeworms can live in the intestine 30 years or longer. Eosinophilia is often present, but the duration and magnitude vary. The incubation period (time for eggs to appear in stool) is 8–10 weeks for *T. solium* and 10–14 weeks for *T. saginata*.

DIAGNOSIS

Adult tapeworm infection is identified by eggs, proglottids (segments), or tapeworm antigens in the feces or on anal swabs. Differentiation of *T. solium* from *T. saginata* is based on morphology of the scolex and gravid proglottids.

TREATMENT

Praziquantel is used to treat intestinal infections with *T. solium* or *T. saginata*. Niclosamide is an alternative but is not as widely available.

PREVENTIVE MEASURES FOR TRAVELERS

Cook meat to safe temperatures (≥150°F [65°C] throughout). Freezing (23°F [–5°C]) meat for ≥4 days will kill cysticerci. For more on the prevention of cysticercosis, see the Cysticercosis section earlier in this chapter.

BIBLIOGRAPHY

1. Abramowicz M. Drugs for Parasitic Infections. New Rochelle (NY): The Medical Letter, Inc; 2007.
2. CDC. Cysticercosis. Atlanta: CDC; 2009 [updated 2009 Jul 20; cited 2010 Oct 22]. Available from: http://www.dpd.cdc.gov/dpdx/HTML/Cysticercosis.htm.
3. CDC. Taeniasis. Atlanta: CDC; 2009 [updated 2009 Jul 20; cited 2010 Oct 22]. Available from: http://www.dpd.cdc.gov/dpdx/HTML/Taeniasis.htm.
4. Wittner M, Tanowitz HB. Taenia and other tapeworms. In: Guerrant RL, Walker DH, Weller PF, editors. Tropical Infectious Diseases: Principles, Pathogens, and Practice. 2nd ed. Philadelphia: Churchill Livingstone; 2006. p. 1327–30.

TETANUS

Ryan T. Novak, Cynthia G. Thomas

INFECTIOUS AGENT

Clostridium tetani, the tetanus bacillus, is a spore-forming, anaerobic, gram-positive bacterium. Clinical disease is caused by a potent neurotoxin produced by the vegetative state of the bacterium growing in contaminated wounds.

MODE OF TRANSMISSION

C. tetani spores are ubiquitous in the environment and can be introduced into the body through nonintact skin, usually via injuries from contaminated objects. Lesions that are considered "tetanus prone" are wounds contaminated with dirt, feces, or saliva; punctures; burns; crush injuries; or injuries with necrotic tissue. However, tetanus has also been associated with apparently clean superficial wounds, surgical procedures, insect bites, dental infections, compound fractures, chronic sores and infections, and intravenous drug use. In 10% of reported cases in the United States, no antecedent wound was identified. Tetanus is not transmitted from person to person.

EPIDEMIOLOGY

Tetanus occurs everywhere in the world, almost exclusively in people who are inadequately immunized. Travel does not increase risk of disease. In the United States, tetanus occurs rarely in people who have completed the primary series and received appropriate boosters. In 2006, an estimated 290,000 people worldwide died of tetanus, most of them in Asia, Africa, and South America.

A reservoir of tetanus bacteria exists in the intestines of horses and other animals, including humans, in which the organism is a harmless normal inhabitant. Soil or fomites contaminated with animal and human feces propagate transmission. Worldwide, the disease is more common in agricultural regions and in areas where contact with soil or animal excreta is more likely and immunization is inadequate. In developing countries, tetanus in neonates born to unvaccinated mothers

(neonatal tetanus) is the most common form of the disease.

There is no increased risk to travelers who are adequately vaccinated. With or without travel, inadequately vaccinated people are at risk when they are injured by a contaminated object, use injection drugs, or require surgery or dental care in unhygienic conditions. In addition, there may be an increased risk of neonatal tetanus for infants of inadequately vaccinated mothers who deliver outside the United States, if the birth occurs in an unhygienic environment.

CLINICAL PRESENTATION

Acute manifestations of tetanus are characterized by muscle rigidity and painful spasms, often starting in the muscles of the jaw and neck. Severe tetanus can lead to respiratory failure and death. The incubation period is usually 3–21 days (average 10 days), although it may range from 1 day to several months, depending on the character, extent, and location of the wound. Most cases occur within 14 days. In general, shorter incubation periods are associated with more heavily contaminated wounds, more severe disease, and a worse prognosis.

Generalized Tetanus

Generalized tetanus is the most common form, accounting for more than 80% of cases. Neonatal tetanus usually occurs because of umbilical stump infections. The most common initial sign is trismus (spasm of the muscles of mastication or "lockjaw"). Trismus may be followed by painful spasms in other muscle groups in the neck, trunk, and extremities and by generalized, tonic, seizurelike activity or frank convulsions in severe cases. Generalized tetanus can be accompanied by autonomic nervous system abnormalities, as well as a variety of complications related to severe spasm and prolonged hospitalization. The clinical course of generalized tetanus is variable and depends on the degree of prior immunity, the amount of toxin present, and the age and general health of the patient. Even with modern intensive care, generalized tetanus is associated with death rates of 10%–20%.

Localized Tetanus

Localized tetanus is an unusual form of the disease consisting of muscle spasms in a confined area close to the site of the injury. Although localized tetanus often occurs in people with partial immunity and is usually mild, progression to generalized tetanus can occur.

Cephalic Tetanus

The rarest form, cephalic tetanus, is associated with lesions of the head or face and has been described in association with ear infections (otitis media). The incubation period is short, usually 1–2 days. Unlike generalized and localized tetanus, cephalic tetanus results in flaccid cranial nerve palsies rather than spasm. Trismus may also be present. Like localized tetanus, cephalic tetanus can progress to the generalized form.

DIAGNOSIS

The diagnosis is made clinically, since tetanus is a clinical syndrome without confirmatory laboratory tests. The disease is characterized by painful muscular contractions, primarily of the masseter and neck muscles, secondarily of trunk muscles. A common first sign suggestive of tetanus in older children and adults is abdominal rigidity, although rigidity is sometimes confined to the region of injury. Generalized spasms occur, frequently induced by sensory stimuli; typical features of the tetanic spasm are the position of opisthotonos and the facial expression known as "risus sardonicus." History of an injury or apparent portal of entry may be lacking. The organism is rarely recovered from the site of infection, and usually there is no detectable antibody response.

TREATMENT

Tetanus is a medical emergency requiring hospitalization, immediate treatment with human tetanus immune globulin (TIG) (or equine antitoxin if human immune globulin is not available), a tetanus toxoid booster, agents to control muscle spasm, and aggressive wound care and antibiotics as indicated. TIG is administered intramuscularly in doses of 3,000–6,000 IU. If immunoglobulin is not available, tetanus antitoxin (equine origin) in a single large dose should be given intravenously, after testing for hypersensitivity.

Metronidazole is the most appropriate antibiotic. It is associated with the shortest recovery time and lowest case-fatality ratio. It should be given for 7–14 days in large doses, which also allows for a reduction in the amount of muscle relaxants and sedatives required. The wound should be debrided widely and excised if possible. Wide debridement of the umbilical stump in neonates is not indicated.

Depending on the severity of disease, mechanical ventilation and agents to control autonomic nervous system instability may be required. An adequate airway should be maintained, and sedation should be used as indicated; muscle relaxant drugs, together with tracheostomy or nasotracheal intubation and mechanically assisted respiration, may be lifesaving. Active immunization should be initiated concurrently with treatment.

PREVENTIVE MEASURES FOR TRAVELERS
Personal Protection Measures

Universal active immunization with adsorbed tetanus toxoid gives durable protection for ≥10 years; after the initial basic series has been completed, single booster doses elicit high levels of immunity. Travelers should ensure they have adequate immunity to tetanus provided by completion of the 3-dose tetanus toxoid primary series and a booster if it has been >10 years since the last dose. Infants of actively immunized mothers acquire passive immunity that protects them from neonatal tetanus. Recovery from tetanus may not result in immunity; second attacks can occur, and primary immunization is indicated after recovery.

Prophylaxis in Wound Management

Tetanus prophylaxis in wounded patients is based on careful assessment of whether the wound is clean or contaminated, the immunization status of the patient, proper use of tetanus toxoid or TIG, wound cleaning, and where required, surgical debridement and the proper use of antibiotics. Table 3-18 provides recommendations on provision of Td (tetanus and diphtheria toxoids vaccine) or TIG on the

Table 3-18. Summary guide to tetanus prophylaxis in routine wound management

HISTORY OF TETANUS IMMUNIZATION (DOSES)	CLEAN, MINOR WOUNDS		ALL OTHER WOUNDS	
	Td[1]	TIG	Td[1]	TIG[2]
Uncertain or <3 doses	Yes	No	Yes	Yes
≥3 doses	No, unless >10 years since last dose	No	No, unless >5 years since last dose[3]	No

[1] For children aged <7 years, DTaP (DT, if pertussis vaccine contraindicated) is preferred to tetanus toxoid alone. For children aged 7–10 years who are not fully vaccinated against pertussis and for whom no contraindication to pertussis vaccine exists, a single dose of Tdap should be given to provide protection against pertussis. If additional doses of tetanus and diphtheria toxoid-containing vaccines are needed, then children aged 7–10 years should be vaccinated according to catch-up guidance, with Tdap preferred as the first dose. For adolescents and adults aged 10–64 years, a single dose of Tdap should be provided in place of one Td booster if the patient has not previously been vaccinated with Tdap. Adults aged ≥65 years who have or who anticipate having close contact with an infant aged <12 months and who have not previously received Tdap should receive a single dose of Tdap to protect against pertussis and reduce the likelihood of transmission; all other adults ≥65 years who have not previously received Tdap may be given a single dose of Tdap instead of Td.

[2] Passive immunization with ≥250 IU of TIG intramuscularly (or 1,500–5,000 IU of antitoxin of animal origin, if globulin is not available), regardless of the patient's age, is indicated for patients with other than clean, minor wounds and a history of no, unknown, or fewer than 3 previous tetanus toxoid doses. When tetanus toxoid and TIG or antitoxin are given concurrently, separate syringes and separate sites must be used.

[3] More frequent boosters are not needed and can accentuate side effects.

basis of the circumstances of the wound and immunization status of the patient. However, it may be difficult to determine whether a clean, minor wound is tetanus prone. In those circumstances, providers should consider giving Td as a booster dose to people with ≥3 previous doses if it has been >5 years since the last dose.

Vaccine

Complete vaccination of children aged <7 years with 5 doses of acellular pertussis vaccine in combination with diphtheria and tetanus toxoids (DTaP) is recommended; an accelerated schedule of doses may be used to complete the DTaP series. When contraindications to pertussis vaccine exist, a double (DT) antigen vaccine can be used. Children aged 7–10 years who are not fully vaccinated against pertussis and for whom no contraindication to pertussis vaccine exists should receive a single dose of Tdap to provide protection against pertussis.

If additional doses of tetanus and diphtheria toxoid-containing vaccines are needed, then children aged 7–10 years should be vaccinated according to catch-up guidance, with Tdap preferred as the first dose. Adolescents aged 11–18 years should receive a single dose of Tdap instead of Td for booster immunization against tetanus, diphtheria, and pertussis if they have completed the recommended childhood DTwP/DTaP vaccination series and they have not previously received Tdap. Tdap should also be used instead of Td as wound prophylaxis in adolescents who have not previously received Tdap.

Adults aged 19–64 years who have not previously received Tdap should receive a single dose of Tdap to replace a single dose of Td for booster immunization against tetanus, diphtheria, and pertussis regardless of interval since their last tetanus toxoid-containing vaccine (such as Td). Adults aged ≥65 years who have or who anticipate having close contact with an infant aged <12 months and who have not previously received Tdap should receive a single dose of Tdap to protect against pertussis and reduce the likelihood of transmission; all other adults aged ≥65 years who have not previously received Tdap may be given a single dose of Tdap instead of Td.

Adolescents and adults who have never been immunized against pertussis, tetanus, or diphtheria, who have incomplete immunization, or whose immunity is uncertain should follow the catch-up schedule established for Td/Tdap. Tdap can be substituted for any of the Td doses in the series.

For children and adults who are severely immunocompromised or infected with HIV, tetanus toxoid is indicated in the same schedule and dose as for immunocompetent people, even though the immune response may be suboptimal.

BIBLIOGRAPHY

1. American Academy of Pediatrics. Tetanus (lockjaw). In: Pickering LK, Baker CJ, Kimberlin DW, Long SS, editors. Red Book: 2009 Report of the Committee on Infectious Diseases. 28th ed. Elk Grove Village, IL: American Academy of Pediatrics; 2009. p. 655–60.
2. Broder KR, Cortese MM, Iskander JK, Kretsinger K, Slade BA, Brown KH, et al. Preventing tetanus, diphtheria, and pertussis among adolescents: use of tetanus toxoid, reduced diphtheria toxoid and acellular pertussis vaccines. Recommendations of the Advisory Committee on Immunization Practices (ACIP). MMWR Recomm Rep. 2006 Mar 24;55(RR-3):1–34.
3. CDC. Updated recommendations for use of tetanus toxoid, reduced diphtheria toxoid and acellular pertussis (Tdap) vaccine from the Advisory Committee on Immunization Practices, 2010. MMWR Morb Mortal Wkly Rep. 2011 Jan 14;60(1):13–5.
4. Farrar JJ, Yen LM, Cook T, Fairweather N, Binh N, Parry J, et al. Tetanus. J Neurol Neurosurg Psychiatry. 2000 Sep;69(3):292–301.
5. Hsu SS, Groleau G. Tetanus in the emergency department: a current review. J Emerg Med. 2001 May;20(4):357–65.
6. Kretsinger K, Broder KR, Cortese MM, Joyce MP, Ortega-Sanchez I, Lee GM, et al. Preventing tetanus, diphtheria, and pertussis among adults: use of tetanus toxoid, reduced diphtheria toxoid and acellular pertussis vaccine recommendations of the Advisory Committee on Immunization Practices (ACIP) and recommendation of ACIP, supported by the Healthcare Infection Control Practices Advisory Committee (HICPAC), for use of Tdap among healthcare personnel. MMWR Recomm Rep. 2006 Dec 15;55(RR-17):1–37.
7. Murphy TV, Slade BA, Broder KR, Kretsinger K, Tiwari T, Joyce PM, et al. Prevention of pertussis, tetanus, and diphtheria among pregnant and postpartum women and their infants recommendations of the Advisory Committee on Immunization Practices (ACIP). MMWR Recomm Rep. 2008 May 30;57(RR-4):1–51.
8. Pascual FB, McGinley EL, Zanardi LR, Cortese MM, Murphy TV. Tetanus surveillance—United States, 1998–2000. MMWR Surveill Summ. 2003 Jun 20;52(3):1–8.
9. Roper MH, Vandelaer JH, Gasse FL. Maternal and neonatal tetanus. Lancet. 2007 Dec 8;370(9603):1947–59.
10. Wassilak SGF, Roper MH, Kretsinger K, Orenstein WA. Tetanus toxoid. In: Plotkin SA, Orenstein WA, Offit PA, editors. Vaccines. 5th ed. Philadelphia: Saunders Elsevier; 2008. p. 805–39.

TICKBORNE ENCEPHALITIS
Marc Fischer, Katherine B. Gibney, Adam MacNeil

INFECTIOUS AGENT
Tickborne encephalitis virus (TBEV) is a single-stranded RNA virus that belongs to the genus *Flavivirus* and is closely related to Powassan virus. TBEV has 3 subtypes: European, Siberian, and Far Eastern.

MODE OF TRANSMISSION
TBEV is transmitted to humans through the bite of an infected tick of the *Ixodes* species, primarily *I. ricinus* (European subtype) or *I. persulcatus* (Siberian and Far Eastern subtypes). The virus is maintained in discrete

areas of deciduous forests. Ticks act as both vector and virus reservoir, and small rodents are the primary amplifying host. Tickborne encephalitis (TBE) can also be acquired by ingesting unpasteurized dairy products (such as milk and cheese) from infected goats, sheep, or cows. TBEV transmission has infrequently been reported through laboratory exposure and slaughtering viremic animals. Direct person-to-person spread of TBEV occurs only rarely, through blood transfusion or breastfeeding.

EPIDEMIOLOGY

TBE is endemic in temperate regions of Europe and Asia (from eastern France to northern Japan and from northern Russia to Albania) and up to about 4,921 ft (1,500) m in altitude. Russia has the highest number of reported TBE cases, and western Siberia has the highest incidence of TBE in the world. Other countries where the incidence is high include the Czech Republic, Estonia, Germany, Hungary, Latvia, Lithuania, Poland, Slovenia, Sweden, and Switzerland. High vaccination rates in Austria have reduced the incidence of TBE; however, unvaccinated travelers to this country are still at risk. European countries with no reported cases are Belgium, Iceland, Ireland, Luxembourg, the Netherlands, Portugal, Spain, and the United Kingdom. Asian countries known to be endemic for TBE include China, Japan, Mongolia, and South Korea.

Most cases occur from April through November, with peaks in early and late summer when ticks are active. The incidence and severity of disease are highest in people aged ≥50 years. In the last 30 years, the geographic range of TBEV and the number of reported TBE cases have increased significantly. These trends are likely due to a complex combination of changes in the ecology and climate, increased human activity in affected areas, and increased recognition.

The overall risk of acquiring TBE for an unvaccinated visitor to a highly endemic area during the TBEV transmission season has been estimated at 1 case per 10,000 person-months of exposure. Most TBEV infections result from tick bites acquired in forested areas through activities such as camping, hiking, fishing, bicycling, outdoor occupations such as forestry or military training, and collecting mushrooms, berries, or flowers. The risk is negligible for people who remain in urban or unforested areas and who do not consume unpasteurized dairy products.

Vector tick population density and infection rates in TBEV-endemic foci are highly variable. For example, TBEV infection rates in I. ricinus in central Europe vary from <0.1% to approximately 5%, depending on geographic location and time of year, while rates of up to 40% have been reported in I. persulcatus in Siberia. The number of TBE cases reported from a country depends on the ecology and geographic distribution of TBEV, the intensity of diagnosis and surveillance, and the vaccine coverage in the population. Therefore, the number of human TBE cases reported from an area may not be a reliable predictor of a traveler's risk for infection.

Since 2000, 5 cases of TBE among US travelers to Europe and China have been reported. TBE is not a nationally notifiable disease in the United States, and additional cases may have occurred. The same ticks that transmit TBEV can also transmit other pathogens, including Borrelia burgdorferi (the agent for Lyme disease), Anaplasma phagocytophilum (anaplasmosis), and Babesia spp. (babesiosis). Therefore, simultaneous infection with multiple organisms is possible.

CLINICAL PRESENTATION

Approximately two-thirds of infections are asymptomatic. The median incubation period for TBE is 8 days (range, 4–28 days). The incubation period for milkborne exposure is usually shorter (3–4 days). Acute neuroinvasive disease is the most commonly recognized clinical manifestation of TBEV infection. However, TBE disease often presents with milder forms of the disease or a biphasic course:

- First phase: nonspecific febrile illness with headache, myalgia, and fatigue. Usually lasts for several days and may be followed by an afebrile and relatively asymptomatic period. Up to two-thirds of patients may recover without any further illness.
- Second phase: central nervous system involvement resulting in aseptic meningitis, encephalitis, or myelitis. Cranial nerve involvement, bulbar syndrome, and acute flaccid paralysis of the upper extremities have also been described.

Among patients with central nervous system involvement, approximately 10% require intensive care and 5% need mechanical ventilation. Clinical course and long-term outcome vary by subtype of TBEV:

- The European subtype is associated with milder disease, a case-fatality ratio of <2%, and neurologic sequelae in up to 30% of patients.
- The Far Eastern subtype is often associated with a more severe disease course, including a case-fatality ratio of 20%–40% and higher rates of severe neurologic sequelae.
- The Siberian subtype is more frequently associated with chronic or progressive disease and has a case-fatality ratio of 2%–3%.

DIAGNOSIS

TBE should be suspected in travelers who develop a nonspecific febrile illness that progresses to neuroinvasive disease within 4 weeks of arriving from an endemic area. A history of tick bite may be a clue to this diagnosis; however, approximately 30% of TBE patients do not recall a tick bite.

Serology is typically used for laboratory diagnosis. IgM-capture ELISA performed on serum or cerebrospinal fluid is virtually always positive during the neuroinvasive phase of the illness. Vaccination history, date of onset of symptoms, and information regarding other flaviviruses known to circulate in the geographic area that may cross-react in serologic assays need to be considered when interpreting results. During the first phase of the illness, TBEV or TBEV RNA can sometimes be detected in serum samples by virus isolation or RT-PCR. However, by the time neurologic symptoms are recognized, the virus or viral RNA is usually undetectable. Therefore, virus isolation and RT-PCR should not be used to rule out a diagnosis of TBE. Clinicians should contact their state or local health department, CDC's Viral Special Pathogens Branch (404-639-1115), or CDC's Division of Vector-Borne Diseases (970-221-6400) for assistance with diagnostic testing.

TREATMENT

There is no specific antiviral treatment for TBE; therapy consists of supportive care and management of complications.

PREVENTIVE MEASURES FOR TRAVELERS
Personal Protection Measures

Travelers should avoid consuming unpasteurized dairy products and use all measures to avoid tick bites (see Chapter 2, Protection against Mosquitoes, Ticks, and Other Insects and Arthropods).

Vaccine

No TBE vaccines are licensed or available in the United States. Two safe, effective inactivated TBE vaccines are available in Europe, in adult and pediatric formulations: FSME-IMMUN (Baxter, Austria) and Encepur (Novartis, Germany). The adult formulation of FSME-IMMUN is also licensed in Canada. At least one other TBE vaccine is produced in Russia, but little information is available in the English literature regarding its safety and efficacy.

Immunogenicity studies suggest that the European vaccines, produced using the TBEV European subtype, should also provide cross-protection against the Far Eastern subtype. For both FSME-IMMUN and Encepur, the primary vaccination series consists of 3 doses (Table 3-19). The specific recommended intervals between doses vary by country and vaccine. Although no formal efficacy trials of these vaccines have been conducted, indirect evidence suggests that their efficacy is >95%. Vaccine failures have been reported, particularly in people aged ≥50 years. Regardless of age, the first booster dose should be given 3 years after the primary series. Recommended intervals for subsequent booster doses vary by age; boosters should be given every 5 years for people aged <50 years and every 3 years for those aged ≥50 years.

Because the routine primary vaccination series requires ≥6 months for completion, most travelers to TBE-endemic areas will find avoiding tick bites to be more practical than vaccination. However, an accelerated vaccination schedule has been evaluated for both European vaccines, and results in seroconversion rates are similar to those observed with the standard vaccination schedule. The first booster dose is administered at 3 years, according to the conventional schedule. Travelers anticipating high-risk exposures, such as working or camping in forested areas or farmland, adventure travel, or living in TBE-endemic countries for an extended period of time, may wish to be vaccinated in Canada or Europe.

Table 3-19. Tickborne encephalitis vaccination schedules[1,2]

| VACCINATION | AGE | VACCINATION SCHEDULES | | |
| | | CONVENTIONAL | ACCELERATED | |
			FSME-IMMUN[3]	ENCEPUR[4]
Primary series (3 doses)	≥1 year	0, 1–3 months, 6–15 months[5]	0, 14 days, 5–12 months[5]	0, 7, 21 days
First booster	≥1 year	3 years	3 years	12–18 months
Subsequent boosters	<50 years	5 years	5 years	5 years
	≥50 years	3 years	3 years	3 years

[1] Modified from Rendi-Wagner P. Advances in vaccination against tick-borne encephalitis. Expert Rev Vaccines. 2008 Jul;7(5):589–96.
[2] No TBE vaccines are licensed or available in the United States.
[3] Different formulation and dose for children aged 1–15 years.
[4] Different formulation and dose for children aged 1–11 years.
[5] Recommended interval for the third dose varies by country and vaccine.

BIBLIOGRAPHY

1. Barrett PN, Plotkin SA, Ehrlich HJ. Tick-borne encephalitis virus vaccines. In: Plotkin SA, Orenstein WA, Offit PA, editors. Vaccines. 5th ed. Philadelphia: Elsevier; 2008. p. 841–56.

2. CDC. Tick-borne encephalitis among US travelers to Europe and Asia—2000–2009. MMWR Morb Mortal Wkly Rep. 2010 Mar 26;59(11):335–8.

3. Committee to Advise on Tropical Medicine and Travel (CATMAT). Statement on tick-borne encephalitis. An Advisory Committee Statement (ACS). Can Commun Dis Rep. 2006 Apr 1;32(ACS-3):1–18.

4. Dumpis U, Crook D, Oksi J. Tick-borne encephalitis. Clin Infect Dis. 1999 Apr;28(4):882–90.

5. Haglund M, Gunther G. Tick-borne encephalitis—pathogenesis, clinical course and long-term follow-up. Vaccine. 2003 Apr 1;21 Suppl 1:S11–8.

6. Holzmann H. Diagnosis of tick-borne encephalitis. Vaccine. 2003 Apr 1;21 Suppl 1:S36–40.

7. Kaiser R. The clinical and epidemiological profile of tick-borne encephalitis in southern Germany 1994–98: a prospective study of 656 patients. Brain. 1999 Nov;122 (Pt 11):2067–78.

8. Kunz C. TBE vaccination and the Austrian experience. Vaccine. 2003 Apr 1;21 Suppl 1:S50–5.

9. Kunze U. Tick-borne encephalitis: from childhood to golden age does increased mobility mean increased risk? Conference report of the 11th meeting of the International Scientific Working Group on Tick-Borne Encephalitis (ISW-TBE). Vaccine. 2010 Jan 22;28(4):875–6.

10. Leonova GN, Ternovoi VA, Pavlenko EV, Maistrovskaya OS, Protopopova EV, Loktev VB. Evaluation of vaccine Encepur Adult for induction of human neutralizing antibodies against recent Far Eastern subtype strains of tick-borne encephalitis virus. Vaccine. 2007 Jan 15;25(5):895–901.

11. Lindquist L, Vapalahti O. Tick-borne encephalitis. Lancet. 2008 May 31;371(9627):1861–71.

12. Loew-Baselli A, Konior R, Pavlova BG, Fritsch S, Poellabauer E, Maritsch F, et al. Safety and immunogenicity of the modified adult tick-borne encephalitis vaccine FSME-IMMUN: results of two large phase 3 clinical studies. Vaccine. 2006 Jun 12;24(24):5256–63.

13. Lu Z, Broker M, Liang G. Tick-borne encephalitis in mainland China. Vector Borne Zoonotic Dis. 2008 Oct;8(5):713–20.

14. Rendi-Wagner P. Advances in vaccination against tick-borne encephalitis. Expert Rev Vaccines. 2008 Jul;7(5):589–96.

15. Rendi-Wagner P. Risk and prevention of tick-borne encephalitis in travelers. J Travel Med. 2004 Sep–Oct;11(5):307–12.

16. Schoendorf I, Ternak G, Oroszlan G, Nicolay U, Banzhoff A, Zent O. Tick-born encephalitis (TBE) vaccination in children: advantage of the rapid immunization schedule (ie, days 0, 7, 21). Hum Vaccin. 2007 Mar–Apr;3(2):42–7.

17. Schondorf I, Beran J, Cizkova D, Lesna V, Banzhoff A, Zent O. Tick-borne encephalitis (TBE) vaccination: applying the most suitable vaccination schedule. Vaccine. 2007 Feb 9;25(8):1470–5.

18. Suss J. Tick-borne encephalitis in Europe and beyond—the epidemiological situation as of 2007. Euro Surveill. 2008 Jun 26;13(26).

19. Zent O, Broker M. Tick-borne encephalitis vaccines: past and present. Expert Rev Vaccines. 2005 Oct;4(5):747–55.

TOXOPLASMOSIS
Jeffrey L. Jones

③

INFECTIOUS AGENT

Toxoplasma gondii is an intracellular coccidian protozoan parasite of humans and warm-blooded animals that completes the sexual phase of its life cycle in cats.

MODE OF TRANSMISSION

Toxoplasmosis is transmitted by the following:

- Ingestion of oocysts in cat feces or soil or water contaminated with cat feces
- Ingestion of undercooked meat
- Congenitally when a woman becomes infected during pregnancy
- Blood transfusion and organ transplantation

EPIDEMIOLOGY

Human infection with *T. gondii* occurs worldwide. The prevalence in adults ranges from <10% to >90%; higher prevalences tend to occur at lower elevations and in latitudes closer to the equator. The risk for infection is higher in many developing and tropical countries, especially when people eat undercooked meat, drink untreated water, or are extensively exposed to soil.

CLINICAL PRESENTATION

The incubation period is 5–23 days. Acute infection in children and adults with normal immunity is often asymptomatic. When illness occurs, it is usually mild with influenzalike symptoms (such as tender lymph nodes and muscle aches) that last for several weeks. An infectious mononucleosislike syndrome has been described in febrile returning travelers, characterized by prolonged fever, lymphadenopathy, elevated liver enzymes, lymphocytosis, and weakness. Among acutely infected people, 0.5%–2% develop ocular disease, usually retinochoroiditis; symptoms include blurred vision, pain, photophobia, tearing, and loss of vision. Higher rates of ocular disease have been described in southern Brazil.

In severely immunosuppressed people, including those with HIV infection, severe and even fatal toxoplasmic encephalitis, pneumonitis, and other systemic illnesses can occur, most often from reactivation of a previous infection. Immunosuppressed people with HIV infection are routinely prescribed prophylactic medication active against *T. gondii*.

In 70%–90% of cases, infants with congenital toxoplasmosis are asymptomatic or have mild symptoms not recognized at birth. However, learning disabilities, mental retardation, or visual impairment often occur later in life. Congenital infection can result in maculopapular rash, generalized lymphadenopathy, hepatomegaly, splenomegaly, jaundice, and thrombocytopenia. In addition, hydrocephalus, microcephaly, seizures, retinochoroiditis, and deafness can occur. Cerebral calcifications may be seen on radiography or ultrasonography of the head.

DIAGNOSIS

Acutely infected children and adults are diagnosed by serologic testing for *T. gondii* antibodies (*Toxoplasma*-specific IgM and IgG). Ocular disease is diagnosed by characteristic retinal lesions and serum testing for *T. gondii* antibodies; ocular fluid can also be tested for *T. gondii* antibodies.

Immunosuppressed people are diagnosed by serologic testing (usually but not always

Toxoplasma IgG positive), typical clinical course, and identification of 1 or more mass lesions by CT, MRI, or other radiographic testing. Biopsy may be needed to make a definitive diagnosis.

To determine infection status and help estimate the timing of infection in pregnant women, serologic testing at a *Toxoplasma* reference laboratory is recommended (for example, IgM, IgG, avidity, and at some laboratories, differential agglutination [AC/HS test], IgA, and IgE). Some commercial IgM tests have high false-positive rates. Fetal and congenital infections often require PCR and reference laboratory assistance for diagnosis.

TREATMENT

Pyrimethamine and sulfadiazine are the mainstays of treatment in adults. Ocular disease should be treated in consultation with an ophthalmologist. Corticosteroids may be added to regimens of pyrimethamine, sulfadiazine, and leucovorin (or other combinations of drugs active against *T. gondii*) when retinochoroiditis threatens vision. Immunosuppressed people with active toxoplasmosis should be treated in consultation with a physician experienced in treating immunosuppressed people. Toxoplasmosis during pregnancy and congenital infection in the infant should be treated in consultation with fetal medicine and pediatric specialists.

PREVENTIVE MEASURES FOR TRAVELERS

Travelers should be advised to do the following:

- Cook meat to safe temperatures (≥160°F [71°C] throughout).

- Peel or wash fruits and vegetables thoroughly before eating.
- Wash cutting boards, dishes, counters, utensils, and hands with hot, soapy water after contact with raw meat or with unwashed fruits or vegetables.
- Freeze meat for several days before cooking to reduce chance of infection.
- Wear gloves when gardening and during any contact with soil or sand, because soil or sand might be contaminated with cat feces that contain *T. gondii*. Wash hands thoroughly after gardening or contact with soil or sand.
- Avoid drinking untreated water. *T. gondii* is not killed by chlorine levels used for water treatment, so in developing countries water must be treated and adequately filtered or boiled; alternatively, use safe bottled water.
- Change the litter box daily. *T. gondii* does not become infectious until 1–5 days after it is shed in a cat's feces.

Pregnant or immunocompromised people should take the following additional precautions:

- Avoid changing cat litter if possible. If no one else can perform the task, wear disposable gloves and wash hands thoroughly with soap and water afterward.
- Keep cats indoors.
- Do not adopt or handle stray cats, especially kittens. While pregnant, do not get a new cat.
- Feed cats only canned or dried commercial food or well-cooked table food, not raw or undercooked meats.
- Keep outdoor sandboxes covered.

BIBLIOGRAPHY

1. Abramowicz M. Drugs for Parasitic Infections. New Rochelle (NY): The Medical Letter, Inc; 2007.
2. Bottieau E, Clerinx J, Van den Enden E, Van Esbroeck M, Colebunders R, Van Gompel A, et al. Infectious mononucleosis-like syndromes in febrile travelers returning from the tropics. J Travel Med. 2006 Jul–Aug;13(4):191–7.
3. CDC. Toxoplasmosis. Atlanta: CDC. Available from: http://www.cdc.gov/toxoplasmosis.
4. Kaplan JE, Benson C, Holmes KH, Brooks JT, Pau A, Masur H. Guidelines for prevention and treatment of opportunistic infections in HIV-infected adults and adolescents: recommendations from CDC, the National Institutes of Health, and the HIV Medicine Association of the Infectious Diseases Society of America. MMWR Recomm Rep. 2009 Apr 10;58(RR-4):1–207.
5. Montoya JG, Liesenfeld O. Toxoplasmosis. Lancet. 2004 Jun 12;363(9425):1965–76.
6. Montoya JG, Remington JS. Management of *Toxoplasma gondii* infection during pregnancy. Clin Infect Dis. 2008 Aug 15;47(4):554–66.

TRYPANOSOMIASIS, AFRICAN (HUMAN AFRICAN TRYPANOSOMIASIS, AFRICAN SLEEPING SICKNESS)

Anne Moore

INFECTIOUS AGENT

Two subspecies of the protozoan parasite *Trypanosoma brucei* (*T. b. rhodesiense* and *T. b. gambiense*) cause infection.

MODE OF TRANSMISSION

Infection occurs through vectorborne transmission by the bite of an infected tsetse fly (*Glossina* spp.). Transmission via bloodborne or congenital routes can occur but is rarely reported.

EPIDEMIOLOGY

Human African trypanosomiasis (HAT), or African sleeping sickness, is transmitted only in rural sub-Saharan Africa. The 2 human-infective subspecies of *T. brucei* do not overlap in geographic distribution. *T. b. rhodesiense* is found in eastern and southeastern Africa. More than 95% of the cases of *T. b. rhodesiense* infection occur in Tanzania, Uganda, Malawi, and Zambia. *T. b. gambiense* is found predominately in central Africa and in limited areas of West Africa. More than 95% of the cases of *T. b. gambiense* infection are reported from the Democratic Republic of the Congo, Angola, Sudan, Central African Republic, Republic of the Congo, Chad, and northern Uganda.

Infection of international travelers occurs but is rare. On average, a single case per year is reported among US travelers. Most infections in US travelers are caused by *T. b. rhodesiense* and are acquired in East Africa game parks.

Tsetse flies inhabit rural areas, living in the woodlands and thickets of the savannah and the dense vegetation along streams. Less than 1% of flies are infected in a typical endemic area. Tsetse flies bite during daylight hours. Most bites that occur on the African savannah are quite painful, and travelers often recall the bite. Travelers to urban areas are not at risk.

CLINICAL PRESENTATION

Presentation is variable and depends on the infecting subspecies. Infection with *T. b. rhodesiense* is more acute clinically and progresses more rapidly than *T. b. gambiense*. Symptoms and signs of *T. b. rhodesiense* infection generally appear within 1–3 weeks of the infective bite. These may include high fever, a chancre at the site of the infective bite, skin rash, headache, myalgia, thrombocytopenia, and less commonly, splenomegaly, renal failure, or cardiac dysfunction. Central nervous system involvement can occur within the first month of infection.

Symptoms of *T. b. gambiense* infection are nonspecific, and patients may remain paucisymptomatic for many months after infection. Symptoms and signs may include fever, headache, malaise, myalgia, facial edema, pruritus, lymphadenopathy, and weight loss. Central nervous system involvement occurs after months of infection and is characterized by somnolence, severe headache, and a wide range of neurologic manifestations, including mood disorders, behavior change, focal deficits, and endocrine disorders. Untreated HAT is eventually fatal.

DIAGNOSIS

Diagnosis is made by microscopic identification of parasites in specimens of blood, chancre fluid or tissue, lymph node aspirate, or cerebrospinal fluid. Buffy-coat preparations concentrate the parasite. Parasitemias are higher in *T. b. rhodesiense* than in *T. b. gambiense* infection. Serologic tests are not helpful for diagnosis of *T. b. rhodesiense*. CDC can help arrange serologic testing for *T. b. gambiense*, which is not available in the United States. Diagnostic assistance is available through CDC's Division of Parasitic Diseases and Malaria (www.dpd.cdc.gov/dpdx).

TREATMENT

Travelers who sustain tsetse fly bites and become ill with high fever or other manifestations of HAT are advised to seek early medical attention. The infection can usually be cured by a course of antitrypanosomal therapy. Imported HAT is rare in the United States, and inexperienced physicians should consult with an infectious disease or tropical medicine specialist for diagnosis and treatment. Physicians can consult with CDC for assistance with diagnosis and clinical management (770-488-7775, ncidpbdpi@cdc.gov). Treatment drugs (suramin, melarsoprol, eflornithine) are provided by CDC under investigational protocols.

PREVENTIVE MEASURES FOR TRAVELERS

No vaccine or drug for prophylaxis is available. Preventive measures are aimed at reducing contact with tsetse flies. Areas of heavy infestation tend to be sporadically distributed and are usually well known to local residents. Avoidance of these areas is the best means of protection.

Tsetse flies are attracted to moving vehicles and bright, dark colors. The flies can bite through light-weight clothing. Travelers are advised to wear clothing of wrist and ankle length made of medium-weight fabric in neutral colors that blend with the background environment for the best means of protection. Data are limited but suggest that permethrin-impregnated clothing and use of DEET repellent may minimally reduce the number of fly bites. Regardless, use of repellents can reduce bites of mosquitoes and other insects and arthropods, which helps protect against other infectious diseases.

BIBLIOGRAPHY

1. Braakman HM, van de Molengraft FJ, Hubert WW, Boerman DH. Lethal African trypanosomiasis in a traveler: MRI and neuropathology. Neurology. 2006 Apr 11;66(7):1094–6.
2. Brun R, Blum J, Chappuis F, Burri C. Human African trypanosomiasis. Lancet. 2010 Jan 9;375(9709):148–59.
3. Moore AC, Ryan ET, Waldron MA. Case records of the Massachusetts General Hospital. Weekly clinicopathological exercises. Case 20-2002. A 37-year-old man with fever, hepatosplenomegaly, and a cutaneous foot lesion after a trip to Africa. N Engl J Med. 2002 Jun 27;346(26):2069–76.
4. Moore DA, Edwards M, Escombe R, Agranoff D, Bailey JW, Squire SB, et al. African trypanosomiasis in travelers returning to the United Kingdom. Emerg Infect Dis. 2002 Jan;8(1):74–6.
5. Sholdt LL, Schreck CE, Mwangelwa MI, Nondo J, Siachinji VJ. Evaluations of permethrin-impregnated clothing and three topical repellent formulations of deet against tsetse flies in Zambia. Med Vet Entomol. 1989 Apr;3(2):153–8.

TRYPANOSOMIASIS, AMERICAN (CHAGAS DISEASE)

Alicia I. Hidron, Carlos Franco-Paredes

INFECTIOUS AGENT

American trypanosomiasis is caused by the protozoan parasite, *Trypanosoma cruzi*.

MODE OF TRANSMISSION

Infection occurs through vectorborne transmission in endemic countries via the feces of the triatomine insect (reduviid bug), which may be inadvertently inoculated into the skin or the mucosa of the eyes, nose, or mouth when the insect's bite is scratched and rubbed. Infection may also be transmitted through blood transfusion or organ transplantation, from mother to infant, by consuming contaminated food or beverages (including fruit juices), and through occupational exposure in laboratory workers.

EPIDEMIOLOGY

Approximately 7.6 million people have Chagas disease, according to the most recent estimates.

The disease is endemic in Mexico and Central and South America. Rare cases of Chagas disease attributed to local vectorborne transmission have been reported in the United States, but it is more commonly found in nonendemic areas as a result of immigration. In fact, Chagas disease is considered a globalized disease because of immigration from endemic to nonendemic zones; it has been identified through blood banks or other screening programs.

No cases have been documented of Chagas disease acquired during travel; the risk of acquiring Chagas disease while traveling is assumed to be extremely low. Travelers could be at risk for Chagas disease if staying in poor-quality housing (for example, mud walls with cracks) in endemic areas. Chagas disease could be acquired through blood transfusion in areas with poor screening or by consuming contaminated food or beverages.

CLINICAL PRESENTATION

The acute phase of Chagas disease lasts up to 90 days, followed by asymptomatic chronic infection, usually undetectable by parasitologic methods. Most infected people never develop symptoms but remain infected throughout their lives. People with chronic infection but without signs or symptoms are considered to have the indeterminate form of Chagas disease. This is the most common clinical presentation in nonendemic areas where patients are incidentally diagnosed through blood donation. Those who develop acute illness will do so 1 week or more after exposure. A chagoma may develop, which is an area of edema and erythema at the site of infection; the classic picture is the Romaña sign, which presents as edema of the eyelid and ocular tissues when the entry site was the conjunctiva. Approximately 20%–30% of infected patients will develop manifestations of chronic Chagas disease, usually involving the heart. Clinical signs include conduction system abnormalities, ventricular arrhythmias, and in late-stage disease, congestive cardiomyopathy. Less commonly, chronic gastrointestinal problems may ensue when Chagas causes megaesophagus or megacolon. Reactivation disease can occur in immunocompromised patients.

DIAGNOSIS

Diagnosis requires consideration of both test results and patient exposure history. During the acute phase, parasites may be detectable in fresh preparations of buffy coat or stained peripheral blood specimens. After the acute phase, diagnosis relies on the use of 2 or more different serologic tests (most commonly, ELISA and the immunofluorescent antibody test). Infected people should be evaluated for symptoms and signs of cardiac and gastrointestinal disease.

TREATMENT

Clinicians should consult with an infectious disease or tropical medicine specialist to diagnose and treat Chagas disease. Antitrypanosomal drug treatment is always recommended for acute, early congenital, and reactivated T. cruzi infection and for chronic T. cruzi infection in children up to 18 years old. In adults, treatment is usually recommended, based on recent data suggesting that a course of antitrypanosomal treatment delays progression of cardiomyopathy and decreases mortality.

In the United States, the only source of the antitrypanosomal drugs, benznidazole and nifurtimox, is through CDC. The drugs are not licensed in the United States and are provided only under investigational new drug protocols. Clinicians should contact the CDC's Parasitic Diseases public inquiries line (770-448-7775), the CDC Drug Service (404-639-3670), or outside business hours, the CDC Emergency Operations Center (770-488-7100). CDC also provides guidance on diagnostic testing and clinical evaluation.

PREVENTIVE MEASURES FOR TRAVELERS

No vaccine is available. Preventive measures include insecticide spraying of sleeping quarters or infested houses. Travelers who cannot avoid camping, sleeping outdoors, or sleeping in poorly constructed houses in endemic areas should use insecticide-impregnated bed nets and tuck in the edges to provide a physical barrier to the vectors. Compliance with food and water precautions in endemic areas is also recommended to prevent the extremely rare occurrence of foodborne Chagas disease. Blood transfusion and organ transplantation should be avoided in travelers visiting or living in endemic countries, if at all possible, unless urgently or emergently required (see Chapter 2, Medical Tourism).

BIBLIOGRAPHY

1. Bern C, Montgomery SP, Herwaldt BL, Rassi A Jr, Marin-Neto JA, Dantas RO, et al. Evaluation and treatment of Chagas disease in the United States: a systematic review. JAMA. 2007 Nov 14;298(18):2171–81.
2. CDC. Chagas disease after organ transplantation—United States, 2001. MMWR Morb Mortal Wkly Rep. 2002 Mar 15;51(10):210–2.
3. Dias JC. The indeterminate form of human chronic Chagas' disease A clinical epidemiological review. Rev Soc Bras Med Trop. 1989 Jul–Sep;22(3):147–56.
4. Dorn PL, Perniciaro L, Yabsley MJ, Roellig DM, Balsamo G, Diaz J, et al. Autochthonous transmission of *Trypanosoma cruzi*, Louisiana. Emerg Infect Dis. 2007 Apr;13(4):605–7.
5. Magill AJ, Reed SG. American trypanosomiasis. In: Strickland GT, editor. Hunter's Tropical Medicine and Emerging Infectious Diseases. 8th ed. Philadelphia: WB Saunders Company; 2000. p. 653–64.
6. ProMED-mail. Trypanosomiasis, foodborne—Brazil (Santa Catarina). 2005 [updated Mar 27]. Available from: http://www.promedmail.org.
7. Rassi A Jr, Rassi A, Little WC. Chagas' heart disease. Clin Cardiol. 2000 Dec;23(12):883–9.
8. Rassi A Jr, Rassi A, Marin-Neto JA. Chagas disease. Lancet. 2010 Apr 17;375(9723):1388–402.
9. Schmunis GA. Epidemiology of Chagas disease in non-endemic countries: the role of international migration. Mem Inst Oswaldo Cruz. 2007 Oct 30;102 Suppl 1:75–85.
10. Schmunis GA, Cruz JR. Safety of the blood supply in Latin America. Clin Microbiol Rev. 2005 Jan;18(1):12–29.

TUBERCULOSIS
Philip LoBue

INFECTIOUS AGENT

Mycobacterium tuberculosis is a rod-shaped, nonmotile, acid-fast bacterium.

MODE OF TRANSMISSION

Tuberculosis (TB) transmission occurs when a contagious patient coughs, spreading bacilli through the air. Bovine TB (caused by the closely related *Mycobacterium bovis*) can be transmitted by consuming contaminated, unpasteurized dairy products from infected cattle.

EPIDEMIOLOGY

Globally, more than 9 million new TB cases and nearly 2 million TB-related deaths occur each year. TB occurs throughout the world, but the incidence varies (see Map 3-15). In the United States, the annual incidence is approximately 4 per 100,000 population, but in some countries in sub-Saharan Africa and Asia, the annual incidence is several hundred per 100,000.

Drug-resistant TB is of increasing concern. Multidrug-resistant (MDR) TB is resistant to the 2 most effective drugs, isoniazid and rifampin. Extensively drug-resistant (XDR) TB is resistant to isoniazid and rifampin, any fluoroquinolone, and at least 1 of 3 injectable second-line drugs (amikacin, kanamycin, or capreomycin). MDR TB is less common than drug-susceptible TB, but nearly 500,000 new cases of MDR TB are diagnosed each year, and some countries have proportions of MDR TB as high as 20% (see Map 3-16). MDR and XDR TB are of particular concern among HIV-infected or other immunocompromised people. As of early 2010, XDR TB had been reported in 58 countries (see Map 3-17).

Travelers who anticipate possible prolonged exposure to TB (such as those who would spend time in hospitals, prisons, or homeless shelters) or those who stay for years in an endemic country should have a 2-step tuberculin skin test (TST) or a single interferon-γ release assay (IGRA), either the QuantiFERON TB test (Gold or Gold In-Tube versions) or T-SPOT.TB test, before leaving the United States (see Chapter 3, Perspectives: Tuberculin Skin Testing of Travelers). If the predeparture test result is negative, a single TST or IGRA should be repeated 8–10 weeks after returning from travel. Because people with HIV infection or other immunocompromising conditions are more likely to have an impaired response to the test, travelers should inform their physicians about such conditions. Except for travelers with impaired immunity, travelers who have already been infected are unlikely to be reinfected.

The risk of TB transmission on an airplane does not appear to be higher than in any other enclosed space. To prevent TB transmission on airplanes, people who have infectious TB should not travel by commercial airplanes or other commercial conveyances. The World Health Organization (WHO) has issued guidelines for notifying passengers who might have been exposed to TB aboard airplanes. Passengers concerned about possible exposure to TB should see their primary health care provider for evaluation.

Bovine TB (M. bovis) is a risk in travelers who consume unpasteurized dairy products in countries where M. bovis in cattle is common. Mexico is a common place of infection for US travelers.

CLINICAL PRESENTATION

TB disease can affect any organ but most commonly occurs in the lungs (70%–80%). Common TB symptoms include prolonged cough, fever, anorexia, weight loss, night sweats, and hemoptysis. The most common types of extrapulmonary disease include lymphadenitis, pleuritis, bone and joint disease, meningitis, and genitourinary disease.

Infection is manifested by a positive TST or IGRA result, which usually occurs 8–10 weeks after exposure. Overall, only 5%–10% people progress from infection to disease during their lifetime. In the remainder, the infection remains in a latent state (latent TB infection or LTBI). However, the risk of progression is much higher in immunosuppressed people (8%–10% per year in HIV-infected people not receiving antiretroviral therapy). In recent years, people who are receiving tumor necrosis factor α inhibitors to treat rheumatoid arthritis and other chronic inflammatory conditions have also been found to be at increased risk for disease progression. LTBI is an asymptomatic condition, and people with LTBI do not transmit TB. Progression to disease can occur weeks to decades after initial infection.

DIAGNOSIS

Diagnosis of TB disease is confirmed by culturing M. tuberculosis from sputum or other respiratory specimens for pulmonary TB and from other affected body tissues or fluids for extrapulmonary TB. On average, it takes about 2 weeks to culture and identify M. tuberculosis, even with rapid culture techniques. A preliminary diagnosis of TB can be made when acid-fast bacilli are seen on sputum smear or in other body tissues or fluids. However, microscopy cannot distinguish between M. tuberculosis and nontuberculous mycobacteria. This is particularly problematic in countries such as the United States where the incidence is low. Nucleic acid amplification tests are more rapid than culture and specific for M. tuberculosis. They are also more sensitive than the acid-fast bacilli smear but less sensitive than culture. A diagnosis of TB disease can be made by using clinical criteria in the absence of microbiologic confirmation. LTBI is diagnosed by a positive TST or IGRA.

TREATMENT

People with LTBI can be treated to prevent progression to TB disease. American Thoracic Society (ATS)/CDC guidelines for treatment of LTBI recommend 9 months of isoniazid as the preferred treatment and suggest that 4 months of rifampin is a reasonable alternative. Travelers who suspect that they have been exposed to TB should inform their health care provider of the possible exposure and receive medical evaluation. CDC and ATS have published guidelines for targeted testing and treatment of LTBI. Recent data from WHO suggest that drug resistance is relatively common in some parts of the world. Travelers who have TST or IGRA conversion associated with international travel should consult experts in infectious diseases or pulmonary medicine.

TB disease is treated with a multiple-drug regimen for 6–9 months (usually isoniazid, rifampin, ethambutol, and pyrazinamide for 2 months, followed by isoniazid and rifampin for 4 months) if the TB is not MDR TB. MDR TB treatment is more difficult, requiring 4–6 drugs for 18–24 months; it should be managed by an expert in MDR TB. ATS/CDC/Infectious Diseases Society of America have published guidelines on TB treatment.

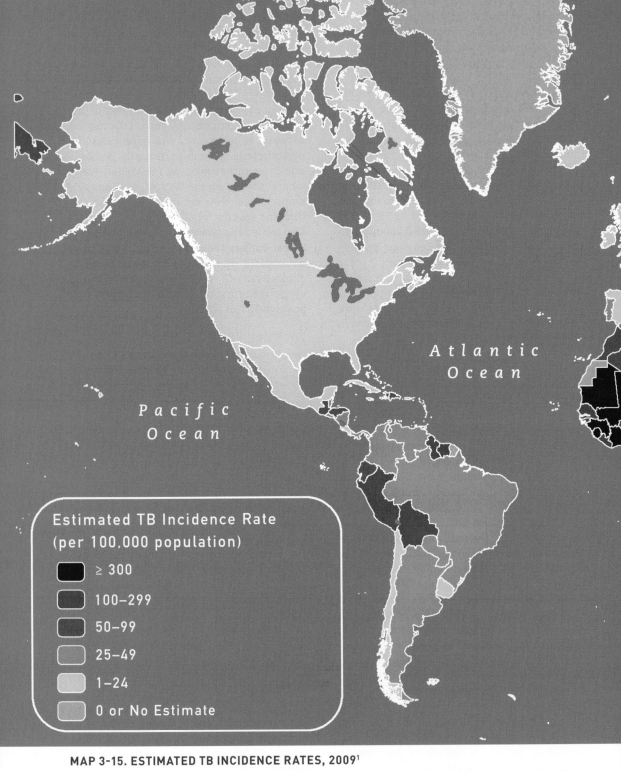

**Estimated TB Incidence Rate
(per 100,000 population)**

- ≥ 300
- 100–299
- 50–99
- 25–49
- 1–24
- 0 or No Estimate

MAP 3-15. ESTIMATED TB INCIDENCE RATES, 2009[1]

[1] Data from World Health Organization. Global tuberculosis control: WHO report 2010. Geneva: World Health Organization; 2010.

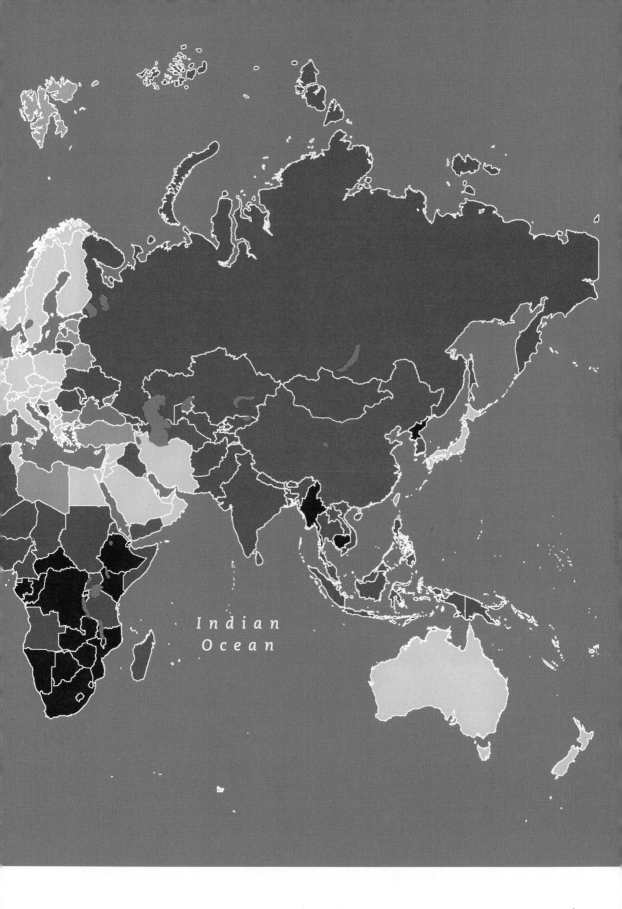

Indian
Ocean

INFECTIOUS DISEASES RELATED TO TRAVEL

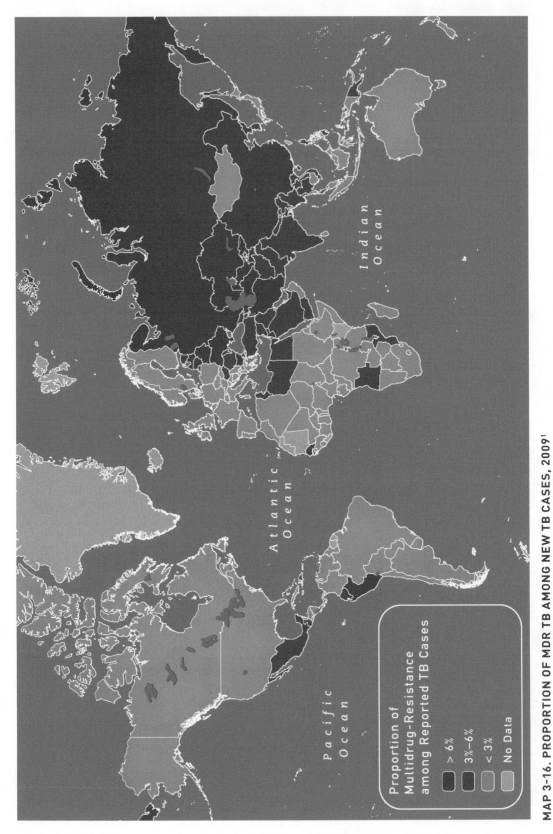

MAP 3-16. PROPORTION OF MDR TB AMONG NEW TB CASES, 2009[1]

[1] Data from the World Health Organization's Global tuberculosis database. Available from: www.who.int/tb/country/data/download/en/index.html.

TUBERCULIN SKIN TESTING OF TRAVELERS
Philip LoBue

Screening for asymptomatic tuberculosis (TB) infections should only be carried out among travelers who will be at significant risk of acquiring TB (see the preceding section on Tuberculosis). Screening with a tuberculin skin test (TST) in a very low-risk population may result in a false-positive test, leading to unnecessary additional screening or unnecessary treatment. Using even highly sensitive and specific tests in very low-prevalence populations will produce more false positives than true positives.

Therefore, the TST should be considered only for travelers who are spending years in a country with a high risk of TB, or for those traveling for any length of time who will come in contact routinely with hospital, prison, or homeless shelter populations. The general recommendation is that people at low risk for TB, which includes most travelers, do not need to be screened before or after travel.

For travelers who anticipate a long stay or contact with a high-risk population, careful pre-travel screening should be carried out, with use of 2-step TST screening. For 2-step TSTs, people whose baseline TSTs yield a negative result are retested 1–3 weeks after the initial test; if the second test result is negative, they are considered not infected. If the second test result is positive, they are classified as having had previous TB infection. The 2-step TST is recommended in this population for the following reasons:

- The use of 2-step testing can reduce the number of positive TSTs that would otherwise be misclassified as recent skin test conversions during future periodic screenings.
- Certain people who were infected with *Mycobacterium tuberculosis* years earlier exhibit waning delayed-type hypersensitivity to tuberculin. When they are skin tested years after infection, they might have a false-negative TST result (even though they are truly infected). However, the first TST might stimulate the ability to react to subsequent tests, resulting in a "booster" reaction. When the test is repeated, the reaction might be misinterpreted as a new infection (recent conversion) rather than a boosted reaction.

Two-step testing is important for travelers who will have potential prolonged TB exposure. Two-step testing before travel will detect boosting and potentially prevent "false conversions"—positive TST results that appear to indicate infection acquired during travel, but which are really the result of previous TB infection. This distinction is particularly important if the traveler is going to a country where extensively drug-resistant TB (XDR TB) is rampant: it would be critical to know whether the person's skin test had been positive before travel.

If the 2-step TST result is negative, the traveler should have a repeat TST 8–10 weeks after returning from the trip, or as part of a periodic screening examination for those who remain at high risk. Two-step testing should be considered for the baseline testing of people who report no history of a recent TST and who will receive repeated TSTs as part of ongoing monitoring.

People who have had repeat TSTs must be tested with the same commercial antigen, since switching antigens can also lead to false TST conversions. Two commercial tuberculin skin test antigens are approved by the Food and Drug Administration (FDA) and are commercially available in the United States: Aplisol (JHP Pharmaceuticals) and Tubersol (Sanofi Pasteur).

An alternative to 2-step TST is a single FDA-approved interferon-γ release assay (IGRA), either the QuantiFERON TB test (Gold or Gold In-Tube versions) or T-SPOT.TB test. IGRAs are approximately as specific as TST in people who are not vaccinated with Bacillus Calmette-Guérin and much more specific in vaccinated populations. For a traveler whose time before departure is short, a single-step TST would be an acceptable alternative if there were insufficient time for the 2-step TST and the IGRAs were not available.

In general, it is best not to mix tests. There is approximately 15% discordance between TST and IGRA, usually with the TST positive and the IGRA negative. There are multiple reasons for the discordance, and in any person it is often difficult to be confident about the reason for discordance. However, if the clinician decides to mix tests, it is better to go from TST to IGRA than the other way around, because the likelihood of having a discordant result with the TST negative and the IGRA positive is much lower. Such discordant results may become unavoidable as more medical establishments switch from TSTs to IGRAs.

The use of TST among those visiting friends and relatives in TB-endemic areas should take into account the high rate of TST positivity in this population. In a study among 53,000 adults in Tennessee, the prevalence of a positive TST among the foreign born was 11 times that of the US born (34% vs 3%). Confirming TST status before travel would prevent the conclusion that a positive TST after travel was due to recent conversion.

BIBLIOGRAPHY

1. Al-Jahdali H, Memish ZA, Menzies D. Tuberculosis in association with travel. Int J Antimicrob Agents. 2003 Feb;21(2):125–30.

2. Cobelens FG, van Deutekom H, Draayer-Jansen IW, Schepp-Beelen AC, van Gerven PJ, van Kessel RP, et al. Risk of infection with Mycobacterium tuberculosis in travellers to areas of high tuberculosis endemicity. Lancet. 2000 Aug 5;356(9228):461–5.

3. Haley CA, Cain KP, Yu C, Garman KF, Wells CD, Laserson KF. Risk-based screening for latent tuberculosis infection. South Med J. 2008 Feb;101(2):142–9.

4. Johnston VJ, Grant AD. Tuberculosis in travellers. Travel Med Infect Dis. 2003 Nov;1(4):205–12.

5. Jung P, Banks RH. Tuberculosis risk in US Peace Corps volunteers, 1996 to 2005. J Travel Med. 2008 Mar–Apr;15(2):87–94.

6. Leder K, Tong S, Weld L, Kain KC, Wilder-Smith A, von Sonnenburg F, et al. Illness in travelers visiting friends and relatives: a review of the GeoSentinel Surveillance Network. Clin Infect Dis. 2006 Nov 1;43(9):1185–93.

7. Mancuso JD, Tobler SK, Keep LW. Pseudoepidemics of tuberculin skin test conversions in the US Army after recent deployments. Am J Respir Crit Care Med. 2008 Jun 1;177(11):1285–9.

8. Mazurek M, Jereb J, Vernon A, LoBue P, Goldberg S, Castro K. Updated guidelines for using interferon gamma release assays to detect Mycobacterium tuberculosis infection—United States, 2010. MMWR Recomm Rep. 2010 Jun 25;59(RR-5):1–25.

9. Villarino ME, Burman W, Wang YC, Lundergan L, Catanzaro A, Bock N, et al. Comparable specificity of 2 commercial tuberculin reagents in persons at low risk for tuberculous infection. JAMA. 1999 Jan 13;281(2):169–71.

TYPHOID & PARATYPHOID FEVER

Achuyt Bhattarai, Eric Mintz

INFECTIOUS AGENT

Typhoid fever is an acute, life-threatening febrile illness caused by the bacterium *Salmonella enterica* serotype Typhi. Paratyphoid fever is a similar illness caused by S. Paratyphi A, B, or C.

MODE OF TRANSMISSION

Humans are the only source of these bacteria; no animal or environmental reservoirs have been identified. Typhoid and paratyphoid fever are most often acquired through consumption of water or food that has been contaminated by feces of an acutely infected or convalescent person or a chronic, asymptomatic carrier. Transmission through sexual contact, especially among men who have sex with men, has rarely been documented.

EPIDEMIOLOGY

An estimated 22 million cases of typhoid fever and 200,000 related deaths occur worldwide each year; an additional 6 million cases of paratyphoid fever are estimated to occur annually. Approximately 300 cases of typhoid fever and 150 cases of paratyphoid fever are reported each year in the United States, most of which are in recent travelers. The risk of typhoid fever is highest for travelers to southern Asia (6–30 times higher than for all other destinations). Other areas of risk include East and Southeast Asia, Africa, the Caribbean, and Central and South America. The risk of paratyphoid fever is also increasing among travelers to southern and Southeast Asia.

Travelers to southern Asia are at highest risk for infections that are nalidixic acid–resistant or multidrug-resistant (resistant to ampicillin, chloramphenicol, and trimethoprim-sulfamethoxazole). Travelers who are visiting friends and relatives (VFRs) are at increased risk (see Chapter 8, Immigrants Returning Home to Visit Friends and Relatives). Although the risk of acquiring typhoid or paratyphoid fever increases with the duration of stay, travelers have acquired typhoid fever even during visits <1 week to countries where the disease is endemic.

CLINICAL PRESENTATION

The incubation period of typhoid and paratyphoid infections is 6–30 days. The onset of illness is insidious, with gradually increasing fatigue and a fever that increases daily from low-grade to as high as 102°F–104°F (38°C–40°C) by the third to fourth day of illness. Headache, malaise, and anorexia are nearly universal. Hepatosplenomegaly can often be detected. A transient, macular rash of rose-colored spots can occasionally be seen on the trunk. Fever is commonly lowest in the morning, reaching a peak in late afternoon or evening. Untreated, the disease can last for a month. The serious complications of typhoid fever generally occur after 2–3 weeks of illness and may include intestinal hemorrhage or perforation, which can be life threatening.

DIAGNOSIS

Infection with typhoid or paratyphoid fever results in a very low-grade septicemia. A single blood culture is positive in only half the cases. Stool culture is not usually positive during the acute phase of the disease. Bone marrow culture increases the diagnostic yield to about 80% of cases.

The Widal test is an old serologic assay for detecting IgM and IgG to the O and H antigens of salmonella. The test is unreliable but is widely used in developing countries because of its low cost. Newer serologic assays are somewhat more sensitive and specific than the Widal test but are infrequently available.

Because there is no definitive serologic test for typhoid or paratyphoid fever, the diagnosis often has to be made clinically. The combination of a history of risk for infection and a gradual onset of fever that increases in severity over several days should raise suspicion of typhoid or paratyphoid fever.

TREATMENT

Specific antimicrobial therapy shortens the clinical course of typhoid fever and reduces the risk for death. Empiric treatment in most parts of the world would use a fluoroquinolone, most often ciprofloxacin. However, resistance to fluoroquinolones is highest in the Indian subcontinent and increasing in other areas. Injectable third-generation cephalosporins are often the empiric drug of choice when the possibility of fluoroquinolone resistance is high.

Patients treated with an appropriate antibiotic may still require 3–5 days to defervesce completely, although the height of the fever decreases each day. Patients may actually feel worse when the fever starts to go away. If fever does not subside within 5 days, alternative antimicrobial agents or other foci of infection should be considered.

PREVENTIVE MEASURES FOR TRAVELERS
Vaccine
Indications for Use

CDC recommends typhoid vaccine for travelers to areas where there is an increased risk of exposure to S. Typhi. The typhoid vaccines do not protect against S. Paratyphi infection. Both typhoid vaccines protect 50%–80% of recipients; travelers should be reminded that typhoid immunization is not 100% effective, and typhoid fever could still occur. Two typhoid vaccines are available in the United States:

- Oral live, attenuated vaccine (Vivotif vaccine, manufactured from the Ty21a strain of S. Typhi by Crucell/Berna)
- Vi capsular polysaccharide vaccine (ViCPS) (Typhim Vi, manufactured by Sanofi Pasteur) for intramuscular use

Vaccine Administration

Table 3-20 provides information on vaccine dosage, administration, and revaccination. The time required for primary vaccination differs for the 2 vaccines, as do the lower age limits.

Primary vaccination with oral Ty21a vaccine consists of 4 capsules, 1 taken every other day. The capsules should be kept refrigerated (not frozen), and all 4 doses must be taken to achieve maximum efficacy. Each capsule should be taken with cool liquid no warmer than 98.6°F (37°C), approximately 1 hour before a meal. This regimen should be completed 1 week before potential exposure. The vaccine manufacturer recommends that Ty21a not be administered to infants or children aged <6 years.

Primary vaccination with ViCPS consists of one 0.5-mL (25-mg) dose administered intramuscularly. One dose of this vaccine should be given ≥2 weeks before expected exposure. The manufacturer does not recommend the vaccine for infants and children aged <2 years.

Vaccine Safety and Adverse Reactions

Adverse reactions to Ty21a vaccine are rare and mainly consist of abdominal discomfort, nausea, vomiting, and rash. ViCPS vaccine is most often associated with headache (16%–20%) and injection-site reactions (7%). No information is available on the safety of these vaccines in pregnancy; it is prudent on theoretical grounds to avoid vaccinating pregnant women. Live, attenuated Ty21a vaccine should not be given to immunocompromised travelers, including those infected with HIV. The intramuscular vaccine presents a theoretically safer alternative for this group. The only contraindication to vaccination with ViCPS vaccine is a history of severe local or systemic reactions after a previous dose. Neither of the available vaccines should be given to people with an acute febrile illness.

Precautions and Contraindications

Theoretical concerns have been raised about the immunogenicity of live, attenuated Ty21a vaccine in people concurrently receiving antimicrobials (including antimalarial chemoprophylaxis), viral vaccines, or immune globulin. The growth of the live Ty21a strain is inhibited in vitro by various antibacterial agents, and vaccination with Ty21a should be delayed for >72 hours after the administration of any antibacterial agent. Available data do not suggest that simultaneous administration of oral polio or yellow fever vaccine decreases the immunogenicity of Ty21a. If typhoid vaccination is warranted, it should not be delayed because of administration of viral vaccines. Simultaneous administration of Ty21a and immune globulin does not appear to pose a problem.

Table 3-20. Dosage and schedule for typhoid fever vaccination

VACCINATION	AGE (y)	DOSE/MODE OF ADMINISTRATION	NUMBER OF DOSES	DOSING INTERVAL	BOOSTING INTERVAL
Oral, Live, Attenuated Ty21a Vaccine (Vivotif)[1]					
Primary series	≥6	1 capsule,[2] oral	4	48 hours	Not applicable
Booster	≥6	1 capsule,[2] oral	4	48 hours	Every 5 years
Vi Capsular Polysaccharide Vaccine (Typhim Vi)					
Primary series	≥2	0.5 mL, intramuscular	1	Not applicable	Not applicable
Booster	≥2	0.5 mL, intramuscular	1	Not applicable	Every 2 years

[1] The vaccine must be kept refrigerated (35.6°F–46.4°F, 2°C–8°C).
[2] Administer with cool liquid no warmer than 98.6°F (37°C).

BIBLIOGRAPHY

1. Ackers ML, Puhr ND, Tauxe RV, Mintz ED. Laboratory-based surveillance of *Salmonella* serotype Typhi infections in the United States: antimicrobial resistance on the rise. JAMA. 2000 May 24–31;283(20):2668–73.
2. Beeching NJ, Clarke PD, Kitchin NR, Pirmohamed J, Veitch K, Weber F. Comparison of two combined vaccines against typhoid fever and hepatitis A in healthy adults. Vaccine. 2004 Nov 15;23(1):29–35.
3. CDC. Typhoid immunization: recommendations of the Advisory Committee on Immunization Practices (ACIP). MMWR Recomm Rep. 1994 Dec 9;43(RR-14):1–7.
4. Crump JA, Luby SP, Mintz ED. The global burden of typhoid fever. Bull World Health Organ. 2004 May;82(5):346–53.
5. Gupta SK, Medalla F, Omondi MW, Whichard JM, Fields PI, Gerner-Smidt P, et al. Laboratory-based surveillance of paratyphoid fever in the United States: travel and antimicrobial resistance. Clin Infect Dis. 2008 Jun 1;46(11):1656–63.
6. Klugman KP, Gilbertson IT, Koornhof HJ, Robbins JB, Schneerson R, Schulz D, et al. Protective activity of Vi capsular polysaccharide vaccine against typhoid fever. Lancet. 1987 Nov 21;2(8569):1165–9.
7. Kollaritsch H, Que JU, Kunz C, Wiedermann G, Herzog C, Cryz SJ, Jr. Safety and immunogenicity of live oral cholera and typhoid vaccines administered alone or in combination with antimalarial drugs, oral polio vaccine, or yellow fever vaccine. J Infect Dis. 1997 Apr;175(4):871–5.
8. Lynch MF, Blanton EM, Bulens S, Polyak C, Vojdani J, Stevenson J, et al. Typhoid fever in the United States, 1999–2006. JAMA. 2009 Aug 26;302(8):859–65.
9. Parry CM, Hien TT, Dougan G, White NJ, Farrar JJ. Typhoid fever. N Engl J Med. 2002 Nov 28;347(22):1770–82.
10. Simanjuntak CH, Paleologo FP, Punjabi NH, Darmowigoto R, Soeprawoto, Totosudirjo H, et al. Oral immunisation against typhoid fever in Indonesia with Ty21a vaccine. Lancet. 1991 Oct 26;338(8774):1055–9.
11. Steinberg EB, Bishop R, Haber P, Dempsey AF, Hoekstra RM, Nelson JM, et al. Typhoid fever in travelers: who should be targeted for prevention? Clin Infect Dis. 2004 Jul 15;39(2):186–91.

VARICELLA (CHICKENPOX)

Kathleen H. Harriman, Gilberto F. Chavez

INFECTIOUS AGENT

Varicella zoster virus is a member of the herpesvirus family. Humans are the only reservoir of the virus, and disease occurs only in humans.

MODE OF TRANSMISSION

Varicella is transmitted from person to person by direct contact, inhalation of aerosols from vesicular fluid of skin lesions of varicella (chickenpox) or herpes zoster (shingles), which is a reactivation of latent varicella, or from infected respiratory tract secretions that might also be aerosolized. The varicella zoster virus enters the host through the upper respiratory tract or the conjunctiva.

In utero infection can also occur as a result of transplacental passage of virus during maternal varicella infection.

EPIDEMIOLOGY

Varicella occurs worldwide. In temperate climates, varicella tends to be a childhood disease, with peak incidence during late winter and early spring. In tropical climates, infection tends to occur at older ages, resulting in higher susceptibility among adults than in temperate climates.

Varicella vaccine is routinely used to vaccinate healthy children in only some countries, including the United States, Australia, Canada, Costa Rica, Dominican Republic, Germany, Mexico, Qatar, Spain, South Korea, Switzerland, United Arab Emirates, and Uruguay. Although varicella is still widely circulating in the United States, the risk of exposure to varicella zoster virus is higher in most other parts of the world than it is currently in the United States. Additionally, exposure to herpes zoster poses a risk for varicella infection in susceptible travelers, although localized herpes zoster has been shown to be much less infectious than varicella. Travelers at highest risk for severe varicella disease are immunocompromised people or pregnant women without a history of varicella disease or vaccination (see below for postexposure prophylaxis recommendations).

CLINICAL PRESENTATION

Varicella is generally a mild disease in children. Infection is often characterized by a short (1 or 2 days) prodromal period (low-grade fever, malaise), although this may be absent, and by pruritic rash consisting of crops of macules, papules, and vesicles (typically 250–500 lesions), which appear in 3 or more successive waves and resolve by crusting. Serious complications are the exception, but they can occur, most commonly in infants, adolescents, and adults. Complications include secondary bacterial infections of skin lesions, pneumonia, cerebellar ataxia, and encephalitis.

The average incubation period for varicella is 14–16 days (range, 10–21 days). The period of communicability is estimated to begin 1–2 days before the onset of rash and end when all lesions are crusted, typically 4–7 days after onset of rash in immunocompetent people, but this period may be longer in immunocompromised people.

Although varicella vaccine is 70%–90% effective in preventing all varicella, modified varicella, also known as breakthrough varicella, can occur in vaccinated people. In breakthrough varicella, which is often mild, the rash is often atypical in appearance with less than 50 vesicles and a predominance of maculopapular lesions; a fever is less common or of shorter duration. Breakthrough varicella is infectious, although less so than varicella in unvaccinated people. People with breakthrough varicella should be isolated for as long as lesions persist.

DIAGNOSIS

Skin lesions are the preferred specimen for laboratory confirmation of varicella disease. Vesicular swabs or scraping and scabs from crusted lesions can be used to identify varicella zoster virus by polymerase chain reaction or direct fluorescent antibody. In the absence of vesicles or scabs, scrapings of maculopapular lesions can be collected for testing.

Serologic tests may also be used to confirm disease:

- In the absence of skin lesions, a significant rise in serum varicella IgG from acute- and convalescent-phase samples by any standard serologic assay can confirm a diagnosis retrospectively but may not be reliable in immunocompromised people.
- Commercially available tests may not be sufficiently sensitive to reliably demonstrate vaccine-induced immunity.

POSTEXPOSURE PROPHYLAXIS
Vaccine
Varicella vaccine is recommended for postexposure administration for healthy unvaccinated people aged ≥12 months without other evidence of immunity. Administration of varicella vaccine to exposed susceptible people aged ≥12 months, as soon as possible within 72 hours and possibly up to 120 hours after exposure, may prevent or modify disease and is recommended, if there are no contraindications to use. In several studies, protective efficacy was reported as ≥90% when children were vaccinated within 3 days of exposure.

Varicella Zoster Immune Globulin
In certain circumstances, postexposure prophylaxis with varicella zoster immune globulin (VZIG) is recommended. People at high risk for severe complications include immunocompromised people, pregnant women without evidence of immunity, and some infants. If the vaccine is contraindicated in a person from one of these groups, he or she may benefit from postexposure prophylaxis with VZIG.

The VZIG product in use in the United States is available under an investigational new drug protocol and can be obtained from the sole authorized US distributor, FFF Enterprises (Temecula, California) at 800-843-7477 or www.fffenterprises.com.

VZIG provides maximum benefit when administered as soon as possible after exposure but may be effective if administered as late as 96 hours after exposure. If VZIG cannot be administered within 96 hours of exposure, administration of immune globulin intravenous should be considered as an alternative (also within 96 hours of exposure).

CDC does not officially recommend using acyclovir as prophylaxis. However, if VZIG is not available or >96 hours have passed since exposure, some experts recommend prophylaxis with acyclovir (80 mg/kg/day, administered 4 times/day for 7 days; maximum dose, 800 mg, 4 times/day) beginning 7–10 days after exposure for immunocompromised people without evidence of immunity. Similarly, a 7-day course of acyclovir also may be given to adults without evidence of immunity if vaccine is contraindicated.

TREATMENT
Oral acyclovir is not recommended for routine use in healthy children with varicella but should be considered for otherwise healthy people at increased risk for moderate to severe disease, such as people aged >12 years, people with chronic cutaneous or pulmonary disorders, people who are receiving long-term salicylate therapy, and people who are receiving short, intermittent, or aerosolized courses of corticosteroids. Intravenous antiviral therapy, when administered within 24 hours of onset of rash, is recommended for immunocompromised people, including patients being treated with chronic corticosteroids.

PREVENTIVE MEASURES FOR TRAVELERS
Vaccine
Indications for Use
Although vaccination against varicella is not a requirement for entry into any country (including the United States), people traveling or living abroad should ensure that they are immune. Evidence of immunity to varicella includes any of the following:

- Documentation of age-appropriate vaccination:
  > Preschool-age children aged ≥12 months: 1 dose
  > School-age children, adolescents, and adults: 2 doses
- Laboratory evidence of immunity or laboratory confirmation of disease
- Birth in the United States before 1980 (not a criterion for health care personnel, pregnant women, and immunocompromised people)
- A health care provider's diagnosis of varicella or a health care provider's verification of a history of varicella disease
- A health care provider's diagnosis of herpes zoster or a health care provider's verification of a history of herpes zoster disease

Vaccine Administration

Varicella vaccine contains live, attenuated varicella zoster virus. Two doses of varicella-containing vaccine are now recommended for all people aged ≥12 months without evidence of immunity to varicella who do not have contraindications to the vaccine. The first dose should be administered at age 12–15 months and the second dose at 4–6 years of age. A second catch-up dose of varicella vaccination is recommended for children, adolescents, and adults who have received only 1 dose. The minimum interval between doses for children <13 years is 3 months, and those aged ≥13 years can be vaccinated at an interval of 4–8 weeks. In cases of uncertainty, prior varicella disease is not a contraindication to varicella vaccination.

Vaccine Safety and Adverse Reactions

The 2-dose single-antigen varicella vaccine regimen is generally well tolerated. The most common adverse events after varicella vaccine are self-limited injection site reactions (pain, soreness, redness, and swelling). Fever was reported in uncontrolled trials in 15% of children and 10% of adolescents and adults. A varicella-like rash, usually consisting of a few lesions at the injection site, was reported in 3% and 1% of people receiving the first and second dose, respectively, with generalized rashes with a small number of lesions reported even less frequently.

Contraindications
Allergy

People with severe allergy (hives, swelling of the mouth or throat, difficulty breathing, hypotension, and shock) to gelatin or neomycin or who have had a severe allergic reaction to a prior dose of vaccine should not be vaccinated.

Single-antigen varicella vaccine does not contain egg protein or preservative.

For the combination MMRV vaccine, live measles and live mumps vaccine are produced in chick embryo culture. However, the risk for serious allergic reactions after administration of measles- or mumps-containing vaccines in people who are allergic to eggs is low.

Altered immunity

People with immunosuppression of cellular immune function resulting from leukemia, lymphomas of any type, generalized malignancy, immunodeficiency disease, or immunosuppressive therapy should not be vaccinated. Treatment with low-dose prednisone (<2 mg/kg of body weight per day or <20 mg/day) or aerosolized steroid preparations is not a contraindication to varicella vaccination. People whose immunosuppressive therapy with steroids has been stopped for 1 month (3 months for chemotherapy) may be vaccinated. In addition, people with impaired humoral immunity may be vaccinated. Because HIV-infected children are at greater risk of morbidity from varicella and herpes zoster than healthy children, the Advisory Committee on Immunization Practices recommends considering varicella vaccine for HIV-infected children aged ≥12 months who have CD4+ T-lymphocyte percentages of ≥15% and who do not have evidence of varicella immunity. Eligible children should receive 2 doses of single-antigen varicella vaccine, with a minimum 3-month interval between doses. Vaccination (2 doses, administered 3 months apart) may be considered for HIV-infected older children, adolescents, and adults with CD4+ T-lymphocyte count ≥200 cells/mL, after the risks and benefits are weighed.

Pregnancy

Women who are pregnant or attempting to become pregnant should not receive varicella vaccine. Pregnancy should be avoided for 1 month after varicella vaccination. Breastfeeding is not a contraindication to varicella vaccination.

Precautions
Illness

People who have acute severe illness, including untreated, active tuberculosis, should not be vaccinated until they have recovered.

Recent administration of blood, plasma, or immune globulin

The effect of immune globulin on the response to varicella virus vaccine is unknown. Because passively transferred antibodies may inhibit the antibody response, varicella vaccines should not be administered for 3–11 months, depending on the dose, after administration of blood (except washed red cells), plasma, or immune globulin.

Use of salicylates

No adverse events after varicella vaccination have been reported related to the use of salicylates (such as aspirin). However, the manufacturer recommends that vaccine recipients avoid the use of salicylates for 6 weeks after receiving varicella vaccine because of the association between aspirin use and Reye syndrome after varicella.

BIBLIOGRAPHY

1. American Academy of Pediatrics. Varicella. In: Pickering LK, Baker CJ, Kimberlin DW, Long SS, editors. Red Book: Report of the Committee on Infectious Diseases. 28th ed. Elk Grove Village, IL: American Academy of Pediatrics; 2009. p. 714–27.
2. CDC. A new product (VariZIG) for postexposure prophylaxis of varicella available under an investigational new drug application expanded access protocol. MMWR Morb Mortal Wkly Rep. 2006 Mar 3;55(8):209–10.
3. Gershon AA, Takahasi M, Seward J. Varicella vaccine. In: Plotkin SA, Orenstein WA, Offit PA, editors. Vaccines. Philadelphia: Saunders Elsevier; 2008. p. 915–58.
4. Guris D, Jumaan AO, Mascola L, Watson BM, Zhang JX, Chaves SS, et al. Changing varicella epidemiology in active surveillance sites—United States, 1995–2005. J Infect Dis. 2008 Mar 1;197 Suppl 2:S71–5.
5. Harpaz R, Ortega-Sanchez IR, Seward JF. Prevention of herpes zoster: recommendations of the Advisory Committee on Immunization Practices (ACIP). MMWR Recomm Rep. 2008 Jun 6;57(RR-5):1–30.
6. Marin M, Guris D, Chaves SS, Schmid S, Seward JF. Prevention of varicella: recommendations of the Advisory Committee on Immunization Practices (ACIP). MMWR Recomm Rep. 2007 Jun 22;56 (RR-4):1–40.
7. World Health Organization. Immunization summary: the 2007 edition. 2007 Feb [cited 2008 Apr 14]. Available from: http://www.unicef.org/publications/files/Immunization_Summary_2007.pdf.

VIRAL HEMORRHAGIC FEVERS
Pierre E. Rollin

INFECTIOUS AGENT

Viral hemorrhagic fevers (VHFs) are caused by several families of enveloped RNA viruses: filoviruses (Ebola and Marburg viruses), arenaviruses (Lassa fever, Lujo, Guanarito, Machupo, Junin, Sabia, and Chapare viruses), bunyaviruses (Rift Valley fever [RVF], Crimean-Congo hemorrhagic fever [CCHF], and hantaviruses), and flaviviruses (dengue, yellow fever, Omsk hemorrhagic fever, Kyasanur Forest disease, and Alkhurma viruses) (see the Dengue Fever and Yellow Fever sections in this chapter).

MODE OF TRANSMISSION

Some VHFs are spread person to person through direct contact with symptomatic patients, body fluids, or cadavers or through inadequate infection control (filoviruses, arenaviruses, CCHF virus). Zoonotic spread includes the following:

- Livestock via slaughter or consumption of raw milk or meat from infected animals (CCHF, RVF, Alkhurma viruses)
- Bushmeat, likely via slaughter or consumption of infected animals (Ebola, Marburg viruses)
- Rodent (arenaviruses, hantaviruses) via inhalation of or contact with materials contaminated with rodent excreta
- Other reservoir species, such as bats (Ebola, Marburg viruses)
- Vectorborne transmission also occurs via mosquito (RVF virus) or tick (CCHF, Omsk, Kyasanur Forest disease, Alkhurma viruses) bites or by crushing ticks

EPIDEMIOLOGY

The viruses that cause VHF are distributed over much of the globe. Each virus is associated with 1 or more nonhuman host or vector species, restricting the virus and the initial contamination to the areas inhabited by these species. The diseases caused by these viruses are seen in people living in or having visited these areas. Humans are incidental hosts for these enzootic diseases; however, person-to-person transmission of some viruses can result in large human outbreaks. Specific viruses are addressed below.

Ebola and Marburg: Filoviral Diseases

Ebola and Marburg viruses cause hemorrhagic fever in humans and nonhuman primates. Five species of Ebola virus have been identified: Côte d'Ivoire, Sudan, Zaire, Bundibugyo, and Reston. Ebola-Reston has not been shown to cause human disease. These diseases occur in tropical regions in Africa. Countries with confirmed human cases of Ebola hemorrhagic fever include Republic of the Congo, Côte d'Ivoire, Democratic Republic of the Congo, Gabon, Sudan, and Uganda. Countries with confirmed human cases of Marburg hemorrhagic fever include Uganda, Kenya, Democratic Republic of the Congo, Angola, and possibly Zimbabwe. Growing evidence indicates that fruit bats are the natural reservoir for filoviruses. Outbreaks occur when a person becomes infected after exposure to the reservoir species or an infected nonhuman primate and then transmits the virus to other people in the community.

Four cases of Marburg hemorrhagic fever have occurred in travelers visiting caves harboring bats, including Kitum cave in Kenya and Python cave in Maramagambo Forest, Uganda. Miners have also acquired Marburg infection from working in underground mines harboring bats in the Democratic Republic of the Congo and Uganda.

Lassa Fever and Other Arenaviral Diseases

Arenaviruses are transmitted from rodents to humans, except Tacaribe virus, which is found in bats. Most infections are mild, but some result in hemorrhagic fever with high death rates. Old World (Eastern Hemisphere) and New World (Western Hemisphere) viruses cause the following diseases:

- Old World viruses: Lassa virus (Lassa fever), Lymphocytic choriomeningitis virus (meningitis, encephalitis, and congenital fetal infection in normal hosts, hemorrhagic fever in organ transplant recipients). Lassa fever occurs in rural West Africa, with hyperendemic areas in Sierra Leone, Guinea, Liberia, and Nigeria. Lujo virus has been recently described in Zambia and the Republic of South Africa during a nosocomial outbreak.
- New World viruses: Junin (Argentine hemorrhagic fever), Machupo (Bolivian hemorrhagic fever), Guanarito (Venezuelan hemorrhagic fever), Sabia (Brazilian hemorrhagic fever), and the recently discovered Chapare virus (single case in Bolivia).

Reservoir host species are New World rats and mice (family Muridae, subfamily Sigmodontinae) and Old World rats and mice (family Muridae, subfamily Murinae). These rodent types are found worldwide, including Europe, Asia, Africa, and the Americas. Virus is transmitted through inhalation of aerosols from rodent urine, ingestion of rodent-contaminated food, or direct contact of broken skin with rodent excreta. Risk of Lassa virus infection is associated with peridomestic rodent exposure. Inappropriate food storage increases the risk for exposure. Nosocomial transmission of Lassa, Lujo, and Machupo viruses has occurred through droplet and contact. One anecdotal report of possible airborne transmission exists. Several cases of Lassa fever have been confirmed in international travelers living in traditional dwellings in the countryside.

Rift Valley Fever and Other Bunyaviral Diseases

RVF causes fever, hemorrhage, encephalitis, and retinitis in humans, but primarily affects livestock. RVF is endemic to sub-Saharan Africa. Sporadic outbreaks have occurred in humans in Egypt, Madagascar, and Mauritania. Large epidemics occurred in Kenya, Somalia, and Tanzania in 1997–1998 and 2006–2007, Saudi Arabia and Yemen in 2000, Madagascar in 2008, and South Africa in 2010. RVF virus is transmitted by mosquito, percutaneous inoculation, and slaughter or consumption of infected animals.

CCHF is endemic where ticks of the genus *Hyalomma* are found in Africa and Eurasia, including South Africa, the Balkans, the Middle East, Russia, and western China, and is highly endemic in Afghanistan, Iran,

Pakistan, and Turkey. CCHF virus is transmitted to humans by infected ticks or direct handling and preparation of fresh carcasses of infected animals, usually domestic livestock. Nosocomial transmission often occurs.

Hantaviruses cause hantavirus pulmonary syndrome (HPS) and hemorrhagic fever with renal syndrome (HFRS). The viruses that cause HPS are present in the New World; those that cause HFRS occur worldwide. The viruses that cause both HPS and HFRS are transmitted to humans through contact with urine, feces, or saliva of infected rodents. Travelers staying in rodent-infested dwellings are at risk for HPS and HFRS. Human-to-human transmission has been reported only with Andes virus in Chile and Argentina.

CLINICAL PRESENTATION

Signs and symptoms vary by disease, but in general, patients with VHF present with abrupt onset of fever, myalgias, and prostration, followed in severe forms by coagulopathy with a petechial rash or ecchymoses and sometimes overt bleeding. Vascular endothelial damage leads to shock and pulmonary edema, and liver injury is common. Signs seen with specific viruses include renal failure (HFRS), ecchymoses (CCHF), hearing loss, anasarca and shock in newborns (Lassa fever), and spontaneous abortion (Lassa and lymphocytic choriomeningitis viruses). Because the incubation period may be as long as 21 days, patients may not develop illness until returning from travel; therefore, a thorough travel and exposure history is critical.

DIAGNOSIS

US-based clinicians should notify CDC's Viral Special Pathogens Branch immediately of any suspected cases of VHF occurring in patients residing in or requiring evacuation to the United States: 404-639-1115 or the CDC Emergency Operations Center at 770-488-7100 after hours. CDC also provides consultation for international clinicians and health ministries. Whole blood or serum may be tested for virologic (RT-PCR, antigen detection, virus isolation) and immunologic (IgM, IgG) evidence of infection. Tissue may be tested by immunohistochemistry, RT-PCR, and virus isolation. Postmortem skin biopsies fixed in formalin and blood collected within a few hours after death by cardiac puncture can be used for diagnosis. Samples should be sent for testing to a reference laboratory with biosafety level 3 and 4 capability.

TREATMENT

Ribavirin is effective for treating Lassa fever, New World arenaviruses, and likely CCHF, but it is not approved by the Food and Drug Administration (FDA) for these indications. Convalescent-phase plasma is effective in treating Argentine hemorrhagic fever. Intravenous ribavirin can be obtained for compassionate use through FDA from Valeant Pharmaceuticals (Aliso Viejo, California). Requests should be initiated by the provider through FDA (301-443-1240), with simultaneous notification to Valeant: 800-548-5100, extension 5 (domestic telephone) or 949-461-6971 (international telephone). The process is explained on FDA's website (www.fda.gov/Drugs/DevelopmentApprovalProcess/HowDrugsareDevelopedandApproved/ApprovalApplications/InvestigationalNewDrugIND Application/default.htm).

PREVENTIVE MEASURES FOR TRAVELERS

The risk of acquiring VHF is very low for international travelers. Travelers at increased risk for exposure include those engaging in animal research, health care workers, and others providing care for patients in the community, particularly where outbreaks of VHF are occurring.

Prevention should focus on avoiding contact with host or vector species. Travelers should not visit locations where an outbreak is occurring. Contact with rodents should be avoided. Travelers should avoid contact with livestock in RVF- and CCHF-endemic areas, and they should use insecticide-treated bed nets and insect repellent to prevent vectorborne disease.

Standard precautions and contact and droplet precautions for suspected VHF case-patients are recommended to avoid transmission. Direct contact should be avoided with corpses of patients suspected of having died of Ebola, Marburg, or Old World arenavirus infection. Contact with or consumption of primates, bats, and other bushmeat should be avoided. Bat-inhabited caves or mines should be avoided. Investigational vaccines exist for Argentine hemorrhagic fever and RVF; however, neither is approved by FDA or commonly available in the United States.

BIBLIOGRAPHY

1. Bausch DG, Borchert M, Grein T, Roth C, Swanepoel R, Libande ML, et al. Risk factors for Marburg hemorrhagic fever, Democratic Republic of the Congo. Emerg Infect Dis. 2003 Dec;9(12):1531–7.

2. Bausch DG, Ksiazek TG. Viral hemorrhagic fevers including hantavirus pulmonary syndrome in the Americas. Clin Lab Med. 2002 Dec;22(4):981–1020, viii.

3. de Manzione N, Salas RA, Paredes H, Godoy O, Rojas L, Araoz F, et al. Venezuelan hemorrhagic fever: clinical and epidemiological studies of 165 cases. Clin Infect Dis. 1998 Feb;26(2):308–13.

4. Feldmann H, Jones SM, Schnittler HJ, Geisbert T. Therapy and prophylaxis of Ebola virus infections. Curr Opin Investig Drugs. 2005 Aug;6(8):823–30.

5. Geisbert TW, Jahrling PB. Exotic emerging viral diseases: progress and challenges. Nat Med. 2004 Dec;10(12 Suppl):S110–21.

6. Gunther S, Lenz O. Lassa virus. Crit Rev Clin Lab Sci. 2004;41(4):339–90.

7. Madani TA, Al-Mazrou YY, Al-Jeffri MH, Mishkhas AA, Al-Rabeah AM, Turkistani AM, et al. Rift Valley fever epidemic in Saudi Arabia: epidemiological, clinical, and laboratory characteristics. Clin Infect Dis. 2003 Oct 15;37(8):1084–92.

8. Marty AM, Jahrling PB, Geisbert TW. Viral hemorrhagic fevers. Clin Lab Med. 2006 Jun;26(2):345–86, viii.

9. Ozkurt Z, Kiki I, Erol S, Erdem F, Yilmaz N, Parlak M, et al. Crimean-Congo hemorrhagic fever in eastern Turkey: clinical features, risk factors and efficacy of ribavirin therapy. J Infect. 2006 Mar;52(3):207–15.

10. Paweska JT, Sewlall NH, Ksiazek TG, Blumberg LH, Hale MJ, Lipkin WI, et al. Nosocomial outbreak of novel arenavirus infection, southern Africa. Emerg Infect Dis. 2009 Oct;15(10):1598–602.

11. Peters CJ, Jahrling PB, Khan AS. Patients infected with high-hazard viruses: scientific basis for infection control. Arch Virol Suppl. 1996;11:141–68.

12. Peters CJ, Zaki SR. Overview of viral hemorrhagic fevers. In: Guerrant RL, Walker DH, Weller PF, editors. Tropical infectious diseases: principles, pathogens & practice. 2nd ed. Philadelphia: Churchill Livingstone; 2006. p. 726–33.

13. Rouquet P, Froment JM, Bermejo M, Kilbourn A, Karesh W, Reed P, et al. Wild animal mortality monitoring and human Ebola outbreaks, Gabon and Republic of Congo, 2001–2003. Emerg Infect Dis. 2005 Feb;11(2):283–90.

14. Vapalahti O, Mustonen J, Lundkvist A, Henttonen H, Plyusnin A, Vaheri A. Hantavirus infections in Europe. Lancet Infect Dis. 2003 Oct;3(10):653–61.

15. Wahl-Jensen V, Feldman H, Sanchez A. Filovirus infections. In: Guerrant RL, Walker DH, Weller PF, editors. Tropical infectious diseases: principles, pathogens & practice. 2nd ed. Philadelphia: Churchill Livingstone; 2006. p. 784–96.

16. Watts DM, Flick R, Peters CJ. Rift valley fever and Crimean-Congo hemorrhagic fever. In: Guerrant RL, Walker DH, Weller PF, editors. Tropical infectious diseases: principles, pathogens & practice. 2nd ed. Philadelphia: Churchill Livingstone; 2006. p. 756–61.

YELLOW FEVER

Mark Gershman, J. Erin Staples

INFECTIOUS AGENT

Yellow fever virus (YFV) is a single-stranded RNA virus that belongs to the genus *Flavivirus*.

MODE OF TRANSMISSION

Vectorborne transmission occurs via the bite of an infected mosquito, primarily *Aedes* or *Haemagogus* spp. Nonhuman and human primates are the main reservoirs of the virus, with anthroponotic (human-to-vector-to-human) transmission occurring. There are 3 transmission cycles for yellow fever: sylvatic (jungle), intermediate (savannah), and urban.

- The sylvatic (jungle) transmission cycle involves transmission of the virus between nonhuman primates and mosquito species found in the forest canopy. The virus is transmitted via mosquitoes from monkeys to humans when the humans encroach into the jungle during occupational or recreational activities.

- In Africa, an intermediate (savannah) cycle involves transmission of YFV from tree hole-breeding *Aedes* spp. to humans living or working in jungle border areas. In this cycle, the virus may be transmitted from monkeys to humans or from human to human via these mosquitoes.

- The urban transmission cycle involves transmission of the virus between humans and urban mosquitoes, primarily *Aedes aegypti*.

Humans infected with YFV experience the highest levels of viremia and can transmit the virus to mosquitoes shortly before onset of fever and for the first 3–5 days of illness. Given the high level of viremia, bloodborne transmission theoretically can occur via transfusion or needlesticks.

EPIDEMIOLOGY

Yellow fever occurs in sub-Saharan Africa and tropical South America, where it is endemic and intermittently epidemic (see Tables 3-21 and 3-22 for a list of countries with risk of YFV transmission). Most yellow fever disease in humans is due to sylvatic or intermediate transmission cycles. However, urban yellow fever occurs periodically in Africa and sporadically in the Americas. In Africa, natural immunity accumulates with age, and thus, infants and children are at highest risk for disease. In South America, yellow fever occurs most frequently in unimmunized young men who are exposed to mosquito vectors through their work in forested or transitional areas.

RISK FOR TRAVELERS

A traveler's risk for acquiring yellow fever is determined by various factors, including immunization status, location of travel, season, duration of exposure, occupational and recreational activities while traveling, and local rate of virus transmission at the time of travel. Although reported cases of human disease are the principal indicator of disease risk, case reports may be absent because of a low level of transmission, a high level of immunity in the population (because of vaccination, for example), or failure of local surveillance systems to detect cases. This "epidemiologic silence" does not equate to absence of risk and should not lead to travel without the protection provided by vaccination.

YFV transmission in rural West Africa is seasonal, with an elevated risk during the end of the rainy season and the beginning of the dry season (usually July–October). However, YFV may be episodically transmitted by *Ae. aegypti* even during the dry season in both rural and densely settled urban areas.

The risk for infection in South America is highest during the rainy season (January–May, with a peak incidence in February and March). Given the high level of viremia that may occur in infected humans and the

Table 3-21. Countries with risk of yellow fever virus (YFV) transmission[1]

AFRICA			CENTRAL AND SOUTH AMERICA
Angola	Ethiopia[2]	Nigeria	Argentina[2]
Benin	Gabon	Rwanda	Bolivia[2]
Burkina Faso	The Gambia	Senegal	Brazil[2]
Burundi	Ghana	Sierra Leone	Colombia[2]
Cameroon	Guinea	Sudan[2]	Ecuador[2]
Central African Republic	Guinea-Bissau	Togo	French Guiana
	Kenya[2]	Uganda	Guyana
Chad[2]	Liberia		Panama[2]
Congo, Republic of the	Mali[2]		Paraguay
Côte d'Ivoire	Mauritania[2]		Peru[2]
Democratic Republic of the Congo[2]	Niger[2]		Suriname
			Trinidad and Tobago[2]
Equatorial Guinea			Venezuela[2]

[1] Countries/areas where "a risk of yellow fever transmission is present," as defined by the World Health Organization, are countries or areas where "yellow fever has been reported currently or in the past, plus vectors and animal reservoirs currently exist" (see the current country list within the *International Travel and Health* publication (Annex 1) at www.who.int/ith/en/index.html).

[2] These countries are not holoendemic (only a portion of the country has risk of yellow fever transmission). See Maps 3-18 and 3-19 and yellow fever vaccine recommendations (Yellow Fever and Malaria Information, by Country) for details.

Table 3-22. Countries with low potential for exposure to yellow fever virus (YFV)[1]

AFRICA
Eritrea[2]
São Tomé and Príncipe[3]
Somalia[2]
Tanzania[3]
Zambia

[1] Countries listed in this table are not contained on the official WHO list of countries with risk of YFV transmission (Table 3-21). Therefore, proof of yellow fever vaccination should not be required if traveling from one of these countries to another country with a vaccination entry requirement (unless that country requires proof of yellow fever vaccination from all arriving travelers; see Table 3-24).

[2] These countries are classified as "low potential for exposure to YFV" in only some areas; the remaining areas of these countries are classified as having no risk of exposure to YFV.

[3] The entire area of these countries is classified as "low potential for exposure to YFV."

widespread distribution of *Ae. aegypti* in many towns and cities, South America is at risk for a large-scale urban epidemic.

From 1970 through 2010, a total of 9 cases of yellow fever were reported in unvaccinated travelers from the United States and Europe who traveled to West Africa (5 cases) or South America (4 cases). Eight (88%) of these 9 travelers died. There has been only 1 documented case of yellow fever in a vaccinated traveler. This nonfatal case occurred in a traveler from Spain who visited several West African countries during 1988.

The risk of acquiring yellow fever is difficult to predict because of variations in ecologic determinants of virus transmission. For a 2-week stay, the risks for illness and death due to yellow fever for an unvaccinated traveler traveling to an endemic area in:

- West Africa are 50 per 100,000 and 10 per 100,000, respectively
- South America are 5 per 100,000 and 1 per 100,000, respectively

These estimates are a rough guideline based on the risk to indigenous populations, often during peak transmission season. Thus, these risk estimates may not accurately reflect the true risk to travelers, who may have a different immunity profile, take precautions against getting bitten by mosquitoes, and have less outdoor exposure.

The risk of acquiring yellow fever in South America is lower than that in Africa, because the mosquitoes that transmit the virus between monkeys in the forest canopy in South America do not often come in contact with humans. Additionally, there is a relatively high level of immunity in local residents because of vaccine use, which might reduce the risk of transmission.

CLINICAL PRESENTATION

Asymptomatic or clinically inapparent infection is believed to occur in most people infected with YFV. For people who develop symptomatic illness, the incubation period is typically 3–6 days. The initial illness presents as a nonspecific influenzalike syndrome with sudden onset of fever, chills, headache, backache, myalgias, prostration, nausea, and vomiting. Most patients improve after the initial presentation. After a brief remission of hours to a day, approximately 15% of patients progress to a more serious or toxic form of the disease characterized by jaundice, hemorrhagic symptoms, and eventually shock and multisystem organ failure. The case-fatality ratio for severe cases with hepatorenal dysfunction is 20%–50%.

DIAGNOSIS

The preliminary diagnosis is based on the patient's clinical features, places and dates of travel, and activities. Laboratory diagnosis is best performed by:

- Serologic assays to detect virus-specific IgM and IgG antibodies. Because of cross-reactivity between antibodies raised against other flaviviruses, more specific antibody testing, such as a plaque reduction neutralization test, should be done to confirm the infection.

- Virus isolation or nucleic acid amplification tests performed early in the illness for YFV or yellow fever viral RNA. However, by the time more overt symptoms are recognized, the virus or viral RNA is usually undetectable. Therefore, virus isolation and nucleic acid amplification should not be used for ruling out a diagnosis of yellow fever.

Clinicians should contact their state or local health department or call 800-CDC-INFO (800-232-4636) for assistance with diagnostic testing for yellow fever infections and for questions about antibody response to vaccination.

TREATMENT

Treatment is for symptoms. Rest, fluids, and use of analgesics and antipyretics may relieve symptoms of fever and aching. Care should be taken to avoid certain medications, such as aspirin or nonsteroidal anti-inflammatory drugs, which may increase the risk for bleeding. Infected people should be protected from further mosquito exposure (staying indoors or under a mosquito net) during the first few days of illness, so they do not contribute to the transmission cycle.

PREVENTIVE MEASURES FOR TRAVELERS
Personal Protection Measures

The best way to prevent mosquitoborne diseases, including yellow fever, is to avoid mosquito bites (see Chapter 2, Protection against Mosquitoes, Ticks, and Other Insects and Arthropods).

Vaccine

Yellow fever is preventable by a relatively safe, effective vaccine. All yellow fever vaccines currently manufactured are live-attenuated viral vaccines. YF-Vax, the only yellow fever vaccine licensed for use in the United States, is manufactured by Sanofi Pasteur. Studies comparing the reactogenicity and immunogenicity of various yellow fever vaccines, including those manufactured outside the United States, suggest that there is no significant difference in the reactogenicity or immune response generated by the various vaccines.

Thus, people who receive yellow fever vaccines in other countries should be considered protected against yellow fever.

Indications for Use

Yellow fever vaccine is recommended for people aged ≥9 months who are traveling to or living in areas at risk for VFV transmission in South America and Africa. In addition, some countries require proof of yellow fever vaccination for entry. See the Yellow Fever and Malaria Information, by Country section at the end of this chapter for more detailed information on the requirements and recommendations for yellow fever vaccination for specific countries.

Because of the risk of serious adverse events that can occur after yellow fever vaccination, clinicians should only vaccinate people who 1) are at risk of exposure to YFV or 2) require proof of vaccination to enter a country. To further minimize the risk of serious adverse events, clinicians should carefully observe the contraindications and consider the precautions to vaccination before administering yellow fever vaccine (Table 3-23). For additional information, refer to the yellow fever vaccine recommendations of the Advisory Committee on Immunization Practices (ACIP) at www.cdc.gov/vaccines/pubs/ACIP-list.htm.

Vaccine Administration

For all eligible people, a single injection of 0.5 mL of reconstituted vaccine should be administered subcutaneously. The International Health Regulations (IHR) published by the World Health Organization (WHO) require revaccination at 10-year intervals.

Vaccine Safety and Adverse Reactions
Common adverse reactions

Reactions to yellow fever vaccine are generally mild; 10%–30% of vaccinees report mild systemic adverse events. Reported events typically include low-grade fever, headache, and myalgias that begin within days after vaccination and last 5–10 days. Approximately 1% of vaccinees temporarily curtail their regular activities because of these reactions.

Severe adverse reactions
Hypersensitivity

Immediate hypersensitivity reactions, characterized by rash, urticaria, bronchospasm,

Table 3-23. Contraindications and precautions to yellow fever vaccine administration

CONTRAINDICATIONS	PRECAUTIONS
• Allergy to vaccine component • Age <6 months • Symptomatic HIV infection or CD4 T-lymphocytes <200/mm^3 (or <15% of total in children aged <6 years)[1] • Thymus disorder associated with abnormal immune-cell function • Primary immunodeficiencies • Malignant neoplasms • Transplantation • Immunosuppressive and immunomodulatory therapies	• Age 6–8 months • Age ≥60 years • Asymptomatic HIV infection and CD4 T-lymphocytes 200–499/mm^3 (or 15%–24% of total in children aged <6 years)[1] • Pregnancy • Breastfeeding

[1] Symptoms of HIV are classified in 1) Adults and Adolescents, Table 1. CDC. 1993 Revised classification system for HIV infection and expanded surveillance case definition for AIDS among adolescents and adults.MMWR Recomm Rep 1992 Dec 18: 41(RR-17). Available from: www.cdc.gov/mmwr/preview/mmwrhtml/00018871.htm and 2) Panel on Antiretroviral Therapy and Medical Management of HIV-Infected Children. Guidelines for the use of antiretroviral agents in pediatric HIV infection. 2010. Available from: http://aidsinfo.nih.gov/ContentFiles/PediatricGuidelines.pdf. p. 20–2.

or a combination of these, are uncommon. Anaphylaxis after yellow fever vaccine is reported to occur at a rate of 1.8 cases per 100,000 doses administered.

Yellow fever vaccine–associated neurologic disease (YEL-AND)

YEL-AND represents a conglomerate of different clinical syndromes, including meningo-encephalitis, Guillain-Barré syndrome, acute disseminated encephalomyelitis, bulbar palsy, and Bell palsy. Historically, YEL-AND was seen primarily among infants as encephalitis, but more recent reports have been among people of all ages.

The onset of illness for documented cases is 3–28 days after vaccination, and almost all cases were in first-time vaccine recipients. YEL-AND is rarely fatal. The incidence of YEL-AND in the United States is 0.8 per 100,000 doses administered. The rate is higher in people aged ≥60 years, with a rate of 1.6 per 100,000 doses in people aged 60–69 and 2.3 per 100,000 doses in people aged ≥70 years.

Yellow fever vaccine–associated viscerotropic disease (YEL-AVD)

YEL-AVD is a severe illness similar to wild-type disease, with vaccine virus proliferating in multiple organs and often leading to multisystem organ failure and death. Since the initial cases of YEL-AVD were published in 2001, more than 50 confirmed and suspected cases have been reported throughout the world.

YEL-AVD appears to occur after the first dose of yellow fever vaccine, rather than with booster doses. The onset of illness for YEL-AVD cases averaged 3 days (range, 1–8 days) after vaccination. The case-fatality ratio for reported YEL-AVD cases is 65%. The incidence of YEL-AVD in the United States is 0.4 cases per 100,000 doses of vaccine administered. The rate is higher for people aged ≥60 years, with a rate of 1.0 per 100,000 doses in people aged 60–69 years and 2.3 per 100,000 doses in people aged ≥70 years.

Contraindications

Infants younger than 6 months

Yellow fever vaccine is contraindicated for infants aged <6 months. This contraindication was instituted in the late 1960s in response to a high rate of YEL-AND documented in vaccinated young infants (50–400 per 100,000). The mechanism of increased neurovirulence in infants is unknown but may be due to the immaturity of the blood-brain barrier, higher or more prolonged viremia, or immune system immaturity.

Hypersensitivity

Yellow fever vaccine is contraindicated for people with a history of hypersensitivity to any of the vaccine components, including eggs, egg products, chicken proteins, or gelatin. The stopper used in vials of vaccine also contains dry latex rubber, which may cause an allergic reaction.

If vaccination of a person with a questionable history of hypersensitivity to one of the vaccine components is considered essential because of a high risk for acquiring yellow fever, skin testing, as described in the vaccine package insert, should be performed under close medical supervision. If a person has a positive skin test to the vaccine or has a severe egg sensitivity and the vaccination is recommended, desensitization, as described in the package insert, can be performed under direct supervision of a physician experienced in the management of anaphylaxis.

Altered immune status
Thymus disorder

Yellow fever vaccine is contraindicated for people with a thymus disorder that is associated with abnormal immune cell function, such as thymoma or myasthenia gravis. If travel to a yellow fever–endemic area cannot be avoided in a person with a thymus disorder that is associated with abnormal immune cell function, a medical waiver should be provided and counseling on protective measures against mosquito bites should be emphasized. Because there is no evidence of immune dysfunction or increased risk of yellow fever vaccine–associated serious adverse events in people who have undergone incidental surgical removal of their thymus or have had indirect radiation therapy in the distant past, these people can be given yellow fever vaccine if recommended or required.

HIV infection

Yellow fever vaccine is contraindicated for people with AIDS or other clinical manifestations of HIV, including people with CD4 T-lymphocyte values <200/mm³ or <15% of total lymphocytes for children less than <6 years. This recommendation is based on a theoretical increased risk of encephalitis in this population (see HIV infection under the following section, Precautions).

If travel to a yellow fever–endemic area cannot be avoided in a person with severe immune suppression based on CD4 counts (<200/mm³ or <15% total for children less than <6 years) or symptomatic HIV, a medical waiver should be provided, and counseling on protective measures against mosquito bites should be emphasized. See the following section, Precautions, for other HIV-infected people not meeting the above criteria.

Immunodeficiencies (other than thymus disorder or HIV infection)

Yellow fever vaccine is contraindicated for people with primary immunodeficiencies, malignant neoplasms, and transplantation. While there are no data on the use of yellow fever vaccine in these people, they presumably are at increased risk for yellow fever vaccine–associated serious adverse events (see the section in Chapter 8, Immunocompromised Travelers).

If someone with an immunodeficiency cannot avoid travel to a yellow fever–endemic area, a medical waiver should be provided, and counseling on protective measures against mosquito bites should be emphasized.

Immunosuppressive and immunomodulatory therapies

Yellow fever vaccine is contraindicated for people whose immunologic response is either suppressed or modulated by current or recent radiation therapies or drugs. Drugs with known immunosuppressive or immunomodulatory properties include, but are not limited to, high-dose systemic corticosteroids, alkylating drugs, antimetabolites, tumor necrosis factor α inhibitors (such as etanercept), interleukin-1 blocking agents (such as anakinra), or other monoclonal antibodies targeting immune cells (such as rituximab or alemtuzumab). There are no specific data on the use of yellow fever vaccine in people receiving these therapies. However, these people are presumed to be at increased risk for yellow fever vaccine–associated serious adverse events, and the use of live attenuated vaccines is contraindicated in the package insert for most of these therapies (see the section in Chapter 8, Immunocompromised Travelers).

Live viral vaccines should be deferred in people who have discontinued these therapies until immune function has improved. If travel to a yellow fever–endemic area cannot be avoided for someone receiving immunosuppressive or immunomodulatory therapies, a medical waiver should be provided and counseling on protective measures against mosquito bites should be emphasized.

Family members of people with an altered immune status who themselves have no contraindications can receive yellow fever vaccine.

Precautions
Infants aged 6–8 months
Age 6–8 months is a precaution for yellow fever vaccination. Two cases of YEL-AND have been reported among infants aged 6–8 months. In infants <6 months of age, the rates of YEL-AND are significantly elevated (50–400 per 100,000). By 9 months of age, risk for YEL-AND is believed to be substantially lower. ACIP generally recommends that, whenever possible, travel to yellow fever-endemic countries should be postponed or avoided for children aged 6–8 months. If travel is unavoidable, the decision of whether to vaccinate these infants needs to balance the risks of YFV exposure with the risk for adverse events after vaccination.

Adults 60 years of age or older
Age ≥60 years is a precaution for yellow fever vaccination, particularly if this is the first dose of the yellow fever vaccine given. A recent analysis of adverse events passively reported to VAERS from 2000 through 2006 indicates that people aged ≥60 years are at increased risk for any serious adverse event after vaccination, compared with younger people. The rate of serious adverse events in people aged ≥60 years was 8.3 per 100,000 doses distributed, compared with 4.7 per 100,000 for all vaccine recipients. The risk of YEL-AND and YEL-AVD is also increased in this age group, at 1.8 and 1.4 per 100,000 doses, respectively, compared with 0.8 and 0.4 per 100,000 for all vaccine recipients. Given that YEL-AND and YEL-AVD are seen almost exclusively in primary vaccine recipients, more caution should be exercised with older travelers who may be receiving yellow fever vaccine for the first time. If travel is unavoidable, the decision to vaccinate travelers aged ≥60 years needs to weigh the risks and benefits of the vaccination

in the context of their destination-specific risk for exposure to YFV.

HIV infection
Asymptomatic HIV infection with CD4 T-lymphocyte values 200–499/mm³ or 15%–24% of total lymphocytes for children aged <6 years is a precaution for yellow fever vaccination (see also the HIV infection in the Contraindications section above). Large prospective, randomized trials have not been performed to adequately address the safety and efficacy of yellow fever vaccine among this group. Several retrospective and prospective studies including approximately 450 people infected with HIV have reported no serious adverse events among patients considered moderately immunosuppressed based on their CD4 counts. However, HIV infection has been associated with a reduced immunologic response to a number of inactivated and live attenuated vaccines, including yellow fever vaccine. The mechanisms for the diminished immune response in HIV-infected people are uncertain but appear to be correlated with HIV RNA levels and CD4 T-cell counts.

Because vaccinating asymptomatic HIV-infected people might be less effective than vaccinating people not infected with HIV, their neutralizing antibody response to vaccination should be measured before travel. Contact the appropriate state health department or the CDC Arboviral Diseases Branch (970-221-6400) to further discuss serologic testing.

If an asymptomatic HIV-infected person with moderate immune suppression (CD4 T-lymphocyte values 200–499/mm³ or 15%–24% of total lymphocytes for children aged <6 years) is traveling to a yellow fever–endemic area, vaccination may be considered. Vaccinated people should be monitored closely after vaccination for evidence of adverse events, and the state health department or CDC should be notified if an adverse event occurs.

If international travel requirements—not risk of yellow fever—are the only reason to vaccinate an HIV-infected person, the person should be excused from immunization and issued a medical waiver to fulfill health regulations. If an asymptomatic HIV-infected person has no evidence of immune suppression based on CD4 counts (CD4 T-lymphocyte values ≥500/mm³ or ≥25% of total lymphocytes for children aged <6 years), yellow fever vaccine can be administered if recommended.

Pregnancy

Pregnancy is a precaution for yellow fever vaccine administration. The safety of yellow fever vaccination during pregnancy has not been studied in a large prospective trial. However, a recent study of women who were vaccinated with yellow fever vaccine early in their pregnancies found no major malformations in their infants. A slight increased risk was noted for minor, mostly skin, malformations in infants. A higher rate of spontaneous abortions in pregnant women receiving the vaccine was reported but not substantiated. The proportion of women vaccinated during pregnancy who develop yellow fever IgG-specific antibodies is variable depending on the study (39% or 98%) and may be correlated with the trimester in which they received the vaccine. Because pregnancy may affect immunologic function, serologic testing can be considered to document a protective immune response to the vaccine.

If travel is unavoidable and the vaccination risks are felt to outweigh the risks of YFV exposure, pregnant women should be excused from immunization and issued a medical waiver to fulfill health regulations. Pregnant women who must travel to areas where YFV exposure is likely should be vaccinated. Although there are no specific data, ACIP recommends that a woman wait 4 weeks after receiving the yellow fever vaccine before conceiving.

Breastfeeding

Breastfeeding is a precaution for yellow fever vaccine administration. Two YEL-AND cases have been reported in exclusively breastfed infants whose mothers were vaccinated with yellow fever vaccine. Both infants were aged <1 month at the time of exposure. Further research is needed to document the risk of potential vaccine exposure through breastfeeding. Until more information is available, yellow fever vaccine should be avoided in breastfeeding women. However, when travel of nursing mothers to a yellow fever–endemic area cannot be avoided or postponed, these women should be vaccinated.

Other Considerations

Chronic medical conditions that may be associated with varying degrees of immune deficit include, but are not limited to, chronic renal disease, chronic liver disease (including hepatitis C), and diabetes mellitus. Because no information is available regarding possible increased adverse events or decreased vaccine efficacy after administration of yellow fever vaccine to patients with these diseases, caution should be used if considering vaccination of such patients. Factors to consider in assessing patients' general level of immune competence include disease severity, duration, clinical stability, complications, and comorbidities.

Simultaneous Administration of Other Vaccines and Drugs

Determination of whether to administer yellow fever vaccine and other immunobiologics simultaneously (administration on the same day but at a different injection site) should be made on the basis of convenience to the traveler in completing the desired vaccinations before travel and on information regarding potential immune interference. No evidence exists that inactivated vaccines interfere with the immune response to yellow fever vaccine. Therefore, inactivated vaccines can be administered either simultaneously or at any time before or after yellow fever vaccination. ACIP recommends that yellow fever vaccine be given at the same time as other live-virus vaccines. Otherwise, the clinician should wait 30 days between vaccinations, as the immune response to one live-virus vaccine might be impaired if administered within 30 days of another live-virus vaccine. Because of the different routes of administration, oral Ty21a typhoid vaccine can be administered simultaneously or at any interval before or after yellow fever vaccine.

INTERNATIONAL CERTIFICATE OF VACCINATION OR PROPHYLAXIS (ICVP)

The IHRs allow countries to require proof of yellow fever vaccination as a condition of entry for travelers arriving from certain countries, even if only in transit, to prevent importation and indigenous transmission of YFV. Some countries require evidence of vaccination from all entering travelers, which includes direct travel from the United States (Table 3-24). Travelers who arrive in a country with a yellow fever vaccination entry requirement without proof of yellow fever vaccination

Table 3-24. Countries that require proof of yellow fever vaccination from all arriving travelers[1]

Angola	Ghana
Benin	Guinea-Bissau
Burkina Faso	Liberia
Burundi	Mali
Cameroon	Niger
Central African Republic	Rwanda
Congo, Republic of the	São Tomé and Príncipe
Côte d'Ivoire	Sierra Leone
Democratic Republic of the Congo	Togo
French Guiana	
Gabon	

[1] Country requirements for yellow fever vaccination are subject to change at any time; therefore, CDC encourages travelers to check with the destination country's embassy or consulate before departure.

may be quarantined for up to 6 days, refused entry, or vaccinated on site. A traveler who has a specific contraindication to yellow fever vaccine and who cannot avoid travel to a country requiring vaccination should request a waiver from a physician before embarking on travel (see the Medical Waivers section).

Authorization to Provide Vaccinations and to Validate the ICVP

Under the revised IHR (2005), effective December 15, 2007, all state parties (countries) are required to issue a new ICVP. This is intended to replace the former International Certificate of Vaccination against Yellow Fever (ICV). People who received a yellow fever vaccination after December 15, 2007, must provide proof of vaccination on the new ICVP. If the person received the vaccine before December 15, 2007, the original ICV card is still valid, provided that the vaccination was given <10 years previously. Vaccinees should receive a completed ICVP (Figure 3-1), validated (stamped and signed) with the center's stamp where the vaccine was given (see below). An ICVP must be complete in every detail; if incomplete or inaccurate, it is not valid. Failure to secure validations can cause a traveler to be quarantined, denied entry, or possibly revaccinated at the point of entry to a country. Revaccination at the point of entry is not a recommended option for the traveler.

Clinics may purchase ICVPs, CDC 731 (formerly PHS 731), from the US Government Printing Office (http://bookstore.gpo.gov/, 866-512-1800). The stock number is 017-001-00567-3 for 25 copies and 017-001-00566-5 for 100 copies. This certificate of vaccination is valid for a period of 10 years, beginning 10 days after the date of vaccination. When a booster dose of the vaccine is given within this 10-year period, the certificate is considered valid from the date of revaccination.

People Authorized to Sign the ICVP and Designated Yellow Fever Vaccination Centers

The ICVP must be signed by a medical provider, who may be a licensed physician or a health care worker designated by the physician, supervising the administration of the vaccine (Figure 3-1). A signature stamp is not acceptable. Yellow fever vaccination must be given at a certified center in possession of an official "uniform stamp," which can be used to validate the ICVP.

State health departments are responsible for designating nonfederal yellow fever vaccination centers and issuing uniform stamps to clinicians. Information about the location and hours of yellow fever vaccination centers may be obtained by visiting CDC's website at wwwnc.cdc.gov/travel/yellow-fever-vaccination-clinics-search.aspx.

Medical Waivers (Exemptions)

Some countries do not require an ICVP for infants younger than a certain age (<6 months, <9 months, or <1 year of age, depending on the country). Age requirements for vaccination

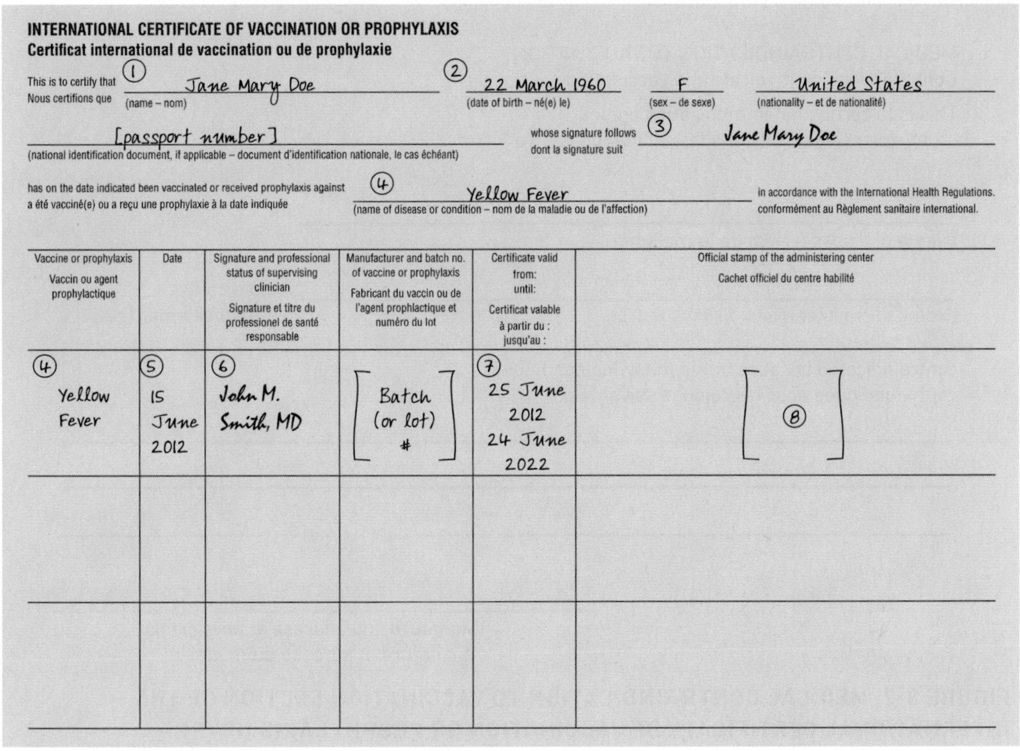

3

INTERNATIONAL CERTIFICATE OF VACCINATION OR PROPHYLAXIS
Certificat international de vaccination ou de prophylaxie

This is to certify that / Nous certifions que (1) _Jane Mary Doe_ (name – nom) (2) _22 March 1960_ (date of birth – né(e) le) _F_ (sex – de sexe) _United States_ (nationality – et de nationalité)

[passport number]
(national identification document, if applicable – document d'identification nationale, le cas échéant)

whose signature follows / dont la signature suit (3) _Jane Mary Doe_

has on the date indicated been vaccinated or received prophylaxis against / a été vacciné(e) ou a reçu une prophylaxie à la date indiquée (4) _Yellow Fever_ (name of disease or condition – nom de la maladie ou de l'affection) in accordance with the International Health Regulations. / conformément au Règlement sanitaire international.

Vaccine or prophylaxis / Vaccin ou agent prophylactique	Date	Signature and professional status of supervising clinician / Signature et titre du professionel de santé responsable	Manufacturer and batch no. of vaccine or prophylaxis / Fabricant du vaccin ou de l'agent prophylactique et numéro du lot	Certificate valid from: until: / Certificat valable à partir du : jusqu'au :	Official stamp of the administering center / Cachet officiel du centre habilité
(4) Yellow Fever	(5) 15 June 2012	(6) John M. Smith, MD	Batch (or lot) #	(7) 25 June 2012 / 24 June 2022	(8)

FIGURE 3-1. EXAMPLE INTERNATIONAL CERTIFICATE OF VACCINATION OR PROPHYLAXIS (ICVP)

(1) Name should appear exactly as on the patient's passport.
(2, 5, 7) All dates should be entered with the day in numerals, followed by the month in letters, then the year. For example: in the above example, the patient's date of birth is 22 March 1960.
(3) This space is for the patient's signature.
(4) For a yellow fever vaccination, 'Yellow Fever' should be written in both spaces. Should the ICVP be used for a required vaccination or prophylaxis against another disease or condition (following an amendment to the International Health Regulations or by recommendation of WHO), that disease or condition should be written in this space. Other vaccinations may be listed on the other side.
(5) The date on which the vaccination is given should be entered as shown above.
(6) A handwritten signature of the clinician—either the stamp holder or another health care provider authorized by the stamp holder—administering or supervising the administration of the vaccine (or prophylaxis) should appear in this box. A signature stamp is not acceptable.
(7) The certificate of yellow fever vaccination is valid for 10 years, beginning 10 days after the date of primary vaccination. The ending date for a valid vaccination recorded on the ICVP is 1 calendar day prior to the calendar day on which the vaccine became valid. For example, a vaccination given on 15 June 2012 will be valid on 25 June 2012 and will expire on 24 June 2022. In the case of revaccination, the certificate of yellow fever vaccination is valid immediately if documentation exists on an ICVP demonstrating that the previous yellow fever vaccination was given within the last 10 years.
(8) The Uniform Stamp of the vaccinating center should appear in this box.

for individual countries can be found in the Yellow Fever and Malaria Information, by Country section in this chapter. For medical contraindications, a physician who has decided to issue a waiver should fill out and sign the Medical Contraindications to Vaccination section of the ICVP (Figure 3-2). The clinician should also do the following:

- Give the traveler a signed and dated exemption letter on the physician's letterhead stationery, clearly stating the contraindications to vaccination and bearing the stamp used by the yellow fever vaccination centers to validate the ICVP.
- Inform the traveler of any increased risk for yellow fever infection associated with non-vaccination and how to minimize this risk by avoiding mosquito bites.

Reasons other than medical contraindications are not acceptable for exemption from vaccination. The traveler should be advised that issuance of a waiver does not guarantee its acceptance by the destination country. On arrival at the destination, the traveler may be faced with quarantine, refusal of entry, or

MEDICAL CONTRAINDICATION TO VACCINATION
Contre-indication médicale à la vaccination

This is to certify that immunization against
Je soussigné(e) certifie que la vaccination contre

_____   for
(Name of disease–Nom de la maladie)   pour

_____   is medically
(Name of traveler–Nom du voyageur)   est médicalement

contraindicated because of the following conditions:
contre-indiquée pour les raisons suivantes:

_____

_____

_____

_____
(Signature and address of physician)
(Signature et adresse du médecin)

FIGURE 3-2. MEDICAL CONTRAINDICATION TO VACCINATION SECTION OF THE INTERNATIONAL CERTIFICATE OF VACCINATION OR PROPHYLAXIS (ICVP)

vaccination on site. To improve the likelihood that the waiver will be accepted at the destination country, clinicians can suggest that the traveler take the following additional measures before beginning travel:

- Obtain specific and authoritative advice from the embassy or consulate of the destination country or countries.
- Request documentation of requirements for waivers from embassies or consulates and retain these along with the completed Medical Contraindication to Vaccination section of the ICVP.

REQUIREMENTS VERSUS RECOMMENDATIONS

Country entry requirements for proof of yellow fever vaccination under the IHRs are different from CDC's recommendations. Yellow fever vaccine entry requirements are established by countries to prevent the importation and transmission of YFV and are allowed under the IHRs. Travelers must comply with these to enter the country, unless they have been issued a medical waiver. Certain countries require vaccination from travelers arriving from all countries, while some countries require vaccination only for travelers coming from "a country with risk of yellow fever transmission" (see the Yellow Fever and Malaria Information, by Country section in this chapter). WHO defines those areas "with risk of yellow fever transmission" as countries or areas where yellow fever has been reported currently or in the past, plus where vectors and animal reservoirs exist. Country requirements are subject to change at any time; therefore, CDC encourages travelers to check with the appropriate embassy or consulate before departure.

The information in the section on yellow fever vaccine recommendations is advice given by CDC to prevent yellow fever infections among travelers. Recommendations are subject to change at any time if disease conditions change; therefore, CDC encourages travelers to check the destination pages for up-to-date vaccine information and to check for relevant travel notices on the CDC website before departure (www.cdc.gov/travel).

NEW CHANGES TO YELLOW FEVER RISK CLASSIFICATION AND CDC VACCINE RECOMMENDATIONS

CDC, WHO, and other yellow fever experts recently completed a comprehensive review of available data and revised the criteria and global maps designating the risk of YFV

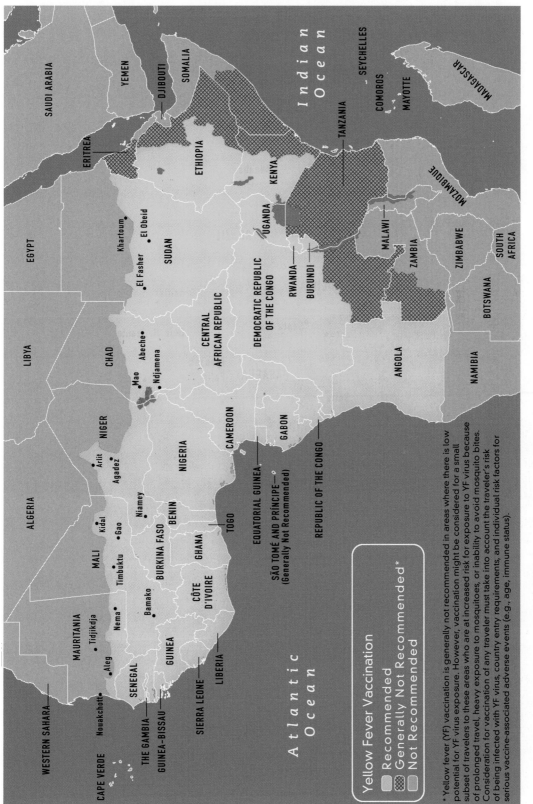

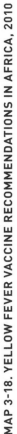

Yellow Fever Vaccination
- Recommended
- Generally Not Recommended*
- Not Recommended

* Yellow fever (YF) vaccination is generally not recommended in areas where there is low potential for YF virus exposure. However, vaccination might be considered for a small subset of travelers to these areas who are at increased risk for exposure to YF virus because of prolonged travel, heavy exposure to mosquitoes, or inability to avoid mosquito bites. Consideration for vaccination of any traveler must take into account the traveler's risk of being infected with YF virus, country entry requirements, and individual risk factors for serious vaccine-associated adverse events (e.g., age, immune status).

MAP 3-18. YELLOW FEVER VACCINE RECOMMENDATIONS IN AFRICA, 2010

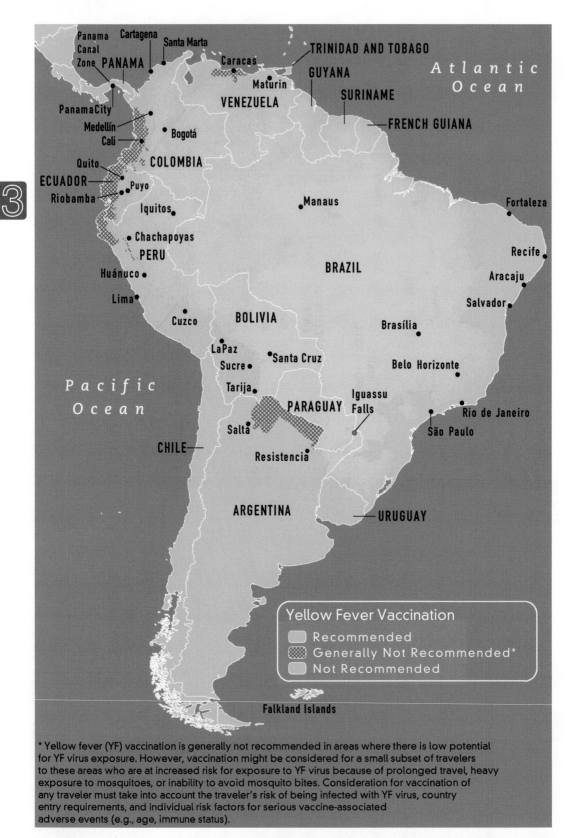

MAP 3-19. YELLOW FEVER VACCINE RECOMMENDATIONS IN THE AMERICAS, 2010

transmission. The new criteria establish 4 categories of risk for YFV transmission that apply to all geographic areas: endemic, transitional, low potential for exposure, and no risk.

Yellow fever vaccination is recommended for travel to endemic and transitional areas. Although vaccination is generally not recommended for travel to areas with low potential for exposure, it might be considered for a small subset of travelers whose itinerary could place them at increased risk for exposure to YFV (such as prolonged travel, heavy exposure to mosquitoes, or inability to avoid mosquito bites).

Based on the revised criteria for yellow fever risk classification, the current maps (Maps 3-18 and 3-19) and country-specific information (see the Yellow Fever and Malaria Information, by Country later in this chapter) designate 3 levels of yellow fever vaccine recommendations: recommended, generally not recommended, and not recommended. Note: *The revised yellow fever Maps 3-18 and 3-19 now depict vaccination recommendations rather than yellow fever risk.*

Countries that only contain areas with low potential for exposure to YFV (Table 3-22) are not included on the official WHO list of countries with risk of YFV transmission (Table 3-21). Therefore, proof of yellow fever vaccination should not be required if traveling from a country with low potential for exposure to YFV to a country with a vaccination entry requirement (unless that country requires proof of yellow fever vaccination from all arriving travelers; see Table 3-24).

VACCINATION FOR TRAVEL ON MILITARY ORDERS

Because military requirements may exceed those indicated in this publication, any person who plans to travel on military orders (civilians and military personnel) should contact the nearest military medical facility to determine the requirements for his or her trip.

BIBLIOGRAPHY

1. Barwick R. History of thymoma and yellow fever vaccination. Lancet. 2004 Sep 11–17;364(9438):936.

2. Cavalcanti DP, Salomao MA, Lopez-Camelo J, Pessoto MA. Early exposure to yellow fever vaccine during pregnancy. Trop Med Int Health. 2007 Jul;12(7): 833–7.

3. CDC. General recommendations on immunization: recommendations of the Advisory Committee on Immunization Practices (ACIP). MMWR Recomm Rep. 2010.

4. CDC. Transmission of yellow fever vaccine virus through breast-feeding—Brazil, 2009. MMWR Morb Mortal Wkly Rep. 2010 Feb 12;59(5):130–2.

5. Fletcher MA, Fabre P, Debois H, Saliou P. Vaccines administered simultaneously: directions for new combination vaccines based on an historical review of the literature. Int J Infect Dis. 2004 Nov;8(6): 328–38.

6. Hayes EB. Acute viscerotropic disease following vaccination against yellow fever. Trans R Soc Trop Med Hyg. 2007 Oct;101(10):967–71.

7. Lindsey NP, Schroeder BA, Miller ER, Braun MM, Hinckley AF, Marano N, et al. Adverse event reports following yellow fever vaccination. Vaccine. 2008 Nov 11;26(48):6077–82.

8. McMahon AW, Eidex RB, Marfin AA, Russell M, Sejvar JJ, Markoff L, et al. Neurologic disease associated with 17D-204 yellow fever vaccination: a report of 15 cases. Vaccine. 2007 Feb 26;25(10):1727–34.

9. Monath TP, Cetron MS. Prevention of yellow fever in people traveling to the tropics. Clin Infect Dis. 2002 May 15;34(10):1369–78.

10. Monath TP, Nichols R, Archambault WT, Moore L, Marchesani R, Tian J, et al. Comparative safety and immunogenicity of two yellow fever 17D vaccines (ARILVAX and YF-VAX) in a phase III multicenter, double-blind clinical trial. Am J Trop Med Hyg. 2002 May;66(5):533–41.

11. Monath TP, Teuwen D, Cetron MS. Yellow fever vaccine. In: Plotkin S, Orenstein WA, Offit PA, editors. Vaccines. 5th ed. Philadelphia: WB Saunders; 2008. p. 959–1055.

12. Nasidi A, Monath TP, Vandenberg J, Tomori O, Calisher CH, Hurtgen X, et al. Yellow fever vaccination and pregnancy: a four-year prospective study. Trans R Soc Trop Med Hyg. 1993 May–Jun;87(3):337–9.

13. Nishioka SD, Nunes-Araujo FRF, Pires WP, Silva FA, Costa HL. Yellow fever vaccination during pregnancy and spontaneous abortion: a case-control study. Trop Med Int Health. 1998 Jan;3(1):29–33.

14. Pan American Health Organization. Yellow fever in Paraguay: mobilization continues. 2008 [cited 2010 Oct 19]. Available from: http://www.paho.org/English/ad/dpc/cd/eid-eer-2008-02-25.htm.

15. Staples JE, Gershman M, Fischer M. Yellow fever vaccine: recommendations of the Advisory Committee on Immunization Practices (ACIP). MMWR Recomm Rep. 2010 Jul 30;59(RR-7):1–27.

16. Suzano CES, Amaral E, Sato HK, Papaiordanou PM, Fever CGY. The effects of yellow fever immunization (17DD) inadvertently used in early pregnancy during a mass campaign in Brazil. Vaccine. 2006 Feb 27;24(9):1421–6.

17. Tomori O. Yellow fever: the recurring plague. Crit Rev Clin Lab Sci. 2004;41(4):391–427.

18. Whittembury A, Ramirez G, Hernandez H, Ropero AM, Waterman S, Ticona M, et al. Viscerotropic disease following yellow fever vaccination in Peru. Vaccine. 2009 Oct 9;27(43):5974–81.

19. World Health Organization. International Health Regulations, 2005. 2008 [cited 2010 Oct 19]. Available from: http://whqlibdoc.who.int/publications/2008/9789241580410_eng.pdf.

20 World Health Organization. Yellow fever vaccine. WHO position paper. WklyEpidemiol Rec. 2003 Oct 3;78(40):349–59.

YERSINIOSIS

Kanyin L. Ong, Amy L. Boore, L. Hannah Gould

INFECTIOUS AGENT

Yersiniosis is caused by facultative anaerobic gram-negative coccobacilli of the genus *Yersinia*. Most known human infections are associated with *Yersinia enterocolitica* serogroups O:3, O:5,27, O:8, and O:9. Infection with *Y. pseudotuberculosis* can also occur but is uncommon; *Y. pseudotuberculosis* infections tend to be more severe.

MODE OF TRANSMISSION

Y. enterocolitica is transmitted by consumption or handling of contaminated food products (most commonly raw or undercooked pork products), unpasteurized or inadequately pasteurized milk, untreated water, or by direct or indirect contact with animals. The epidemiology of other species has been less studied. However, these infections are generally thought to be transmitted through fecal contamination of food or water.

EPIDEMIOLOGY

Yersiniosis is more common in cooler months in temperate climates. The highest incidence is reported in northern Europe (particularly Scandinavia), Japan, and Canada. The incidence of microbiologically confirmed yersiniosis was estimated to be 8 per 10,000 international travelers who sought care at travel clinics throughout the world.

People with high iron levels, such as those with chronic hemolysis, sickle cell disease, or β-thalassemia, or who are using iron-chelating agents such as deferoxamine, are at higher risk of infection and severe disease. The incidence among travelers to developing countries has been low in the few studies that specifically looked for *Yersinia*.

CLINICAL PRESENTATION

The incubation period is typically 4–6 days (range, 1–14 days). Common symptoms include fever, abdominal pain, and diarrhea, which may be bloody. The duration of diarrhea varies, but it can persist for several weeks. Abdominal pain in yersiniosis may mimic appendicitis. Necrotizing enterocolitis has been described in young infants. Bacteremia is rare and occurs most commonly in young children and infants with predisposing conditions such as excessive iron storage and immunosuppressive states.

Focal manifestations may occur rarely, including pharyngitis, meningitis, osteomyelitis, pyomyositis, conjunctivitis, pneumonia, empyema, endocarditis, acute peritonitis, abscesses of the liver and spleen, and primary cutaneous infection. Postinfectious sequelae are sometimes reported, predominantly in adults. Reactive arthritis affecting the wrists, knees, and ankles can occur, with onset usually 1 month after the initial diarrhea episode and symptoms typically resolving after 1–6 months. Erythema nodosum can also occur, manifesting as painful, raised red or purple lesions along the trunk and legs. This condition is more commonly reported among women; symptoms usually resolve spontaneously within 1 month.

DIAGNOSIS

Definitive diagnosis is made by isolating the organism from stool, blood, bile, wound, throat swab, mesenteric lymph node, cerebrospinal fluid, or peritoneal fluid. Most laboratories do not routinely test for *Y. enterocolitica*. If yersiniosis is suspected, the clinical laboratory should be notified and instructed to culture on CIN agar. Postinfectious sequelae, including reactive arthritis and erythema nodosum, are diagnosed clinically and serologically. Serologic tests for *Y. enterocolitica* serogroup O:9 may cross-react with tests for *Brucella* and *Escherichia coli* O157:H7.

TREATMENT

Antibiotic treatment may reduce the duration of fecal shedding. However, the benefit of antibiotic therapy in uncomplicated cases is not well established. Antibiotic treatment should be given for severe cases, including patients with septicemia, metastatic focal infections, or underlying immunosuppression. *Y. enterocolitica* isolates are usually susceptible to trimethoprim-sulfamethoxazole, aminoglycosides, cefotaxime, fluoroquinolones, tetracycline, doxycycline, and chloramphenicol. *Y. enterocolitica* isolates typically are resistant to first-generation and most second-generation cephalosporins and most penicillins. Antimicrobial therapy has no effect on postinfectious sequelae.

PREVENTIVE MEASURES FOR TRAVELERS

No vaccine is available. Drugs for preventing infection are not recommended. Travelers should avoid raw or undercooked pork products, unpasteurized milk products, and untreated water (see Chapter 2, Food and Water Precautions).

BIBLIOGRAPHY

1. Adamkiewicz TV, Berkovitch M, Krishnan C, Polsinelli C, Kermack D, Olivieri NF. Infection due to *Yersinia enterocolitica* in a series of patients with beta-thalassemia: incidence and predisposing factors. Clin Infect Dis. 1998 Dec;27(6):1362–6.
2. Cover TL, Aber RC. *Yersinia enterocolitica*. N Engl J Med. 1989 Jul 6;321(1):16–24.
3. Nuorti JP, Niskanen T, Hallanvuo S, Mikkola J, Kela E, Hatakka M, et al. A widespread outbreak of *Yersinia pseudotuberculosis* O:3 infection from iceberg lettuce. J Infect Dis. 2004 Mar 1;189(5):766–74.
4. Ostroff SM, Kapperud G, Hutwagner LC, Nesbakken T, Bean NH, Lassen J, et al. Sources of sporadic *Yersinia enterocolitica* infections in Norway: a prospective case-control study. Epidemiol Infect. 1994 Feb;112(1):133–41.
5. Perdikogianni C, Galanakis E, Michalakis M, Giannoussi E, Maraki S, Tselentis Y, et al. *Yersinia enterocolitica* infection mimicking surgical conditions. Pediatr Surg Int. 2006 Jul;22(7):589–92.
6. Swaminathan A, Torresi J, Schlagenhauf P, Thursky K, Wilder-Smith A, Connor BA, et al. A global study of pathogens and host risk factors associated with infectious gastrointestinal disease in returned international travellers. J Infect. 2009 Jul;59(1):19–27.
7. Tauxe RV, Vandepitte J, Wauters G, Martin SM, Goossens V, De Mol P, et al. *Yersinia enterocolitica* infections and pork: the missing link. Lancet. 1987 May 16;1(8542):1129–32.
8. Vantrappen G, Geboes K, Ponette E. *Yersinia* enteritis. Med Clin North Am. 1982 May;66(3):639–53.

Yellow Fever & Malaria Information, by Country

Mark Gershman, Emily S. Jentes, Theresa Sommers,
J. Erin Staples (YELLOW FEVER)

Kathrine R. Tan, Paul M. Arguin, Stefanie F. Steele (MALARIA)

The following pages present country-specific information on yellow fever vaccine requirements and recommendations and malaria transmission information and prophylaxis recommendations. Reference maps of 13 countries are included within the country-specific list to aid in interpreting the recommendations. The information was accurate at the time of publication; however, this information is subject to change at any time as a result of changes in disease transmission or, in the case of yellow fever, changing country entry requirements. Updated information, reflecting changes since publication, can be found in the online version of this book (www.cdc.gov/yellowbook) and on the CDC Travelers' Health website (www.cdc.gov/travel).

Yellow Fever

Yellow fever vaccination recommendations have changed substantially since the 2010 edition of *CDC Health Information for International Travel*. From 2008 through 2010, CDC, the World Health Organization (WHO), and other yellow fever and travel medicine experts reviewed available data and revised the criteria and maps that describe the risk of yellow fever virus (YFV) transmission. Based on the review, updated recommendations have been made for Argentina, Brazil, Colombia, Democratic Republic of the Congo, Ecuador, Eritrea, Ethiopia, Kenya, Panama, Paraguay, Peru, São Tomé and Príncipe, Somalia, Tanzania, Trinidad and Tobago, Venezuela, and Zambia (see the country-specific information in this section and Maps 3-18 and 3-19).

The review process also resulted in the creation of 3 categories of recommendations regarding yellow fever vaccination. See Table 3-25 for definitions of these recommendation categories. ***Note****: The format of the yellow fever maps (Maps 3-18 and 3-19) has been revised to depict vaccination recommendations rather than yellow fever risk.*

Ultimately, the clinician's decision whether or not to vaccinate any traveler must take into account the traveler's risk of being infected with YFV, country entry requirements, and individual risk factors for serious adverse events after yellow fever vaccination (such as age and immune status). For a thorough discussion of yellow fever and guidance for appropriate vaccination, see the Yellow Fever section earlier in this chapter.

Malaria

The recommendations for malaria prevention have also been extensively updated since the 2010 edition and now include estimates of malaria risk to US travelers. These estimates are based on numbers of malaria cases reported in US travelers and the estimated volume of travel to these countries. In some instances, the risk may be low because the actual intensity of transmission is low in that country. In other instances, significant malaria transmission may occur only in small focal areas of the country where US travelers seldom go. Thus, even though the risk for the average traveler to that country may be low, the risk for the rare traveler going to the areas with higher transmission intensity will be higher. For some countries rarely visited by US travelers, insufficient information exists to make a risk estimate. Information about malaria species present in each country is based on the best available data from multiple sources.

Several medications are available for malaria chemoprophylaxis. When deciding on which drug to use, clinicians should consider the specific itinerary, length of trip, cost of the drugs, previous adverse reactions to antimalarials, drug allergies, and medical history.

For a thorough discussion of malaria and guidance for appropriate prophylaxis, see the Malaria section earlier in this chapter.

348 INFECTIOUS DISEASES RELATED TO TRAVEL

Table 3-25. Categories of recommendations for yellow fever vaccination

YELLOW FEVER VACCINATION CATEGORY	RATIONALE FOR RECOMMENDATION
Recommended	Vaccination recommended for all travelers ≥9 months of age to areas with endemic or transitional yellow fever risk, as determined by persistent or periodic YFV transmission.
Generally not recommended	Vaccination generally not recommended in areas where the potential for YFV exposure is low, as determined by absence of reports of human yellow fever and past evidence suggestive of only low levels of YFV transmission. However, vaccination might be considered for a small subset of travelers who are at increased risk for exposure to YFV because of prolonged travel, heavy exposure to mosquitoes, or inability to avoid mosquito bites.
Not recommended	Vaccination not recommended in areas where there is no risk of YFV transmission, as determined by absence of past or present evidence of YFV circulation in the area or environmental conditions not conducive to YFV transmission.

Abbreviation: YFV, yellow fever virus.

Country-Specific Information

AFGHANISTAN
Yellow Fever
Requirements: Required if traveling from a country with risk of YFV transmission.[a]
Recommendations: None

Malaria
Areas with malaria: April–December in all areas <2,000 m (6,561 ft).
Estimated relative risk of malaria for US travelers: High[b]
Drug resistance[c]: Chloroquine
Malaria species: *P. vivax* 80%–90%, *P. falciparum* 10%–20%.
Recommended chemoprophylaxis: Atovaquone-proguanil, doxycycline, or mefloquine.

ALBANIA
Yellow Fever
Requirements: Required if traveling from a country with risk of YFV transmission and ≥1 year of age.[a]
Recommendations: None

Malaria
No malaria transmission.

ALGERIA
Yellow Fever
Requirements: Required if traveling from a country with risk of YFV transmission and ≥1 year of age.[a]
Recommendations: None

Malaria
No malaria transmission.

AMERICAN SAMOA (US)
Yellow Fever
No requirements or recommendations.

Malaria
No malaria transmission.

ANDORRA
Yellow Fever
No requirements or recommendations.

Malaria
No malaria transmission.

ANGOLA
Yellow Fever
Requirements: Required upon arrival from all countries if traveler is ≥1 year of age.
Recommendations: *Recommended* for all travelers ≥9 months of age.

Malaria
Areas with malaria: All
Estimated relative risk of malaria for US travelers: Moderate
Drug resistance[c]: Chloroquine
Malaria species: *P. falciparum* 90%, *P. ovale* 5%, *P. vivax* 5%.
Recommended chemoprophylaxis: Atovaquone-proguanil, doxycycline, or mefloquine.

ANGUILLA (UK)
Yellow Fever
Requirements: Required if traveling from a country with risk of YFV transmission and ≥1 year of age.[a]
Recommendations: None

Malaria
No malaria transmission.

ANTARCTICA
Yellow Fever
No requirements or recommendations.

Malaria
No malaria transmission.

ANTIGUA AND BARBUDA
Yellow Fever
Requirements: Required if traveling from a country with risk of YFV transmission and ≥1 year of age.[a]
Recommendations: None

Malaria
No malaria transmission.

FOOTNOTES:
[a] The official WHO list of countries with risk of YFV transmission can be found in Table 3-21. Proof of yellow fever vaccination should be required only if traveling from a country on the WHO list, unless otherwise specified. The following countries, containing only areas with low potential for exposure to YFV, are not on the WHO list: Eritrea, São Tomé and Príncipe, Somalia, Tanzania, Zambia.

ARGENTINA (See Map 3-20.)

Yellow Fever

Requirements: None

Recommendations:

Recommended for all travelers ⩾9 months of age who are going to northern and northeastern forested areas of Argentina bordering Brazil and Paraguay <2,300 m in elevation[d] (see Map 3-19). Travelers to designated departments in the following provinces should be vaccinated: Corrientes (Berón de Astrada, Capital, General Alvear, General Paz, Itatí, Ituzaingó, Paso de los Libres, San Cosme, San Martín, San Miguel, Santo Tomé) and Misiones (all departments). Vaccination is also recommended for travelers visiting Iguassu Falls.

Generally not recommended for travelers whose itinerary is limited to the designated departments in the following provinces <2,300 m in elevation[d]: Chaco (Bermejo), Formosa (all departments), Jujuy (Ledesma, San Pedro, Santa Bárbara, Valle Grande), and Salta (Anta, General José de San Martín, Oran, Rivadavia) (see Map 3-19).

Not recommended for travelers whose itineraries are limited to areas >2,300 m in elevation[d] and all provinces and departments not listed above.

Malaria

Areas with malaria: Rural areas of northern Salta Province (along Bolivian border). Rare cases reported in the city of Puerto Iguazú in Misiones Province. No transmission at Iguassu Falls.

Estimated relative risk of malaria for US travelers: Very low

Drug resistance[c]: None

Malaria species: *P. vivax* 100%.

Recommended chemoprophylaxis:

Salta province: Atovaquone-proguanil, chloroquine, doxycycline, mefloquine, or primaquine.[e]

Misiones province: Mosquito avoidance only.

ARMENIA

Yellow Fever

No requirements or recommendations.

Malaria

No malaria transmission.

ARUBA

Yellow Fever

Requirements: Required if traveling from a country with risk of YFV transmission and ⩾6 months of age.[a]

Recommendations: None

Malaria

No malaria transmission.

AUSTRALIA

Yellow Fever

Requirements: Required for all people ⩾1 year of age who enter Australia within 6 days of having stayed overnight or longer in a country with risk of YFV transmission,[a] including São Tomé and Príncipe, Somalia, and Tanzania, but excluding Galápagos Islands in Ecuador and limited to Misiones Province in Argentina.

Recommendations: None

Malaria

No malaria transmission.

AUSTRIA

Yellow Fever

No requirements or recommendations.

Malaria

No malaria transmission.

AZERBAIJAN

Yellow Fever

No requirements or recommendations.

Malaria

Areas with malaria: May–October in rural areas <1,500 m (4,921 ft). None in Baku.

Estimated relative risk of malaria for US travelers: Very low

Drug resistance[c]: None

Malaria species: *P. vivax* 100%.

---

[b] This risk estimate is based largely on cases occurring in US military personnel who travel for extended periods of time with unique itineraries that likely do not reflect the risk for the average US traveler.

[c] Refers to *P. falciparum* malaria unless otherwise noted.

[d] An elevation of 2,300 m is equivalent to 7,546 ft.

[e] Primaquine can cause hemolytic anemia in people with glucose-6-phosphate dehydrogenase (G6PD) deficiency. Patients must be screened for G6PD deficiency before starting primaquine.

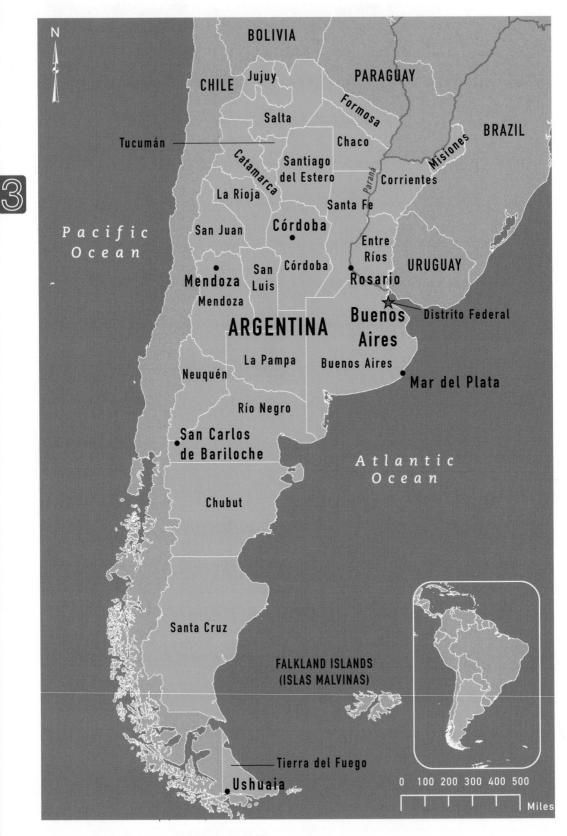

MAP 3-20. ARGENTINA REFERENCE MAP

INFECTIOUS DISEASES RELATED TO TRAVEL

Recommended chemoprophylaxis:
Atovaquone-proguanil, chloroquine,
doxycycline, mefloquine, or primaquine.[e]

AZORES (PORTUGAL)
Yellow Fever
No requirements or recommendations.

Malaria
No malaria transmission.

BAHAMAS, THE
Yellow Fever
Requirements: Required if traveling from a
country with risk of YFV transmission and ≥1
year of age.[a]
Recommendations: None

Malaria
No malaria transmission.

BAHRAIN
Yellow Fever
Requirements: Required if traveling from a
country with risk of YFV transmission and ≥1
year of age.[a]
Recommendations: None

Malaria
No malaria transmission.

BANGLADESH
Yellow Fever
Requirements: Required if traveling from a
country with risk of YFV transmission and ≥1
year of age.[a]
Recommendations: None

Malaria
Areas with malaria: All areas, except in the
city of Dhaka.
**Estimated relative risk of malaria for US
travelers:** Moderate
Drug resistance[c]: Chloroquine

Malaria species: *P. falciparum* 77%, *P. vivax*
23%.
Recommended chemoprophylaxis:
Atovaquone-proguanil, doxycycline, or
mefloquine.

BARBADOS
Yellow Fever
Requirements: Required if ≥1 year of age
and traveling from a country with risk of YFV
transmission,[a] except Guyana and Trinidad
and Tobago.
Recommendations: None

Malaria
No malaria transmission.

BELARUS
Yellow Fever
No requirements or recommendations.

Malaria
No malaria transmission.

BELGIUM
Yellow Fever
No requirements or recommendations.

Malaria
No malaria transmission.

BELIZE
Yellow Fever
Requirements: Required if traveling from a
country with risk of YFV transmission and ≥1
year of age.[a]
Recommendations: None

Malaria
Areas with malaria: All areas, especially the
districts of Cayo, Stann Creek, and Toledo.
None in Belize City and islands frequented by
tourists.
**Estimated relative risk of malaria for US
travelers:** Low

FOOTNOTES:
[a] The official WHO list of countries with risk of YFV transmission can be found in Table 3-21. Proof of yellow fever vaccination should be required only if traveling from a country on the WHO list, unless otherwise specified. The following countries, containing only areas with low potential for exposure to YFV, are not on the WHO list: Eritrea, São Tomé and Príncipe, Somalia, Tanzania, Zambia.
[c] Refers to *P. falciparum* malaria unless otherwise noted.
[e] Primaquine can cause hemolytic anemia in people with glucose-6-phosphate dehydrogenase (G6PD) deficiency. Patients must be screened for G6PD deficiency before starting primaquine.

Drug resistance[c]: None
Malaria species: *P. vivax* 100%.
Recommended chemoprophylaxis:
Districts of Cayo, Stann Creek, and Toledo:
Atovaquone-proguanil, chloroquine,
doxycycline, mefloquine, or primaquine.[e]
All other areas with malaria: Mosquito
avoidance only.

BENIN
Yellow Fever
Requirements: Required upon arrival from
all countries if traveler is ≥1 year of age.
Recommendations: *Recommended* for all
travelers ≥9 months of age.

Malaria
Areas with malaria: All
**Estimated relative risk of malaria for US
travelers:** High
Drug resistance[c]: Chloroquine
Malaria species: *P. falciparum* 85%, *P. ovale*
5%–10%, *P. vivax* rare.
Recommended chemoprophylaxis:
Atovaquone-proguanil, doxycycline, or
mefloquine.

BERMUDA (UK)
Yellow Fever
No requirements or recommendations.

Malaria
No malaria transmission.

BHUTAN
Yellow Fever
Requirements: Required if traveling from a
country with risk of YFV transmission.[a]
Recommendations: None

Malaria
Areas with malaria: Rural areas <1,700 m
(5,577 ft) of the southern belt districts along
the border with India: Chirang, Geylegphug,
Jongkhar, Samchi, Samdrup, and Shemgang.
**Estimated relative risk of malaria for US
travelers:** Very low

Drug resistance[c]: Chloroquine
Malaria species: *P. falciparum* 60%, *P. vivax*
40%.
Recommended chemoprophylaxis:
Atovaquone-proguanil, doxycycline, or
mefloquine.

BOLIVIA (See Map 3-21.)
Yellow Fever
Requirements: Required for travelers ≥1
year of age arriving from countries with risk
of YFV transmission.[a]
Recommendations:
Recommended for all travelers ≥9 months of
age traveling to the following areas east of
the Andes Mountains <2,300 m in elevation[d]:
the entire departments of Beni, Pando, Santa
Cruz, and designated areas (see Map 3-19) of
Chuquisaca, Cochabamba, La Paz, and Tarija.
Not recommended for travelers whose
itineraries are limited to areas >2,300 m in
elevation[d] and all areas not listed above,
including the cities of La Paz and Sucre.

Malaria
Areas with malaria: All areas <2,500 m
(8,202 ft). None in the city of La Paz.
**Estimated relative risk of malaria for US
travelers:** Low
Drug resistance[c]: Chloroquine
Malaria species: *P. vivax* 91%, *P. falciparum* 9%.
Recommended chemoprophylaxis:
Atovaquone-proguanil, doxycycline,
mefloquine, or primaquine.[e]

BOSNIA AND HERZEGOVINA
Yellow Fever
No requirements or recommendations.

Malaria
No malaria transmission.

BOTSWANA
Yellow Fever
Requirements: Required for travelers
≥1 year of age arriving from or having

FOOTNOTES:
[a] The official WHO list of countries with risk of YFV transmission can be found in Table 3-21. Proof of yellow fever
vaccination should be required only if traveling from a country on the WHO list, unless otherwise specified. The
following countries, containing only areas with low potential for exposure to YFV, are not on the WHO list: Eritrea,
São Tomé and Príncipe, Somalia, Tanzania, Zambia.

passed through countries with risk of YFV transmission.[a]
Recommendations: None

Malaria

Areas with malaria: Present in the following districts: Central, Chobe, Ghanzi, Northeast, and Northwest. None in the cities of Francistown and Gaborone.
Estimated relative risk of malaria for US travelers: Very low
Drug resistance[c]: Chloroquine
Malaria species: *P. falciparum* 90%, *P. vivax* 5%, *P. ovale* 5%.
Recommended chemoprophylaxis: Atovaquone-proguanil, doxycycline, or mefloquine.

BRAZIL (See Map 3-22.)

Yellow Fever
Requirements: None
Recommendations:
Recommended for all travelers ≥9 months of age going to the following areas: the entire states of Acre, Amapá, Amazonas, Distrito Federal (including the capital city of Brasília), Goiás, Maranhão, Mato Grosso, Mato Grosso do Sul, Minas Gerais, Pará, Rondônia, Roraima, Tocantins, and designated areas (see Map 3-19) of the following states: Bahia, Paraná, Piauí, Rio Grande do Sul, Santa Catarina, and São Paulo. Vaccination is also recommended for travelers visiting Iguassu Falls.

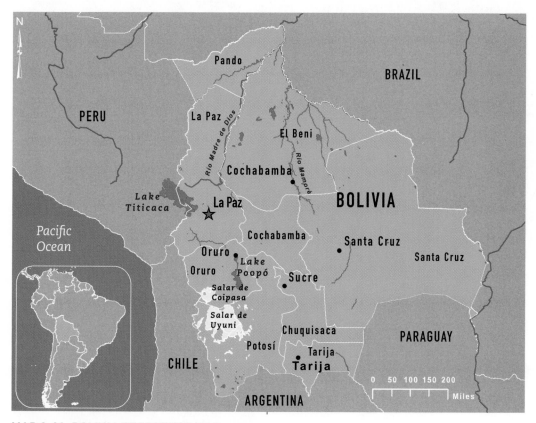

MAP 3-21. BOLIVIA REFERENCE MAP

[c] Refers to *P. falciparum* malaria unless otherwise noted.
[d] An elevation of 2,300 m is equivalent to 7,546 ft.
[e] Primaquine can cause hemolytic anemia in people with glucose-6-phosphate dehydrogenase (G6PD) deficiency. Patients must be screened for G6PD deficiency before starting primaquine.

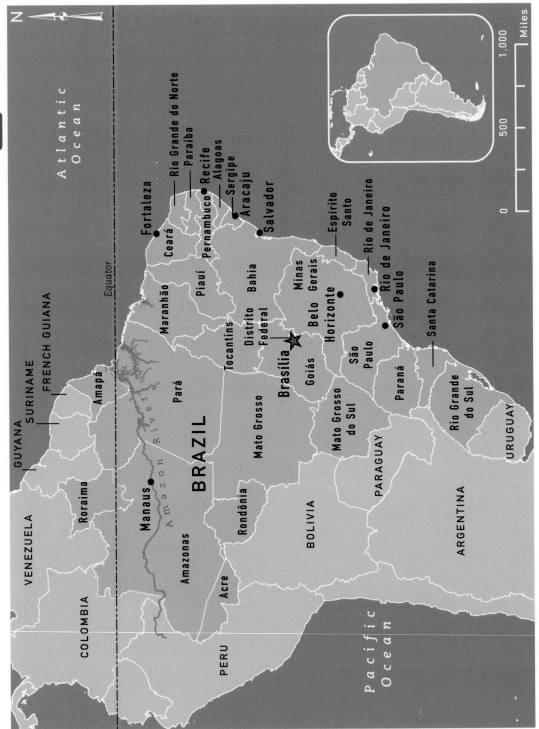

MAP 3-22. BRAZIL REFERENCE MAP

Not recommended for travelers whose itineraries are limited to areas not listed above, including the cities of Fortaleza, Recife, Rio de Janeiro, Salvador, and São Paulo (see Map 3-19).

Malaria
Areas with malaria: States of Acre, Amapá, Amazonas, Mato Grosso, Para, Rondonia, Roraima, Tocantins, and the western part of Maranhaõ. Also present in urban areas, including cities such as Boa Vista, Macapa, Manaus, Maraba, Porto Velho, and Santarem. Rare cases in Belem. No transmission at Iguassu Falls.
Estimated relative risk of malaria for US travelers: Low
Drug resistance[c]: Chloroquine
Malaria species: *P. vivax* 75%, *P. falciparum* 25%.
Recommended chemoprophylaxis:
Areas with malaria: Atovaquone-proguanil, doxycycline, or mefloquine.
Belem City: Mosquito avoidance only.

BRITISH INDIAN OCEAN TERRITORY, INCLUDES DIEGO GARCIA (UK)
Yellow Fever
No requirements or recommendations.

Malaria
No malaria transmission.

BRUNEI
Yellow Fever
Requirements: Required for travelers ≥1 year of age arriving from countries with risk of YFV transmission[a] or having passed through areas partly or wholly at risk of YFV transmission within the preceding 6 days.
Recommendations: None

Malaria
No malaria transmission.

BULGARIA
Yellow Fever
No requirements or recommendations.

Malaria
No malaria transmission.

BURKINA FASO
Yellow Fever
Requirements: Required upon arrival from all countries if traveler is ≥1 year of age.
Recommendations: *Recommended* for all travelers ≥9 months of age.

Malaria
Areas with malaria: All
Estimated relative risk of malaria for US travelers: High
Drug resistance: Chloroquine
Malaria species: *P. falciparum* 80%, *P. ovale* 5%–10%, *P. vivax* rare.
Recommended chemoprophylaxis:
Atovaquone-proguanil, doxycycline, or mefloquine.

BURMA (MYANMAR)
Yellow Fever
Requirements: Required if traveling from a country with risk of YFV transmission.[a] Required also for nationals and residents of Burma (Myanmar) departing for a country with risk of YFV transmission.
Recommendations: None

Malaria
Areas with malaria: Rural areas throughout the country at altitudes <1,000 m (3,281 ft). None in the cities of Mandalay and Rangoon (Yangon).
Estimated relative risk of malaria for US travelers: Moderate
Drug resistance[c]: Chloroquine, mefloquine (see Map 3-11).
Malaria species: *P. falciparum* 80%, *P. vivax* 20%.
Recommended chemoprophylaxis:
In the provinces of Bago, Kachin, Kayah, Kayin, Shan, and Tanintharyi: Atovaquone-proguanil or doxycycline.
All other areas with malaria: Atovaquone-proguanil, doxycycline, or mefloquine.

FOOTNOTES:
[a] The official WHO list of countries with risk of YFV transmission can be found in Table 3-21. Proof of yellow fever vaccination should be required only if traveling from a country on the WHO list, unless otherwise specified. The following countries, containing only areas with low potential for exposure to YFV, are not on the WHO list: Eritrea, São Tomé and Príncipe, Somalia, Tanzania, Zambia.
[c] Refers to *P. falciparum* malaria unless otherwise noted.

BURUNDI
Yellow Fever
Requirement: Required upon arrival from all countries if traveler is ≥1 year of age.
Recommendations: *Recommended* for all travelers ≥9 months of age.

Malaria
Areas with malaria: All
Estimated relative risk of malaria for US travelers: Moderate
Drug resistance[c]: Chloroquine
Malaria species: *P. falciparum* 86%, *P. malariae* 12%, remainder *P. ovale* and *P. vivax*.
Recommended chemoprophylaxis: Atovaquone-proguanil, doxycycline, or mefloquine.

CAMBODIA
Yellow Fever
Requirements: Required if traveling from a country with risk of YFV transmission and ≥1 year of age.[a]
Recommendations: None

Malaria
Areas with malaria: Present throughout the country, except none at the temple complex at Angkor Wat, Phnom Penh, and around Lake Tonle Sap.
Estimated relative risk of malaria for US travelers: Moderate
Drug resistance[c]: Chloroquine, mefloquine (see Map 3-11).
Malaria species: *P. falciparum* 86%, *P. vivax* 12%, *P. malariae* 2%.
Recommended chemoprophylaxis:
In the provinces of Banteay Meanchey, Battambang, Koh Kong, Odder Meanchey, Pailin, Kampot, Preah Vihear, Pursat, and Siemreap bordering Thailand: Atovaquone-proguanil or doxycycline.
All other areas with malaria: Atovaquone-proguanil, doxycycline, or mefloquine.

CAMEROON
Yellow Fever
Requirements: Required upon arrival from all countries if traveler is ≥1 year of age.
Recommendations: *Recommended* for all travelers ≥9 months of age.

Malaria
Areas with malaria: All
Estimated relative risk of malaria for US travelers: High
Drug resistance[c]: Chloroquine
Malaria species: *P. falciparum* 80%, *P. ovale* 5%–10%, *P. vivax* rare.
Recommended chemoprophylaxis: Atovaquone-proguanil, doxycycline, or mefloquine.

CANADA
Yellow Fever
No requirements or recommendations.

Malaria
No malaria transmission.

CANARY ISLANDS (SPAIN)
Yellow Fever
No requirements or recommendations.

Malaria
No malaria transmission.

CAPE VERDE
Yellow Fever
Requirements: Required if traveling from a country with risk of YFV transmission and ≥1 year of age.[a]
Recommendations: None

Malaria
Areas with malaria: Limited cases in São Tiago Island.
Estimated relative risk of malaria for US travelers: Very low
Drug resistance[c]: Chloroquine
Malaria species: Primarily *P. falciparum*.
Recommended chemoprophylaxis: Mosquito avoidance only.

FOOTNOTES:
[a] The official WHO list of countries with risk of YFV transmission can be found in Table 3-21. Proof of yellow fever vaccination should be required only if traveling from a country on the WHO list, unless otherwise specified. The following countries, containing only areas with low potential for exposure to YFV, are not on the WHO list: Eritrea, São Tomé and Príncipe, Somalia, Tanzania, Zambia.

CAYMAN ISLANDS (UK)
Yellow Fever
No requirements or recommendations.

Malaria
No malaria transmission.

CENTRAL AFRICAN REPUBLIC
Yellow Fever
Requirements: Required upon arrival from all countries if traveler is ⩾1 year of age.
Recommendations: *Recommended* for all travelers ⩾9 months of age.

Malaria
Areas with malaria: All
Estimated relative risk of malaria for US travelers: High
Drug resistance^c: Chloroquine
Malaria species: *P. falciparum* 85%; *P. malariae, P. ovale,* and *P. vivax* 15% combined.
Recommended chemoprophylaxis:
Atovaquone-proguanil, doxycycline, or mefloquine.

CHAD
Yellow Fever
Requirements: Required if traveling from a country with risk of YFV transmission.^a
Recommendations:
Recommended for all travelers ⩾9 months of age traveling to areas south of the Sahara Desert (see Map 3-18).
Not recommended for travelers whose itineraries are limited to areas in the Sahara Desert (see Map 3-18).

Malaria
Areas with malaria: All
Estimated relative risk of malaria for US travelers: High
Drug resistance^c: Chloroquine
Malaria species: *P. falciparum* 85%; *P. malariae, P. ovale,* and *P. vivax* 15% combined.
Recommended chemoprophylaxis:
Atovaquone-proguanil, doxycycline, or mefloquine.

CHILE
Yellow Fever
No requirements or recommendations.

Malaria
No malaria transmission.

CHINA (See Map 3-23.)
Yellow Fever
Requirements: Required if traveling from a country with risk of YFV transmission and ⩾9 months of age.^a
Recommendations: None

Malaria
Areas with malaria: Rural parts of Anhui, Guizhou, Hainan, Henan, Hubei, and Yunnan Provinces. Rare cases occur in other rural parts of the country <1,500 m (4,921 ft) May–December. None in urban areas. Some major river cruises may go through malaria-endemic areas in Anhui and Hubei Provinces.
Estimated relative risk of malaria for US travelers: Low
Drug resistance^c: Chloroquine, mefloquine (see Map 3-11).
Malaria species: Primarily *P. vivax, P. falciparum* in select locations.
Recommended chemoprophylaxis:
Along China-Burma (Myanmar) border in the western part of Yunnan Province: Atovaquone-proguanil or doxycycline.
Hainan and other parts of Yunnan Province: Atovaquone-proguanil, doxycycline, or mefloquine.
Anhui, Guizhou, Henan, and Hubei provinces: Atovaquone-proguanil, chloroquine, doxycycline, mefloquine, or primaquine.^e
All other areas with malaria, including river cruises that pass through malaria-endemic provinces: Mosquito avoidance only.

CHRISTMAS ISLAND (AUSTRALIA)
Yellow Fever
Requirements: Required for all people ⩾1 year of age who enter Australia within 6 days of having stayed overnight or longer

---

^c Refers to *P. falciparum* malaria unless otherwise noted.
^e Primaquine can cause hemolytic anemia in people with glucose-6-phosphate dehydrogenase (G6PD) deficiency. Patients must be screened for G6PD deficiency before starting primaquine.

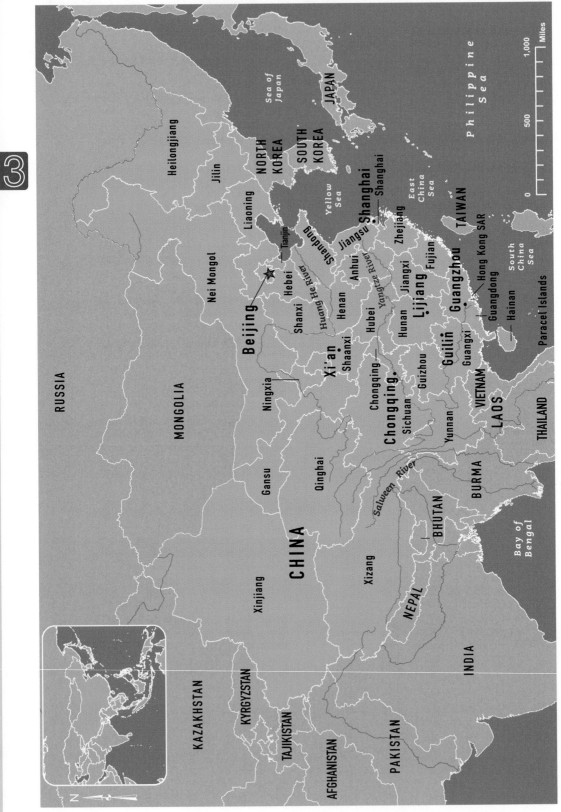

MAP 3-23. CHINA REFERENCE MAP

in a country with risk of YFV transmission,[a] including São Tomé and Príncipe, Somalia, and Tanzania, but excluding Galápagos Islands in Ecuador and limited to Misiones Province in Argentina.
Recommendations: None

Malaria
No malaria transmission.

COCOS (KEELING) ISLANDS (AUSTRALIA)
Yellow Fever
Requirements: Required for all people ≥1 year of age who enter Australia within 6 days of having stayed overnight or longer in a country with risk of YFV transmission,[a] including São Tomé and Príncipe, Somalia, and Tanzania, but excluding Galápagos Islands in Ecuador and limited to Misiones Province in Argentina.
Recommendations: None

Malaria
No malaria transmission.

COLOMBIA (See Map 3-24.)
Yellow Fever
Requirements: None
Recommendations:
Recommended for all travelers ≥9 months of age traveling to the following departments <2,300 m in elevation[d] (see Map 3-19): Amazonas, Antioquia, Arauca, Atlántico, Bolivar, Boyacá, Caldas, Caquetá, Casanare, Cauca, Cesar, Choco (only the municipalities of Acandí, Juradó, Riosucio, and Unguía), Códoba, Cundinamarca, Guainía, Guaviare, Huila, La Guajira (only the municipalities of Albania, Barrancas, Dibulla, Distracción, El Molino, Fonseca, Hatonuevo, La Jagua del Pilar, Maicao, Manaure, Riohacha, San Juan del Cesar, Urumita, and Villanueva), Magdalena, Meta, Norte de Santander, Putumayo, Quindio, Risaralda, San Andrés and Providencia, Santander, Sucre, Tolima, Vaupés, and Vichada.

Generally not recommended for travelers whose itinerary is limited to the following areas west of the Andes <2,300 m in elevation[d]: the departments of Cauca, Nariño, Valle de Cauca, and central and southern Choco, and the cities of Barranquilla, Cali, Cartagena, and Medellín (see Map 3-19).
Not recommended for travelers whose itineraries are limited to all areas >2,300 m in elevation,[d] including the city of Bogotá, and also the municipality of Uribia in the La Guajira department.

Malaria
Areas with malaria: All areas <1,700 m (5,577 ft). None in Bogotá and Cartagena.
Estimated relative risk of malaria for US travelers: Low
Drug resistance[c]: Chloroquine
Malaria species: *P. falciparum* 35%–40%, *P. vivax* 60%–65%.
Recommended chemoprophylaxis: Atovaquone-proguanil, doxycycline, or mefloquine.

COMOROS
Yellow Fever
No requirements or recommendations.

Malaria
Areas with malaria: All
Estimated relative risk of malaria for US travelers: No data
Drug resistance[c]: Chloroquine
Malaria species: Primarily *P. falciparum*.
Recommended chemoprophylaxis: Atovaquone-proguanil, doxycycline, or mefloquine.

CONGO, REPUBLIC OF THE (CONGO-BRAZZAVILLE)
Yellow Fever
Requirements: Required upon arrival from all countries for travelers ≥1 year of age.
Recommendations: *Recommended* for all travelers ≥9 months of age.

FOOTNOTES:
[a] The official WHO list of countries with risk of YFV transmission can be found in Table 3-21. Proof of yellow fever vaccination should be required only if traveling from a country on the WHO list, unless otherwise specified. The following countries, containing only areas with low potential for exposure to YFV, are not on the WHO list: Eritrea, São Tomé and Príncipe, Somalia, Tanzania, Zambia.
[c] Refers to *P. falciparum* malaria unless otherwise noted.
[d] An elevation of 2,300 m is equivalent to 7,546 ft.

Malaria

Areas with malaria: All

Estimated relative risk of malaria for US travelers: High

Drug resistance[c]: Chloroquine

Malaria species: *P. falciparum* 90%, *P. ovale* 5%–10%, *P. vivax* rare.

Recommended chemoprophylaxis: Atovaquone-proguanil, doxycycline, or mefloquine.

COOK ISLANDS (NEW ZEALAND)

Yellow Fever

No requirements or recommendations.

Malaria

No malaria transmission.

COSTA RICA

Yellow Fever

Requirements: Required for travelers ≥9 months of age arriving from countries with risk of YFV transmission,[a] with the exception of Argentina, Panama, and Trinidad and Tobago.

Recommendations: None

Malaria

Areas with malaria: Limón Province, but not in Limón City (Puerto Limón). Rare cases in other parts of the country.

Estimated relative risk of malaria for US travelers: Low

Drug resistance[c]: None

Malaria species: *P. vivax* 100%.

Recommended chemoprophylaxis: Limón Province: Atovaquone-proguanil, chloroquine, doxycycline, mefloquine, or primaquine.[e]

All other areas: Mosquito avoidance only.

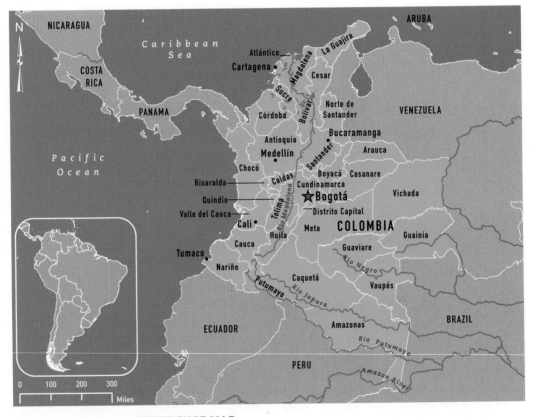

MAP 3-24. COLOMBIA REFERENCE MAP

FOOTNOTES:

[a] The official WHO list of countries with risk of YFV transmission can be found in Table 3-21. Proof of yellow fever vaccination should be required only if traveling from a country on the WHO list, unless otherwise specified. The following countries, containing only areas with low potential for exposure to YFV, are not on the WHO list: Eritrea, São Tomé and Príncipe, Somalia, Tanzania, Zambia.

CÔTE D'IVOIRE (IVORY COAST)
Yellow Fever
Requirements: Required upon arrival from all countries for travelers ≥1 year of age.
Recommendations: *Recommended* for all travelers ≥9 months of age.

Malaria
Areas with malaria: All
Estimated relative risk of malaria for US travelers: High
Drug resistance[c]: Chloroquine
Malaria species: *P. falciparum* 85%, *P. ovale* 5%–10%, *P. vivax* rare.
Recommended chemoprophylaxis: Atovaquone-proguanil, doxycycline, or mefloquine.

CROATIA
Yellow Fever
No requirements or recommendations.

Malaria
No malaria transmission.

CUBA
Yellow Fever
No requirements or recommendations.

Malaria
No malaria transmission.

CYPRUS
Yellow Fever
No requirements or recommendations.

Malaria
No malaria transmission.

CZECH REPUBLIC
Yellow Fever
No requirements or recommendations.

Malaria
No malaria transmission.

DEMOCRATIC REPUBLIC OF THE CONGO (CONGO-KINSHASA)
Yellow Fever
Requirements: Required upon arrival from all countries for travelers ≥1 year of age.
Recommendations:
Recommended for all travelers ≥9 months of age, except as mentioned below.
Generally not recommended for travelers whose itinerary is limited to Katanga Province.

Malaria
Areas with malaria: All
Estimated relative risk of malaria for US travelers: No data
Drug resistance[c]: Chloroquine
Malaria species: *P. falciparum* 90%, *P. ovale* 5%, *P. vivax* rare.
Recommended chemoprophylaxis: Atovaquone-proguanil, doxycycline, or mefloquine.

DENMARK
Yellow Fever
No requirements or recommendations.

Malaria
No malaria transmission.

DJIBOUTI
Yellow Fever
Requirements: Required if traveling from a country with risk of YFV transmission and ≥1 year of age.[a]
Recommendations: None

Malaria
Areas with malaria: All
Estimated relative risk of malaria for US travelers: No data
Drug resistance[c]: Chloroquine
Malaria species: *P. falciparum* 90%, *P. vivax* 5%–10%.
Recommended chemoprophylaxis: Atovaquone-proguanil, doxycycline, or mefloquine.

[c] Refers to *P. falciparum* malaria unless otherwise noted.
[e] Primaquine can cause hemolytic anemia in people with glucose-6-phosphate dehydrogenase (G6PD) deficiency. Patients must be screened for G6PD deficiency before starting primaquine.

DOMINICA

Yellow Fever
Requirements: Required if traveling from a country with risk of YFV transmission and ≥1 year of age.[a]
Recommendations: None

Malaria
No malaria transmission.

DOMINICAN REPUBLIC

Yellow Fever
No requirements or recommendations.

Malaria
Areas with malaria: All areas (including resort areas), except none in the cities of Santiago and Santo Domingo.
Estimated relative risk of malaria for US travelers: Low
Drug resistance[c]: None
Malaria species: *P. falciparum* 100%.
Recommended chemoprophylaxis: Atovaquone-proguanil, chloroquine, doxycycline, or mefloquine.

EASTER ISLAND (CHILE)

Yellow Fever
Requirements: Required if traveling from a country with risk of YFV transmission.[a]
Recommendations: None

Malaria
No malaria transmission.

ECUADOR, INCLUDING THE GALÁPAGOS ISLANDS (See Map 3-25.)

Yellow Fever
Requirements: Required for travelers ≥1 year of age arriving from a country with risk of YFV transmission.[a] Nationals and residents of Ecuador are required to possess certificates of vaccination on their departure to an area with risk of YFV transmission.
Recommendations:
Recommended for all travelers ≥9 months of age traveling to the following provinces east of the Andes Mountains <2,300 m in elevation[d]: Morona-Santiago, Napo, Orellana, Pastaza, Sucumbios, and Zamora-Chinchipe (see Map 3-19).
Generally not recommended for travelers whose itinerary is limited to the following provinces west of the Andes and <2,300 m in elevation[d]: Esmeraldas, Guayas, Los Rios, Manabi, and designated areas of Azuay, Bolivar, Canar, Carchi, Chimborazo, Cotopaxi, El Oro, Imbabura, Loja, Pichincha, and Tungurahua (see Map 3-19).
Not recommended for travelers whose itineraries are limited to all areas >2,300 m in elevation,[d] the cities of Guayaquil and Quito, or the Galápagos Islands (see Map 3-19).

Malaria
Areas with malaria: All areas <1,500 m (4,921 ft). Not present in the cities of Guayaquil and Quito or the Galápagos Islands.
Estimated relative risk of malaria for US travelers: Low
Drug resistance[c]: Chloroquine
Malaria species: *P. vivax* 90%, *P. falciparum* 10%.
Recommended chemoprophylaxis: Atovaquone-proguanil, doxycycline, mefloquine, or primaquine.[e]

EGYPT

Yellow Fever
Requirements: Required if traveling from countries with risk of YFV transmission and ≥1 year of age.[a] All travelers arriving from Sudan are required to have a vaccination certificate or a location certificate issued by a Sudanese official center that states that they have not been in Sudan south of 15°N within the previous 6 days.
Recommendations: None

Malaria
No malaria transmission.

FOOTNOTES:
[a] The official WHO list of countries with risk of YFV transmission can be found in Table 3-21. Proof of yellow fever vaccination should be required only if traveling from a country on the WHO list, unless otherwise specified. The following countries, containing only areas with low potential for exposure to YFV, are not on the WHO list: Eritrea, São Tomé and Príncipe, Somalia, Tanzania, Zambia.

EL SALVADOR

Yellow Fever

Requirements: Required if traveling from a country with risk of YFV transmission and ≥1 year of age.[a]

Recommendations: None

Malaria

Areas with malaria: Rural areas of Ahuachapán, La Unión, and Santa Ana Departments.

Estimated relative risk of malaria for US travelers: Low

Drug resistance[c]: None

Malaria species: *P. vivax* 99%, *P. falciparum* <1%.

Recommended chemoprophylaxis: Atovaquone-proguanil, chloroquine, doxycycline, mefloquine, or primaquine.[e]

EQUATORIAL GUINEA

Yellow Fever

Requirements: Required if traveling from a country with risk of YFV transmission.[a]

Recommendations: *Recommended* for all travelers ≥9 months of age.

Malaria

Areas with malaria: All

Estimated relative risk of malaria for US travelers: High

Drug resistance[c]: Chloroquine

Malaria species: *P. falciparum* 85%; *P. malariae*, *P. ovale*, and *P. vivax* 15% combined.

Recommended chemoprophylaxis: Atovaquone-proguanil, doxycycline, or mefloquine.

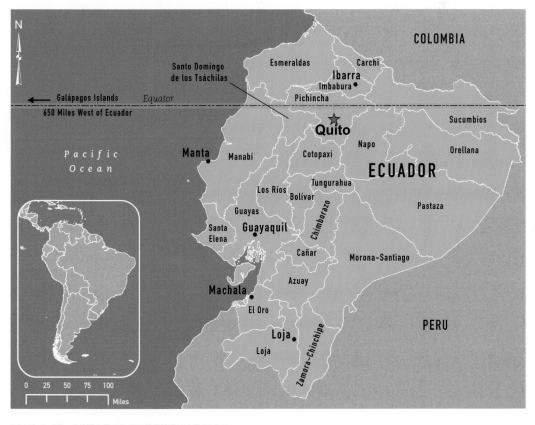

MAP 3-25. ECUADOR REFERENCE MAP

[c] Refers to *P. falciparum* malaria unless otherwise noted.
[d] An elevation of 2,300 m is equivalent to 7,546 ft.
[e] Primaquine can cause hemolytic anemia in people with glucose-6-phosphate dehydrogenase (G6PD) deficiency. Patients must be screened for G6PD deficiency before starting primaquine.

ERITREA
Yellow Fever
Requirements: Required if traveling from a country with risk of YFV transmission.[a]
Recommendations:
Generally not recommended for travelers going to the following states: Anseba, Debub, Gash Barka, Mae Kel, and Semenawi Keih Bahri.
Not recommended for all areas not listed above, including the Dahlak Archipelago (see Map 3-18).

Malaria
Areas with malaria: All areas <2,200 m (7,218 ft). None in Asmara.
Estimated relative risk of malaria for US travelers: No data
Drug resistance[c]: Chloroquine
Malaria species: *P. falciparum* 85%, *P. vivax* 10%–15%, *P. ovale* rare.
Recommended chemoprophylaxis: Atovaquone-proguanil, doxycycline, or mefloquine.

ESTONIA
Yellow Fever
No requirements or recommendations.

Malaria
No malaria transmission.

ETHIOPIA (See Map 3-26.)
Yellow Fever
Requirements: Required if traveling from a country with risk of YFV transmission and ≥1 year of age.[a]
Recommendations:
Recommended for all travelers ≥9 months of age, except as mentioned below.
Generally not recommended for travelers whose itinerary is limited to the Afar and Somali Provinces (see Map 3-18).

Malaria
Areas with malaria: All areas <2,500 m (8,202 ft), except none in Addis Ababa.

Estimated relative risk of malaria for US travelers: Moderate
Drug resistance[c]: Chloroquine
Malaria species: *P. falciparum* 76%, *P. vivax* 24%, *P. malariae* and *P. ovale* rare.
Recommended chemoprophylaxis: Atovaquone-proguanil, doxycycline, or mefloquine.

FALKLAND ISLANDS (UK)
Yellow Fever
No requirements or recommendations.

Malaria
No malaria transmission.

FAROE ISLANDS (DENMARK)
Yellow Fever
No requirements or recommendations.

Malaria
No malaria transmission.

FIJI
Yellow Fever
Requirements: Required if traveling from a country with risk of YFV transmission and ≥1 year of age.[a]
Recommendations: None

Malaria
No malaria transmission.

FINLAND
Yellow Fever
No requirements or recommendations.

Malaria
No malaria transmission.

FRANCE
Yellow Fever
No requirements or recommendations.

Malaria
No malaria transmission.

FOOTNOTES:
[a] The official WHO list of countries with risk of YFV transmission can be found in Table 3-21. Proof of yellow fever vaccination should be required only if traveling from a country on the WHO list, unless otherwise specified. The following countries, containing only areas with low potential for exposure to YFV, are not on the WHO list: Eritrea, São Tomé and Príncipe, Somalia, Tanzania, Zambia.

FRENCH GUIANA

Yellow Fever

Requirements: Required upon arrival from all countries for travelers ⩾1 year of age.
Recommendations: *Recommended* for all travelers ⩾9 months of age.

Malaria

Areas with malaria: All areas, except none in the city of Cayenne or Devil's Island (Ile du Diable).
Estimated relative risk of malaria for US travelers: Moderate
Drug resistance[c]: Chloroquine
Malaria species: *P. falciparum* <50%, remainder *P. vivax*, *P. malariae* rare.
Recommended chemoprophylaxis: Atovaquone-proguanil, doxycycline, or mefloquine.

FRENCH POLYNESIA, INCLUDING THE ISLAND GROUPS OF SOCIETY ISLANDS (TAHITI, MOOREA, AND BORA-BORA), MARQUESAS ISLANDS (HIVA OA AND UA HUKA), AND AUSTRAL ISLANDS (TUBUAI AND RURUTU)

Yellow Fever

No requirements or recommendations.

Malaria

No malaria transmission.

GABON

Yellow Fever

Requirements: Required upon arrival from all countries for travelers ⩾1 year of age.

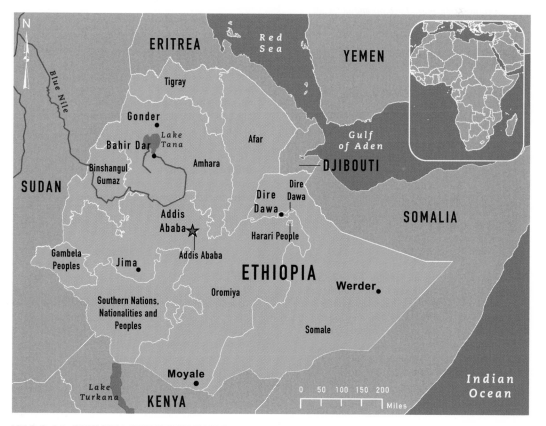

MAP 3-26. ETHIOPIA REFERENCE MAP

[c] Refers to *P. falciparum* malaria unless otherwise noted.

Recommendations: *Recommended* for all travelers ≥9 months of age.

Malaria
Areas with malaria: All
Estimated relative risk of malaria for US travelers: High
Drug resistance[c]: Chloroquine
Malaria species: *P. falciparum* 95%; *P. malariae*, *P. ovale*, and *P. vivax* 5% combined.
Recommended chemoprophylaxis: Atovaquone-proguanil, doxycycline, or mefloquine.

GAMBIA, THE
Yellow Fever
Requirements: Required if traveling from a country with risk of YFV transmission and ≥1 year of age.[a]
Recommendations: *Recommended* for all travelers ≥9 months of age.

Malaria
Areas with malaria: All
Estimated relative risk of malaria for US travelers: High
Drug resistance[c]: Chloroquine
Malaria species: *P. falciparum* 85%; *P. malariae*, *P. ovale*, and *P. vivax* 15% combined.
Recommended chemoprophylaxis: Atovaquone-proguanil, doxycycline, or mefloquine.

GEORGIA
Yellow Fever
No requirements or recommendations.

Malaria
Areas with malaria: Present June–October in the southeastern part of the country near the Azerbaijan border, mainly in the Kakheti and Kveno Kartli regions. None in Tbilisi.
Estimated relative risk of malaria for US travelers: Very low
Drug resistance[c]: None
Malaria species: *P. vivax* 100%.

Recommended chemoprophylaxis: Atovaquone-proguanil, chloroquine, doxycycline, mefloquine, or primaquine.[e]

GERMANY
Yellow Fever
No requirements or recommendations.

Malaria
No malaria transmission.

GHANA
Yellow Fever
Requirements: Required upon arrival for all travelers ≥9 months of age.
Recommendations: *Recommended* for all travelers ≥9 months of age.

Malaria
Areas with malaria: All
Estimated relative risk of malaria for US travelers: High
Drug resistance[c]: Chloroquine
Malaria species: *P. falciparum* 85%, *P. ovale* 5%–10%, *P. vivax* rare.
Recommended chemoprophylaxis: Atovaquone-proguanil, doxycycline, or mefloquine.

GIBRALTAR (UK)
Yellow Fever
No requirements or recommendations.

Malaria
No malaria transmission.

GREECE
Yellow Fever
No requirements or recommendations.

Malaria
No malaria transmission.

FOOTNOTES:
[a] The official WHO list of countries with risk of YFV transmission can be found in Table 3-21. Proof of yellow fever vaccination should be required only if traveling from a country on the WHO list, unless otherwise specified. The following countries, containing only areas with low potential for exposure to YFV, are not on the WHO list: Eritrea, São Tomé and Príncipe, Somalia, Tanzania, Zambia.

GREENLAND (DENMARK)
Yellow Fever
No requirements or recommendations.

Malaria
No malaria transmission.

GRENADA
Yellow Fever
Requirements: Required if traveling from a country with risk of YFV transmission and ≥1 year of age.[a]
Recommendations: None

Malaria
No malaria transmission.

GUADELOUPE, INCLUDING SAINT-BARTHÉLEMY AND SAINT MARTIN (FRANCE)
Yellow Fever
Requirements: Required if traveling from a country with risk of YFV transmission and ≥1 year of age.[a]
Recommendations: None

Malaria
No malaria transmission.

GUAM (US)
Yellow Fever
No requirements or recommendations.

Malaria
No malaria transmission.

GUATEMALA
Yellow Fever
Requirements: Required if traveling from a country with risk of YFV transmission and ≥1 year of age.[a]
Recommendations: None

Malaria
Areas with malaria: Rural areas only at altitudes <1,500 m (4,921 ft). None in Antigua, Guatemala City, or Lake Atitlán.

Estimated relative risk of malaria for US travelers: Moderate
Drug resistance[c]: None
Malaria species: *P. vivax* 97%, *P. falciparum* 3%.
Recommended chemoprophylaxis: Atovaquone-proguanil, chloroquine, doxycycline, mefloquine, or primaquine.[e]

GUINEA
Yellow Fever
Requirements: Required if traveling from a country with risk of YFV transmission and ≥1 year of age.[a]
Recommendations: *Recommended* for all travelers ≥9 months of age.

Malaria
Areas with malaria: All
Estimated relative risk of malaria for US travelers: High
Drug resistance[c]: Chloroquine
Malaria species: *P. falciparum* 85%, *P. ovale* 5%–10%, *P. vivax* rare.
Recommended chemoprophylaxis: Atovaquone-proguanil, doxycycline, or mefloquine.

GUINEA-BISSAU
Yellow Fever
Requirements: Required upon arrival from all countries for travelers ≥1 year of age.
Recommendations: *Recommended* for all travelers ≥9 months of age.

Malaria
Areas with malaria: All
Estimated relative risk of malaria for US travelers: No data
Drug resistance[c]: Chloroquine
Malaria species: *P. falciparum* 85%, *P. ovale* 5%–10%, *P. vivax* rare.
Recommended chemoprophylaxis: Atovaquone-proguanil, doxycycline, or mefloquine.

GUYANA
Yellow Fever
Requirements: Required for travelers ≥1 year of age arriving from a country with risk

[c] Refers to *P. falciparum* malaria unless otherwise noted.
[e] Primaquine can cause hemolytic anemia in people with glucose-6-phosphate dehydrogenase (G6PD) deficiency. Patients must be screened for G6PD deficiency before starting primaquine.

of YFV transmission,[a] with the exception of Argentina, Paraguay, Suriname, and Trinidad and Tobago.

Recommendations: *Recommended* for all travelers ≥9 months of age.

Malaria
Areas with malaria: Present in all areas <900 m (2,953 ft), including Georgetown.
Estimated relative risk of malaria for US travelers: Moderate
Drug resistance[c]: Chloroquine
Malaria species: *P. falciparum* 50%, *P. vivax* 50%.
Recommended chemoprophylaxis: Atovaquone-proguanil, doxycycline, or mefloquine.

HAITI
Yellow Fever
Requirements: Required if traveling from a country with risk of YFV transmission.[a]
Recommendations: None

Malaria
Areas with malaria: All (including Port Labadee).
Estimated relative risk of malaria for US travelers: Moderate
Drug resistance[c]: None
Malaria species: *P. falciparum* 100%.
Recommended chemoprophylaxis: Atovaquone-proguanil, chloroquine, doxycycline, or mefloquine.

HONDURAS
Yellow Fever
Requirements: Required for travelers ≥1 year of age coming from countries with risk of YFV transmission.[a]
Recommendations: None

Malaria
Areas with malaria: Present throughout the country at altitudes <1,000 m (3,281 ft) and in Roatán and other Bay Islands. None in San Pedro Sula and Tegucigalpa.

Estimated relative risk of malaria for US travelers: Moderate
Drug resistance[c]: None
Malaria species: *P. vivax* 93%, *P. falciparum* 7%.
Recommended chemoprophylaxis: Atovaquone-proguanil, chloroquine, doxycycline, mefloquine, or primaquine.[e]

HONG KONG SAR (CHINA)
Yellow Fever
No requirements or recommendations.

Malaria
No malaria transmission.

HUNGARY
Yellow Fever
No requirements or recommendations.

Malaria
No malaria transmission.

ICELAND
Yellow Fever
No requirements or recommendations.

Malaria
No malaria transmission.

INDIA (See Map 3-27.)
Yellow Fever
Requirements: Any traveler (except infants ≤6 months old) arriving by air or sea without a certificate is detained in isolation for up to 6 days if that person—

1) arrives within 6 days of departure from an area with risk of YFV transmission,
2) has been in such an area in transit (except those passengers and members of flight crews who, while in transit through an airport in an area with risk of YFV transmission, remained in the airport during their entire stay and

FOOTNOTES:
[a] The official WHO list of countries with risk of YFV transmission can be found in Table 3-21. Proof of yellow fever vaccination should be required only if traveling from a country on the WHO list, unless otherwise specified. The following countries, containing only areas with low potential for exposure to YFV, are not on the WHO list: Eritrea, São Tomé and Príncipe, Somalia, Tanzania, Zambia.
[c] Refers to *P. falciparum* malaria unless otherwise noted.
[e] Primaquine can cause hemolytic anemia in people with glucose-6-phosphate dehydrogenase (G6PD) deficiency. Patients must be screened for G6PD deficiency before starting primaquine.

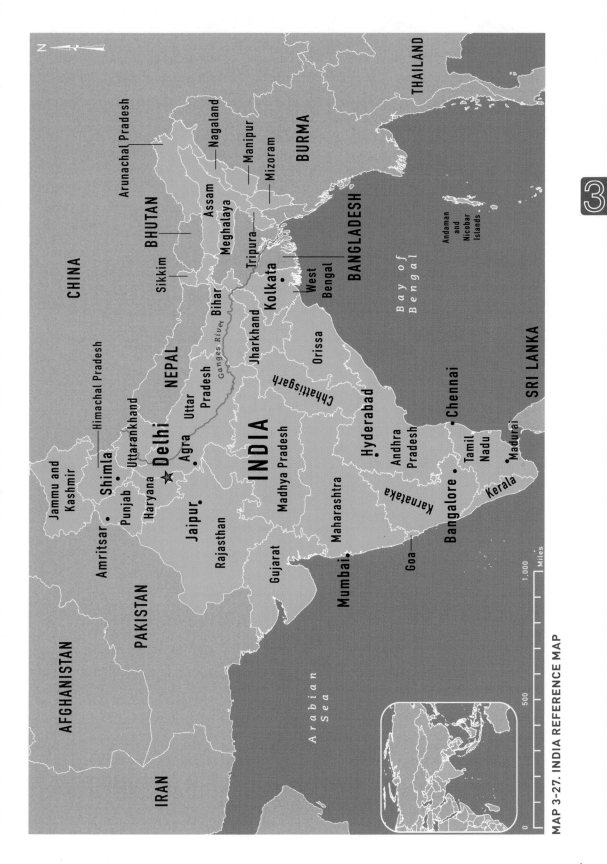

MAP 3-27. INDIA REFERENCE MAP

the health officer agrees to such an exemption),

3) arrives on a ship that started from or touched at any port in an area with risk of YFV transmission up to 30 days before its arrival in India, unless such a ship has been disinsected in accordance with the procedure recommended by WHO, or

4) arrives on an aircraft that has been in an area with risk of YFV transmission and has not been disinsected in accordance with the Indian Aircraft Public Health Rules, 1954, or as recommended by WHO.

The following are regarded as countries and areas with risk of YFV transmission:

Africa: Angola, Bénin, Burkina Faso, Burundi, Cameroon, Central African Republic, Chad, Congo, Côte d'Ivoire, Democratic Republic of the Congo, Equatorial Guinea, Ethiopia, Gabon, The Gambia, Ghana, Guinea, Guinea-Bissau, Kenya, Liberia, Mali, Niger, Nigeria, Rwanda, São Tomé and Príncipe, Senegal, Sierra Leone, Somalia, Sudan, Tanzania, Togo, Uganda, and Zambia

Americas: Bolivia, Brazil, Colombia, Ecuador, French Guiana, Guyana, Panama, Peru, Suriname, Trinidad and Tobago, and Venezuela

Note: When a case of yellow fever is reported from any country, that country is regarded by the government of India as a country with risk of yellow fever transmission and is added to the above list.

Recommendations: None

Malaria
Areas with malaria: All areas throughout the country, including cities of Bombay (Mumbai) and Delhi, except none in areas >2,000 m (6,561 ft) in Himachal, Jammu, Kashmir, Pradesh, and Sikkim.
Estimated relative risk of malaria for US travelers: Moderate
Drug resistance[c]: Chloroquine
Malaria species: *P. vivax* 40%, *P. falciparum* 20%–40%, remainder *P. malariae* and *P. ovale.*

Recommended chemoprophylaxis: Atovaquone-proguanil, doxycycline, or mefloquine.

INDONESIA
Yellow Fever
Requirements: Required if traveling from a country with risk of YFV transmission and ≥9 months of age.[a]
Recommendations: None

Malaria
Areas with malaria: Rural areas of Kalimantan (Borneo), Nusa Tenggara Barat (includes the island of Lombok), Sulawesi, and Sumatra. All areas of eastern Indonesia (provinces of Irian Jaya Barat, Maluku, Maluku Utara, Nusa Tenggara Timur, and Papua Indonesia). None in Jakarta or resort areas of Bali and Java. Low transmission in rural areas of Java.
Estimated relative risk of malaria for US travelers: Moderate
Drug resistance[c]: Chloroquine (*P. falciparum* and *P. vivax*).
Malaria species: *P. falciparum* 66%, remainder primarily *P. vivax.*
Recommended chemoprophylaxis: Atovaquone-proguanil, doxycycline, or mefloquine.

IRAN
Yellow Fever
Requirements: Required if traveling from a country with risk of YFV transmission.[a]
Recommendations: None

Malaria
Areas with malaria: Rural areas of Sistan-Baluchestan Province and southern, tropical parts of Kerman and Hormozgan Provinces. Ardabil and East Azerbaijan Provinces north of the Zagros Mountains during March–November.
Estimated relative risk of malaria for US travelers: Very low
Drug resistance[c]: Chloroquine

FOOTNOTES:
[a] The official WHO list of countries with risk of YFV transmission can be found in Table 3-21. Proof of yellow fever vaccination should be required only if traveling from a country on the WHO list, unless otherwise specified. The following countries, containing only areas with low potential for exposure to YFV, are not on the WHO list: Eritrea, São Tomé and Príncipe, Somalia, Tanzania, Zambia.

Malaria species: *P. vivax* 88%, *P. falciparum* 12%.
Recommended chemoprophylaxis: Atovaquone-proguanil, doxycycline, or mefloquine.

IRAQ
Yellow Fever
Requirements: Required if traveling from a country with risk of YFV transmission.[a]
Recommendations: None

Malaria
No malaria transmission.

IRELAND
Yellow Fever
No requirements or recommendations.

Malaria
No malaria transmission.

ISRAEL
Yellow Fever
No requirements or recommendations.

Malaria
No malaria transmission.

ITALY, INCLUDING HOLY SEE (VATICAN CITY)
Yellow Fever
No requirements or recommendations.

Malaria
No malaria transmission.

JAMAICA
Yellow Fever
Requirements: Required if traveling from a country with risk of YFV transmission and ≥1 year of age.[a]
Recommendations: None

Malaria
Areas with malaria: Rare local cases in Kingston.
Estimated relative risk of malaria for US travelers: Very low
Drug resistance[c]: None
Malaria species: *P. falciparum* 100%.
Recommended chemoprophylaxis: Mosquito avoidance only.

JAPAN
Yellow Fever
No requirements or recommendations.

Malaria
No malaria transmission.

JORDAN
Yellow Fever
Requirements: Required if traveling from a country with risk of YFV transmission and ≥1 year of age.[a]
Recommendations: None

Malaria
No malaria transmission.

KAZAKHSTAN
Yellow Fever
Requirements: Required if traveling from a country with risk of YFV transmission.[a]
Recommendations: None

Malaria
No malaria transmission.

KENYA (See Map 3-28.)
Yellow Fever
Requirements: Required if traveling from a country with risk of YFV transmission and ≥1 year of age.[a]

[c] Refers to *P. falciparum* malaria unless otherwise noted.

Recommendations:
Recommended for all travelers ≥9 months of age, except as mentioned below.
Generally not recommended for travelers whose itinerary is limited to the following areas: the entire North Eastern Province; the states of Kilifi, Kwale, Lamu, Malindi, and Tanariver in the Coastal Province; and the cities of Mombasa and Nairobi (see Map 3-18).

Malaria
Areas with malaria: Present in all areas (including game parks) <2,500 m (<8,202 ft). None in Nairobi.
Estimated relative risk of malaria for US travelers: Moderate
Drug resistance[c]: Chloroquine

Malaria species: *P. falciparum* 85%, *P. vivax* 5%–10%, *P. ovale* up to 5%.
Recommended chemoprophylaxis: Atovaquone-proguanil, doxycycline, or mefloquine.

KIRIBATI (FORMERLY GILBERT ISLANDS), INCLUDES TARAWA, TABUAERAN (FANNING ISLAND), AND BANABA (OCEAN ISLAND)

Yellow Fever
Requirements: Required if traveling from a country with risk of YFV transmission and ≥1 year of age.[a]
Recommendations: None

Malaria
No malaria transmission.

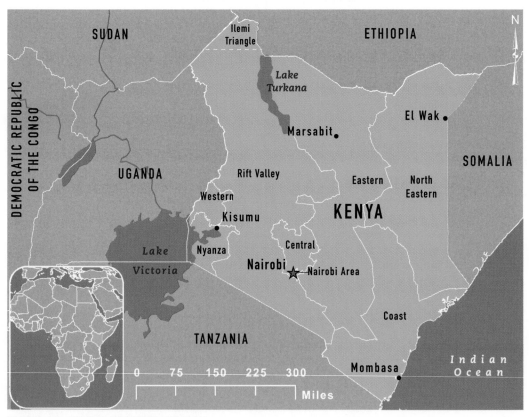

MAP 3-28. KENYA REFERENCE MAP

FOOTNOTES:
[a] The official WHO list of countries with risk of YFV transmission can be found in Table 3-21. Proof of yellow fever vaccination should be required only if traveling from a country on the WHO list, unless otherwise specified. The following countries, containing only areas with low potential for exposure to YFV, are not on the WHO list: Eritrea, São Tomé and Príncipe, Somalia, Tanzania, Zambia.

KOSOVO

Yellow Fever

Requirements: This country has not stated its yellow fever vaccination certificate requirements.
Recommendations: None

Malaria
No malaria transmission.

KUWAIT

Yellow Fever
No requirements or recommendations.

Malaria
No malaria transmission.

KYRGYZSTAN

Yellow Fever
No requirements or recommendations.

Malaria
Areas with malaria: Frequent border crossings between neighboring countries with malaria pose a small risk of malaria transmission along the border with Tajikistan. No malaria transmission reported in Bishkek.
Estimated relative risk of malaria for US travelers: Very low
Drug resistance[c]: None
Malaria species: *P. vivax* 99%, *P. falciparum* rare imported cases.
Recommended chemoprophylaxis: Mosquito avoidance only.

LAOS

Yellow Fever
Requirements: Required if traveling from a country with risk of YFV transmission.[a]
Recommendations: None

Malaria
Areas with malaria: All, except none in the city of Vientiane.
Estimated relative risk of malaria for US travelers: Very low

Drug resistance[c]: Chloroquine, mefloquine (see Map 3-11).
Malaria species: *P. falciparum* 95%, *P. vivax* 4%, *P. malariae* and *P. ovale* 1% combined.
Recommended chemoprophylaxis:
Along the Laos-Burma (Myanmar) border in the provinces of Bokeo and Louang Namtha and along the Laos-Thailand border in the province of Champasak and Saravan: Atovaquone-proguanil or doxycycline.
All other areas with malaria: Atovaquone-proguanil, doxycycline, or mefloquine.

LATVIA

Yellow Fever
No requirements or recommendations.

Malaria
No malaria transmission.

LEBANON

Yellow Fever
Requirements: Required if traveling from a country with risk of YFV transmission and ≥6 months of age.[a]
Recommendations: None

Malaria
No malaria transmission.

LESOTHO

Yellow Fever
Requirements: Required if traveling from a country with risk of YFV transmission and ≥9 months of age.[a]
Recommendations: None

Malaria
No malaria transmission.

LIBERIA

Yellow Fever
Requirements: Required upon arrival from all countries and ≥1 year of age.
Recommendations: *Recommended* for all travelers ≥9 months of age.

[c] Refers to *P. falciparum* malaria unless otherwise noted.

Malaria
Areas with malaria: All
Estimated relative risk of malaria for US travelers: High
Drug resistance[c]: Chloroquine
Malaria species: *P. falciparum* 85%, *P. ovale* 5%–10%, *P. vivax* rare.
Recommended chemoprophylaxis: Atovaquone-proguanil, doxycycline, or mefloquine.

LIBYA
Yellow Fever
Requirements: Required if traveling from a country with risk of YFV transmission.[a]
Recommendations: None

Malaria
No malaria transmission.

LIECHTENSTEIN
Yellow Fever
No requirements or recommendations.

Malaria
No malaria transmission.

LITHUANIA
Yellow Fever
No requirements or recommendations.

Malaria
No malaria transmission.

LUXEMBOURG
Yellow Fever
No requirements or recommendations.

Malaria
No malaria transmission.

MACAU SAR (CHINA)
Yellow Fever
No requirements or recommendations.

Malaria
No malaria transmission.

MACEDONIA
Yellow Fever
No requirements or recommendations.

Malaria
No malaria transmission.

MADAGASCAR
Yellow Fever
Requirements: Required if traveling from a country with risk of YFV transmission.[a]
Recommendations: None

Malaria
Areas with malaria: All
Estimated relative risk of malaria for US travelers: Moderate
Drug resistance[c]: Chloroquine
Malaria species: *P. falciparum* 85%, *P. vivax* 5%–10%, *P. ovale* 5%.
Recommended chemoprophylaxis: Atovaquone-proguanil, doxycycline, or mefloquine.

MADEIRA ISLANDS (PORTUGAL)
Yellow Fever
No requirements or recommendations.

Malaria
No malaria transmission.

MALAWI
Yellow Fever
Requirements: Required if traveling from a country with risk of YFV transmission and ≥1 year of age.[a]
Recommendations: None

Malaria
Areas with malaria: All
Estimated relative risk of malaria for US travelers: Moderate
Drug resistance[c]: Chloroquine

FOOTNOTES:
[a] The official WHO list of countries with risk of YFV transmission can be found in Table 3-21. Proof of yellow fever vaccination should be required only if traveling from a country on the WHO list, unless otherwise specified. The following countries, containing only areas with low potential for exposure to YFV, are not on the WHO list: Eritrea, São Tomé and Príncipe, Somalia, Tanzania, Zambia.

Malaria species: *P. falciparum* 90%;
P. malariae, *P. ovale*, and *P. vivax* 10%
combined.
Recommended chemoprophylaxis:
Atovaquone-proguanil, doxycycline, or
mefloquine.

MALAYSIA
Yellow Fever
Requirements: Required for travelers ≥1 year
of age arriving from countries with risk of YFV
transmission.[a]
Recommendations: None

Malaria
Areas with malaria: Present in rural areas
of Malaysian Borneo (Sabah and Sarawak
Provinces) and to a lesser extent in rural
areas of Peninsular Malaysia.
**Estimated relative risk of malaria for US
travelers:** Low
Drug resistance[c]: Chloroquine
Malaria species: *P. falciparum* 40%; *P. vivax*
50%; remainder *P. malariae, P. knowlesi, and
P. ovale. P. knowlesi* reported to cause 28% of
cases in Sarawak and known to cause cases
in both Malaysian Borneo and Peninsular
Malaysia.
Recommended chemoprophylaxis:
Atovaquone-proguanil, doxycycline, or
mefloquine.

MALDIVES
Yellow Fever
Requirements: Required if traveling from a
country with risk of YFV transmission and ≥1
year of age.[a]
Recommendations: None

Malaria
No malaria transmission.

MALI
Yellow Fever
Requirements: Required upon arrival from
all countries and ≥1 year of age.

Recommendations:
Recommended for all travelers ≥9 months of
age going to areas south of the Sahara Desert
(see Map 3-18).
Not recommended for travelers whose
itineraries are limited to areas in the Sahara
Desert (see Map 3-18).

Malaria
Areas with malaria: All
**Estimated relative risk of malaria for US
travelers:** High
Drug resistance[c]: Chloroquine
Malaria species: *P. falciparum* 85%, *P. ovale*
5%–10%, *P. vivax* rare.
Recommended chemoprophylaxis:
Atovaquone-proguanil, doxycycline, or
mefloquine.

MALTA
Yellow Fever
Requirements: Required if traveling from a
country with risk of YFV transmission and ≥9
months of age.[a] If indicated on epidemiologic
grounds, infants <9 months of age are subject
to isolation or surveillance if coming from an
area with risk of YFV transmission.
Recommendations: None

Malaria
No malaria transmission.

MARSHALL ISLANDS
Yellow Fever
No requirements or recommendations.

Malaria
No malaria transmission.

MARTINIQUE (FRANCE)
Yellow Fever
Requirements: Required if traveling from a
country with risk of YFV transmission and ≥1
year of age.[a]
Recommendations: None

Malaria
No malaria transmission.

[c] Refers to *P. falciparum* malaria unless otherwise noted.

MAURITANIA
Yellow Fever
Requirements: Required if traveling from a country with risk of YFV transmission and ≥1 year of age.[a]

Recommendations:

Recommended for all travelers ≥9 months of age traveling to areas south of the Sahara Desert (see Map 3-18).

Not recommended for travelers whose itineraries are limited to areas in the Sahara Desert (see Map 3-18).

Malaria
Areas with malaria: Present in southern provinces. None in Adrar, Dakhlet-Nouâdhibou, Inchiri, and Tiris Zemmour regions.

Estimated relative risk of malaria for US travelers: No data

Drug resistance[c]: Chloroquine

Malaria species: *P. falciparum* 85%, *P. ovale* 5%–10%, *P. vivax* rare.

Recommended chemoprophylaxis: Atovaquone-proguanil, doxycycline, or mefloquine.

MAURITIUS
Yellow Fever
Requirements: Required if traveling from a country with risk of YFV transmission and ≥1 year of age.[a]

Recommendations: None

Malaria
No malaria transmission.

MAYOTTE (FRANCE)
Yellow Fever
No requirements or recommendations.

Malaria
Areas with malaria: All

Estimated relative risk of malaria for US travelers: No data

Drug resistance[c]: Chloroquine

Malaria species: *P. falciparum* 40%–50%, *P. vivax* 35%–40%, *P. ovale* <1%.

Recommended chemoprophylaxis: Atovaquone-proguanil, doxycycline, or mefloquine.

MEXICO (See Map 3-29.)
Yellow Fever
No requirements or recommendations.

Malaria
Areas with malaria: Present in Chiapas and in rural areas in the states of Nayarit, Oaxaca, and Sinaloa; also present in an area between 24°N and 28°N latitude and 106°W and 110°W longitude, which lies in parts of Chihuahua, Durango, and Sonora. Rare cases in Quintana Roo and Tabasco. No malaria along the United States-Mexico border.

Estimated relative risk of malaria for US travelers: Low

Drug resistance[c]: None

Malaria species: *P. vivax* 100%.

Recommended chemoprophylaxis:

Areas with malaria, except states of Quintana Roo and Tabasco: Atovaquone-proguanil, chloroquine, doxycycline, mefloquine, or primaquine.[e]

States of Quintana Roo and Tabasco: Mosquito avoidance only.

MICRONESIA, FEDERATED STATES OF; INCLUDES YAP ISLANDS, POHNPEI, CHUUK, AND KOSRAE
Yellow Fever
No requirements or recommendations.

Malaria
No malaria transmission.

MOLDOVA
Yellow Fever
No requirements or recommendations.

Malaria
No malaria transmission.

FOOTNOTES:

[a] The official WHO list of countries with risk of YFV transmission can be found in Table 3-21. Proof of yellow fever vaccination should be required only if traveling from a country on the WHO list, unless otherwise specified. The following countries, containing only areas with low potential for exposure to YFV, are not on the WHO list: Eritrea, São Tomé and Príncipe, Somalia, Tanzania, Zambia.

[c] Refers to *P. falciparum* malaria unless otherwise noted.

[e] Primaquine can cause hemolytic anemia in people with glucose-6-phosphate dehydrogenase (G6PD) deficiency. Patients must be screened for G6PD deficiency before starting primaquine.

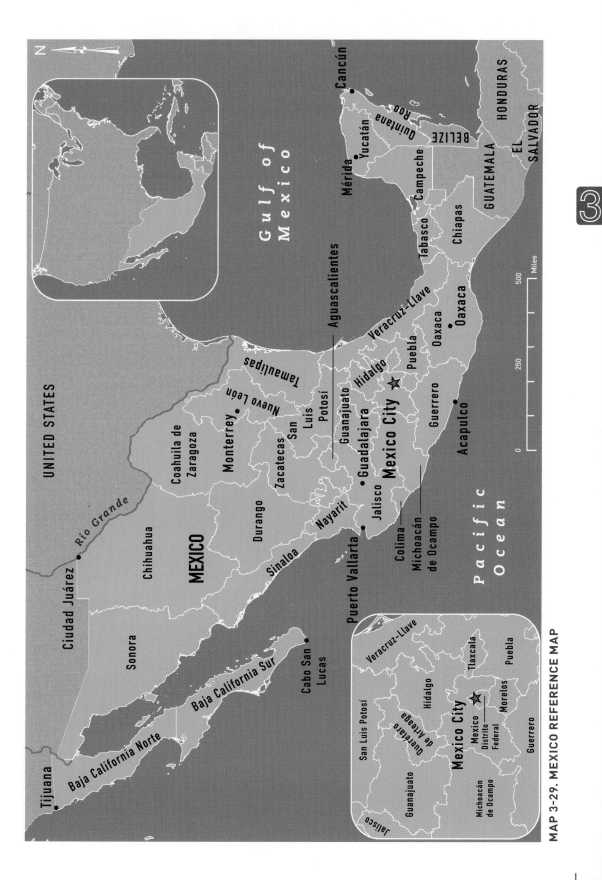

MAP 3-29. MEXICO REFERENCE MAP

MONACO
Yellow Fever
No requirements or recommendations.

Malaria
No malaria transmission.

MONGOLIA
Yellow Fever
No requirements or recommendations.

Malaria
No malaria transmission.

MONTENEGRO
Yellow Fever
No requirements or recommendations.

Malaria
No malaria transmission.

MONTSERRAT (UK)
Yellow Fever
Requirements: Required if traveling from a country with risk of YFV transmission and ≥1 year of age.[a]
Recommendations: None

Malaria
No malaria transmission.

MOROCCO
Yellow Fever
No requirements or recommendations.

Malaria
No malaria transmission.

MOZAMBIQUE
Yellow Fever
Requirements: Required if traveling from a country with risk of YFV transmission and ≥1 year of age.[a]
Recommendations: None

Malaria
Areas with malaria: All
Estimated relative risk of malaria for US travelers: High
Drug resistance[c]: Chloroquine
Malaria species: *P. falciparum* 98%, *P. malariae* and *P. ovale* 2%, *P. vivax* rare.
Recommended chemoprophylaxis: Atovaquone-proguanil, doxycycline, or mefloquine.

NAMIBIA
Yellow Fever
Requirements: Required if traveling from a country with risk of YFV transmission. The countries or parts of countries included in the endemic zones in Africa and South America are regarded as areas with risk of YFV transmission.[a] Travelers on scheduled flights that originated outside the countries with risk of YFV transmission, but who have been in transit through these areas, are not required to possess a certificate provided that they remained at the airport or in the adjacent town during transit. All travelers whose flights originated in countries with risk of YFV transmission or who have been in transit through these countries on unscheduled flights are required to possess a certificate. The certificate is not required for children <1 year of age, but such infants may be subject to surveillance.
Recommendations: None

Malaria
Areas with malaria: Present in the provinces of Kunene, Ohangwena, Okavango, Omaheke, Omusati, Oshana, Oshikoto, and Otjozondjupa and in the Caprivi Strip.
Estimated relative risk of malaria for US travelers: Moderate
Drug resistance[c]: Chloroquine
Malaria species: *P. falciparum* 90%; *P. malariae*, *P. ovale*, and *P. vivax* 10% combined.
Recommended chemoprophylaxis: Atovaquone-proguanil, doxycycline, or mefloquine.

FOOTNOTES:
[a] The official WHO list of countries with risk of YFV transmission can be found in Table 3-21. Proof of yellow fever vaccination should be required only if traveling from a country on the WHO list, unless otherwise specified. The following countries, containing only areas with low potential for exposure to YFV, are not on the WHO list: Eritrea, São Tomé and Príncipe, Somalia, Tanzania, Zambia.

NAURU
Yellow Fever
Requirements: Required if traveling from a country with risk of YFV transmission and ≥1 year of age.[a]
Recommendations: None

Malaria
No malaria transmission.

NEPAL
Yellow Fever
Requirements: Required if traveling from a country with risk of YFV transmission.[a]
Recommendations: None

Malaria
Areas with malaria: Present throughout the country at altitudes <1,200 m (3,937 ft). None in Kathmandu and on typical Himalayan treks.
Estimated relative risk of malaria for US travelers: No data
Drug resistance[c]: Chloroquine
Malaria species: *P. vivax* 88%, *P. falciparum* 12%.
Recommended chemoprophylaxis: Atovaquone-proguanil, doxycycline, or mefloquine.

NETHERLANDS, THE
Yellow Fever
No requirements or recommendations.

Malaria
No malaria transmission.

NETHERLANDS ANTILLES (BONAIRE, CURAÇAO, SABA, SINT EUSTATIUS, AND SINT MAARTEN)
Yellow Fever
Requirements: Required if traveling from a country with risk of YFV transmission and ≥6 months of age.[a]
Recommendations: None

Malaria
No malaria transmission.

NEW CALEDONIA (FRANCE)
Yellow Fever
Requirements: Required if traveling from a country with risk of YFV transmission and ≥1 year of age.[a] *Note:* In the event of an epidemic threat to the territory, a specific vaccination certificate may be required.
Recommendations: None

Malaria
No malaria transmission.

NEW ZEALAND
Yellow Fever
No requirements or recommendations.

Malaria
No malaria transmission.

NICARAGUA
Yellow Fever
Requirements: Required if traveling from a country with risk of YFV transmission and ≥1 year of age.[a]
Recommendations: None

Malaria
Areas with malaria: Present in districts of Chinandega, Leon, Managua, Matagalpa, Región Autónoma Atlántico Norte (RAAN), and Región Autónoma Atlántico Sur (RAAS).
Estimated relative risk of malaria for US travelers: Low
Drug resistance[c]: None
Malaria species: *P. vivax* 95%, *P. falciparum* 5%.
Recommended chemoprophylaxis: Atovaquone-proguanil, chloroquine, doxycycline, mefloquine, or primaquine.[e]

NIGER
Yellow Fever
Requirements: Required upon arrival from all countries if traveler is ≥1 year of age. The government of Niger recommends vaccine for travelers departing Niger.

---

[c] Refers to *P. falciparum* malaria unless otherwise noted.
[e] Primaquine can cause hemolytic anemia in people with glucose-6-phosphate dehydrogenase (G6PD) deficiency. Patients must be screened for G6PD deficiency before starting primaquine.

Recommendations:
Recommended for all travelers ≥9 months of age traveling to areas south of the Sahara Desert (see Map 3-18).
Not recommended for travelers whose itineraries are limited to areas in the Sahara Desert (see Map 3-18).

Malaria
Areas with malaria: All
Estimated relative risk of malaria for US travelers: High
Drug resistance[c]: Chloroquine
Malaria species: *P. falciparum* 85%, *P. ovale* 5%–10%, *P. vivax* rare.
Recommended chemoprophylaxis: Atovaquone-proguanil, doxycycline, or mefloquine.

NIGERIA
Yellow Fever
Requirements: Required if traveling from a country with risk of YFV transmission and ≥1 year of age.[a]
Recommendations: ***Recommended*** for all travelers ≥9 months of age.

Malaria
Areas with malaria: All
Estimated relative risk of malaria for US travelers: High
Drug resistance[c]: Chloroquine
Malaria species: *P. falciparum* 85%, *P. ovale* 5%–10%, *P. vivax* rare.
Recommended chemoprophylaxis: Atovaquone-proguanil, doxycycline, or mefloquine.

NIUE (NEW ZEALAND)
Yellow Fever
Requirements: Required if traveling from a country with risk of YFV transmission and ≥9 months of age.[a]
Recommendations: None

Malaria
No malaria transmission.

NORFOLK ISLAND (AUSTRALIA)
Yellow Fever
Requirements: Required for all people ≥1 year of age who enter Australia within 6 days of having stayed overnight or longer in a country with risk of YFV transmission,[a] including São Tomé and Príncipe, Somalia, and Tanzania, but excluding Galápagos Islands in Ecuador and limited to Misiones Province in Argentina.
Recommendations: None

Malaria
No malaria transmission.

NORTH KOREA
Yellow Fever
Requirements: Required if traveling from a country with risk of YFV transmission and ≥1 year of age.[a]
Recommendations: None

Malaria
Areas with malaria: Present in southern provinces.
Estimated relative risk of malaria for US travelers: No data
Drug resistance[c]: None
Malaria species: Presumed to be 100% *P. vivax*.
Recommended chemoprophylaxis: Atovaquone-proguanil, chloroquine, doxycycline, mefloquine, or primaquine.[e]

NORTHERN MARIANA ISLANDS (US), INCLUDES SAIPAN, TINIAN, AND ROTA ISLAND
Yellow Fever
No requirements or recommendations.

Malaria
No malaria transmission.

NORWAY
Yellow Fever
No requirements or recommendations.

Malaria
No malaria transmission.

FOOTNOTES:
[a] The official WHO list of countries with risk of YFV transmission can be found in Table 3-21. Proof of yellow fever vaccination should be required only if traveling from a country on the WHO list, unless otherwise specified. The following countries, containing only areas with low potential for exposure to YFV, are not on the WHO list: Eritrea, São Tomé and Príncipe, Somalia, Tanzania, Zambia.

OMAN

Yellow Fever

Requirements: Required if traveling from a country with risk of YFV transmission and ≥1 year of age.[a]

Recommendations: None

Malaria

No malaria transmission.

PAKISTAN

Yellow Fever

Requirements: Required for travelers arriving from any part of a country in which there is a risk of YFV transmission[a]; infants <6 months of age are exempt if the mother's vaccination certificate shows that she was vaccinated before the birth of the child.

Recommendations: None

Malaria

Areas with malaria: All areas (including all cities) <2,500 m (8,202 ft).

Estimated relative risk of malaria for US travelers: Moderate

Drug resistance[c]: Chloroquine

Malaria species: *P. falciparum* 70%, *P. vivax* 30%.

Recommended chemoprophylaxis: Atovaquone-proguanil, doxycycline, or mefloquine.

PALAU

Yellow Fever

No requirements or recommendations.

Malaria

No malaria transmission.

PANAMA (See Map 3-30.)

Yellow Fever

Requirements: Required if traveling from a country with risk of YFV transmission.[a]

Recommendations:

Recommended for all travelers ≥9 months of age traveling to all mainland areas east of the Canal Zone, encompassing the entire comarcas (autonomous territories) of Emberá and Kuna Yala, the entire province of Darién, and areas of the provinces of Colón and Panamá that are east of the Canal Zone (see Map 3-19).

Not recommended for travelers whose itineraries are limited to areas west of the Canal Zone, the city of Panama, the Canal Zone itself, the San Blas Islands, and the Balboa Islands (see Map 3-19).

Malaria

Areas with malaria: Most transmission in provinces east of the Panama Canal toward the border with Colombia (provinces of Panamá east of the canal and Darién). Transmission also in provinces of C. Ngöbe-Buglé, Chiriqui, Coclé, Kuna Yala (San Blas), and Veraguas. None in urban areas of Panama City or in the former Canal Zone.

Estimated relative risk of malaria for US travelers: Low

Drug resistance[c]: Chloroquine (east of the Panama Canal).

Malaria species: *P. vivax* 99%, *P. falciparum* 1%.

Recommended chemoprophylaxis: Provinces east of the Panama Canal: Atovaquone-proguanil, doxycycline, mefloquine, or primaquine.[e]

Other areas with malaria: Mosquito avoidance only.

PAPUA NEW GUINEA

Yellow Fever

Requirements: Required if traveling from a country with risk of YFV transmission and ≥1 year of age.[a]

Recommendations: None

Malaria

Areas with malaria: Present throughout the country at altitudes <1,800 m (5,906 ft).

Estimated relative risk of malaria for US travelers: High

Drug resistance[c]: Chloroquine (both *P. falciparum* and *P. vivax*).

Malaria species: *P. falciparum* 65%–80%, *P. vivax* 10%–30%, remainder *P. malariae* and *P. ovale*.

---

[c] Refers to *P. falciparum* malaria unless otherwise noted.

[e] Primaquine can cause hemolytic anemia in people with glucose-6-phosphate dehydrogenase (G6PD) deficiency. Patients must be screened for G6PD deficiency before starting primaquine.

Recommended chemoprophylaxis:
Atovaquone-proguanil, doxycycline, or mefloquine.

PARAGUAY

Yellow Fever

Requirements: Required if traveling from a country with risk of YFV transmission and ≥1 year of age.[a]

Recommendations:

Recommended for all travelers ≥9 months of age, except as mentioned below.

Generally not recommended for travelers whose itinerary is limited to the city of Asunción.

Malaria

Areas with malaria: Present in the departments of Alto Paraná, Caaguazú, and Canendiyú.

Estimated relative risk of malaria for US travelers: Very low

Drug resistance[c]: None

Malaria species: *P. vivax* 95%, *P. falciparum* 5%.

Recommended chemoprophylaxis:
Atovaquone-proguanil, chloroquine, doxycycline, mefloquine, or primaquine.[e]

PERU (See Map 3-31.)

Yellow Fever

Requirements: None

Recommendations:

Recommended for all travelers ≥9 months of age going to the following areas <2,300 m in elevation[d]: the entire regions of Amazonas, Loreto, Madre de Dios, San Martin, and Ucayali and designated areas (see Map 3-19) of the following regions: far northeastern Ancash; northern Apurimac; northern

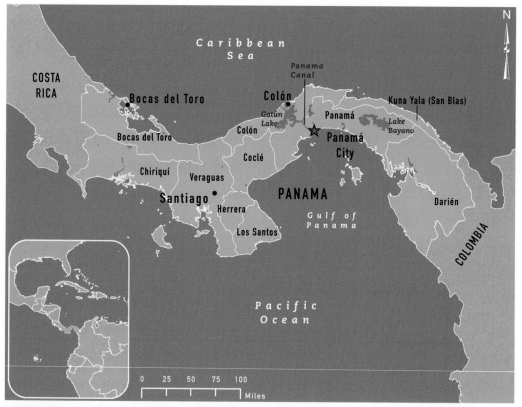

MAP 3-30. PANAMA REFERENCE MAP

FOOTNOTES:

[a] The official WHO list of countries with risk of YFV transmission can be found in Table 3-21. Proof of yellow fever vaccination should be required only if traveling from a country on the WHO list, unless otherwise specified. The following countries, containing only areas with low potential for exposure to YFV, are not on the WHO list: Eritrea, São Tomé and Príncipe, Somalia, Tanzania, Zambia.

and northeastern Ayacucho; northern and eastern Cajamarca; northwestern, northern, and northeastern Cusco; far northern Huancavelica; northern, central, and eastern Huanuco; northern and eastern Junin; eastern La Libertad; central and eastern Pasco; eastern Piura; and northern Puno. ***Generally not recommended*** for travelers whose itinerary is limited to the following areas west of the Andes: the entire regions of Lambayeque and Tumbes and the designated areas of west-central Cajamarca and western Piura (see Map 3-19).

Not recommended for travelers whose itineraries are limited to the following areas: all areas >2,300 m in elevation,[d] areas west of the Andes not listed above, the cities of Cuzco and Lima, Machu Picchu, and the Inca Trail (see Map 3-19).

Malaria

Areas with malaria: All departments <2,000 m (6,561 ft), including the cities of Iquitos and Puerto Maldonado, except none in the cities of Ica, Lima (and coast south of Lima), and Nazca.

None in the highland tourist areas (Cuzco, Machu Picchu, and Lake Titicaca) and southern cities of Arequipa, Moquegua, Puno, and Tacna.

Estimated relative risk of malaria for US travelers: Low

Drug resistance[c]: Chloroquine

Malaria species: *P. vivax* 70%, *P. falciparum* 30%, *P. malariae* <1%.

Recommended chemoprophylaxis: Atovaquone-proguanil, doxycycline, or mefloquine.

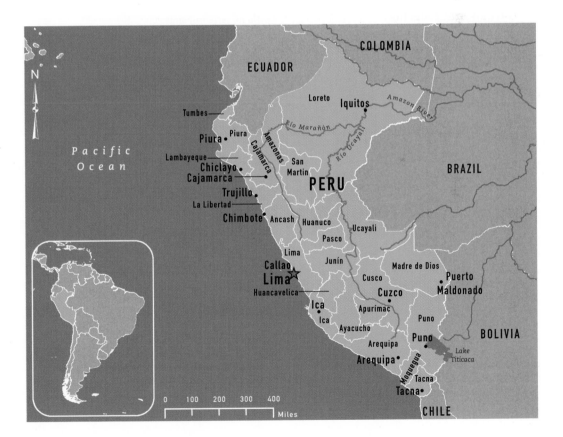

MAP 3-31. PERU REFERENCE MAP

[c] Refers to *P. falciparum* malaria unless otherwise noted.
[d] An elevation of 2,300 m is equivalent to 7,546 ft.
[e] Primaquine can cause hemolytic anemia in people with glucose-6-phosphate dehydrogenase (G6PD) deficiency. Patients must be screened for G6PD deficiency before starting primaquine.

PHILIPPINES
Yellow Fever
Requirements: Required if traveling from a country with risk of YFV transmission and ≥1 year of age.[a]
Recommendations: None

Malaria
Areas with malaria: Present in rural areas <600 m (1,969 ft) on the islands of Luzon, Mindanao, Mindoro, and Palawan. None in urban areas.
Estimated relative risk of malaria for US travelers: Low
Drug resistance[c]: Chloroquine
Malaria species: *P. falciparum* 70%–80%, *P. vivax* 20%–30%.
Recommended chemoprophylaxis: Atovaquone-proguanil, doxycycline, or mefloquine.

PITCAIRN ISLANDS (UK)
Yellow Fever
Requirements: Required if traveling from a country with risk of YFV transmission and ≥1 year of age.[a]
Recommendations: None

Malaria
No malaria transmission.

POLAND
Yellow Fever
No requirements or recommendations.

Malaria
No malaria transmission.

PORTUGAL
Yellow Fever
No requirements or recommendations.

Malaria
No malaria transmission.

PUERTO RICO (US)
Yellow Fever
No requirements or recommendations.

Malaria
No malaria transmission.

QATAR
Yellow Fever
No requirements or recommendations.

Malaria
No malaria transmission.

RÉUNION (FRANCE)
Yellow Fever
Requirements: Required if traveling from a country with risk of YFV transmission and ≥1 year of age.[a]
Recommendations: None

Malaria
No malaria transmission.

ROMANIA
Yellow Fever
No requirements or recommendations.

Malaria
No malaria transmission.

RUSSIA
Yellow Fever
Requirements: Required if traveling from a country with risk of YFV transmission and ≥9 months of age.[a]
Recommendations: None

Malaria
No malaria transmission.

RWANDA
Yellow Fever
Requirements: Required upon arrival from all countries for travelers ≥1 year of age.
Recommendations: *Recommended* for all travelers ≥9 months of age.

FOOTNOTES:
[a] The official WHO list of countries with risk of YFV transmission can be found in Table 3-21. Proof of yellow fever vaccination should be required only if traveling from a country on the WHO list, unless otherwise specified. The following countries, containing only areas with low potential for exposure to YFV, are not on the WHO list: Eritrea, São Tomé and Príncipe, Somalia, Tanzania, Zambia.

Malaria
Areas with malaria: All
Estimated relative risk of malaria for US travelers: Moderate
Drug resistance[c]: Chloroquine
Malaria species: *P. falciparum* >85%, *P. vivax* 5%, *P. ovale* 5%.
Recommended chemoprophylaxis: Atovaquone-proguanil, doxycycline, or mefloquine.

SAINT HELENA (UK)
Yellow Fever
Requirements: Required if traveling from a country with risk of YFV transmission and ≥1 year of age.[a]
Recommendations: None

Malaria
No malaria transmission.

SAINT KITTS (SAINT CHRISTOPHER) AND NEVIS (UK)
Yellow Fever
Requirements: Required if traveling from a country with risk of YFV transmission and ≥1 year of age.[a]
Recommendations: None

Malaria
No malaria transmission.

SAINT LUCIA
Yellow Fever
Requirements: Required if traveling from a country with risk of YFV transmission and ≥1 year of age.[a]
Recommendations: None

Malaria
No malaria transmission.

SAINT PIERRE AND MIQUELON (FRANCE)
Yellow Fever
No requirements or recommendations.

Malaria
No malaria transmission.

SAINT VINCENT AND THE GRENADINES
Yellow Fever
Requirements: Required if traveling from a country with risk of YFV transmission and ≥1 year of age.[a]
Recommendations: None

Malaria
No malaria transmission.

SAMOA (FORMERLY WESTERN SAMOA)
Yellow Fever
Requirements: Required if traveling from a country with risk of YFV transmission and ≥1 year of age.[a]
Recommendations: None

Malaria
No malaria transmission.

SAN MARINO
Yellow Fever
No requirements or recommendations.

Malaria
No malaria transmission.

SÃO TOMÉ AND PRÍNCIPE
Yellow Fever
Requirements: Required upon arrival from all countries for travelers ≥1 year of age.
Recommendations: *Generally not recommended* for travelers to São Tomé and Príncipe.

Malaria
Areas with malaria: All
Estimated relative risk of malaria for US travelers: Very low
Drug resistance[c]: Chloroquine

[c] Refers to *P. falciparum* malaria unless otherwise noted.

Malaria species: *P. falciparum* 85%, *P. malariae* and *P. ovale* 15% combined, *P. vivax* rare.
Recommended chemoprophylaxis: Atovaquone-proguanil, doxycycline, or mefloquine.

SAUDI ARABIA
Yellow Fever
Requirements: Required if traveling from a country with risk of YFV transmission.[a]
Recommendations: None

Malaria
Areas with malaria: Present in emirates by border with Yemen, specifically Asir and Jizan. Transmission also in emirate of Al Bahah. None in the cities of Jiddah, Mecca, Medina, Riyadh, and Ta'if.
Estimated relative risk of malaria for US travelers: Low
Drug resistance[c]: Chloroquine
Malaria species: *P. falciparum* predominantly, remainder *P. vivax*.
Recommended chemoprophylaxis: Atovaquone-proguanil, doxycycline, or mefloquine.

SENEGAL
Yellow Fever
Requirements: Required if traveling from a country with risk of YFV transmission and ≥9 months of age.[a]
Recommendations: *Recommended* for all travelers ≥9 months of age.

Malaria
Areas with malaria: All
Estimated relative risk of malaria for US travelers: High
Drug resistance[c]: Chloroquine
Malaria species: *P. falciparum* >85%, *P. ovale* 5%–10%, *P. vivax* rare.
Recommended chemoprophylaxis: Atovaquone-proguanil, doxycycline, or mefloquine.

SERBIA
Yellow Fever
No requirements or recommendations.

Malaria
No malaria transmission.

SEYCHELLES
Yellow Fever
Requirements: Required if traveling from a country with risk of YFV transmission and ≥1 year of age.[a]
Recommendations: None

Malaria
No malaria transmission.

SIERRA LEONE
Yellow Fever
Requirements: Required upon arrival from all countries.
Recommendations: *Recommended* for all travelers ≥9 months of age.

Malaria
Areas with malaria: All
Estimated relative risk of malaria for US travelers: High
Drug resistance[c]: Chloroquine
Malaria species: *P. falciparum* 85%; *P. malariae*, *P. ovale*, and *P. vivax* 15% combined.
Recommended chemoprophylaxis: Atovaquone-proguanil, doxycycline, or mefloquine.

SINGAPORE
Yellow Fever
Requirements: Required for travelers who are ≥1 year of age and who within the preceding 6 days have been in or passed through any country with risk of YFV transmission.[a]
Recommendations: None

Malaria
No malaria transmission.

FOOTNOTES:
[a] The official WHO list of countries with risk of YFV transmission can be found in Table 3-21. Proof of yellow fever vaccination should be required only if traveling from a country on the WHO list, unless otherwise specified. The following countries, containing only areas with low potential for exposure to YFV, are not on the WHO list: Eritrea, São Tomé and Príncipe, Somalia, Tanzania, Zambia.

SLOVAKIA
Yellow Fever
No requirements or recommendations.

Malaria
No malaria transmission.

SLOVENIA
Yellow Fever
No requirements or recommendations.

Malaria
No malaria transmission.

SOLOMON ISLANDS
Yellow Fever
Requirements: Required if traveling from a country with risk of YFV transmission.[a]
Recommendations: None

Malaria
Areas with malaria: All
Estimated relative risk of malaria for US travelers: High
Drug resistance[c]: Chloroquine
Malaria species: *P. falciparum* 60%, *P. vivax* 35%–40%, *P. ovale* <1%.
Recommended chemoprophylaxis: Atovaquone-proguanil, doxycycline, or mefloquine.

SOMALIA
Yellow Fever
Requirements: Required if traveling from a country with risk of YFV transmission.[a]
Recommendations:
Generally not recommended for travelers going to the following regions: Bakool, Banaadir, Bay, Galguduud, Gedo, Hiiraan, Lower Jubabada, Lower Shabelle, Middle Jubabada, and Middle Shabelle (see Map 3-18).
Not recommended for all other areas not listed above.

Malaria
Areas with malaria: All

Estimated relative risk of malaria for US travelers: No data
Drug resistance[c]: Chloroquine
Malaria species: *P. falciparum* 95%; *P. malariae*, *P. ovale*, and *P. vivax* 5% combined.
Recommended chemoprophylaxis: Atovaquone-proguanil, doxycycline, or mefloquine.

SOUTH AFRICA
Yellow Fever
Requirements: Required if traveling from a country with risk of YFV transmission and ≥1 year of age.[a]
Recommendations: None

Malaria
Areas with malaria: Present in northeastern KwaZulu-Natal Province as far south as the Tugela River, Limpopo (Northern) Province, and Mpumalanga Province. Present in Kruger National Park.
Estimated relative risk of malaria for US travelers: Low
Drug resistance[c]: Chloroquine
Malaria species: *P. falciparum* 90%, *P. vivax* 5%, *P. ovale* 5%.
Recommended chemoprophylaxis: Atovaquone-proguanil, doxycycline, or mefloquine.

SOUTH GEORGIA AND SOUTH SANDWICH ISLANDS (UK)
Yellow Fever
Requirements: These islands have not stated their yellow fever vaccination certificate requirements.
Recommendations: None

Malaria
No malaria transmission.

SOUTH KOREA
Yellow Fever
No requirements or recommendations.

[c] Refers to *P. falciparum* malaria unless otherwise noted.

Malaria

Areas with malaria: Limited to the months of March–December in rural areas in the northern parts of Incheon, Kangwon-do, and Kyônggi-do Provinces, including the demilitarized zone (DMZ).
Estimated relative risk of malaria for US travelers: Low
Drug resistance^c: None
Malaria species: *P. vivax* 100%.
Recommended chemoprophylaxis: Atovaquone-proguanil, chloroquine, doxycycline, mefloquine, or primaquine.^e

SPAIN

Yellow Fever

No requirements or recommendations.

Malaria

No malaria transmission.

SRI LANKA

Yellow Fever

Requirements: Required if traveling from a country with risk of YFV transmission and ≥1 year of age.^a
Recommendations: None

Malaria

Areas with malaria: All areas, except none in the districts of Colombo, Galle, Gampaha, Kalutara, Matara, and Nuwara Eliya.
Estimated relative risk of malaria for US travelers: Very low
Drug resistance^c: Chloroquine
Malaria species: *P. vivax* 88%, *P. falciparum* 12%.
Recommended chemoprophylaxis: Atovaquone-proguanil, doxycycline, or mefloquine.

SUDAN

Yellow Fever

Requirements: Required if traveling from a country with risk of YFV transmission and ≥9 months of age.^a A certificate may be required for travelers departing Sudan.

Recommendations:

Recommended for all travelers ≥9 months of age traveling to areas south of the Sahara Desert (see Map 3-18).
Not recommended for travelers whose itineraries are limited to areas in the Sahara Desert and the city of Khartoum (see Map 3-18).

Malaria

Areas with malaria: All
Estimated relative risk of malaria for US travelers: High
Drug resistance^c: Chloroquine
Malaria species: *P. falciparum* 90%; *P. malariae*, *P. vivax*, and *P. ovale* 10% combined.
Recommended chemoprophylaxis: Atovaquone-proguanil, doxycycline, or mefloquine.

SURINAME

Yellow Fever

Requirements: Required if traveling from a country with risk of YFV transmission and ≥1 year of age.^a
Recommendations: ***Recommended*** for all travelers ≥9 months of age.

Malaria

Areas with malaria: Present in provinces of Brokopondo and Sipaliwini. None in Paramaribo.
Estimated relative risk of malaria for US travelers: Moderate
Drug resistance^c: Chloroquine
Malaria species: *P. falciparum* 70%, *P. vivax* 15%–20%.
Recommended chemoprophylaxis: Atovaquone-proguanil, doxycycline, or mefloquine.

SWAZILAND

Yellow Fever

Requirements: Required if traveling from a country with risk of YFV transmission.^a
Recommendations: None

FOOTNOTES:
^a The official WHO list of countries with risk of YFV transmission can be found in Table 3-21. Proof of yellow fever vaccination should be required only if traveling from a country on the WHO list, unless otherwise specified. The following countries, containing only areas with low potential for exposure to YFV, are not on the WHO list: Eritrea, São Tomé and Príncipe, Somalia, Tanzania, Zambia.

Malaria

Areas with malaria: Present in eastern areas bordering Mozambique and South Africa, including all of Lubombo district and the eastern half of Hhohho and Shiselweni districts.
Estimated relative risk of malaria for US travelers: Very low
Drug resistance[c]: Chloroquine
Malaria species: *P. falciparum* 90%, *P. vivax* 5%, *P. ovale* 5%.
Recommended chemoprophylaxis: Atovaquone-proguanil, doxycycline, or mefloquine.

SWEDEN

Yellow Fever
No requirements or recommendations.

Malaria
No malaria transmission.

SWITZERLAND

Yellow Fever
No requirements or recommendations.

Malaria
No malaria transmission.

SYRIA

Yellow Fever
Requirements: Required if traveling from a country with risk of YFV transmission and ≥6 months of age.[a]
Recommendations: None

Malaria
No malaria transmission.

TAIWAN

Yellow Fever
No requirements or recommendations.

Malaria
No malaria transmission.

TAJIKISTAN

Yellow Fever
No requirements or recommendations.

Malaria
Areas with malaria: All areas <2,000 m (6,561 ft).
Estimated relative risk of malaria for US travelers: Very low
Drug resistance[c]: Chloroquine
Malaria species: *P. vivax* 90%, *P. falciparum* 10%.
Recommended chemoprophylaxis: Atovaquone-proguanil, doxycycline, mefloquine, or primaquine.[e]

TANZANIA

Yellow Fever
Requirements: Required if traveling from a country with risk of YFV transmission and ≥1 year of age.[a]
Recommendations: *Generally not recommended* for travelers to Tanzania.

Malaria
Areas with malaria: All areas <1,800 m (5,906 ft).
Estimated relative risk of malaria for US travelers: Moderate
Drug resistance[c]: Chloroquine
Malaria species: *P. falciparum* >85%, *P. malariae* and *P. ovale* >10% combined, *P. vivax* rare.
Recommended chemoprophylaxis: Atovaquone-proguanil, doxycycline, or mefloquine.

THAILAND

Yellow Fever
Requirements: Required if traveling from a country with risk of YFV transmission and ≥9 months of age.[a]
Recommendations: None

Malaria
Areas with malaria: Rural, forested areas that border Burma (Myanmar), Cambodia,

---

[c] Refers to *P. falciparum* malaria unless otherwise noted.
[e] Primaquine can cause hemolytic anemia in people with glucose-6-phosphate dehydrogenase (G6PD) deficiency. Patients must be screened for G6PD deficiency before starting primaquine.

and Laos. Rare local cases in Phang Nga and Phuket. None in the cities and major tourist resorts. None in the cities of Bangkok, Chiang Mai, Chiang Rai, Koh Phangan, Koh Samui, and Pattaya.
Estimated relative risk of malaria for US travelers: Low
Drug resistance[c]: Chloroquine, mefloquine (see Map 3-11).
Malaria species: *P. falciparum* 50% (up to 75% in some areas), *P. vivax* 50% (up to 60% in some areas), remainder *P. ovale.*
Recommended chemoprophylaxis: Atovaquone-proguanil or doxycycline.

TIMOR-LESTE
Yellow Fever
Requirements: Required if traveling from a country with risk of YFV transmission and ≥1 year of age.[a]
Recommendations: None

Malaria
Areas with malaria: All
Estimated relative risk of malaria for US travelers: No data
Drug resistance[c]: Chloroquine
Malaria Species: *P. falciparum* 50%, *P. vivax* 50%, *P. ovale* <1%, *P. malariae* <1%.
Recommended chemoprophylaxis: Atovaquone-proguanil, doxycycline, or mefloquine.

TOGO
Yellow Fever
Requirements: Required upon arrival from all countries for travelers ≥1 year of age.
Recommendations: *Recommended* for all travelers ≥9 months of age.

Malaria
Areas with malaria: All
Estimated relative risk of malaria for US travelers: High
Drug resistance[c]: Chloroquine
Malaria species: *P. falciparum* 85%, *P. ovale* 5%–10%, remainder *P. vivax.*

Recommended chemoprophylaxis: Atovaquone-proguanil, doxycycline, or mefloquine.

TOKELAU (NEW ZEALAND)
Yellow Fever
No requirements or recommendations.

Malaria
No malaria transmission.

TONGA
Yellow Fever
No requirements or recommendations.

Malaria
No malaria transmission.

TRINIDAD AND TOBAGO
Yellow Fever
Requirements: Required if traveling from a country with risk of YFV transmission and ≥1 year of age.[a]
Recommendations:
Recommended for all travelers ≥9 months of age traveling to the island of Trinidad, except as mentioned below.
Generally not recommended for travelers whose itinerary is limited to the urban areas of Port of Spain, cruise ship passengers who do not disembark from the ship, and airplane passengers in transit.
Not recommended for travelers whose itineraries are limited to the island of Tobago.

Malaria
No malaria transmission.

TUNISIA
Yellow Fever
Requirements: Required if traveling from a country with risk of YFV transmission and ≥1 year of age.[a]
Recommendations: None

Malaria
No malaria transmission.

FOOTNOTES:
[a] The official WHO list of countries with risk of YFV transmission can be found in Table 3-21. Proof of yellow fever vaccination should be required only if traveling from a country on the WHO list, unless otherwise specified. The following countries, containing only areas with low potential for exposure to YFV, are not on the WHO list: Eritrea, São Tomé and Príncipe, Somalia, Tanzania, Zambia.

TURKEY
Yellow Fever
No requirements or recommendations.

Malaria
Areas with malaria: Present in southeastern part of the country. None on the Incerlik US Air Force Base or on typical cruise itineraries.
Estimated relative risk of malaria for US travelers: Very low
Drug resistance[c]: None
Malaria species: *P. vivax* predominantly, *P. falciparum* sporadically.
Recommended chemoprophylaxis: Atovaquone-proguanil, chloroquine, doxycycline, mefloquine, or primaquine.[e]

TURKMENISTAN
Yellow Fever
No requirements or recommendations.

Malaria
No malaria transmission.

TURKS AND CAICOS ISLANDS (UK)
Yellow Fever
Requirements: Required if traveling from a country with risk of YFV transmission and ≥1 year of age.[a]
Recommendations: None

Malaria
No malaria transmission.

TUVALU
Yellow Fever
No requirements or recommendations.

Malaria
No malaria transmission.

UGANDA
Yellow Fever
Requirements: Required if traveling from a country with risk of YFV transmission and ≥1 year of age.[a]

Recommendations: *Recommended* for all travelers ≥9 months of age.

Malaria
Areas with malaria: All
Estimated relative risk of malaria for US travelers: High
Drug resistance[c]: Chloroquine
Malaria species: *P. falciparum* >85%; remainder *P. malariae*, *P. ovale*, and *P. vivax*.
Recommended chemoprophylaxis: Atovaquone-proguanil, doxycycline, or mefloquine.

UKRAINE
Yellow Fever
No requirements or recommendations.

Malaria
No malaria transmission.

UNITED ARAB EMIRATES
Yellow Fever
No requirements or recommendations.

Malaria
No malaria transmission.

UNITED KINGDOM, WITH CHANNEL ISLANDS AND ISLE OF MAN
Yellow Fever
No requirements or recommendations.

Malaria
No malaria transmission.

UNITED STATES
Yellow Fever
No requirements or recommendations.

Malaria
No malaria transmission.

[c] Refers to *P. falciparum* malaria unless otherwise noted.
[e] Primaquine can cause hemolytic anemia in people with glucose-6-phosphate dehydrogenase (G6PD) deficiency. Patients must be screened for G6PD deficiency before starting primaquine.

URUGUAY
Yellow Fever
Requirements: Required if traveling from a country with risk of YFV transmission.[a]
Recommendations: None

Malaria
No malaria transmission.

UZBEKISTAN
Yellow Fever
No requirements or recommendations.

Malaria
Areas with malaria: Previously, rare cases along the Afghanistan and Tajikistan borders. No cases reported in 2009.
Estimated relative risk of malaria for US travelers: Very low
Drug resistance[c]: None
Malaria species: Previously *P. vivax* 100%.
Recommended chemoprophylaxis: Mosquito avoidance only.

VANUATU
Yellow Fever
No requirements or recommendations.

Malaria
Areas with malaria: All
Estimated relative risk of malaria for US travelers: High
Drug resistance[c]: Chloroquine
Malaria species: *P. falciparum* 60%, *P. vivax* 35%–40%, *P. ovale* <1%.
Recommended chemoprophylaxis:
Atovaquone-proguanil, doxycycline, or mefloquine.

VENEZUELA (See Map 3-32.)
Yellow Fever
Requirements: None
Recommendations:
Recommended for all travelers ≥9 months of age, except as mentioned below.
Generally not recommended for travelers whose itinerary is limited to the following

areas: the states of Aragua, Carabobo, Miranda, Vargas, and Yaracuy, and the Distrito Federal (see Map 3-19).
Not recommended for travelers whose itineraries are limited to the following areas: the states of Falcón and Lara, the peninsular section of Paez Municipality in Zulia Province, Margarita Island, and the cities of Caracas and Valencia (see Map 3-19).

Malaria
Areas with malaria: Rural areas of the following states: Amazonas, Anzoátegui, Apure, Bolivar, Delta Amacuro, Monagas, Sucre, and Zulia. Present in Angel Falls. None in Margarita Island.
Estimated relative risk of malaria for US travelers: Low
Drug resistance[c]: Chloroquine
Malaria species: *P. vivax* 83%, *P. falciparum* 17%.
Recommended chemoprophylaxis:
Atovaquone-proguanil, doxycycline, or mefloquine.

VIETNAM
Yellow Fever
Requirements: Required if traveling from a country with risk of YFV transmission and ≥1 year of age.[a]
Recommendations: None

Malaria
Areas with malaria: Rural only, except none in the Red River Delta and the coast north of Nha Trang. Rare cases in the Mekong Delta. None in Da Nang, Haiphong, Hanoi, Ho Chi Minh City (Saigon), Nha Trang, and Qui Nhon.
Estimated relative risk of malaria for US travelers: Low
Drug resistance[c]: Chloroquine, mefloquine (see Map 3-11).
Malaria species: *P. falciparum* 50%–90%, remainder *P. vivax*.
Recommended chemoprophylaxis:
Southern part of the country in the provinces of Dac Lac, Gia Lai, Khanh Hoa, Kon Tum, Lam Dong, Ninh Thuan, Song Be, Tay Ninh: Atovaquone-proguanil or doxycycline.

FOOTNOTES:
[a] The official WHO list of countries with risk of YFV transmission can be found in Table 3-21. Proof of yellow fever vaccination should be required only if traveling from a country on the WHO list, unless otherwise specified. The following countries, containing only areas with low potential for exposure to YFV, are not on the WHO list: Eritrea, São Tomé and Príncipe, Somalia, Tanzania, Zambia.

Other areas with malaria except Mekong Delta: Atovaquone-proguanil, doxycycline, or mefloquine.
Mekong Delta: Mosquito avoidance only.

VIRGIN ISLANDS, BRITISH
Yellow Fever
No requirements or recommendations.

Malaria
No malaria transmission.

VIRGIN ISLANDS, US
Yellow Fever
No requirements or recommendations.

Malaria
No malaria transmission.

WAKE ISLAND, US
Yellow Fever
No requirements or recommendations.

Malaria
No malaria transmission.

WALLIS AND FUTUNA ISLANDS (FRANCE)
Yellow Fever
Requirements: These islands have not stated their yellow fever vaccination certificate requirements.
Recommendations: None

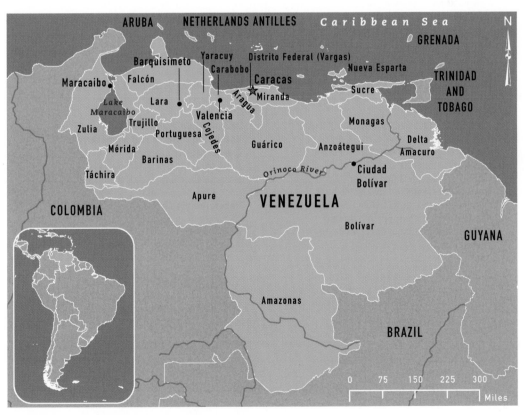

MAP 3-32. VENEZUELA REFERENCE MAP

ᶜ Refers to *P. falciparum* malaria unless otherwise noted.

Malaria
No malaria transmission.

WESTERN SAHARA
Yellow Fever
Requirements: This territory has not stated its yellow fever vaccination certificate requirements.
Recommendations: None

Malaria
Areas with malaria: Rare cases
Estimated relative risk of malaria for US travelers: No data
Drug resistance[c]: Chloroquine
Malaria species: Unknown
Recommended chemoprophylaxis: Mosquito avoidance only.

YEMEN
Yellow Fever
Requirements: Required if traveling from a country with risk of YFV transmission and ⩾1 year of age.[a]
Recommendations: None

Malaria
Areas with malaria: All areas <2,000 m (6,561 ft). None in Sana'a.
Estimated relative risk of malaria for US travelers: Moderate
Drug resistance[c]: Chloroquine
Malaria species: *P. falciparum* 95%; *P. malariae, P. vivax,* and *P. ovale* 5% combined.
Recommended chemoprophylaxis: Atovaquone-proguanil, doxycycline, or mefloquine.

ZAMBIA
Yellow Fever
Requirements: None
Recommendations:
Generally not recommended for travelers going to the North West and Western Provinces.
Not recommended in all other areas not listed above.

Malaria
Areas with malaria: All
Estimated relative risk of malaria for US travelers: Moderate
Drug resistance[c]: Chloroquine
Malaria species: *P. falciparum* >90%, *P. vivax* up to 5%, *P. ovale* up to 5%.
Recommended chemoprophylaxis: Atovaquone-proguanil, doxycycline, or mefloquine.

ZIMBABWE
Yellow Fever
Requirements: Required if traveling from a country with risk of YFV transmission.[a]
Recommendations: None

Malaria
Areas with malaria: All
Estimated relative risk of malaria for US travelers: Moderate
Drug resistance[c]: Chloroquine
Malaria species: *P. falciparum* >90%, *P. vivax* up to 5%, *P. ovale* up to 5%.
Recommended chemoprophylaxis: Atovaquone-proguanil, doxycycline, or mefloquine.

FOOTNOTES:
[a] The official WHO list of countries with risk of YFV transmission can be found in Table 3-21. Proof of yellow fever vaccination should be required only if traveling from a country on the WHO list, unless otherwise specified. The following countries, containing only areas with low potential for exposure to YFV, are not on the WHO list: Eritrea, São Tomé and Príncipe, Somalia, Tanzania, Zambia.
[c] Refers to *P. falciparum* malaria unless otherwise noted.

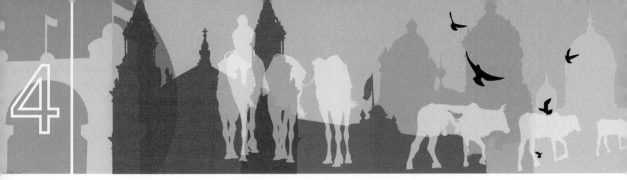

Select Destinations

RATIONALE FOR SELECT DESTINATIONS
David R. Shlim

The quality of travel health advice is based on trying to reduce risks for the traveler in a particular destination. Our ability to counsel travelers is improved when we have visited a particular destination ourselves, or at least are familiar with typical itineraries and the specifics of health risks. However, one's travel experiences rarely encompass all the destinations that one's clients seek to visit. Thus, this chapter of the Yellow Book was created to allow experts who have lived in or visited particular destinations frequently to share their insider's knowledge of these places.

These sections should be considered a personal perspective on these areas. Preventive recommendations that are covered elsewhere in the book are usually not repeated in these chapters, other than to address controversies or to emphasize important points.

The destination sections proved to be the most popular addition to the 2010 Yellow Book. In this edition, the chapter has expanded to include 6 new destinations. The goal of these sections is to allow travel health providers to feel more comfortable giving advice about specific destinations that he or she may have never visited, and to provide a level of detail about the attractions and health risks that have not been provided elsewhere in this book.

THE CARIBBEAN
Clive M. Brown

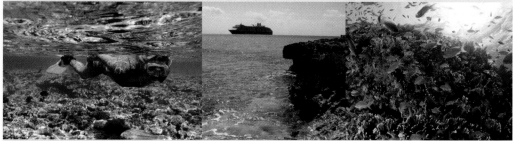

DESTINATION OVERVIEW

The Caribbean is an arc-shaped group of islands that separate the Gulf of Mexico and the Caribbean Sea from the Atlantic Ocean. Historically, politically, culturally, and geographically, the Caribbean region can be divided as follows:

> Greater Antilles: Cuba, Jamaica, Cayman Islands, Hispaniola (Haiti and Dominican Republic), and Puerto Rico
> Lesser Antilles: Virgin Islands, Anguilla, Saint Kitts and Nevis, Dominica, Barbuda, Montserrat, Guadeloupe, Martinique, Saint Lucia, Saint Vincent and the Grenadines, Barbados, and Grenada
> Atlantic Ocean islands: Bermuda, The Bahamas, and the Turks and Caicos Islands
> South American shelf islands: Trinidad and Tobago, Aruba, Curacao, and Bonaire

In addition, coastal areas of the mainland countries of Belize in Central America and Guyana, Suriname, and French Guiana in South America are often considered part of the Caribbean.

The islands and mainland countries vary in geography, from sandy and dry islands with fantastic beaches to volcanic, lush rainforests. Ah, the beaches! For many tourists, this is the Caribbean's raison d'être, and with over a thousand islands to chose from, choices are almost limitless. The dazzling beaches on the islands and mainland coasts of the Caribbean Sea, the Gulf of Mexico, and the Atlantic Ocean provide a vacation experience that broadens the mind and provides a travel destination with luxury, excitement, tranquility, and relaxation.

Coral reefs are among the most diverse and beautiful of all marine habitats, and the Caribbean has about 7% of the world's coral reefs. With reefs surrounding virtually the entire border of the Cuban marine shelf, the Belize barrier reef complex is the largest continuous reef system in the western Atlantic. Jamaican reefs are among the most species-rich in the Caribbean, and The Bahamas offers over 1,000 dives, including specialty dives such as shark close-ups and diving with dolphins. The Caribbean is one of the world's top diving destinations: travelers can dive year round, and water temperatures average 74°F–81°F (23°C–27°C).

The Caribbean climate is tropical, with daytime temperatures in most of the region in the low- to mid-80s°F (26°C–30°C) during North America's winter months and in the upper 80s to low 90s°F (lower 30s°C) in the summer months. Nighttime temperatures are around 10°F (5°C) cooler. Bermuda has similar summertime temperatures, but in the cooler months the nighttime low is in the upper 50s°F (12°C–15°C). Temperatures fluctuate depending on altitude, especially in the mountainous countries of Cuba (Pico Real del Turquino: 6,476 ft; 1,974 m), Jamaica (Blue Mountain Peak: 7,402 ft; 2,256 m), Haiti (Morne de la Selle: 8,959 ft; 2,731 m), and the Dominican Republic (Pico Duarte: 10,164 ft; 3,098 m). The sunny climate and recreational resources make the Caribbean a major winter vacation destination. The Caribbean is considered "a tropical paradise," and tourism is an extremely important economic activity for the region. Tourist arrivals were recorded by the Caribbean Tourism Organization as slightly over 22 million in 2009 for their 33 member countries. In 2007, the United States accounted for almost 12 million tourist arrivals.

HEALTH ISSUES

Immunizations

Everyone should be up to date with routine vaccinations, whether or not they travel. In addition, hepatitis A and B vaccination is recommended for all unvaccinated travelers. Typhoid vaccine is recommended for some travelers to the Caribbean, especially if they are staying long-term, staying with friends or relatives, or visiting smaller cities, villages, or rural areas where exposure might occur through food or water. Preexposure rabies vaccination may be recommended for some travelers in rare instances.

Malaria

Malaria caused by chloroquine-sensitive *Plasmodium falciparum* is endemic in Haiti. Travelers to Haiti should take appropriate chemoprophylactic and preventive measures to minimize the risk of acquiring malaria. Forty-five years after it had been eradicated, autochthonous malaria transmission has been reported in Jamaica (rare local cases in Kingston) and The Bahamas (Great Exuma). There have not been ongoing reports of malaria in travelers to Great Exuma, suggesting no sustained transmission; therefore, there are no specific recommendations for travel to The Bahamas, although measures to avoid mosquitoes are recommended to prevent dengue. Mosquito avoidance measures are recommended for travel to Jamaica, particularly Kingston. In addition, malaria occurs in the Dominican Republic (see Chapter 3, Yellow Fever and Malaria Information, by Country). Endemic malaria occurs in the 3 mainland countries of Guyana, Suriname, and Belize, and appropriate prophylaxis is recommended when visiting these countries.

Other Vectorborne Diseases

Dengue

The Caribbean is among the most common regions from which US travelers acquire dengue. Dengue is endemic in most Caribbean countries because the vector, the *Aedes* mosquito, is ubiquitous. Outbreaks are being reported more frequently, and the numbers of cases of dengue hemorrhagic fever (DHF) and dengue shock syndrome (DSS) reported in these countries are increasing. All 4 dengue serotypes have been isolated in the Caribbean. Although the overall transmission of dengue fever was not reported to be unusually high across the region, reports of dengue fever, DHF, and DSS increased during 2009 and 2010, with larger increases reported in 2010 than in 2009 by some islands (notably Jamaica, Trinidad and Tobago, and the French islands Martinique and Guadeloupe). During 2009, the predominant dengue serotypes identified were types 2 and 3, although predominantly types 1 and 2 were identified during 2010. Suriname reported serotype 4 both years and type 1 in 2010, and Saint Lucia also reported serotypes 1 and 2. Residents of the United States traveling to the Caribbean should take appropriate prevention measures to protect themselves from dengue.

Yellow Fever

Trinidad and Tobago and the mainland countries of French Guiana, Guyana, and Suriname are areas with risk of yellow fever virus transmission, but it is not holoendemic in Trinidad and Tobago. Vaccine is recommended for travelers aged ≥9 months to the 3 mainland countries and the island of Trinidad (except the urban areas of Port of Spain), but not the island of Tobago.

Other Diseases
Travelers' Diarrhea and Foodborne Diseases
Caribbean cuisine is a fusion of spices and cooking styles from African, Amerindian, British, Spanish, French, Dutch, Indian, and Chinese cultures. Whether jerked chicken or ackee and salt fish in Jamaica, cracked (deep fried) conch or conch fritters in The Bahamas, or *roti* with curried meat or vegetables in Trinidad and Tobago, travelers will want to experience the culinary excitement of Caribbean cuisine. However, travelers should stick to legitimate eating establishments and avoid itinerant vendors. Travelers' diarrhea is one of the most common travel-related illnesses, and some countries in the Caribbean fall into the intermediate-risk group, with attack rates of 8%–20%. Central America falls into the high-risk group, with attack rates of 20%–50%. Jamaica is unique among tourist destinations for having a hotel-based surveillance system of illness and injuries in travelers and for doing occasional exit surveys among travelers at its airport to estimate the risk of travelers' diarrhea. Since interventions to prevent and control diarrhea in visitors were implemented, Jamaica reported a 72% reduction in diarrhea in the visitor population from 1996 to 2002. Outbreaks of ciguatera poisoning, which results from eating toxin-containing reef fish, have also occurred on many islands (see Chapter 2, Food Poisoning from Marine Toxins).

Histoplasmosis
Outbreaks of histoplasmosis have occurred in travelers to some Caribbean islands and to mainland French Guinea. For ecotourism enthusiasts, spelunking and trekking are possible activities that may put travelers at higher risk for exposure.

Physical Concerns for the Traveler
Crime and Drugs
The crime rate is high in some countries of the Caribbean; however, the Department of State reports often note that even in the most troubled countries, violent crime rarely affects tourists. A 2007 report from the World Bank estimated that the overall murder rate in the Caribbean was 30 per 100,000 inhabitants, 4 times that in North America. Jamaica has one of the highest rates of violent crime in the world but a relatively low rate of property crime. Visitors are rarely the victims of violent crime, but are most often victims of property crimes and may be targeted in locations frequented by tourists. Statistics suggest lower crime rates in the Caribbean countries of Montserrat, the Cayman Islands, Saint-Barthélemy, the British Virgin Islands, Bonaire, and Dominica. Travelers from the United States who are visiting friends and relatives in the Caribbean will most likely enter communities that the average tourist will not. These travelers should be reminded that they are not immune to crime and injury in these communities.

Travelers are reminded that while illegal drug use is prevalent in some tourist areas, possession or use of marijuana or other illicit drugs is illegal, including in Jamaica. In addition to the health risks associated with illicit drug use, each year, many American citizens are arrested and incarcerated for drug-related crimes in Jamaica.

Traffic
Road traffic accidents are the leading cause of injury death among US citizens in foreign countries. Tourists will encounter road conditions that differ significantly from those in the United States. In some countries, roads may vary from 2-lane paved roads to dirt tracks, and some may lack markings or reflectors. Although many Caribbean countries have areas with well paved roads and even highways, many countries and many areas within countries have long, curvy roads with steep stretches where some parts of the road are in disrepair. This is especially true in rural and mountainous areas. In a few of the smaller Caribbean islands, such as Bermuda, motor vehicle rentals may be limited to motorbikes, since cars are not often available. Unlike in the United States, drivers drive on the left in the English-speaking Caribbean countries.

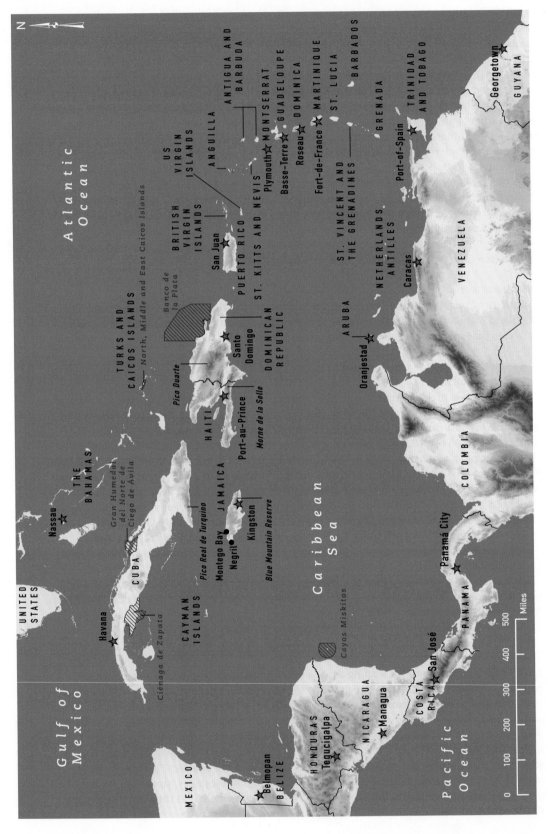

MAP 4-1. CARIBBEAN DESTINATION MAP

Natural Disasters

The Atlantic hurricane season runs from June through November and peaks between August and October, when the waters of the Caribbean are warmest. Many of the Caribbean islands are in the path of Atlantic hurricanes through the Atlantic Ocean, the Caribbean Sea, and the Gulf of Mexico. The southernmost islands (Aruba, Barbados, Curaçao, Bonaire, Grenada, and Trinidad and Tobago) are rarely hit by hurricanes.

The Caribbean is also an area of major earthquake activity (magnitude ≥7.0) with the potential for generating tsunamis. On January 12, 2010, Haiti was hit by a magnitude 7.0 earthquake, resulting in more than 200,000 estimated deaths.

Beaches, Rafting, Diving, and Snorkeling

Even in the cooler months of the year, travelers are at risk for sunburn, which can be more severe with alcohol use. Travelers should use adequate sun protection and keep hydrated. Drowning is the third leading cause of injury death among US citizens in foreign countries, so travelers should ensure that they are fit and healthy to undertake water-related activities and always have company when doing them. Dives should not be done within 24 hours before a flight or before mountain hikes to avoid the risk of decompression sickness. Jamaica has a decompression facility in Discovery Bay on its north coast near many of the diving areas.

Cutaneous larva migrans is a risk for travelers on some beaches in the Caribbean. Leptospirosis is common in many areas, most notably some regions in Jamaica, and poses a risk to travelers engaged in recreational freshwater activities. Such activities may include whitewater rafting, kayaking, adventure racing, or hiking. Travelers can reduce their risk for leptospirosis by avoiding activities that expose them to contaminated fresh surface water.

BIBLIOGRAPHY

1. Ashley DV, Walters C, Dockery-Brown C, McNab A, Ashley DE. Interventions to prevent and control food-borne diseases associated with a reduction in traveler's diarrhea in tourists to Jamaica. J Travel Med. 2004 Nov–Dec;11(6):364–7.
2. Caribbean Epidemiology Center and Pan American Health Organization. CAREC surveillance report. 2010. Available from: http://new.paho.org/carec/dmdocuments/CSR_August_2010.pdf.
3. Caribbean Tourism Organization. Caribbean Tourism Overview—2009. Caribbean Tourism Organization; 2010 [updated Feb 8]. Available from: http://www.onecaribbean.org/content/files/ctomediaConf.Feb82010Caribbean TourismOverview2009%281%29.pdf.
4. de Luna Martinez J. Workers' remittances to developing countries: a survey with central banks on selected public policy issues. Washington, DC: The World Bank; 2005. Available from: http://econ.worldbank.org/external/default/main?pagePK=64165259&theSitePK=469372&piPK=64165421&menuPK=64166093&entityID=000012009_2 0050608121914.
5. Freedman DO, Weld LH, Kozarsky PE, Fisk T, Robins R, von Sonnenburg F, et al. Spectrum of disease and relation to place of exposure among ill returned travelers. N Engl J Med. 2006 Jan 12;354(2):119–30.
6. Greenwood Z, Black J, Weld L, O'Brien D, Leder K, Von Sonnenburg F, et al. Gastrointestinal infection among international travelers globally. J Travel Med. 2008 Jul–Aug;15(4):221–8.
7. Mohammed HP, Ramos MM, Rivera A, Johansson M, Munoz-Jordan JL, Sun W, et al. Travel-associated dengue infections in the United States, 1996 to 2005. J Travel Med. 2010 Jan–Feb;17(1):8–14.
8. Rawlins SC, Hinds A, Rawlins JM. Malaria and its vectors in the Caribbean: the continuing challenge of the disease forty-five years after eradication from the Islands. West Indian Med J. 2008 Nov;57(5):462–9.
9. ScienceDaily. Major Caribbean earthquakes and tsunamis a real risk. ScienceDaily; 2005. Available from: http://www.sciencedaily.com/releases/2005/02/050205102502.htm.
10. Swaminathan A, Torresi J, Schlagenhauf P, Thursky K, Wilder-Smith A, Connor BA, et al. A global study of pathogens and host risk factors associated with infectious gastrointestinal disease in returned international travellers. J Infect. 2009 Jul;59(1):19–27.
11. United Nations and the World Bank. Crime, violence, and development: trends, costs, and policy options in the Caribbean. Report no. 37820. Geneva: United Nations and the World Bank; 2007. Available from: http://www.unodc.org/pdf/research/Cr_and_Vio_Car_E.pdf.

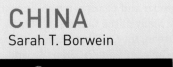

CHINA
Sarah T. Borwein

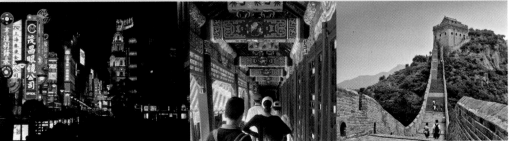

DESTINATION OVERVIEW

China, with more than 1.3 billion people, is the most populous country in the world and the fourth largest geographically, behind Russia, Canada, and the United States. It shares a border with 14 other countries. China is divided into 23 provinces, 5 autonomous regions, and 4 municipalities. This large landmass is home to diverse topography, languages, and customs. The climate varies from tropical in the south to subarctic in the north, with wide variations between regions and seasons. Natural hazards include typhoons along the southern and eastern seaboards, dust storms in the north, floods, earthquakes, and landslides. Six of the 10 deadliest natural disasters in history occurred in China, including the 1956 Shaanxi earthquake, which killed more than 800,000 people, making it the most lethal earthquake in history. More recently, devastating earthquakes have struck the western provinces of Sichuan in 2008 and Qinghai in 2010. Torrential rain, floods, and landslides plagued large areas of China in the summer of 2010.

China has one of the world's oldest continuous civilizations, dating back more than 5,000 years. It has the world's longest continuously used written language system and is the source of many major inventions, including the "four great inventions of Ancient China:" paper, the compass, gunpowder, and printing. Today, China is considerably more advanced (with the ability to put men in space, for example) and wealthier than many other developing countries, yet rural poverty and underdevelopment are still significant problems, particularly in the western part of the country.

Approximately 700 million Chinese live in rural areas. Urban areas are growing rapidly, however, and China is now home to many of the world's largest megacities. Shanghai and Beijing each have at least 20 million inhabitants, and Chongqing, with a metropolitan population exceeding 30 million, is the fastest-growing urban center in the world. Rivers play a central role in China's economy, history, and culture. The Yangtze River basin, stretching 4,000 miles from the Tibetan plateau to the East China Sea near Shanghai, is home to >5% of the world's population.

In 2007, about 55 million tourists visited China, and by 2020, China is widely predicted to be both the largest tourist destination and the largest source of tourists to other countries. China's 5,000 years of continuous civilization and varied natural beauty can be traced in its 38 UNESCO World Heritage Sites, from the imperial grandeur of the Forbidden City and the Temple of Heaven, to the marvel of the Great Wall, the Terracotta Warriors in Xi'an, and the spectacular mountainous sanctuaries of the west. Popular itineraries often include Beijing and the Great Wall, Xi'an, and the Yangtze River. Other important tourist destinations include the following:

> Shanghai and Hong Kong, with their futuristic architecture and East-meets-West mystique

> Lijiang in the province of Yunnan, where many ethnic minorities are concentrated
> Sichuan province, home to China's iconic symbol, the panda
> Guilin, famous for its uniquely shaped limestone Karst mountains that are often featured in Chinese paintings
> Tibet, accessible now by the world's highest railroad directly to Lhasa, with a maximum altitude of 16,640 ft (5,072 m)

Specialized itineraries are increasingly being offered, including hiking, mountain climbing, village tours, the Silk Road, and other more remote regions. Aside from tourism, increasing numbers of people travel to China to visit friends and relatives, to study, or to adopt children. These groups may be at particularly high risk of illness because they underestimate their risks, are less likely to seek pre-travel advice, and stay in more local or rural accommodations. People traveling to China to adopt children often worry about the health of the child but neglect their own health.

HEALTH ISSUES

Although China is now the world's second-largest economy, in per capita terms it is still a low-income country, with wide disparity in income and development between rural and urban and east and west. Health risks vary accordingly.

Immunizations
Routine vaccinations should be up to date, including tetanus/diphtheria, measles, mumps, rubella, varicella, influenza, and pneumococcal vaccines, as indicated. In addition, hepatitis A, hepatitis B, and typhoid vaccinations are usually recommended. Measles and rubella immunity is particularly important. Despite an extensive national immunization program, China continues to report well over 100,000 measles cases annually. A few travelers have made news headlines by triggering outbreaks in their own countries on return from trips to China. While limited data exist on rubella in China, it was not part of the national immunization program until 2008, and incidence is believed to be high.

Rabies Vaccine
Rabies is a serious problem in China, as in much of Asia, with more than 3,000 human deaths per year reported in recent years. Animal bites in any area of China, including urban areas, must be considered high risk for rabies. As international standard rabies immune globulin is generally unavailable, animal bites are often trip-enders, requiring evacuation to Hong Kong, Bangkok, or home for postexposure prophylaxis. Bites are surprisingly common in tourists; dog bites were the most common dermatologic problem seen after China travel in a recent analysis of data from the GeoSentinel Network. Rabies risk and prevention should be discussed in pre-travel consultations, and a strategy for dealing with a possible exposure should be developed. Long-term travelers and expatriates living in China should consider the preexposure vaccination series.

Japanese Encephalitis Vaccine
Japanese encephalitis (JE) occurs in all regions except Qinghai, Xinjiang, and Xizang (Tibet) (Map 3-8). China has greatly reduced the incidence of JE through vaccination, and as of 2008, included JE in its expanded national immunization program; however, the disease remains a threat to unimmunized travelers. Although the JE season varies by region, most human cases are reported from June through October. The risk of JE for most travelers to China is low but varies based on season, destination, duration, and activities. Risk is highest among travelers to rural areas during the transmission season. JE vaccine is recommended for travelers who

plan to spend significant time in endemic areas or shorter-term travelers who plan rural or outdoor activities. However, rare sporadic cases have occurred on an unpredictable basis in short-term travelers, including in periurban Beijing and Shanghai.

Malaria

Malaria is very rarely a consideration for travelers to China, with the exception of those visiting rural parts of southern Yunnan Province or Hainan Island. For these areas, chemoprophylaxis should be considered. Mefloquine resistance in southern Yunnan means that prophylaxis should be with doxycycline or atovaquone-proguanil in this area. For travelers to other regions, the risk is too low to warrant chemoprophylaxis. Rare cases occur in other rural parts of the country <1,500 m (4,921 ft) from May through December, and only insect precautions are recommended.

Other Health Risks
Foodborne Illnesses

The risk for travelers' diarrhea appears to be low in deluxe accommodations in China but moderate elsewhere. Usual food and water precautions should apply, and travelers should carry an antibiotic for empiric self-treatment. Tap water is not drinkable even in major cities. Most hotels provide bottled or boiled water, and bottled water is easily available. In addition, there have been several well-publicized episodes of contamination of food with pesticides and other substances. Travelers should strictly avoid undercooked fish and shellfish and unpasteurized milk.

Sexually Transmitted Diseases

Sexually transmitted diseases, including syphilis, HIV, gonorrhea, and chlamydia, are a growing problem in China, particularly along the booming eastern seaboard. Travel is associated with loosened inhibitions and increased casual sexual liaisons. In addition to risk-reduction counseling, consider hepatitis B vaccination for those who might be at risk.

Air Pollution

Air pollution is a problem in most major cities in China. There is significant potential for exacerbation of respiratory conditions, including asthma and chronic obstructive pulmonary disease (COPD), and heightened risk for respiratory infections. Susceptible travelers should receive influenza and pneumococcal vaccination and bring any inhaled medications they may use.

Medical Care in China

Western-style medical facilities that meet international standards are available in Beijing, Shanghai, and Hong Kong. Some hospitals in other cities have "VIP wards" (*gaogan bingfang*), which may have English-speaking staff. The standard of care in such facilities is somewhat unpredictable, and cultural and regulatory differences can cause difficulties for travelers. In rural areas, only rudimentary medical care may be available. Hepatitis B transmission from poorly sterilized medical equipment remains a risk outside major centers.

Ambulances are not staffed with trained paramedics and often have little or no medical equipment. Therefore, injured travelers may need to take taxis or other immediately available vehicles to the nearest major hospital rather than waiting for ambulances to arrive.

Pharmacies often sell prescription medications over the counter. Such medications have sometimes been counterfeit, substandard, or even contaminated. Travelers should carry all their regular medications in sufficient quantity; if more or other medications are required, it is advisable to visit a reputable clinic or hospital.

Some travelers wish to try traditional Chinese medicine and acupuncture. Although most do so uneventfully, there is a risk of infection from acupuncture needles, and traditional medicine products may be contaminated with heavy metals or pharmaceutical agents. Acupressure may be preferable to acupuncture.

Travelers are strongly advised to purchase travel health care and evacuation insurance before travel. Most hospitals will not directly accept foreign medical insurance, however, and patients will often be expected to pay a deposit before care to cover the expected cost of the treatment.

Language and Culture

Language will be a problem for many travelers to China. Outside major tourist destinations, English speakers may be rare, and most signs will be in Chinese characters. In general, people are helpful and friendly to tourists, and personal safety is rarely an issue. Cultural sensitivity is essential, however. Chinese will often ask near strangers about their weight, their age, and their income, subjects that are taboo in many Western cultures. Travelers should try to avoid taking offense. In turn, Westerners may offend Chinese by raising their voice, losing their temper, or otherwise bringing conflict into the open. Whatever the problem, patience, firmness, and sensitivity to "face" will almost always work better in China than open confrontation.

Sporadic domestic unrest, particularly in the Xinjiang Autonomous Region of northwestern China, can disrupt travel and interrupt access to the Internet, international telephone lines, and text messaging. Travelers need to stay informed about local demonstrations and travel advisories. Foreigners are required to carry their passports at all times and may be subject to random checks.

Finally, it is worth noting that although China covers a geographic area the equivalent of 5 time zones, the entire country operates officially on only one time, China Standard Time or Beijing Time. Some parts of western China also have an unofficial time, usually 2 hours earlier than Beijing Time. This can cause some confusion. Official schedules, such as airline and train times and bank opening hours, will generally operate on Beijing time, while some restaurants and shops may follow the unofficial time.

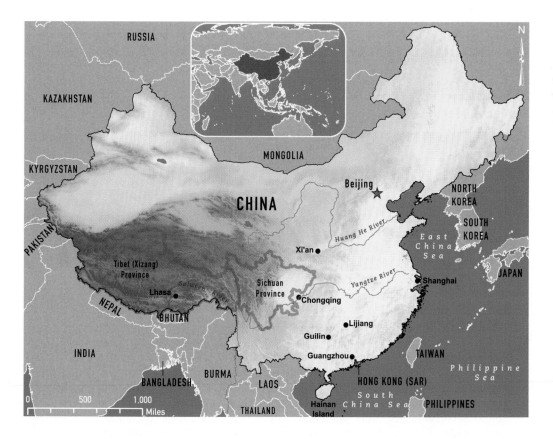

MAP 4-2. CHINA DESTINATION MAP

BIBLIOGRAPHY

1. CDC. Measles among adults associated with adoption of children in China—California, Missouri, and Washington, July–August 2006. MMWR Morb Mortal Wkly Rep. 2007 Feb 23;56(7):144–6.
2. Chen XS, Gong XD, Liang GJ, Zhang GC. Epidemiologic trends of sexually transmitted diseases in China. Sex Transm Dis. 2000 Mar;27(3):138–42.
3. Cutfield NJ, Anderson NE, Brickell K, Hueston L, Pikholz C, Roxburgh RH. Japanese encephalitis acquired during travel in China. Intern Med J. 2005 Aug;35(8):497–8.
4. Davis XM, MacDonald S, Borwein S, Freedman DO, Kozarsky PE, von Sonnenburg F, et al. Health risks in travelers to China: the GeoSentinel experience and implications for the 2008 Beijing Olympics. Am J Trop Med Hyg. 2008 Jul;79(1):4–8.
5. Hills SL, Griggs AC, Fischer M. Japanese encephalitis in travelers from non-endemic countries, 1973–2008. Am J Trop Med Hyg. 2010 May;82(5):930–6.
6. Shaw MT, Leggat PA, Borwein S. Travelling to China for the Beijing 2008 Olympic and Paralympic games. Travel Med Infect Dis. 2007 Nov;5(6):365–73.
7. Shlim DR, Solomon T. Japanese encephalitis vaccine for travelers: exploring the limits of risk. Clin Infect Dis. 2002 Jul 15;35(2):183–8.
8. Tang X, Luo M, Zhang S, Fooks AR, Hu R, Tu C. Pivotal role of dogs in rabies transmission, China. Emerg Infect Dis. 2005 Dec;11(12):1970–2.
9. World Health Organization. Measles bulletin: Western Pacific region. Geneva: World Health Organization; 2010. Available from: http://www.wpro.who.int/NR/rdonlyres/F84088A7-4855-4FDE-811B-1ECAA6172171/0/MeasBulletinVol4Issue1.pdf.
10. Zhang YZ, Xiong CL, Xiao DL, Jiang RJ, Wang ZX, Zhang LZ, et al. Human rabies in China. Emerg Infect Dis. 2005 Dec;11(12):1983–4.

CUZCO–MACHU PICCHU, PERU
Alan J. Magill

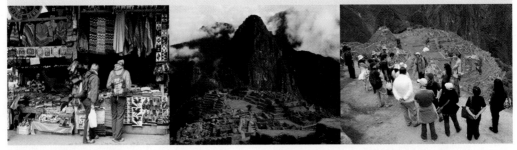

DESTINATION OVERVIEW

Peru is approximately twice the size of the state of Texas, with a population of almost 30 million people. Thousands of tourists are drawn to Peru every year to enjoy the country's magnificent geographic, biologic, and cultural diversity. The primary destination for most travelers is the remarkable Incan ruins of Machu Picchu, recently named as one of the modern Seven Wonders of the World and a UNESCO World Heritage site. Machu Picchu stands in the middle of a tropical mountain forest, in an extraordinarily beautiful setting. It was probably the most amazing urban creation of the Inca Empire at its height; its giant walls, terraces, and ramps seem as if they have been cut naturally in the continuous rock escarpments. The natural setting, on the eastern slopes of the Andes, is in the upper Amazon Basin, with its rich diversity of flora and fauna.

A typical visit to Peru includes arrival at the capital city of Lima, a megacity the size of the state of Rhode Island, with approximately one-third of Peru's population. Interestingly, many people think Lima is a high-altitude Incan city, but it is actually located on the Pacific coast at sea level. After a few days in Lima, one takes an hour-long flight to Cuzco, the gateway to Machu Picchu and a worthwhile destination of its own. Tourists can visit multiple Inca-era ruins and Peruvian mountain villages and markets in the Valle Sagrado before taking the train to Machu Picchu. One of the world's most popular and best-known treks, the Inca Trail, begins classically at kilometer 82 (7,700 ft; 2,600 m) on the Cuzco–Machu Picchu railway. This moderate 26-mile (43-km) trek is usually done in 4 days and 3 nights, and most fit people should be able to complete the hike. Nevertheless it is quite challenging, with 3 high mountain passes; the highest is Warminanusca at 13,779 ft (4,200 m), before ending in the ruins of Machu Picchu (7,970 ft; 2,430 m).

Many people also wish to add a tropical rainforest experience to their Cuzco trip and take the 30-minute flight from Cuzco to Puerto Maldonado, 34 miles (55 km) west of the Bolivian border, on the confluence of the Rio Tambopata with the Madre de Dios River, a major tributary of the Amazon River. Most travelers take a boat up the Rio Tambopata to one of several rustic lodges. Visitors wanting to see the Amazon rainforest may also go to Manu National Park in the south, also reached via Cuzco. The northern Amazon rainforest can be visited by traveling to the lodges around Iquitos or by journeying on the increasingly popular Amazon River cruises that go both upstream and downstream from Iquitos. As elsewhere, ecotourism is a growing activity in Peru. Peru is also home to the Cordillera Blanca, a several hundred-mile range of spectacular snow-covered peaks that form the backbone of the Andes Mountains in Peru.

HEALTH ISSUES

Important pre-travel information for Peru includes advice on preventing high-altitude illness, the risk for cutaneous leishmaniasis, appropriate use of yellow fever vaccine, and the risk of malaria for travelers visiting popular jungle lodges.

Altitude and Acute Mountain Sickness (AMS)

All travelers to Machu Picchu will arrive and transit through Cuzco, 11,203 ft (3,395 m) above sea level. Many arriving travelers will find that the near 11,400-ft (3,500-m) elevation leads to some degree of AMS, with the initial symptoms of headache, nausea, and loss of appetite beginning 4–8 hours after arrival. The hypoxemia of high altitude can also affect the quality of sleep in the first few nights in Cuzco, causing restless sleep, frequent awakening, and periodic breathing (irregular breathing patterns, often alternating periods of deep breathing and shallow breathing), even in those who appear to be doing well during the day. A few travelers may progress to severe forms of altitude illness, including high-altitude pulmonary edema and high-altitude cerebral edema. The symptoms of AMS can markedly impair the traveler and prevent enjoyment of the sights of Cuzco.

Surveys have shown that most travelers arrive in Cuzco with limited or no knowledge of AMS or the fact that AMS can be prevented to a large degree by prophylactic use of acetazolamide. **Every traveler to Cuzco should be counseled about AMS pre-travel and be prepared to prevent or self-treat AMS.** (More information about prevention and treatment of altitude illness can be found in Chapter 2, Altitude Illness.) Locals refer to AMS as *soroche* and will almost always offer the new arrival a cup of hot coca tea (*mate de coca*) when checking in to the hotel. Although many believe *mate de coca* can prevent and treat *soroche*, no data support its use in the prevention or treatment of AMS. Perhaps of concern to some who may experience random drug screening as a condition of employment, people who drink a single cup of coca tea will test positive for cocaine metabolites in standard drug toxicology screens for several days. However, sitting quietly and resting while enjoying a cup of tea is a most civilized activity and a pleasant memory.

New arrivals may also find it helpful to transit directly from Cuzco to the Valle Sagrado (Sacred Valley) of the Rio Urubamba to spend the first few days and nights at a somewhat lower altitude. This spectacular river valley begins 15 miles (24 km) northeast of Cuzco in the town of Pisac (9,751 ft; 2,972 m), known for its colorful Sunday markets, and continues downstream toward the northwest for another 37 miles (60 km) to reach the town of Ollantaytambo (9,337 ft; 2,846 m). One can board the train to Machu Picchu in Ollantaytambo, at the northwest end of the Valle Sagrado, and the not-to-be-missed visit to Cuzco can be made on return from Machu Picchu, when people are better acclimatized. The train follows the Rio Urubamba north and northwest (downstream) to Aguas Calientes (6,600 ft; 2,000 m). Machu Picchu (7,970 ft; 2,430 m) is located on a ridge above the town.

Cutaneous Leishmaniasis

Many areas in the Pacific valleys of the Andes and the Amazon tropical rainforest are endemic for cutaneous leishmaniasis (CL), a parasitic infection transmitted by bites of sand flies (see Chapter 3, Leishmaniasis, Cutaneous). While this disease is widespread in southeastern Peru, the highest risk for travelers seems to be the Manu Park area in Madre de Dios. In Manu, CL is most often caused by *Leishmania braziliensis*, and there is a risk of both simple CL and mucosal leishmaniasis. There is no visceral leishmaniasis in Peru. Travelers should be counseled to be meticulous about vector precautions, as there is no vaccine or chemoprophylaxis to prevent leishmaniasis. Any person with a skin lesion persisting more than a few weeks should be evaluated for CL.

Yellow Fever

Proof of yellow fever vaccination is not required for entry into Peru. Travelers who are limiting travel to the cities of Lima, Cuzco, and Machu Picchu do not need yellow fever vaccination. Peru recommends vaccination for those who intend to visit any jungle areas of the country <2,300 m (7,546 ft).

Malaria

In general, the risk of malaria in travelers visiting Peru is low. There are, on average, <5 cases reported in the United States each year that were acquired in Peru. Both *Plasmodium vivax* malaria and *P. falciparum* malaria are found in the Peruvian Amazon.

There is no malaria risk for travelers visiting only Lima and vicinity, coastal areas south of Lima, or the popular highland tourist areas (Cuzco, Machu Picchu, and Lake Titicaca). The malaria risk areas for most tourists are the neotropical rainforests of the Amazon. There are 2 major destinations. The city of Iquitos in the northern rainforest is a frequent arrival destination for those traveling to jungle lodges around the city or for boarding river cruise boats for rainforest travel. Malaria transmission occurs in the areas in and around Iquitos. Malaria transmission is seasonal, with peak activity between January and May that correlates with the rainy season and the height of the Amazon River. Chemoprophylaxis is recommended for most travelers.

The city of Puerto Maldonado is a 30-minute flight from Cuzco and a popular arrival destination for those visiting the rainforest lodges on the Rio Tambopata. Newly arrived travelers usually transit directly from the airport to the boats that take them up the river to numerous lodges. Peruvian Ministry of Health data document that malaria transmission occurs in Puerto Maldonado. Most cases reported in the region occur in local loggers and gold miners in the forests. Travelers transiting Puerto Maldonado for a short 2- to 3-day visit to lodges on the Rio Tambopata may not need chemoprophylaxis.

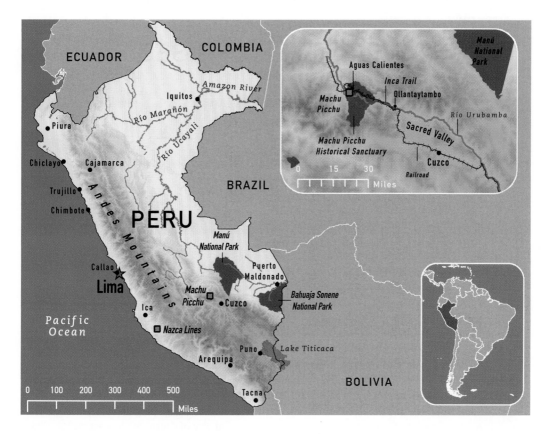

MAP 4-3. PERU DESTINATION MAP

Risk for the traveler varies with itinerary, style of travel, and location of accommodations. Malaria in the Peruvian Amazon is unpredictable from season to season; *P. falciparum* epidemics occasionally occur. When making a decision on whether to recommend chemoprophylaxis or simply mosquito precautions, all these factors and data need to be taken into consideration.

BIBLIOGRAPHY

1. Behrens RH, Carroll B, Beran J, Bouchaud O, Hellgren U, Hatz C, et al. The low and declining risk of malaria in travellers to Latin America: is there still an indication for chemoprophylaxis? Malar J. 2007;6:114.
2. Cabada MM, Maldonado F, Quispe W, Serrano E, Mozo K, Gonzales E, et al. Pretravel health advice among international travelers visiting Cuzco, Peru. J Travel Med. 2005 Mar–Apr;12(2):61–5.
3. Mazor SS, Mycyk MB, Wills BK, Brace LD, Gussow L, Erickson T. Coca tea consumption causes positive urine cocaine assay. Eur J Emerg Med. 2006 Dec;13(6):340–1.
4. Merritt AL, Camerlengo A, Meyer C, Mull JD. Mountain sickness knowledge among foreign travelers in Cuzco, Peru. Wilderness Environ Med. 2007 Spring;18(1):26–9.

EGYPT & NILE RIVER CRUISES

Ann M. Buff

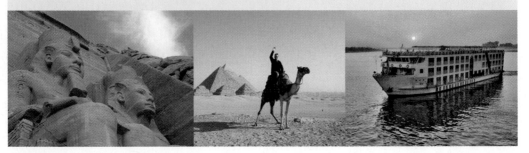

DESTINATION OVERVIEW

The Arab Republic of Egypt covers a land area of over 1,000,000 km², approximately the same size as Texas and New Mexico combined, and >95% of the country is desert. With an estimated 80 million people, Egypt accounts for one-fourth of the Arab world's population. Egypt has long been considered the cradle of civilization and may be the oldest tourist destination on earth. Throughout the world, Egypt is synonymous with the legends of the Pharaohs, the Great Pyramids, treasure-laden tombs, and hieroglyphs. Millions of travelers visit Egypt each year to see the ancient monuments and timeless river vistas along the Nile Valley.

A typical visit to Egypt includes arrival in the capital city of Cairo, the largest city in Africa and the Middle East, with a population of over 16 million. Considered the "Mother of the World" by Arabs, Cairo today is a modern, cosmopolitan mix of Arab, African, and European influences. Travelers generally spend at least a few days in Cairo seeing the Egyptian Antiquities Museum, the Pyramids at Giza, the Citadel and Mosque of Al-Azhar, and Khan al-Khalili bazaar.

Most travelers include an Upper Nile River cruise as part of their itineraries. Nile River cruises are usually 3–7 days, with embarkation in either Luxor or Aswan. Riverboats do not sail through Middle Egypt because of security concerns; therefore, most travelers take short domestic flights or trains from Cairo to Luxor or Aswan. Approximately 200 large riverboats cruise the Nile, and the average boat accommodates 120 passengers. The largest boats accommodate upwards of 300 passengers; chartered yachts might have just a few cabins. Riverboats have a range of accommodations from basic to 5-star luxury, and nights aboard are generally spent cruising from one port to the next.

Virtually all Nile cruises sail between Luxor and Aswan. There are 3 usual Nile cruise durations and itineraries: a 3-night cruise from Aswan to Luxor, a 4-night cruise from Luxor to Aswan, and a 7-night cruise roundtrip from Luxor. A standard itinerary is as follows:

> Day 1: Fly from Cairo to Aswan or Luxor. Stay in a hotel for the first night and spend the afternoon and early the next morning visiting the sites (High Dam and Abu Simbel temple in Aswan or Karnak Temple, Luxor Temple, Valley of the Kings, and Hapshepsut Temple in Luxor).
> Day 2: Board the Nile riverboat and begin cruise.
> Days 3–6: Visit temples of Edfu, Esna, and Kom Ombo and enjoy the passing riverside scenes of ancient villages, minarets, farmers in white *galabiyas*, and traditional *feluccas*. Most travelers have an early breakfast aboard and then depart the boat for sightseeing early in the day to avoid the crowds and heat. Most travelers will be back aboard by early afternoon. Dinner and entertainment follow in the evening.
> Day 5–9: Disembark and spend the night in a hotel. Return to Cairo via air or train.

Egypt is also a beach destination, with thousands of kilometers of Mediterranean and Red Sea coastlines. Alexandria, Egypt's second largest city, is located on the Mediterranean Sea and has a string of beaches and wonderful seafood restaurants. The World War II battlefield of El-Alamein lies along the Mediterranean coast, and divers will find an array of sunken cities and wartime wrecks to explore offshore. Edged by coral reefs and teeming with tropical fish, the Sinai Peninsula has excellent diving, snorkeling, and palm-fringed beaches. Visits to Mount Sinai (7,500 ft [2,285 m] above sea level) and Saint Catherine's Monastery in the mountainous interior are also popular destinations. Egypt's Red Sea coast has more reefs offshore, with diving and snorkeling traditionally centered around Hurghada.

Popular among adventure travelers are desert jeep safaris and camel treks to remote oases and spectacular *wadis*. Many travelers start in Cairo or Assyut and follow the "Great Desert Circuit" through 4 oases and the White Desert.

HEALTH ISSUES

Hepatitis A and B and typhoid vaccines are recommended for travelers to Egypt. There is no risk of malaria. The prevalence of HCV infection is >15% in Egypt; travelers should be reminded to protect themselves from bloodborne pathogens, including HCV.

Travelers' Diarrhea

In most large international tourist hotels, the tap water is heavily chlorinated and generally safe to drink but unpalatable. Tap water is not safe to drink in other locations. Eating thoroughly cooked meat and vegetables in tourist hotels, on Nile River cruise ships, and in tourist restaurants is generally safe. Eating raw or undercooked ground meat or shellfish should be avoided. As in many developing countries, the safety of uncooked vegetables and salads may be in question. The risk of diarrhea in Egypt is high. Travelers to Egypt should be provided with an antibiotic for empiric self-treatment of diarrhea.

Schistosomiasis

Schistosoma mansoni and *S. haematobium* are endemic in Egypt. Travelers to Egypt should avoid wading, swimming, or other contact with freshwater, including the Nile River and irrigation canals. Swimming in saline pools of desert oases, chlorinated swimming pools, and the Mediterranean Sea or Red Sea is virtually always safe.

Rabies

As in most other developing countries, rabies is endemic throughout Egypt. For most travelers on a packaged tour, the risk will be minimal. However, travelers should be aware that there are large numbers of stray dogs and cats in urban areas. Modern hospitals and travel clinics cater to the large expatriate communities in Cairo and Alexandria. Rabies vaccine is readily available for preexposure and postexposure, and human rabies immunoglobulin (HRIG) is also available. Both rabies vaccine and HRIG are produced locally, but it is also possible to find imported rabies vaccine and HRIG (manufactured in the United States or Europe).

Environmental Concerns

Temperature and weather conditions vary widely in Egypt. The desert is extremely hot in the summer (>100°F; >38°C) and can be cold in the winter (32°F; 0°C). Thirst is a late indicator of mild dehydration, and travelers should drink fluids regularly in the heat. Because sweat evaporates immediately, people can become dehydrated without realizing it. Travelers who are elderly or take diuretic, anticholinergic, or neuroleptic medications are at increased risk of heat-associated illnesses. To stay cool and protect themselves from sun exposure, travelers should wear a hat and lightweight, loose-fitting clothing and use sunscreen.

Sandstorms occur sporadically in the desert. Desert sand, dust, and smog can cause eye irritation and exacerbate asthma or other lung disorders. Travelers who wear contact lenses should make sure that they are carrying glasses and all their contact lens care supplies.

Motion Sickness

Generally, the Nile is a slow, smooth river. However, a variety of boats are employed for Nile cruises, and traffic on the Nile can be heavy. The combination of diesel fuel, heat, and motion can cause distress for travelers. Most travelers do not consider the possibility of motion sickness on a river, so they are unprepared. Medical services vary greatly aboard. Travelers who know that they are sensitive to motion should carry anti–motion sickness medication.

Insects

Even without the risk of malaria, mosquitoes and other biting insects can be problematic for travelers to Egypt, particularly in the summer months. Avoiding insect bites can minimize the risk of West Nile virus infection and dengue fever.

ACKNOWLEDGMENT

The author thanks Dr. Mohammad Abdel Sabour Diab, Professor of Pulmonary Medicine, Ain Shams University and Regional Staff Physician, Eastern Mediterranean Regional Office, World Health Organization, Cairo, Egypt, for his valuable contributions and insightful review.

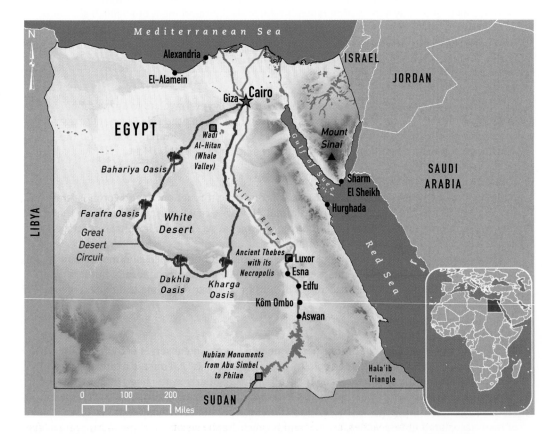

MAP 4-4. EGYPT DESTINATION MAP

BIBLIOGRAPHY

1. Diemert DJ. Prevention and self-treatment of traveler's diarrhea. Clin Microbiol Rev. 2006 Jul;19(3):583–94.
2. Fradin MS, Day JF. Comparative efficacy of insect repellents against mosquito bites. N Engl J Med. 2002 Jul 4;347(1):13–8.
3. Gautret P, Adehossi E, Soula G, Soavi MJ, Delmont J, Rotivel Y, et al. Rabies exposure in international travelers: do we miss the target? Int J Infect Dis. 2010 Mar;14(3):e243–6.
4. Gautret P, Schwartz E, Shaw M, Soula G, Gazin P, Delmont J, et al. Animal-associated injuries and related diseases among returned travellers: a review of the GeoSentinel Surveillance Network. Vaccine. 2007 Mar 30;25(14):2656–63.
5. Golan Y, Onn A, Villa Y, Avidor Y, Kivity S, Berger SA, et al. Asthma in adventure travelers: a prospective study evaluating the occurrence and risk factors for acute exacerbations. Arch Intern Med. 2002 Nov 25;162(21):2421–6.
6. Hajat S, O'Connor M, Kosatsky T. Health effects of hot weather: from awareness of risk factors to effective health protection. Lancet. 2010 Mar 6;375(9717):856–63.
7. Nicolls DJ, Weld LH, Schwartz E, Reed C, von Sonnenburg F, Freedman DO, et al. Characteristics of schistosomiasis in travelers reported to the GeoSentinel Surveillance Network 1997-2008. Am J Trop Med Hyg. 2008 Nov;79(5):729–34.
8. Sherman CR. Motion sickness: review of causes and preventive strategies. J Travel Med. 2002 Sep–Oct;9(5):251–6.

GUATEMALA & BELIZE

Ava W. Navin, Emily S. Jentes

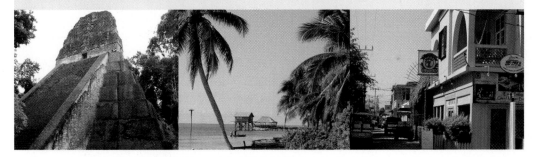

DESTINATION OVERVIEW

Guatemala, known as the Land of Eternal Spring for the temperate climate and lush foliage of its highlands, is located in Central America, with Mexico to the north, Belize to the east, and Honduras and El Salvador to the south and east. In an area the size of Tennessee, Guatemala offers a wide variety of topography: from active volcanoes to the black sand beach and mangrove swamp of Monterrico and the cloud forest reserve of the Biotopo del Quetzal. The visitor to the bustling market town of Chichicastenango in the highlands (7,125 ft; 2,171 m) will need preparation different from that for the visitor to the Mayan temples of Tikal in the hot lowlands of the Petén (636 ft; 193 m). Belize, an equally beautiful tropical paradise, is roughly the size of the state of Massachusetts. Northern Belize is characterized by coastal plains with pockets of dense forest, whereas the west and south are predominantly coastal plains/savannas and low mountains, respectively. To the east, Belize's coastline with the Caribbean Sea boasts sandy white beaches, numerous islands, and the second-longest barrier reef in the world.

Tourists interested in the Ruta Maya often visit sites in both Guatemala and Belize. Temples and ball courts, the remnants of the Mayan civilization that flourished in the Yucatán 1,000 years ago, have been reclaimed from the jungle. In Belize, the Mayan ruins of Xunantunich (Cayo District), Caracol (Cayo District), and Lamanai (Orange Walk District), among others, provide impressive excavated examples of the cities and leave the visitors wondering what else might be hidden underneath the trees and hills.

The colonial capital of Antigua, Guatemala (5,193 ft; 1,582 m), a UNESCO World Heritage site, was founded in 1543 by Spanish conquistadors and destroyed by an earthquake in 1773. The ruins of the cathedral, government buildings, and monasteries provide a hint of colonial grandeur. Holy Week, when the images from the churches are carried through the streets in colorful processions, is an especially popular time to visit Antigua.

Travelers visiting Belize's inland regions will enjoy a variety of adventure activities, including climbing the ruins, zip-lining through jungle canopies, cave tubing, hiking, and canoeing. However, most visitors to Belize are drawn to the sandy white beaches and to the barrier reefs off the coast, which boast some of the best scuba diving in the Caribbean. Near Ambergris Caye, The Hol Chan Marine Reserve and the Great Blue Hole (a UNESCO World Heritage site) are popular sites for both scuba divers and snorkelers, who will be delighted by the variety of fish, eels, and coral living in the clear blue-green water.

Guatemala's tremendous geographic variety extends to its linguistic richness: in addition to Spanish, 21 distinct Mayan languages and many more dialects are spoken. In rural areas, Spanish is more often a second language, and Mayan customs and rituals are still observed. Guatemala, especially Antigua, is noted for immersion language schools; students can live with a family while they attend classes. Belize is similarly linguistically diverse. Although the official language of Belize is English, Belizean Creole, Spanish, Mayan languages, and Plautdietsch (a variety of German spoken by Mennonite settlers) are also spoken.

HEALTH ISSUES

Immunizations

All travelers should always be up to date on routine vaccinations. Hepatitis A and B vaccines are recommended for visitors to both countries. Typhoid vaccination is also recommended for all travelers. Countries in Central America have been the source of many cases of typhoid fever that continue to be imported into the United States.

Rabies vaccination should be considered for travelers who will be involved in outdoor activities or have occupational exposure to animals. It is particularly recommended for long-term travelers such as missionaries and their children. Although yellow fever is not a disease risk in Guatemala or Belize, the governments of both countries require travelers arriving from countries where yellow fever is endemic to present proof of yellow fever vaccination.

Malaria

Malaria is found throughout Belize, except for Belize City. In Guatemala, malaria is found only in rural areas at altitudes <4,921 ft (1,500 m); therefore, the specific destination is important to know. Travelers who plan to visit only the capital and highlands do not need prophylaxis. Travelers who mention plans to scuba dive or visit Mayan ruins, though, will be at risk for malaria. Some clinicians feel that primaquine is the preferred antimalarial drug (only after G6PD testing) due to the amount of *Plasmodium vivax*, although atovaquone-proguanil, chloroquine, doxycycline, and mefloquine are alternative choices.

Other Vectorborne Diseases

Mosquito and insect precautions are important. Dengue infections have been on the rise in most areas of Central America. GeoSentinel data show that the most common cause of febrile illness in travelers returning from this area is dengue. Cutaneous leishmaniasis has been reported in travelers to these countries as well. Although transmission can occur to any part of the body, frequently it occurs while walking on contaminated beaches, so shoes may be protective. Filariasis, onchocerciasis (river blindness), and American trypanosomiasis (Chagas disease) are other diseases carried by insects that also occur in this region, mostly in rural areas and mostly in the indigenous populations.

Travelers' Diarrhea

Diarrhea in travelers is common throughout both Guatemala and Belize and is the most common complaint in returning travelers who seek medical attention at GeoSentinel clinics. Travelers should be reminded of precautions for safe food and water and carry an antibiotic for self-treatment.

Other Health and Safety Risks
Safety and Security

For much of the last 30 years, Guatemala's geologic instability was paralleled by its political unrest. Since the peace accord was signed in 1996, safety concerns are more likely to stem from economic conditions and drug-related violence. Although petty crime such as burglary and pickpocketing can be a serious problem in Belize as well, safety concerns in Guatemala's neighbor more often involve road, boating, and diving accidents. Visitors to both countries are advised to travel in groups and stay on the main roads.

International Adoptions

Guatemala at one time was second only to China as a source country for international adoptions; 4,728 children were adopted by US families in 2007. In early 2008, after allegations of

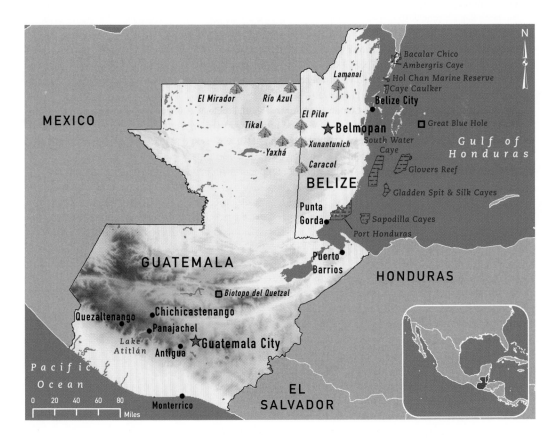

MAP 4-5. GUATEMALA AND BELIZE DESTINATION MAP

fraud and exploitation, adoptions were suspended until the country's procedures could be made compliant with the Hague Convention on Intercountry Adoption. The National Council for Adoptions (CNA), established to oversee adoptions of Guatemalan children, published new procedures in July 2010 to implement the December 2007 adoption law. Concerns about child trafficking have led to suspicion and occasional hostility toward foreigners seen with Guatemalan children. The Department of State advises visitors to avoid close contact with children, especially in rural areas.

Medical Tourism

Travel to obtain medical care has increased in popularity in recent years, and Guatemala, which boasts specialists trained in the United States, has benefited from this trend. Popular procedures sought by medical tourists to this region include cosmetic and bariatric surgery, fertility treatments, and dental procedures. The Internet abounds with sites that promote medical tourism and offer help with transportation, accommodations, and language issues. A government initiative called "International Health City" (*Ciudad Salud Internacional*) has been established under the Tourism and Health Commission to promote medical tourism at a number of health facilities in Guatemala City, including private hospitals, diagnostic centers, clinics, spas, and laboratories. For guidelines for travelers seeking care abroad, see Chapter 2, Medical Tourism.

BIBLIOGRAPHY

1. Central Intelligence Agency. World Factbook: Guatemala. Washington, DC: Central Intelligence Agency; 2010 [updated Sep 22; cited 2010 Aug 6]. Available from: https://www.cia.gov/library/publications/the-world-factbook/geos/gt.html.
2. Lynch MF, Blanton EM, Bulens S, Polyak C, Vojdani J, Stevenson J, et al. Typhoid fever in the United States, 1999–2006. JAMA. 2009 Aug 26;302(8):859–65.
3. Miller L, Chan W, Comfort K, Tirella L. Health of children adopted from Guatemala: comparison of orphanage and foster care. Pediatrics. 2005 Jun;115(6):e710–7.
4. Pan American Health Organization. Guatemala, Country Health Profile. Washington, DC: Pan American Health Organization; 2001 [cited 2010 Oct 22]. Available from: http://www.paho.org/English/SHA/prflgut.htm.
5. UNICEF. At a glance: Guatemala. Geneva: UNICEF; 2010 [updated Aug 5; cited 2010 Oct 22]. Available from: http://www.unicef.org/infobycountry/guatemala.html.
6. US Department of State. Guatemala. Washington, DC: US Department of State. Available from: http://www.state.gov/p/wha/ci/gt/.

HAJJ PILGRIMAGE, SAUDI ARABIA

Qanta Ahmed, Victor Balaban

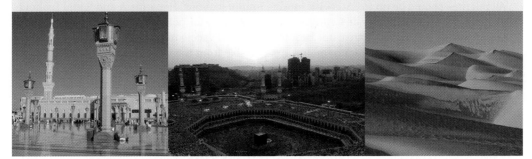

DESTINATION OVERVIEW

They will come to thee on foot and (mounted) on every kind of camel, lean on account of journeys through deep and distant mountain highways ... (Quran 22:27)

The Hajj is the annual pilgrimage to Mecca, Saudi Arabia, and the largest mass gathering in the world. Every able-bodied adult Muslim who can afford to do so is required to make Hajj at least once in his or her lifetime. Hajj takes place from the 8th through the 12th of Dhu al-Hijja, the last month of the Islamic year. Because the Islamic calendar is lunar, the timing of Hajj varies with respect to the Gregorian calendar (for example, it will be November 4–7 in 2011, and October 24–27 in 2012).

From around the world, more than 2 million Muslims make Hajj each year (2.5 million in 2009), and more than 11,000 are travelers from the United States. From the United States, most pilgrims fly into Jiddah and take a bus to Mecca. After arriving in Mecca, pilgrims go to the Grand Mosque, which contains the Ka'aba, the most sacred site in Islam, and perform a *tawaf*, circling the Ka'aba 7 times counterclockwise. Because of the vast number of people (each floor of the 3-level mosque has a capacity of 750,000), a single *tawaf* can take hours. In addition to *tawaf*, pilgrims perform *sa'i*, walking or running 7 times between the hills of Safa and Marwah. This route used to be in open air but is now enclosed by the Grand Mosque and can be traversed via air-conditioned tunnels, with separate sections for walkers, runners, and disabled pilgrims. These safety measures were put in place to prevent stampedes.

Hajj culminates on the Plain of Arafat, a few miles east of Mecca, where the Prophet Muhammad delivered his final sermon. Pilgrims spend the day in supplication, praying and reading the Quran; it is the pinnacle of most pilgrims' spiritual lives. The following day's ritual, the Stoning of the Devil at Jamaraat, is the site of some of the densest crowds during Hajj. Pilgrims throw 7 tiny pebbles (specifically, no larger than a chickpea) at each of 3 white pillars. Because of the sheer number of people crowding around the pillars, panic can easily trigger crowd turbulence and stampede. In 2004, after 251 pilgrims were killed and another 244 injured, the Saudi government replaced the round pillars with wide, elliptical columns to reduce crowd densities. After a stampede in 2006 that killed 380 pilgrims and injured 289, the Jamaraat pedestrian bridge was demolished and replaced with a wider, multilevel bridge.

After Jamaraat, pilgrims traditionally sacrificed an animal to symbolize the ram that Abraham sacrificed instead of his son. In modern times, however, pilgrims often purchase a "sacrifice voucher" in Mecca. Centralized, licensed abattoirs then perform the sacrifice on behalf of the pilgrim, and meat is immediately donated to charity, often reaching international locations. After a final *tawaf*, pilgrims leave Mecca, ending Hajj. Although it is not required as part of Hajj, many pilgrims extend their trips to travel to Medina to visit the Mosque of the Prophet, which contains the tomb of Mohammed and is the second holiest site in Islam.

Immunizations

All pilgrims should be up to date with routine immunizations. Hepatitis A and B and typhoid vaccines are also recommended. Although a requirement for polio vaccine does not include pilgrims from the United States, it is best to ensure full vaccination against polio before travel. Current vaccination requirements are available from the website of the Saudi Arabian Ministry of Health (www.moh.gov.sa/english).

Meningococcal Vaccine

Because of the intensely crowded conditions of the Hajj and high carrier rates of *Neisseria meningitidis* among pilgrims, outbreaks of meningococcal disease have historically been a problem during Hajj. In the aftermath of outbreaks in 2000 and 2001 that affected 1,300 and 1,109 people, respectively, the Saudi Ministry of Health began requiring all pilgrims and local at-risk populations to receive the meningococcal vaccine—Hajj visas cannot be issued without proof of vaccination. All adults and children aged >2 years must have received a single dose of quadrivalent A/C/Y/W-135 vaccine and must show proof of vaccination on a valid International Certificate of Vaccination or Prophylaxis. Hajj pilgrims must have had the meningococcal vaccine ≤3 years and ≥10 days before arriving in Saudi Arabia.

Respiratory Infections

Respiratory tract infections are common during Hajj, and the most common cause of hospital admission is pneumonia. These risks underscore the need to follow the Advisory Committee on Immunization Practices recommendations for pneumococcal polysaccharide vaccine for pilgrims aged ≥65 years and for younger pilgrims with comorbidities. Seasonal influenza vaccine is recommended for all pilgrims.

Other Health and Safety Risks

Communicable Diseases

Diarrheal disease is common during Hajj, and travelers should be educated on usual prevention measures and self-treatment.

Long rituals of standing and walking, heat, sweating, and obesity contribute to the risk for skin infections. Travelers should be advised to keep skin dry, use talcum powder, and be aware of any pain or soreness caused by garments. Any sores or blisters that develop should be disinfected and kept covered.

At the end of Hajj, Muslim men shave their heads, and unclean blades can transmit bloodborne pathogens, such as hepatitis B, hepatitis C, and HIV. Licensed barbers are tested for these bloodborne pathogens and are required to use disposable, single-use blades. Unfortunately, unlicensed barbers continue to operate by the roadside, where they use nonsterile blades on multiple men. Male travelers should be advised to be shaved only at officially designated centers, which are clearly marked.

Noncommunicable Diseases and Other Hazards

Cardiovascular disease is the primary cause of death during Hajj. Hajj is arduous even for young, healthy pilgrims, and many Muslims wait until they are older before making Hajj. Pilgrims who are caught up in the spiritual experience of Hajj may forget to take their usual medications. Consequently, travelers with preexisting cardiovascular disease should consult with their doctors before leaving, ensure that they have an adequate supply of medication, adhere to their usual regimen, and immediately report to the nearest health center if they notice symptoms of cardiac decompensation.

Heat exhaustion and heatstroke are leading causes of death, particularly when Hajj occurs during the summer. Pilgrims should stay hydrated, wear sunscreen, and seek shade when possible. Some rituals may also be performed at night to avoid daytime heat.

Fire is a potential risk at Hajj. In 1997, open stoves set tents on fire, and the resulting blaze killed 343 pilgrims and injured more than 1,500. As a result, makeshift tents were replaced with permanent fiberglass structures; no pilgrim is allowed to set up his own tent. Cooking in the tents is also prohibited.

Trauma

Trauma is a major cause of injury and death during Hajj. Pilgrims may walk long distances through or near dense traffic, and motor vehicle accidents are inevitable. The most feared trauma hazard, however, is stampede, and in such dense crowds, little can be done to avoid or escape a stampede once it has begun. They usually begin as minor incidents; the 2006 Hajj stampede, for example, began when some pilgrims tripped over fallen luggage, but it resulted in hundreds of injuries and deaths. Death usually results from asphyxiation or head trauma, and providing prompt treatment is next to impossible in large crowds.

The Saudi government is committed to mitigating health risks during Hajj, and it has spent >$25 billion to date, in efforts to prevent stampede. The round columns at Jamaraat have been replaced with wider elliptical ones, and a new Jamaraat bridge has been built. The new bridge has a capacity to hold 5 million pilgrims over a 6-hour period. Bottlenecks have been engineered out, and large canopies have been added to protect pilgrims from the sun. To further protect themselves, travelers should try to avoid the most densely crowded areas during Hajj and, when options exist, perform rituals at nonpeak hours. For example, most pilgrims prefer to perform the Stoning of the Devil at midday, but Saudi authorities have decreed that it may be performed anytime between sunrise and sunset.

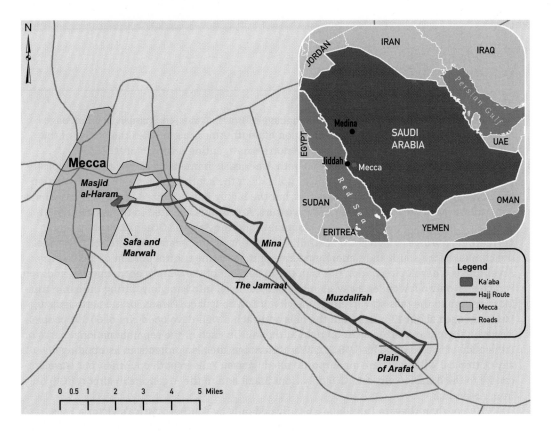

MAP 4-6. HAJJ DESTINATION MAP

BIBLIOGRAPHY

1. Ahmed QA, Arabi YM, Memish ZA. Health risks at the Hajj. Lancet. 2006 Mar 25;367(9515):1008–15.
2. Gatrad AR, Sheikh A. Hajj: journey of a lifetime. BMJ. 2005 Jan 15;330(7483):133–7.
3. Memish ZA, Ahmed QA. Mecca bound: the challenges ahead. J Travel Med. 2002 Jul–Aug;9(4):202–10.
4. Shafi S, Memish ZA, Gatrad AR, Sheikh A. Hajj 2006: communicable disease and other health risks and current official guidance for pilgrims. Euro Surveill. 2005;10(12):E051215.2.
5. World Health Organization. Health conditions for travellers to Saudi Arabia pilgrimage to Mecca (Hajj). Wkly Epidemiol Rec. 2005 Dec 9;80(49–50):431–2.

4 IGUASSU FALLS, BRAZIL/ARGENTINA
David O. Freedman

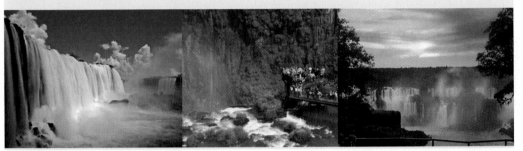

DESTINATION OVERVIEW

Iguassu Falls (*Iguaçu* in Portuguese, the language of Brazil; *Iguazú* in Spanish, the language of Argentina) in the Atlantic rainforest region of South America straddles the border of the southern Brazilian state of Paraná and the northern Argentine province of Misiones.

Brazil, occupying most of eastern South America, is immense and varies from tropical plains and jungle at the equator to cooler uplands in the south. Brazil is a developing nation in the lower half of the world's economies, but the highly industrialized south, which includes São Paulo, is affluent with modern infrastructure. Argentina is located in the southern part of South America, between the Andes Mountains and the Atlantic Ocean. Except for a tiny northernmost fringe, which is tropical, all of Argentina is temperate, characterized by a cool, dry climate in the south and a more moderate climate in the central portion of the country. Argentina is a developing nation but is in the upper half of the world's economies. In addition, Paraguay is only a few miles away, so many people travel into Paraguay during the same trip. Most visitors to the falls stay in either the city of Foz do Iguaçu, Paraná, or in Puerto Iguazú, Misiones, each about 12 miles from the falls and each a well-developed city of 60,000 people. However, there is one sizeable hotel right at the falls in each of the separate national parks on either side of the border. This UNESCO World Heritage site also protects an astounding diversity of tropical wildlife. There are airports called Iguassu Falls in both countries, but travelers can fly to the Brazilian airport (IGU) only from Brazil and to the Argentinean airport (IGR) only from Argentina.

Higher than Niagara Falls, Iguassu is rivaled only by southern Africa's Victoria Falls, which are higher but narrower. Iguassu Falls is a waterfall system consisting of 275 falls along

1.67 miles (2.67 km) of the Iguassu River, varying from 210 to 270 ft (64 to 82 m) in height. The main feature, the Devil's Throat, is a U-shaped cliff, 490 by 2,300 ft (149 by 701 m), which marks the border between Argentina and Brazil. Two-thirds of the falls are on the Argentine side of the gorge, giving the Brazilian side the best view. However, one cannot directly approach the falls from the Brazilian side. Travelers visiting the Argentine side are able to pass over and under the actual falls on a series of catwalks and trails. The bridge connecting the 2 sides of the river is a number of miles away and crosses the Brazil-Argentina border.

US travelers require a visa, which must be obtained in advance, to enter Brazil. Many organized day trips do not stop at the Brazilian immigration post, and this seems to be tolerated. However, a US citizen in Brazil without a visa in his or her passport may face arrest or imprisonment if stopped for any reason by authorities during the short visit. US travelers staying on the Brazilian side on a single-entry Brazilian visa can reenter Brazil after a day trip to Argentina. No visa is required to enter Argentina from Brazil. Ideally, one really should visit both sides, but most people do not, because their stay is too short to deal with the somewhat complicated logistical issues.

HEALTH ISSUES

The infrastructure in tourist accommodations around Iguassu Falls is good, and most travelers are tourists staying only for a short time. Travelers using usual accommodation and dining facilities are at modest risk for enterically transmitted diseases. Travelers should carry an antibiotic to self-treat travelers' diarrhea. Hepatitis A and B vaccines are recommended for all travelers and typhoid vaccine only for those with adventurous dietary habits or who plan to eat away from usual tourist locations.

Yellow Fever

Yellow fever virus circulates in monkeys and mosquitoes in the forested regions along the Iguassu and Paraná rivers. All travelers, even those on a typical 1- to 2-day itinerary, should be vaccinated. Although requirements may change from time to time, at present neither Brazil nor Argentina requires an International Certificate of Vaccination or Prophylaxis for yellow fever for any traveler.

Malaria

Some transmission of *Plasmodium vivax* does occur at the falls and in surrounding areas. In making a decision on whether to recommend chemoprophylaxis or simply mosquito precautions, the itinerary, style of travel, and location of accommodations all need to be taken into consideration. Typical 1- to 2-night travelers on fixed itineraries and staying at the hotels at the falls or in upscale accommodation in the adjacent towns may decide on insect precautions only. Other types of travelers to the area may be at increased risk and may decide to use chemoprophylaxis, in consultation with their travel health provider.

Rabies

Both canine and bat rabies are risks in parts of Brazil, but no cases in animals or humans have been reported around Iguassu Falls. Preexposure vaccine is not necessary for typical travelers, but travelers should be educated about seeking adequate medical care for any bite injuries or bat exposures that occur.

Leishmaniasis

This protozoan disease, transmitted by sandflies, occurs in Brazil and is most common in the Amazonian and northeast regions but is present in Paraná. Cases have not been described in visitors to Iguassu Falls.

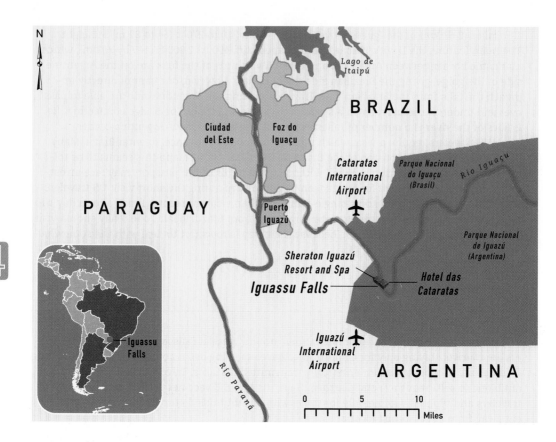

MAP 4-7. IGUASSU FALLS DESTINATION MAP

Chagas Disease (American Trypanosomiasis)
Risk to travelers is unknown but is thought to be negligible. Few travelers stay in houses constructed of mud, adobe brick, or palm thatch, where the vectors live.

Dengue Fever
Dengue occurs in urban and rural areas in the Iguassu Falls region. Daytime insect precautions will reduce risk.

Schistosomiasis
Schistosomiasis, transmitted in freshwater lakes and rivers, is a public health problem in many states in Brazil. Historically, rare cases have been reported from the Iguassu area, but no recent data are available. Cautious travelers should avoid freshwater exposure while visiting the area.

INDIA
Phyllis E. Kozarsky

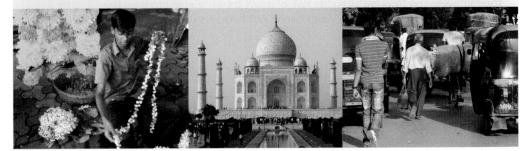

4

DESTINATION OVERVIEW

India is approximately one-third the size of the United States and has 7 times the population (almost 2 billion people). This makes it the second most populous country in the world, behind China. Rich in history, vibrant culture, and diversity, India is the birthplace of 4 world religions: Hinduism, Buddhism, Jainism, and Sikhism. Despite the growth of megacities such as Mumbai and Delhi (both reaching almost 14 million), 70% of the population still resides in rural areas, and 60% work in agriculture. Although India is one of the fastest-growing economies in the world, the literacy rate is only 60%, and the level of poverty is high. The topography is varied, ranging from tropical beaches to foothills, deserts, and the Himalayan Mountains. The north has a more temperate climate, while the south is more tropical year round. Many travelers prefer India during the winter—November through March, when the temperatures are more agreeable—although some, particularly families with children, must travel during the summer vacation time.

India is becoming more popular for US travelers, and rates of travel from the United States are increasing. International businesses are flourishing in India; tourists are flocking to the temples, beaches, and the Taj Mahal. For some new US residents, India remains their homeland, and they make frequent visits to family and friends.

Because tourists could not possibly visit all the tourist sites in India during a 2-week holiday, they usually select a part of India for any given trip. A typical itinerary in the north of India includes Delhi, Agra, and cities in Rajasthan, such as Jaipur (the "pink" city). Agra is the home of the Taj Mahal, a breathtaking monument to lost love. Along the northern travel circle, one can stop to enjoy the magnificent bird sanctuary at Keoladeo Ghana and the tiger reserve at Ran Thambore. Another frequent stop is Goa and its beaches on the western coast, where swaying coconut palms form the backdrop for great parties and old-time hippies. Mumbai, another common entry point to India, hosts Bollywood, the largest film industry in the world. Kolkata is considered the cultural capital of the country. Bengaluru (Bangalore) in the south-central region has become a worldwide information technology center and has managed to meld the very old and traditional India with a new image of a modern hub. Despite the many and varied itineraries, most health recommendations for travelers to India are similar. The incidences of some illnesses, such as those transmitted by mosquitoes, increase during the monsoon season (May–October) with the high temperatures, heavy rains, and the risk of flooding.

Malaria

Although the intensity of malaria may be related to the season, unlike other countries in Asia, malaria is holoendemic in India (except at altitudes >2,000 m [6,561 ft]) and occurs in both rural and urban areas. Rates of *Plasmodium falciparum* have increased in the last 2 decades, and thus chemoprophylaxis is recommended for all destinations. For short-term travelers spending 1–2 days in Delhi in the winter, insect precautions alone may be sufficient to prevent malaria.

Other Infections

Dengue

Large outbreaks have occurred in India, particularly in the north, and particularly at the end of the monsoon season (September–October). Numerous cases in travelers have occurred.

Chikungunya

During the last several years there have been outbreaks of this viral illness, which is transmitted by day-biting mosquitoes. Symptoms are similar to those of dengue and malaria, generally with severe arthralgias.

Hepatitis E

This illness is being recognized more frequently in travelers to India. A traveler who develops symptomatic hepatitis, despite being immunized against hepatitis A, will likely have hepatitis E.

Animal Bites and Wounds

In addition to rabies, other diseases can be transmitted by animal bites and wounds. Cellulitis, fasciitis, and wound infections may result from scratches or bites of any animal. Herpes B virus is carried by Old World monkeys and may be transmitted by active macaques that are kept as pets, inhabit many of the temples, and scatter themselves in many tourist gathering places. Monkeys can be aggressive and often approach travelers because they are commonly fed. When visiting temple areas that have monkeys, travelers should not carry any food in their hands, pockets, or bags. It is important to stress to travelers that monkeys and other animals should not be approached or handled at all.

Travelers' Diarrhea

The risk for travelers' diarrhea is moderate to high in India, with an estimated 30%–50% risk during a 2-week journey. Travelers should practice safe food and water precautions and carry an antibiotic for empiric self-treatment of diarrhea.

Miscellaneous

Arrival in India for the first time may be shocking to travelers who have never ventured into the developing world. The crowds, the intense colors, heat, and smells are striking and invade all the senses at once. It is difficult to enjoy the beauty without being touched by the enormity of the poverty. The close juxtaposition of the old and new is noteworthy. At times this can be overwhelming for travelers. Health care is quite variable in India and dependent on the location.

Transportation in India remains problematic. While traveling through India, travelers should be advised to carry food and beverages with them in the event of delays, almost inevitable no matter the mode of transport. Traveling by train can be harrowing, particularly having to force one's way through the crowd and onto the train. Travelers should make sure to keep passports and valuables safe while in a crowd. Roadways are some of the most hazardous in the world. Animals, rickshaws, motor scooters, people, bicycles, trucks, and overcrowded buses compete for space in an unregulated free-for-all. Rural, nighttime driving should be discouraged, even when a paid driver has been hired.

In general, travelers feel safe while in India. Peddlers and promoters are aggressive with tourists, however, and may require a firm "no." Travelers may want to avoid making eye contact with a peddler or his goods, or they may risk having someone follow them down the street trying to sell them something. The stress of negotiating one's way through India makes this destination a place where having a close traveling companion is important.

It is always wise to pay attention to Department of State advisories in case of issues that arise at some borders or occasional increases in religious tensions or terrorist activities.

BIBLIOGRAPHY

1. Bacaner N, Stauffer B, Boulware DR, Walker PF, Keystone JS. Travel medicine considerations for North American immigrants visiting friends and relatives. JAMA. 2004 Jun 16;291(23):2856–64.
2. Baggett HC, Graham S, Kozarsky PE, Gallagher N, Blumensaadt S, Bateman J, et al. Pretravel health preparation among US residents traveling to India to VFRs: importance of ethnicity in defining VFRs. J Travel Med. 2009 Mar–Apr;16(2):112–8.
3. Chatterjee S. Compliance of malaria chemoprophylaxis among travelers to India. J Travel Med. 1999 Mar;6(1):7–11.
4. Connor BA, Schwartz E. Typhoid and paratyphoid fever in travellers. Lancet Infect Dis. 2005 Oct;5(10): 623–8.
5. Das K, Jain A, Gupta S, Kapoor S, Gupta RK, Chakravorty A, et al. The changing epidemiological pattern of hepatitis A in an urban population of India: emergence of a trend similar to the European countries. Eur J Epidemiol. 2000 Jun;16(6):507–10.
6. Leder K, Tong S, Weld L, Kain KC, Wilder-Smith A, von Sonnenburg F, et al. Illness in travelers visiting friends and relatives: a review of the GeoSentinel Surveillance Network. Clin Infect Dis. 2006 Nov 1;43(9):1185–93.
7. Steinberg EB, Bishop R, Haber P, Dempsey AF, Hoekstra RM, Nelson JM, et al. Typhoid fever in travelers: who should be targeted for prevention? Clin Infect Dis. 2004 Jul 15;39(2):186–91.

KILIMANJARO, TANZANIA

Kevin C. Kain

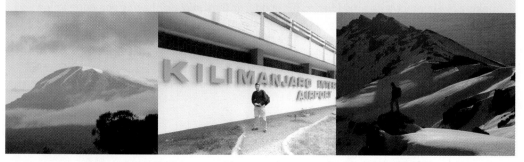

DESTINATION OVERVIEW

As the highest mountain in Africa and one of the largest freestanding volcanoes in the world, Kilimanjaro remains a revered and classic image of East Africa. Its snow-capped peak rising 19,344 ft (5,896 m) above the tropical African savanna is an irresistible draw for trekkers, particularly since no technical climbing is required to reach the summit. Kilimanjaro is one of the "seven summits" representing the highest peaks on each continent. However, because it does not involve technical climbing, the difficulties are often misjudged. Climbing Kilimanjaro is a serious undertaking, requiring serious preparation. Despite being higher than classic trekking destinations in Nepal, such as Kalar Pattar (18,450 ft; 5,625 m) or Everest base camp (17,500 ft; 5,335 m), typical ascent rates on Kilimanjaro are considerably faster (4–6 days vs 8–12 days).

The classic route up Kilimanjaro is the Marangu route (64 km), usually sold as a "5 day/ 4 night" trip. Marangu is frequently nicknamed the "Coca Cola" route, since accommodation and food are provided in bunkhouses and the trail is wide and relatively easy compared with other routes. There are at least 9 other alternative routes, including the stunningly beautiful Machame route (the so-called "whiskey" route, since the days are generally longer, with tougher climbs). This author can vouch for the dramatic rugged beauty of this hike. Machame and other routes involve camping but are usually sold as 6- to 9-day packages, providing more opportunity to acclimatize and greater chances to successfully summit. Kilimanjaro can be climbed throughout the year (March–April is often the wettest), but the weather is unpredictable and the climber must be prepared for extreme weather and rain at any time of the year.

Climbing Kilimanjaro is a dream for many who visit Africa. However, a large number of travelers are ill-prepared, ascend too quickly, and consequently fail to summit. With due preparation and more reasonable ascent rates, climbing "Kili" is an aspiration that can be successfully and safely accomplished by many.

HEALTH ISSUES

The main medical issues for those attempting Kilimanjaro include the prevention and treatment of altitude illness and the potential for drug interactions between medications used for altitude illness and antimalarial or antidiarrheal agents commonly used by travelers to Tanzania.

Altitude and Acute Mountain Sickness (AMS)

Altitude illness is a significant problem on Kilimanjaro and a major contributor to the reason that only 50% of those attempting the standard 4–5 day Marangu route reach the crater rim, known as Gillman's Point (18,600 ft; 5,680 m), and as few as 10% reach the summit, known as Uhuru (Freedom) Peak (19,344 ft; 5,896 m). Prevalence rates of AMS were 75%–77% in recent studies of 4- and 5-day ascents on the Marangu route. Those using acetazolamide were significantly less likely to develop AMS on the 5-day ascents.

Every hiker on Kilimanjaro should receive pre-travel advice on AMS, be able to recognize symptoms, and know how to prevent and treat it. People with certain underlying medical conditions, including pregnancy, cardiac and lung disease, and ocular and neurologic conditions, may be more susceptible to altitude-associated problems or may be taking medications that may interact with altitude medications and should consult a travel health provider with knowledge of altitude illness before travel.

Enjoying the experience and successfully reaching the summit can be significantly enhanced by allowing more time to acclimatize:

> If Ngorongoro crater is part of the planned combined itinerary, try to spend the last few nights of the safari here, because its elevation (7,500 ft; 2,286 m) will aid acclimatization for the Kilimanjaro trek.
> It is strongly encouraged to add at least an extra day or two to the ascent of Kilimanjaro, regardless of the route, but especially on routes normally promoted as 4- to 6-day routes.
> If possible before attempting Kilimanjaro, acclimatize by hiking nearby Mount Meru (14,976 ft; 4,566 m) or Mount Kenya (to Point Lenana, 16,055 ft; 4,895 m). A number of combined climbing trips for Mount Kenya and Kilimanjaro are now offered commercially.

For those with a past history of susceptibility to AMS and for those in whom adequate acclimatization is not possible (most "Kili" clients), the use of medications such as acetazolamide to prevent altitude illness is recommended. Acetazolamide accelerates acclimatization, is effective in preventing (beginning the day before ascent) and treating AMS, and is safe in children.

For those who are intolerant or allergic to acetazolamide, dexamethasone is an alternative for prevention of AMS, but there are cautions involved in using dexamethasone for ascent. Consideration should be given to carrying a treatment course of dexamethasone for high-altitude cerebral edema (HACE). Travelers with symptoms of altitude illness must not continue to ascend and need to descend if symptoms are worsening at the same altitude. A flexible itinerary and having an extra guide who can accompany any member of the group who becomes ill down the mountain are considerations. See Chapter 2, Altitude Illness for more information about prevention and treatment of altitude illness.

Malaria

Kilimanjaro is unique in that its tropical malaria-endemic location means that many trekkers will be on antimalarials and may need to continue them after their climb, particularly if they are also visiting game parks and staying overnight at altitudes <2000 m. Antimalarial prophylaxis is recommended for Tanzania (even if only for a short trip). If a traveler flew directly into Kilimanjaro International Airport (2932 ft; 891 m) and went the same day to an altitude above 2,000 m, there would be no risk of malaria. However, most people will be on safari or traveling before or after their Kilimanjaro trip, and therefore will be on prophylaxis.

Kilimanjaro is also a unique destination in that high altitude will affect everyone and possible interactions should be considered between drugs commonly used for prophylaxis or treatment of AMS, high-altitude pulmonary edema, or high-altitude cerebral edema, such as acetazolamide, dexamethasone, and nifedipine. Fortunately, there are no reported clinically significant drug interactions between common antimalarial prophylaxis agents (atovaquone-proguanil, doxycycline, or mefloquine) and acetazolamide or dexamethasone used to prevent or treat AMS. Nifedipine is metabolized by the CYP3A4 enzyme and concurrent use of CYP3A4 inhibitors, such as doxycycline, could lead to elevated plasma levels of nifedipine and potentially lower blood pressure. Therefore, it would not be advised to take nifedipine as prophylaxis concurrently with doxycycline.

Treatment of Travelers' Diarrhea

There are no reported drug interactions between acetazolamide and the fluoroquinolones (ciprofloxacin, levofloxacin) or macrolides (azithromycin) commonly used to treat travelers' diarrhea. There is a potential increased risk of tendon rupture when dexamethasone is used with fluoroquinolones. Avoid concurrent use of macrolides and nifedipine.

Remote Travel

Treks on Kilimanjaro are physically demanding and require a good level of fitness and preparation for the elements. Kilimanjaro weather is characterized by extremes: be prepared for tropical heat, heavy rains, and bitter cold. Keep gear, especially one's sleeping bag, in waterproof bags. Travelers should have adequate health insurance, including medical evacuation. Travelers are advised to make sure their medical care and medical evacuation policy will cover any potential costs for a rescue or evacuation from the top of the mountain.

Carry a first-aid kit that includes bandages, tape, blister kit, antibacterial and antifungal cream, antibiotics for travelers' diarrhea, antimalarials, antiemetics, antihistamines, analgesics, cold and flu medications, throat lozenges, and altitude medications.

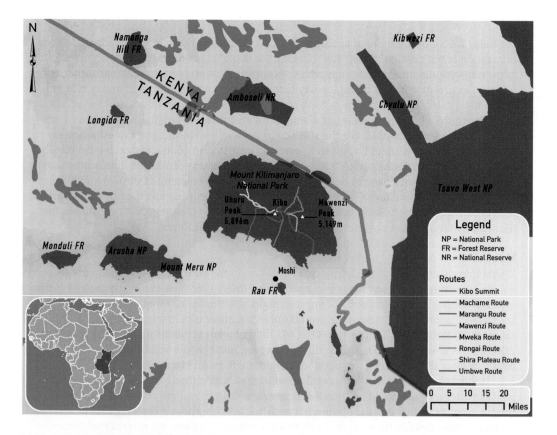

MAP 4-9. KILIMANJARO DESTINATION MAP

BIBLIOGRAPHY

1. Barry PW, Pollard AJ. Altitude illness. BMJ. 2003 Apr 26;326(7395):915–9.
2. Bartsch P, Gibbs JS. Effect of altitude on the heart and the lungs. Circulation. 2007 Nov 6;116(19):2191–202.
3. Basnyat B, Gertsch JH, Holck PS, Johnson EW, Luks AM, Donham BP, et al. Acetazolamide 125 mg BD is not significantly different from 375 mg BD in the prevention of acute mountain sickness: the prophylactic acetazolamide dosage comparison for efficacy (PACE) trial. High Alt Med Biol. 2006 Spring;7(1):17–27.
4. Baumgartner RW, Siegel AM, Hackett PH. Going high with preexisting neurological conditions. High Alt Med Biol. 2007 Summer;8(2):108–16.
5. Davies AJ, Kalson NS, Stokes S, Earl MD, Whitehead AG, Frost H, et al. Determinants of summiting success and acute mountain sickness on Mt Kilimanjaro (5895 m). Wilderness Environ Med. 2009 Winter;20(4):311–7.
6. Hackett PH, Roach RC. High-altitude illness. N Engl J Med. 2001 Jul 12;345(2):107–14.
7. Jean D, Leal C, Kriemler S, Meijer H, Moore LG. Medical recommendations for women going to altitude. High Alt Med Biol. 2005 Spring;6(1):22–31.
8. Karinen H, Peltonen J, Tikkanen H. Prevalence of acute mountain sickness among Finnish trekkers on Mount Kilimanjaro, Tanzania: an observational study. High Alt Med Biol. 2008 Winter;9(4):301–6.
9. Luks AM, Swenson ER. Medication and dosage considerations in the prophylaxis and treatment of high-altitude illness. Chest. 2008 Mar;133(3):744–55.
10. Luks AM, Swenson ER. Travel to high altitude with pre-existing lung disease. Eur Respir J. 2007 Apr;29(4):770–92.
11. Mader TH, Tabin G. Going to high altitude with preexisting ocular conditions. High Alt Med Biol. 2003 Winter;4(4):419–30.
12. Strom BL, Schinnar R, Apter AJ, Margolis DJ, Lautenbach E, Hennessy S, et al. Absence of cross-reactivity between sulfonamide antibiotics and sulfonamide nonantibiotics. N Engl J Med. 2003 Oct 23;349(17):1628–35.

4

MEXICO
Stephen H. Waterman

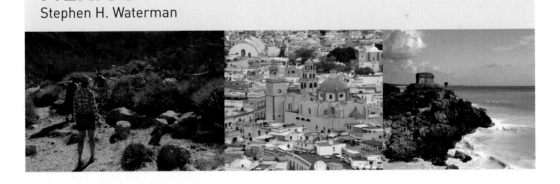

DESTINATION OVERVIEW

Mexico, the second most populous country in Latin America, has a population of over 110 million, with 76% living in urban areas. The United States' second-largest trading partner after Canada, Mexico is now considered a middle-income country. Mexico has a rich history and proud culture that reflect its pre-Columbian civilizations and Hispanic heritage. With one-fifth the area of the United States, Mexico has diverse geographic features. The Sonoran desert is in the northwest, beautiful beaches are available on both coasts, and forested mountain ranges traverse the western and eastern mainland, featuring high volcanic peaks in the interior. The Yucatán Peninsula and southern regions are tropical. The Copper Canyon in Chihuahua is larger than the US Grand Canyon.

Mexico City is one of the world's largest cities, with a population over 20 million. Despite increasing national prosperity, Mexico's large cities contain much urban poverty as well. Extensive migration has taken place from the poor rural south to the northern border for jobs in bustling but drab border cities, such as Ciudad Juárez and Tijuana.

Mexico has the most foreign visitors of any Latin American country and is the country most frequently visited by US tourists. Travel varies from day trips to northern border cities to experience a taste of a foreign culture to longer cultural trips and beach holidays. Popular anthropologic destinations include Teotihuacan outside Mexico City, Chichen Itzá in Yucatán, Monte Alban in Oaxaca, and Palenque in Chiapas. Travel to beach resorts such as Acapulco, Cancún, Cozumel, Puerto Vallarta, and Cabo San Lucas, along with cruise ship tours, makes up a large portion of tourist travel to Mexico. Baja California offers whale watching on the Pacific Coast and sports fishing in the Gulf of California.

HEALTH ISSUES

Immunizations
Hepatitis A is still endemic in Mexico, and all susceptible travelers should be immunized for hepatitis A. Hepatitis B vaccine is also recommended. Other vaccines, such as typhoid and rabies, may be considered, especially if travel is extensive to less developed nontourist areas, by field biologists or missionaries, for example.

Travelers' Diarrhea and Foodborne Infections
Travelers' diarrhea is common among visitors to Mexico. In addition to taking food precautions, travelers should bring along an antibiotic for empiric self-treatment of diarrhea. Travelers who eat raw dairy products and vegetables are at some risk for more serious foodborne infections, including amebiasis, cysticercosis (especially in rural areas where pigs are raised), brucellosis, *Mycobacterium bovis*, and *Listeria*.

Dengue
Dengue is endemic throughout Mexico, except for higher elevations and in Baja California Norte. All 4 dengue serotypes circulate in Mexico, and large outbreaks of dengue hemorrhagic fever have been reported in recent years. Visitors should take precautions to avoid daytime mosquito bites with protective clothing and use of effective repellents.

Malaria
Malaria incidence has decreased dramatically in recent decades in Mexico, and only a few cases are reported among US travelers each year. Major resorts are free of malaria. Malaria prophylaxis is recommended only for low-lying, infrequently visited rural areas of a few states: Sonora, Chihuahua, Durango, Sinaloa, and Nayarit in the west and Oaxaca, Chiapas, Tabasco, and Quintana Roo in the southern region bordering Guatemala and Belize.

Other Infections
Coccidioidomycosis
Coccidioidomycosis, a fungal respiratory disease caused by inhaling spores in the soil, is endemic in northwestern Mexico. Several outbreaks have been reported among missionary groups from the United States doing construction projects in this region.

Parasitic Infections
Onchocerciasis, also known as river blindness, is present in small endemic foci in southern Mexico. Travelers, such as missionaries or field scientists, who spend >3 months in endemic areas are at greater risk for infection. Cutaneous leishmaniasis, transmitted by sandflies, is found in focal areas of coastal and southern Mexico. The risk is higher for ecotourists and long-term

travelers. Vector preventive measures are indicated, including avoiding outdoor activities at night. Chagas disease is also endemic in Mexico, but no cases have been reported among travelers.

Rabies

All travelers should be warned of the risk of acquiring rabies and educated in how to prevent animal bites. Preexposure rabies vaccination should be considered for those who are likely to come into contact with animals or those who will be traveling to areas with limited access to medical care.

Rickettsial Disease

Rickettsial diseases, febrile rash illnesses transmitted by ticks or fleas, in Mexico include Rocky Mountain spotted fever, which is potentially fatal unless treated promptly with antibiotics, and fleaborne typhus, which usually causes an illness similar to dengue. Travelers should take precautions to avoid flea and tick bites when outdoors. An outbreak of Rocky Mountain spotted fever was identified in a neglected urban area in Mexicali, Baja California, in 2009, and endemic transmission has been reported there since then.

Tuberculosis (TB)

Mexico's TB incidence is lower than rates in Asia, Africa, and Eastern Europe but is 5 times that of the United States.

Other Health and Safety Risks

Good health care is available in most sizable Mexican cities, and hotels in tourist resorts usually have well-trained physicians available. Medical tourism has increased in Mexico in recent

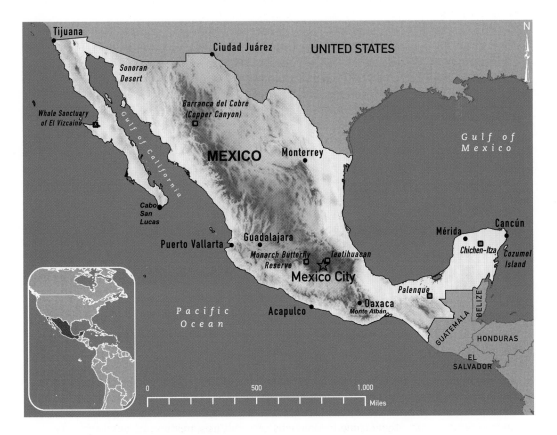

MAP 4-10. MEXICO DESTINATION MAP

years, but adverse events have not been studied. Clinics offering unproven and often dangerous interventions for cancer and other seriously ill patients can operate in northern border cities, such as Tijuana, for varying periods before regulatory authorities intervene.

Mexico's highway system and roads have become increasingly modernized over the years. Toll highways are often of high quality. Nevertheless, driving in traffic in cities and at night through the countryside can be dangerous. Although travel in Mexico is generally safe and enjoyable, there has been a continuing increase in drug-related violence in parts of the country. Department of State advisories should be monitored for alerts in areas where tourists are planning to visit.

A population that requires increasing attention is the large numbers of travelers of Mexican birth or descent who return to visit friends and relatives.

BIBLIOGRAPHY

1. CDC. Coccidioidomycosis in travelers returning from Mexico—Pennsylvania, 2000. MMWR Morb Mortal Wkly Rep. 2000 Nov 10;49(44):1004–6.
2. CDC. Dengue hemorrhagic fever—US-Mexico border, 2005. MMWR Morb Mortal Wkly Rep. 2007 Aug 10;56(31):785–9.
3. CDC. Preventing and controlling tuberculosis along the US-Mexico border. MMWR Recomm Rep. 2001 Jan 19;50(RR-1):1–27.
4. Doyle TJ, Bryan RT. Infectious disease morbidity in the US region bordering Mexico, 1990–1998. J Infect Dis. 2000 Nov;182(5):1503–10.
5. Weinberg M, Hopkins J, Farrington L, Gresham L, Ginsberg M, Bell BP. Hepatitis A in Hispanic children who live along the United States-Mexico border: the role of international travel and food-borne exposures. Pediatrics. 2004 Jul;114(1):e68–73.
6. White AC, Atmar RL. Infections in Hispanic immigrants. Clin Infect Dis. 2002 Jun 15;34(12):1627–32.

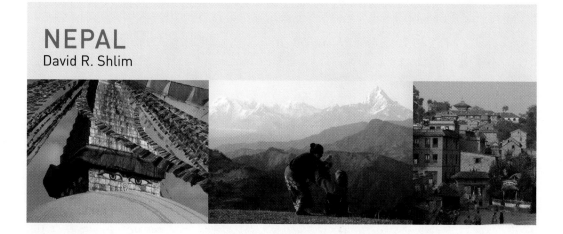

NEPAL
David R. Shlim

DESTINATION OVERVIEW

Nepal is a country of over 27 million people that stretches for 500 miles (805 km) along the Himalayan mountains that form the border of Nepal and Tibet. The topography rises from low plains with an altitude of 200 ft (70 m) to the highest point in the world at 29,135 ft (8,848 m), the summit of Mount Everest. Approximately 30% of tourists come to Nepal to trek into the mountains, while others come to experience the culture and stunning natural beauty. Kathmandu is the capital city, with a population of well over a million people. It sits in a lush valley at 4,300 ft (1,300 m) in altitude. Nepal's latitude of 28° North (the same as Florida) means that the nonmountainous areas are temperate year round. Most of the annual rainfall comes during the monsoon season (June through September). The main tourist seasons are in the spring (March to May) and fall (October and November). The winter months, December through February, are pleasant in the lowlands but can be too cold to make trekking enjoyable in the high mountains.

There are 3 main trekking areas: the Mount Everest region east of Kathmandu, the Annapurna region to the west, and the Langtang region north of Kathmandu. Trekkers into the Mount Everest region routinely sleep at altitudes of >14,000–16,000 ft (4,200–4,900 m) and hike to altitudes >18,000 ft (5,500 m). This prolonged exposure to very high altitudes means that tourists must be knowledgeable about the risks of altitude illness and may need to carry specific medications to prevent and treat the problem (see Chapter 2, Altitude Illness). Most trekkers into the Mount Everest region arrive there by flying to a tiny airstrip at Lukla at 9,000 ft (2,700 m). The following day they reach Namche Bazaar at 11,300 ft (3,500 m). Acetazolamide prophylaxis can substantially decrease the chances of developing acute mountain sickness in Namche.

In the Annapurna region, short-term trekkers may choose to hike to viewpoints in the foothills without reaching any high altitudes. Others may undertake a longer trek around the Annapurna massif, going over a 17,700-ft (5,400-m) pass (the Thorung La). Roads have been constructed up the 2 major valleys of this trek, shortening the overall trekking distance and changing the nature of the experience (cars and motorcycles may be encountered along the trek). The total exposure to high altitude is less in this region than in the Everest region. The Langtang region has a high point of 14,000 ft (4,200 m).

In addition to trekking, Nepal has some of the best rafting and kayaking rivers in the world. Jungle lodges in Chitwan National Park allow tourists to view a wide range of wildlife, including tigers, rhinoceroses, bears, and crocodiles, and a huge variety of exotic birds. It is also possible to travel by road to comfortable lodges in the foothills that afford panoramic views of the Himalayas.

HEALTH ISSUES

Immunizations

Travelers should be up to date with their routine immunizations and are advised to consider hepatitis B vaccine. Travelers to Nepal are at high risk for enterically transmitted diseases. Hepatitis A vaccine and typhoid vaccine are the 2 most important immunizations. The risk of typhoid fever and paratyphoid fever among travelers to Nepal is among the highest in the world, and the prevalence of fluoroquinolone resistance is high.

Japanese encephalitis (JE) is endemic in Nepal, mainly in the Terai region during and immediately after the monsoon season (July through October). JE has been identified in local residents of the Kathmandu Valley, but no cases of JE have been reported in tourists or expatriates in Nepal. JE vaccine is not routinely recommended for those trekking in higher altitude areas or spending short periods in Kathmandu or Pokhara en route to such treks (see Chapter 3, Japanese Encephalitis).

Malaria

Malaria is not a risk for most travelers to Nepal. There is no risk for malaria in Kathmandu or Pokhara, the 2 main cities in Nepal. All the main trekking routes in Nepal are free of malaria transmission. Chitwan National Park is a popular tourist destination for wildlife viewing in the Terai. Although the Nepalese Ministry of Health and other regional organizations regard the Terai to be a malaria transmission area, this author, in 27 years of treating travelers in Nepal, has not seen a single case of malaria in a traveler to Chitwan, including foreign workers living in the park.

Other Health and Safety Risks

Gastrointestinal Issues

Cyclospora cayetanensis is an intestinal protozoal pathogen that is highly endemic in Nepal. The risk for infection is distinctly seasonal: transmission occurs almost exclusively from May through October, with a peak in June and July. Because this is outside the main tourist seasons, the primary effect is on expatriates who stay through the monsoon. Profound anorexia and fatigue are the hallmark symptoms of *Cyclospora* infection. The treatment of choice is trimethoprim-sulfamethoxazole; no highly effective alternatives have been identified.

Since many tourists are heading to remote areas that do not have medical care available, they should be provided with medications for self-treatment. Travelers' diarrhea is a significant risk, and the risk in the spring trekking season (March through May) is double that in the fall trekking season (October and November). All trekkers should have an antibiotic such as ciprofloxacin for empiric treatment of bacterial diarrhea. *Campylobacter* causes as much as 20% of the bacterial diarrhea in Nepal, and up to 70% of the *Campylobacter* isolates are resistant to fluoroquinolones. Although ciprofloxacin remains an excellent choice for empiric treatment of bacterial diarrhea, azithromycin is a good alternative and should be used if the diarrhea does not respond to ciprofloxacin.

Hepatitis E virus is endemic in Nepal, and several cases each year are diagnosed in tourists or expatriates. There is no vaccine commercially available against hepatitis E.

Respiratory Issues

The Kathmandu Valley often has air pollution. People with chronic respiratory diseases, such as asthma and chronic obstructive pulmonary disease (COPD), may suffer exacerbations in Kathmandu, particularly after a viral upper respiratory infection. Exacerbation of asthma has not been a significant problem for tourists outside Kathmandu.

Viral upper respiratory infections are extremely common, and the percentage of these that lead to bacterial sinusitis or bronchitis is high. Trekkers should consider carrying an antibiotic, such as azithromycin, to empirically treat a respiratory infection that lasts >7 days with no sign of improvement. More treks may have been ruined by prolonged respiratory infection than by gastrointestinal illness.

Rabies

Rabies is highly endemic among dogs in Nepal, but in recent years there are fewer stray dogs in Kathmandu. Half of all tourist exposures to a possibly rabid animal occur near Swayambunath, a beautiful hilltop shrine also known as the monkey temple. Tourists should be advised to be extra cautious with dogs and monkeys in this area. The monkeys can be aggressive if approached and can jump on a person's back if they smell food in a backpack. Clinics in Kathmandu that specialize in the care of foreigners almost always have complete postexposure rabies immunoprophylaxis, including human rabies immune globulin. Trekkers who are bitten in the mountains are able to return to Kathmandu within an average of 5 days.

Evacuation and Medical Care

Helicopter evacuation from most areas is readily available. Communication has improved from remote areas because of satellite and cellular telephones, and private helicopter companies accept credit cards and are eager to perform evacuations for profit. Evacuation can often take place on the same day as the request, if weather permits. Helicopter rescue is usually limited to morning hours because of afternoon winds in the mountains. The cost of helicopter evacuation ranges from $3,000 to $5,000.

Two main clinics in Kathmandu specialize in the care of foreigners in Nepal. Contact information is available on the International Society of Travel Medicine website (www.istm. org). Hospital facilities have improved steadily over the years, and general and orthopedic emergency surgery are reliable and available in Kathmandu. The closest evacuation point for definitive care is Bangkok.

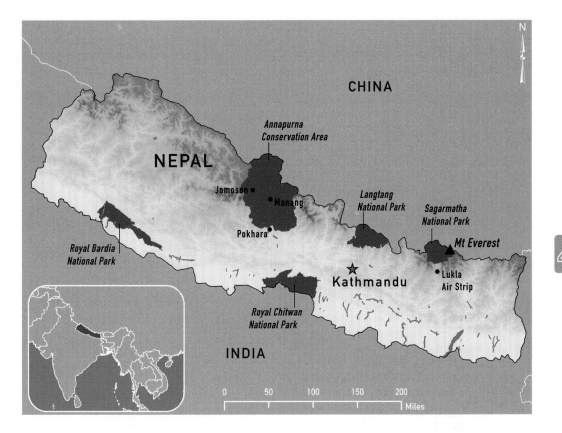

MAP 4-11. NEPAL DESTINATION MAP

The Political Situation

The political situation in Nepal has been in transition since 1990, when a mainly peaceful democratic revolution led to a multiparty parliamentary system under a constitutional monarch. Frustration with the rate of progress in rural areas led to a Maoist insurrection and 10 years of low-grade but violent civil war. A peace agreement was reached in 2008, but an effective government has yet to remain in place. The main effect on tourists can be disruptions to their schedule by demonstrations and strikes, but none of the political tension has been aimed at foreigners, and Nepal remains a safe destination to visit. However, visitors should monitor the political situation while planning their journey.

BIBLIOGRAPHY

1. Cave W, Pandey P, Osrin D, Shlim DR. Chemoprophylaxis use and the risk of malaria in travelers to Nepal. J Travel Med. 2003 Mar–Apr;10(2):100–5.
2. Hoge CW, Shlim DR, Echeverria P, Rajah R, Herrmann JE, Cross JH. Epidemiology of diarrhea among expatriate residents living in a highly endemic environment. JAMA. 1996 Feb 21;275(7):533–8.
3. Schwartz E, Shlim DR, Eaton M, Jenks N, Houston R. The effect of oral and parenteral typhoid vaccination on the rate of infection with *Salmonella typhi* and *Salmonella paratyphi* A among foreigners in Nepal. Arch Intern Med. 1990 Feb;150(2):349–51.

SAFARIS IN EAST & SOUTHERN AFRICA

Karl Neumann

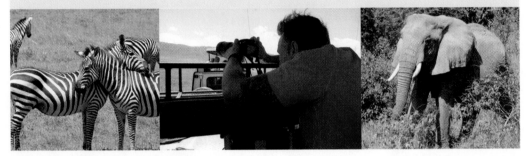

DESTINATION OVERVIEW

Arguably the ultimate in adventure travel, an African safari is also an easily doable family vacation, an experience of a lifetime for people of all ages, and with a little research, not much more difficult to arrange than a week at a Caribbean resort. While the centerpiece of safari-going remains viewing majestic animals in their natural habitats, many tour operators now include programs on local culture, history, geology, and ecosystems, and encourage travelers to get to know the people not merely as subjects of photos. Safaris can also be differentiated by the topography, vegetation, and bird life of the region. There are safaris for families, honeymooners, and people with similar interests (serious photography, for example). Animals can be viewed from open trucks, air-conditioned vans, private aircraft, hot air balloons, or while hiking—where animals are friendly. Accommodations range from crawl-in tents to portable, air-conditioned, walk-in tents with full bathrooms. And there are luxurious 5-star lodges with floodlit water holes to view animals at night. Lunch in the wilderness varies from prepackaged sandwiches eaten sitting on a tree stump to 3-course meals served on tables covered with linen cloths and matching napkins. Some safaris include side trips to exotic places, to see or climb Mount Kilimanjaro, visit Zanzibar, or view Victoria Falls, for example.

Travelers on their first safari often choose game parks in Kenya and Tanzania, in East Africa. The most famous game park in Kenya is the Masai Mara National Reserve, which, in effect, is the northern continuation of the Serengeti National Park game reserve in Tanzania, together forming the home of perhaps the grandest and most complete collection of the large wild animals for which Africa is famous. The Serengeti is the starting point of the annual migration of about 2 million wildebeest and several hundred thousand zebras as they search for pasture and water. Tanzania also has the Ngorongoro Crater, a 100-square mile depression (caldera) formed when a giant volcano, perhaps the size of Mount Kilimanjaro, exploded and collapsed on itself millions of years ago. The crater has most of the same animals as the Masai Mara reserve. In Southern Africa, popular safari destinations are in South Africa, Namibia, and Botswana. South Africa has Kruger National Park, one of the oldest, largest, and most visitor-friendly (much of it handicapped-accessible). Namibia's best-known game reserve is the Etosha National Park, where the terrain consists of a bright white dry lake (salt pan). The Okavango Delta in Botswana is the world's largest inland delta. Seasonally, rivers pour huge amounts of water into this area of the Kalahari Desert. The water has no outlet to the sea and evaporates in the intense heat. For more adventurous travelers, those willing and able to hike through dense rain forests and climb steep slopes, there is gorilla tracking in Rwanda and Uganda, with a good chance (but no promise) that gorillas will be sighted. There are only about 700 of them left in the world. Tours are limited to small groups and have many restrictions: no children and only 1 hour near the gorillas, for example. The major East and Southern African game parks are shown on Map 4-12 and some on Map 4-13.

Travelers should research the optimum time of the year for their safari. The wildebeest migration in the Serengeti is a seasonal event, for example, although the precise time of the migration may vary from year to year. Some parks have a dry season, offering better views of the animals, as the vegetation is sparser. And many areas of Africa have times of the year that are more comfortable for visitors, with cooler weather, less humidity, and less chance of rain.

HEALTH ISSUES

Health and safety issues that safari-goers are likely to encounter are mostly predictable and largely avoidable. The best insurance for carefree trips is a pre-travel consultation with a travel health provider. Advice must be itinerary- and game park-specific. Immunizations and preventive medications necessary for one park may not be necessary for others. Parks are thousands of miles apart and located in countries with different health standards, dissimilar climates, and at various altitudes. And health information for the country may not be sufficiently specific for a park within that country. Malaria, for example, may be a minor problem in South Africa and Namibia, but may be an issue at some parks in these countries, sometimes only seasonally. Generally, proper preparations, common sense precautions, the short duration of most trips (usually ≤2 weeks), experienced guides, leaving the driving to others, and spending little time in the large cities make safaris relatively low-risk undertakings for travelers of all ages.

Food and Water
Travelers' diarrhea appears to be the most common ailment, and most cases are mild. Sensible food and water selections may reduce the incidence. Illness may occur even on deluxe trips. Carrying medication for self-treatment is generally recommended.

Animals
Wild animals are unpredictable. Travelers should follow oral and written instructions provided by safari operators. Animal-related injuries are extremely rare, usually the result of disregarding rules, for example approaching too closely to animals to feed or photograph them.

Rabies exists in most parts of Africa. While most cases result from bites and licks from dogs, all mammals can be rabid. All wounds from animals must be considered rabid until proven otherwise. Licks can result in rabies; the virus can enter through minor breaks in the skin, such as from insect bites, common in the tropics. In addition to rabies, bats can also transmit other diseases, such as viral hemorrhagic fevers, to humans. Travelers should be encouraged to avoid entering caves where bats are known to be present. Recent cases of Marburg fever have occurred in travelers who visited a "python cave" in western Uganda.

Malaria
Malaria transmission occurs in most major game parks. Most infections are caused by *Plasmodium falciparum*, and all *P. falciparum* in sub-Saharan Africa should be considered to be chloroquine-resistant. Safari activities often include sleeping in tents and observing animals at dusk or after dark, sometimes near water holes, all increasing the risk of being bitten by malaria-carrying mosquitoes. Taking appropriate preventive medication and using personal protection techniques—covering up with clothing, using insect repellents, and sleeping under permethrin-impregnated mosquito netting—are essential.

Yellow Fever
Yellow fever vaccination is recommended for virtually all parts of sub-Saharan Africa except those in Southern Africa (see Chapter 3, Yellow Fever and Malaria Information, by Country). Some countries require a valid yellow fever vaccination certificate as a condition of entry.

Moreover, some safaris include more than one country. Travelers must check the requirements of each country on their itinerary. Some may require the certificate even if there is no yellow fever in the country travelers are leaving or entering.

Other Health Risks

Measures to prevent malaria help reduce the risk of 2 other, albeit rare, diseases among travelers: African tickborne fever and African trypanosomiasis. Tickborne fever occurs primarily in rural areas in Southern Africa. Symptoms include fever, localized lymphadenopathy, and rash. Prevention includes tucking pant legs into socks and daily "tick checks." Trypanosomiasis (sleeping sickness) is transmitted by day-biting tsetse flies (*Glossina*). Wearing light-colored clothing seems to deter the flies. Insect repellents are only partially effective. Symptoms include fever, eschar at the site of the bite, headache, and signs of central nervous system involvement.

Myiasis and tungiasis are rare skin diseases. Myiasis is caused by fly larvae penetrating the skin and causing a boil-like lesion with a central aperture. Eggs are usually laid on clothing left to dry outdoors and the larvae enter the skin when the clothing is worn. Clothing should be dried indoors or ironed before wearing. Tungiasis is caused by direct penetration of skin by sand fleas, causing small, painful nodules, often on the foot adjacent to toenails. Prevention includes wearing closed-toed footwear and not walking barefoot.

Schistosomiasis (bilharzia) infection is widespread throughout Africa. The snails exist only in freshwater ponds, lakes, and rivers. All freshwater sources should be considered contaminated. Swimming in the ocean or well-chlorinated pools is safe.

Symptoms of many diseases acquired in Africa may surface weeks and occasionally months later, sometimes long after the traveler has returned home. Informing physicians of recent trips helps them make more prompt diagnoses.

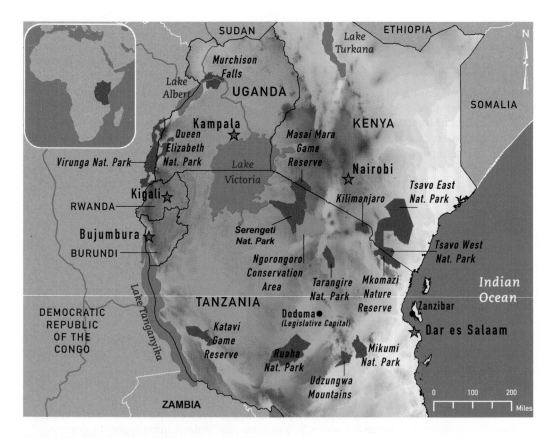

MAP 4-12. EAST AFRICA DESTINATION MAP

Other Safety Risks

Although being a crime victim is an unusual occurrence for those on safari, robbery, muggings, and carjacking may occur in major urban centers, notably Johannesburg, Nairobi, and Mombasa. Street muggings during the day and night are common. The rates of fatal motor vehicle accidents in sub-Saharan Africa are among the highest in the world. Within game parks, serious motor vehicle accidents are rare. The poor roads discourage speeding. However, travel in rural areas between parks is high risk, especially after dark. If at all possible, nighttime driving in sub-Saharan Africa should be avoided.

BIBLIOGRAPHY

1. Durrheim DN, Braack L, Grobler D, Bryden H, Speare R, Leggat PA. Safety of travel in South Africa: the Kruger National Park. J Travel Med. 2001 Jul–Aug;8(4):176–91.
2. Gautret P, Schlagenhauf P, Gaudart J, Castelli F, Brouqui P, von Sonnenburg F, et al. Multicenter EuroTravNet/GeoSentinel study of travel-related infectious diseases in Europe. Emerg Infect Dis. 2009 Nov;15(11):1783–90.
3. Leggat PA, Durrheim DN, Braack L. Traveling in wildlife reserves in South Africa. J Travel Med. 2001 Jan–Feb;8(1):41–5.
4. Meltzer E, Artom G, Marva E, Assous MV, Rahav G, Schwartzt E. Schistosomiasis among travelers: new aspects of an old disease. Emerg Infect Dis. 2006 Nov;12(11):1696–700.
5. Sinha A, Grace C, Alston WK, Westenfeld F, Maguire JH. African trypanosomiasis in two travelers from the United States. Clin Infect Dis. 1999 Oct;29(4):840–4.
6. Thrower Y, Goodyer LI. Application of insect repellents by travelers to malaria endemic areas. J Travel Med. 2006 Jul–Aug;13(4):198–202.
7. United Nations office at Nairobi. Security advice for United Nations visitors to Kenya. Nairobi: United Nations office at Nairobi; 2005 [cited 2008 Jun 30]. Available from: http://www.unon.org/unoncomplex/security_advice.php.
8. World Health Organization. Global status report on road safety: time for action. Geneva: World Health Organization; 2009. Available from: http://www.who.int/violence_injury_prevention/road_safety_status/2009/en/.

SOUTH AFRICA
Gary W. Brunette

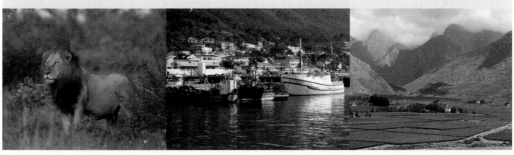

DESTINATION OVERVIEW

South Africa has been called "a world in one country." This refers, in part, to the diversity in the geography, which includes lush subtropical regions, old hardwood forests, sweeping Highveld vistas, and the deep desert of the Kalahari; the splendor of the animal species found throughout the country and protected in expansive games reserves; the diverse origins of the locals (African, European, Indian, and Asian); the cultural, artistic, and culinary variety; and access to the conveniences of a developed infrastructure amid the challenges of Africa.

South Africa has experienced a surge in tourism in the last 2 decades, with visitors from within the African continent as well as those from Europe and North America. Business travelers typically head to the commercial centers of Johannesburg, Cape Town, and Durban. Tourists may be attracted by the game reserves, the largest of which is Kruger National Park, located along the Mozambique border in the northeast. Kwa-Zulu Natal has a number of game parks (Hluhluwe-Umfolozi and Saint Lucia) set inland from Durban, and the Eastern Cape has parks (Addo Elephant Park and Shamwari) easily accessed from Port Elizabeth on the southern coast. Many smaller luxury reserves have emerged to cater to the high-end traveler. Visitors may be attracted to itineraries that include a trip from Cape Town along the south coast through the small scenic towns of Knysna and Plettenberg Bay; a tour of the old gold-mining towns in Mpumalanga, many of which are in near original condition; spectacular drives and fascinating tours of the old wineries along the wine routes in the Western Cape; or visits to the southernmost point of Africa at Cape Agulhas or Cape Point, where the Indian and Atlantic Oceans meet in a roar of foam. South Africa is also a common destination of humanitarian workers, missionaries, and students. A sizable number of South Africans live outside the country and would be considered VFRs (visiting friends and relatives) when returning to the country for a visit.

While there is a wide range of living standards in South Africa, most visitors experience standards comparable to those in developed countries. A smaller number of visitors may go to less developed areas, either the lower-income townships outside most towns and cities or to rural areas. Hikers, adventure-seekers, and missionaries will experience a wider range of living standards. Similarly, the quality and availability of health care are variable. Middle- and upper-income South Africans live in low-risk environments, have a standard of health comparable to that of North Americans, and have access to world-class medical facilities. Poorer South Africans live in areas with few amenities, are exposed to a wide range of diseases, and have limited access to adequate health care.

HEALTH ISSUES

Vaccine-Preventable Diseases

All travelers to South Africa should be up to date with their routine vaccinations. Infectious diseases such as measles and mumps are endemic in the region. In addition, travelers should obtain vaccinations for hepatitis A, hepatitis B, and typhoid.

HIV and Sexually Transmitted Diseases

South Africa has the largest number of people living with HIV of any other country in the world, and the prevalence is approximately 18% among people aged 15–49 years. The commercial sex industry is active, and the prevalence of HIV infection among prostitutes is as high as 33%. Other sexually transmitted diseases are also present at high rates in this population. Travelers should be made aware of these risks and advised to wear condoms if they participate in sexual activities with local residents.

Vectorborne Diseases

The risk for malaria transmission only exists in the northeast of the country in the Mpumalanga and Limpopo Provinces (including Kruger National Park) and in Kwa-Zulu Natal north of the Tugela River. *Plasmodium falciparum* is the predominant species and is universally resistant to chloroquine. Visitors to these areas should be on an appropriate chemoprophylaxis regimen and should be advised about mosquito precautions. Malaria in the northeastern game reserves is seasonal; the highest transmission occurs from October through May, and the period of highest risk is February to early May. The risk to visiting travelers is low. A study conducted in 1999 estimated a case rate of 4.5 cases per 10,000 visitors in April, a high-transmission month. The South African Department of Health recommends chemoprophylaxis for all travelers visiting from September through May and mosquito-avoidance measures for the rest of the year. CDC recommends chemoprophylaxis at all times of the year (see Chapter 3, Yellow Fever and Malaria Information, by Country).

Tick-bite fever caused by rickettsial species is common in South Africa and can result in severe and sometimes fatal complications. Hikers and campers in rural areas who are exposed to ticks are especially at risk. Measures should be taken to prevent tick bites (see Chapter 2, Protection against Mosquitoes, Ticks, and Other Insects and Arthropods). Doxycycline used for malaria prophylaxis will also protect against tick-bite fever. The use of antibiotics after a tick bite is not useful, because it prolongs the incubation period.

Waterborne Diseases

Schistosomiasis, a common parasite throughout Africa, may be present in any body of fresh water, such as lakes, streams, and dams. Travelers should avoid swimming in fresh, unchlorinated water. Those who swim in fresh water should have a serologic test 30 days after their return.

Animal Avoidance

While most travelers avoid wild animals in game reserves, it should be stressed that rabies is common in dogs and other animals throughout the country. Travelers may not be able to tell if an animal is infected and should avoid all contact with dogs and other animals. Any bite or scratch from an animal should be evaluated as soon as possible by a clinician. Rabies vaccine is

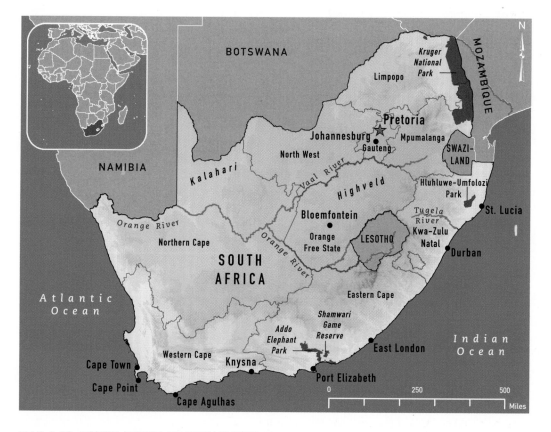

MAP 4-13. SOUTH AFRICA DESTINATION MAP

available throughout South Africa, and human rabies immune globulin is available in major urban medical centers. Appropriate postexposure medical care for rabies exposures can be obtained in South Africa.

Safety and Security

South Africa has struggled with a rise in violent crime, which includes armed robberies, carjackings, home invasions, and rape. Most of these incidents occur in poor areas and, as such, most visitors will not be affected. However, awareness of personal safety and security should be stressed to all visitors.

Although South Africa has a modern road system, drivers should be alert for dangerous driving practices, stray animals, and poor roads in remote rural areas.

BIBLIOGRAPHY

1. Durrheim DN, Braack LE, Waner S, Gammon S. Risk of malaria in visitors to the Kruger National Park, South Africa. J Travel Med. 1998 Dec;5(4):173–7.
2. Kruger National Park. Malaria situation in Kruger National Park. Available from: http://www.krugersafari.com/malaria2.html.
3. South Africa Department of Health. Guidelines for the prevention of malaria in South Africa. 2009. Available from: http://www.doh.gov.za/docs/factsheets/guidelines/prevention_malaria09.pdf.

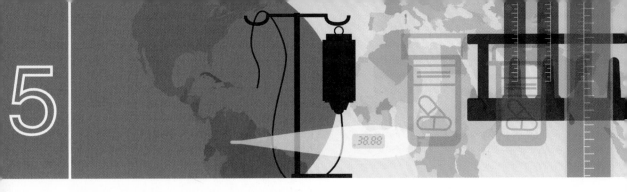

5

Post-Travel Evaluation

GENERAL APPROACH TO THE RETURNED TRAVELER

Carlos Franco-Paredes, Natasha Hochberg

ASSESSING RISK OF ILLNESS IN TRAVELERS

An estimated 15%–70% of international travelers returning to the United States have a travel-related illness. Most travel-related illnesses are mild, but 1%–5% of travelers become sick enough to seek medical care. Although some illnesses may begin during travel, others may occur weeks, months, or even years after return. Therefore, a history of travel, particularly within the previous 6 months, should be part of the routine medical history for every ill patient, especially those with a febrile illness. A detailed history can help assess the risk of illness in a returning traveler (Box 5-1). Clinicians should consider the public health implications of certain infections (such as tuberculosis, measles, and viral hemorrhagic fever) and notify appropriate public health authorities.

A newly returned, ill international traveler should be preferentially evaluated by a physician versed in travel-related illness. For example, a febrile patient should be seen by an infectious disease or tropical medicine specialist. For assistance in finding a provider who practices clinical tropical medicine, access the consultant directory of the American Society of Tropical Medicine and Hygiene website for a listing by country and state/province (www.astmh.org) or the searchable clinic directory of the International Society of Travel Medicine (www.istm.org). For assistance with the diagnosis and management of parasitic infections, the CDC's Division of Parasitic Diseases and Malaria's on-call clinicians can be reached by calling 770-488-7775 (non-malaria parasitic infections) or 770-488-7788 (malaria), during business hours. After business hours, on-call clinicians can be reached by calling CDC's Emergency Operations Center at 770-488-7100.

Particular groups of travelers are considered at higher risk for illness. Travelers visiting friends and relatives are often less likely to seek pre-travel advice, obtain vaccinations, or take antimalarial prophylaxis. Adventure travelers and people visiting friends and relatives are at increased risk for becoming ill, in part because of increased exposure to pathogens. Similarly, people with underlying immunocompromised status may be at increased risk of illness, as well as atypical manifestations of disease.

TYPES OF ILLNESSES AND CLINICAL PRESENTATIONS

The most frequent health problems in ill returned travelers are persistent

5

gastrointestinal illness (10%), skin lesions or rashes (8%), respiratory infections (5%–13%, depending on season of travel), and fever (up to 3%). A recent analysis of the GeoSentinel Surveillance Network has shown substantial regional differences in the morbidity of various syndromic categories in relation to place of exposure among ill returned travelers. For example, dermatologic problems were among the most frequent diagnoses among travelers returning from the Caribbean or Central or South America, but the diagnosis of acute diarrhea was more common for travelers returning from south-central Asia. Fever is a frequently reported complaint among returned travelers; 28% (6,957) of returned travelers seen at GeoSentinel clinics from March 1997 through March 2006 had fever as their chief reason for seeking medical care. Malaria was identified as 1 of the 3 most frequent causes of systemic febrile illness among travelers from any region.

Fever

Febrile illnesses are the most serious illnesses in travelers. Fever in a traveler returned from an area with malaria should be considered a medical emergency. The possibility of malaria as a cause of the fever should be evaluated urgently by appropriate laboratory tests and qualified personnel, and testing should be repeated if the initial result is negative. Every clinician dealing with a febrile returned traveler from an area with malaria should take steps to ensure the patient has serial blood smears evaluated on the day of presentation and should consider if there is any need for hospitalization observation.

The other most frequent "tropical" causes of fever in returned travelers are dengue, invasive bacterial diarrhea, hepatitis A, typhoid, and rickettsial infections. Other than malaria, travelers returning from sub-Saharan Africa were diagnosed most often with rickettsial infections, as well as typhoid and dengue. Nontropical illnesses, such as respiratory or urinary tract infections, also account for a large proportion of febrile illnesses in returned travelers.

In addition to a general physical examination, the clinician should look for any signs that may point to a cause of fever, including dermatologic findings (rash, insect or animal bites, eschar, localized swelling), central nervous system and ocular findings, pulmonary abnormalities, and coagulopathy. The initial evaluation of the febrile traveler should include a prompt evaluation for malaria, as well as other key tests as guided by signs and symptoms, relevant exposures, and duration of illness (Box 5-2). Acute- and convalescent-phase serologies may be needed to confirm particular diagnoses, including many rickettsial infections and dengue.

Empiric treatment for suspected serious illnesses such as malaria, leptospirosis, or rickettsial infections should always be considered when timely and accurate diagnostic testing is not available. All human malarias can be successfully treated by a course of atovaquone-proguanil or artemether-lumefantrine, and all leptospiral or rickettsial infections can be treated with doxycycline (see Chapter 3, Malaria).

Gastrointestinal Disease

Acute bacterial gastroenteritis and parasitic diarrhea, caused mostly by *Giardia*, are overall the most common conditions reported by travelers. Parasitic diarrhea may often present as intermittent diarrhea, nausea, headache, and fatigue but may also present with postprandial rapid expulsions of loose stool.

Persistent gastrointestinal illness in returned travelers is often caused by postinfectious irritable bowel syndrome and postinfectious lactose intolerance after an episode of travelers' diarrhea (see the Persistent Travelers' Diarrhea section later in this chapter). Rarely, postinfectious celiac sprue or postinfectious inflammatory bowel disease may occur after travelers have been ill with travelers' diarrhea. Intestinal parasitic infections are uncommon causes of persistent diarrhea, although infections such as giardiasis or cyclosporiasis are often treated on the basis of clinical findings (without the benefit of laboratory confirmation).

Dermatologic Conditions

Dermatologic conditions are a very common cause of post-travel concerns, as well. Most post-travel skin ailments reported are insect bites, pyoderma, scabies, and cutaneous larva migrans.

Eosinophilia

Marked eosinophilia in a returning traveler usually indicates infection with a helminth. Diagnoses to be considered in travelers with moderate to marked eosinophilia (>1,000 eosinophils/mm³) include acute schistosomiasis or strongyloidiasis, toxocariasis, acute trichinellosis, lymphatic filariasis, loiasis, onchocerciasis, tropical pulmonary eosinophilia, fascioliasis, gnathostomiasis, angiostrongyliasis, and the larval migration of ascariasis, paragonimiasis, and hookworm.

Nonparasitic infectious causes of eosinophilia include HIV, human T-cell lymphotropic virus type 1, coccidioidomycosis, allergic bronchopulmonary aspergillosis, *Mycobacterium tuberculosis*, *Treponema pallidum*, and *Bartonella henselae*.

ASSESSING RISK BY INCUBATION PERIOD

Most travelers infected abroad become ill within 12 weeks after returning to the United States. However, some infections may not cause symptoms for as long as 6–12 months or more after exposure (Table 5-1). When an infectious disease is suspected, calculating an approximate incubation period is a useful step in ruling out possible causes. For example, fever beginning ≥3 weeks after return substantially reduces the probability of

---

BOX 5-2. INITIAL EVALUATION OF FEBRILE RETURNING TRAVELERS

- Multiple peripheral blood smears or rapid diagnostic tests ("dipsticks") for malaria
- Complete blood cell count with differential
- Liver enzymes
- Urinalysis
- Culture of blood, stool, and urine
- Chest radiography
- Consider specific diagnostic assays for diseases such as leptospirosis (serology) and acute HIV infection (RNA viral load)

Table 5-1. Incubation periods of frequent febrile syndromes in returned travelers

INCUBATION PERIOD	SYNDROME	POSSIBLE CAUSE
<2 weeks	Fever with initial nonspecific signs and symptoms	Malaria, dengue, scrub typhus, spotted-fever group rickettsiae, acute HIV, campylobacteriosis, salmonellosis, shigellosis, East African trypanosomiasis, leptospirosis, relapsing fever, typhoid fever
	Fever and coagulopathy	Meningococcemia, leptospirosis and other bacterial pathogens associated with coagulopathy, malaria, viral hemorrhagic fevers
	Fever and central nervous system involvement	Malaria, typhoid fever, rickettsial typhus (epidemic caused by *Rickettsia prowazekii*), meningococcal meningitis, rabies, arboviral encephalitis, East African trypanosomiasis, encephalitis or meningitis due to known pathogens with worldwide distribution, angiostrongyliasis, polio
	Fever and pulmonary involvement	Influenza, pneumonia due to typical pathogens, *Legionella* pneumonia, acute histoplasmosis, acute coccidioidomycosis, Q fever, SARS, malaria
	Fever and skin rash	Viral exanthems (rubella, varicella, measles, mumps, herpes simplex-6), dengue, spotted-fever or typhus group rickettsiosis, typhoid fever, parvovirus B19, HIV infection
2–6 weeks	Various syndromes (fever with pulmonary, dermatologic, central nervous system, or involvement of other sites)	Malaria, tuberculosis, hepatitis A, hepatitis B, acute hepatitis C, hepatitis E, visceral leishmaniasis, acute schistosomiasis, amebic liver abscess, leptospirosis, African trypanosomiasis, viral hemorrhagic fevers, Q fever, acute American trypanosomiasis (Chagas disease), measles, typhoid fever
>6 weeks	Various syndromes (fever with pulmonary, dermatologic, central nervous system, or involvement of other sites)	Malaria, tuberculosis, hepatitis B, acute hepatitis C, hepatitis E, visceral leishmaniasis, filariasis, onchocerciasis, schistosomiasis, amebic liver abscess, chronic mycoses, African trypanosomiasis, rabies

5

dengue, rickettsial infections, and viral hemorrhagic fevers in the differential diagnosis. Late-appearing illnesses include chronic forms of Chagas disease, cutaneous and mucocutaneous leishmaniasis, chronic forms of brucellosis, reactivation of tuberculosis from travel-acquired latent tuberculosis infection, malaria, sequelae of schistosomiasis, and reactivation of chronic systemic mycoses, such as paracoccidioidomycosis or coccidioidomycosis.

BIBLIOGRAPHY

1. Angell SY, Behrens RH. Risk assessment and disease prevention in travelers visiting friends and relatives. Infect Dis Clin North Am. 2005 Mar;19(1):49–65.

2. Bacaner N, Stauffer B, Boulware DR, Walker PF, Keystone JS. Travel medicine considerations for North American immigrants visiting friends and relatives. JAMA. 2004 Jun 16;291(23):2856–64.

3. Basnyat B, Maskey AP, Zimmerman MD, Murdoch DR. Enteric (typhoid) fever in travelers. Clin Infect Dis. 2005 Nov 15;41(10):1467–72.

4. Connor BA. Sequelae of traveler's diarrhea: focus on postinfectious irritable bowel syndrome. Clin Infect Dis. 2005 Dec 1;41 Suppl 8:S577–86.

5. Franco-Paredes C, keystone J. Fever in the returned traveler. In Yu VL, Burdette SD editors. Antimicrobial Therapy and Vaccines: Empiric 2008. Available from: http://www.antimicrobe.org/mycinsearch/atvempiric2.asp.

6. Freedman DO, Leder K. Influenza: changing approaches to prevention and treatment in travelers. J Travel Med. 2005 Jan–Feb;12(1):36–44.

7. Freedman DO, Weld LH, Kozarsky PE, Fisk T, Robins R, von Sonnenburg F, et al. Spectrum of disease and relation to place of exposure among ill returned travelers. N Engl J Med. 2006 Jan 12;354(2):119–30.

8. Hill DR. The burden of illness in international travelers. N Engl J Med. 2006 Jan 12;354(2):115–7.

9. Hill DR. Health problems in a large cohort of Americans traveling to developing countries. J Travel Med. 2000 Sep–Oct;7(5):259–66.

10. Jensenius M, Fournier PE, Raoult D. Rickettsioses and the international traveler. Clin Infect Dis. 2004 Nov 15;39(10):1493–9.

11. Leder K, Sundararajan V, Weld L, Pandey P, Brown G, Torresi J. Respiratory tract infections in travelers: a review of the GeoSentinel surveillance network. Clin Infect Dis. 2003 Feb 15;36(4):399–406.

12. Leder K, Tong S, Weld L, Kain KC, Wilder-Smith A, von Sonnenburg F, et al. Illness in travelers visiting friends and relatives: a review of the GeoSentinel Surveillance Network. Clin Infect Dis. 2006 Nov 1;43(9):1185–93.

13. Mutsch M, Spicher VM, Gut C, Steffen R. Hepatitis A virus infections in travelers, 1988–2004. Clin Infect Dis. 2006 Feb 15;42(4):490–7.

14. Mutsch M, Tavernini M, Marx A, Gregory V, Lin YP, Hay AJ, et al. Influenza virus infection in travelers to tropical and subtropical countries. Clin Infect Dis. 2005 May 1;40(9):1282–7.

15. O'Brien D, Tobin S, Brown GV, Torresi J. Fever in returned travelers: review of hospital admissions for a 3-year period. Clin Infect Dis. 2001 Sep 1;33(5):603–9.

16. Ryan ET, Wilson ME, Kain KC. Illness after international travel. N Engl J Med. 2002 Aug 15;347(7):505–16.

17. Schwartz E, Kozarsky P, Wilson M, Cetron M. Schistosome infection among river rafters on Omo River, Ethiopia. J Travel Med. 2005 Jan–Feb;12(1):3–8.

18. Steffen R, Rickenbach M, Wilhelm U, Helminger A, Schar M. Health problems after travel to developing countries. J Infect Dis. 1987 Jul;156(1):84–91.

19. Wilson ME, Chen LH. Dermatologic infectious diseases in international travelers. Curr Infect Dis Rep. 2004 Feb;6(1):54–62.

20. Wilson ME, Weld LH, Boggild A, Keystone JS, Kain KC, von Sonnenburg F, et al. Fever in returned travelers: results from the GeoSentinel Surveillance Network. Clin Infect Dis. 2007 Jun 15;44(12):1560–8.

FEVER IN RETURNED TRAVELERS

Mary Elizabeth Wilson

INITIAL FOCUS

Fever commonly accompanies serious illness in returned travelers. Because it can signal a rapidly progressive infection, such as malaria, the clinician must initiate early evaluation, especially in people who have visited areas with malaria in recent months (see Chapter 3, Malaria). The initial focus in evaluating a febrile returned traveler should be on identifying infections that are rapidly progressive, treatable, or transmissible. In some instances, public health officials must be alerted if the traveler may have been contagious en route or infected with a pathogen of public health importance (such as yellow fever) at the origin or destination.

USE OF HISTORY, LOCATION OF EXPOSURE, AND INCUBATION TO LIMIT DIFFERENTIAL DIAGNOSIS

Often the list of potential diagnoses is long, but multiple recent studies help to identify more common diagnoses. A significant proportion of illnesses in returned travelers is caused by common, cosmopolitan infections (such as bacterial pneumonia or pyelonephritis), so these must be considered along with unusual infections. Because the geographic area of travel determines the relative likelihood of major causes of fever, it is essential to identify where the febrile patient has traveled and lived (Table 5-2). Details about activities (such as freshwater exposure in

Table 5-2. Common causes of fever, by geographic area

GEOGRAPHIC AREA	MORE COMMON TROPICAL DISEASE CAUSING FEVER	OTHER INFECTIONS CAUSING OUTBREAKS OR CLUSTERS IN TRAVELERS
Caribbean	Dengue, malaria	Acute histoplasmosis, leptospirosis
Central America	Dengue, malaria (primarily *Plasmodium vivax*)	Leptospirosis, histoplasmosis, coccidioidomycosis
South America	Dengue, malaria (primarily *vivax*)	Bartonellosis, leptospirosis
South-central Asia	Dengue, enteric fever, malaria (primarily non-falciparum)	Chikungunya virus infection
Southeast Asia	Dengue, malaria (primarily non-falciparum)	Chikungunya virus infection, leptospirosis
Sub-Saharan Africa	Malaria (primarily *P. falciparum*), tickborne rickettsiae, acute schistosomiasis, filariasis	African trypanosomiasis

schistosomiasis-endemic areas, animal bites, sexual activities, or local medical care with injections) and accommodations in areas with malaria (bed nets, window screens, air conditioning) during travel may provide useful clues. Preparation before travel (such as hepatitis A vaccine or yellow fever vaccine) will markedly reduce the likelihood of some infections, so this is a relevant part of the history.

Because each infection has a characteristic incubation period (although the range is extremely wide with some infections), the time of exposures needs to be defined in different geographic areas (Table 5-3). This knowledge may allow the clinician to exclude some infections from the differential diagnosis. Most serious febrile infections manifest within the first month after return from tropical travel, yet infections related to travel exposures can occasionally occur months or even more than a year after return. In the United States, >90% of reported cases of *Plasmodium falciparum* malaria manifest within 30 days

Table 5-3. Common infections, by incubation periods

DISEASE	USUAL INCUBATION PERIOD (RANGE)	DISTRIBUTION
Incubation <14 Days		
Chikungunya	2–4 days (1–14 days)	Tropics, subtropics (Eastern Hemisphere)
Dengue	4–8 days (3–14 days)	Tropics, subtropics
Encephalitis, arboviral (Japanese encephalitis, tickborne encephalitis, West Nile virus, other)	3–14 days (1–20 days)	Specific agents vary by region
Enteric fever	7–18 days (3–60 days)	Especially in Indian subcontinent
Acute HIV	10–28 days (10 days to 6 weeks)	Worldwide
Influenza	1–3 days	Worldwide, can also be acquired en route
Legionellosis	5–6 days (2–10 days)	Widespread
Leptospirosis	7–12 days (2–26 days)	Widespread, most common in tropical areas
Malaria, *Plasmodium falciparum*	6–30 days (weeks to years)	Tropics, subtropics
Malaria, *P. vivax*	8–30 days (often >1 month)	Widespread in tropics and subtropics
Spotted-fever rickettsiae	Few days to 2–3 weeks	Causative species vary by region

continued

TABLE 5-3. COMMON INFECTIONS, BY INCUBATION PERIODS (continued)

DISEASE	USUAL INCUBATION PERIOD (RANGE)	DISTRIBUTION
Incubation 14 Days to 6 Weeks		
Enteric fever, leptospirosis, malaria	See above incubation periods for relevant diseases	See above distribution for relevant diseases
Amebic liver abscess	Weeks to months	Most common in developing countries
Hepatitis A	28–30 days (15–50 days)	Most common in developing countries
Hepatitis E	26–42 days (2–9 weeks)	Widespread
Acute schistosomiasis (Katayama syndrome)	4–8 weeks	Most common in sub-Saharan Africa
Incubation >6 Weeks		
Amebic liver abscess, hepatitis B, hepatitis E, malaria	See above incubation periods for relevant diseases	See above distribution for relevant diseases
Leishmaniasis, visceral	2–10 months (10 days to years)	Asia, Africa, Latin America, southern Europe, and the Middle East
Tuberculosis	Primary, weeks; reactivation, years	Global distribution, rates and levels of resistance vary widely

5

of return, but almost half of cases of P. vivax malaria manifest >30 days after return. A history of travel and residence should be an integral part of every medical history.

FINDINGS REQUIRING URGENT ATTENTION

Presence of associated signs, symptoms, or laboratory findings can focus attention on specific infections (Table 5-4). Findings that should prompt urgent attention include hemorrhage, neurologic impairment, and acute respiratory distress. Even if an initial physical examination is unremarkable, it is worth repeating the examination, as new findings may appear that will help in the diagnostic process (such as skin lesions or tender liver). Although most febrile illnesses in returned travelers are related to infections, the clinician should bear in mind that other problems, including pulmonary emboli and drug hypersensitivity reactions, can be associated with fever. See Box 5-2 for a list of initial studies for diagnosing patients with unexplained fever.

CDC's Division of Global Migration and Quarantine is responsible for preventing the transmission of illnesses across international borders and, in particular, for preventing transmission of such illnesses into the United

Table 5-4. Common clinical findings and associated infections

COMMON CLINICAL FINDINGS	INFECTIONS TO CONSIDER AFTER TROPICAL TRAVEL
Fever and rash	Dengue, chikungunya, rickettsial infections, enteric fever (skin lesions may be sparse or absent), acute HIV infection, measles
Fever and abdominal pain	Enteric fever, amebic liver abscess
Undifferentiated fever and normal or low white blood cell count	Dengue, malaria, rickettsial infection, enteric fever, chikungunya
Fever and hemorrhage	Viral hemorrhagic fevers (dengue and others), meningococcemia, leptospirosis, rickettsial infections
Fever and eosinophilia	Acute schistosomiasis, drug hypersensitivity reaction, fascioliasis and other parasitic infections (rare)
Fever and pulmonary infiltrates	Common bacterial and viral pathogens, legionellosis, acute schistosomiasis, Q fever
Fever and altered mental status	Cerebral malaria, viral or bacterial meningoencephalitis, African trypanosomiasis
Mononucleosis syndrome	Epstein-Barr virus, cytomegalovirus, toxoplasmosis, acute HIV
Fever persisting >2 weeks	Malaria, enteric fever, Epstein-Barr virus, cytomegalovirus, toxoplasmosis, acute HIV, acute schistosomiasis, brucellosis, tuberculosis, Q fever, visceral leishmaniasis (rare)
Fever with onset >6 weeks after travel	*Plasmodium vivax* malaria, acute hepatitis (B, C, or E), tuberculosis, amebic liver abscess

States. Fever accompanied by any of the following syndromes deserves further scrutiny, because it may indicate a disease of public health importance:

- Skin rash
- Difficulty breathing
- Shortness of breath
- Persistent cough
- Decreased consciousness
- Bruising or unusual bleeding (without previous injury)
- Persistent diarrhea
- Persistent vomiting (other than air or motion sickness)
- Jaundice
- Paralysis of recent onset

People who travel to visit friends and relatives (VFRs) often do not seek pre-travel medical advice. A review of GeoSentinel surveillance data showed that a larger proportion of immigrant VFRs than tourist travelers presented with serious (requiring hospitalization), potentially preventable travel-related illnesses.

CHANGE OVER TIME

Clinicians have access to resources on the Internet that provide information about geographic-specific risks, disease activity, and other useful information, such as drug-susceptibility patterns for pathogens. Infectious diseases are dynamic, as is demonstrated by a review of adult returned travelers with fever and rash seen in 2006 and 2007 at a Paris hospital. The most common diagnosis was chikungunya fever, followed by dengue and African tick-bite fever. In contrast, because of the wide use of vaccine, hepatitis A infection is becoming less common in travelers.

Common infections in returned travelers may be seen at unexpected times of the year. Because influenza transmission can occur throughout the year in tropical areas, and the peak season in the Southern Hemisphere is May to August, clinicians in the Northern Hemisphere must be alert to the possibility of influenza outside the usual influenza season.

The tables in this section identify some common infections by presenting findings or other characteristics by area of travel and by incubation periods. These highlight only the most common infections. The listed references and websites should be consulted for more detailed information. In most studies, a specific cause for fever is not identified in about 25% of returned travelers.

KEEP IN MIND
- Initial symptoms of life-threatening and self-limited infections can be identical.

- Fever in returned travelers is often caused by common, cosmopolitan infections, such as pneumonia and pyelonephritis, which should not be overlooked in the search for more exotic diagnoses.
- Patients with malaria may be afebrile at the time of evaluation but typically give a history of chills.
- Malaria is the most common cause of acute undifferentiated fever after travel to sub-Saharan Africa and to some other tropical areas.
- Malaria, especially *P. falciparum*, can progress rapidly. Diagnostic studies should be done promptly and treatment instituted immediately if malaria is diagnosed (see Chapter 3, Malaria).
- A history of taking malaria chemoprophylaxis does not exclude the possibility of malaria.
- Patients with malaria can have prominent respiratory (including acute respiratory distress syndrome), gastrointestinal, or central nervous system findings.
- Viral hemorrhagic fevers are important to identify but are rare in travelers; bacterial infections, such as leptospirosis, meningococcemia, and rickettsial infections, can also cause fever and hemorrhage and should be always be considered because of the need to institute prompt, specific treatment.
- Sexually transmitted diseases, including acute HIV, can cause acute febrile infections.
- Consider infection control, public health implications, and requirements for reportable diseases.

BIBLIOGRAPHY

1. Bottieau E, Clerinx J, Schrooten W, Van den Enden E, Wouters R, Van Esbroeck M, et al. Etiology and outcome of fever after a stay in the tropics. Arch Intern Med. 2006 Aug 14–28;166(15):1642–8.
2. Bottieau E, Clerinx J, Van den Enden E, Van Esbroeck M, Colebunders R, Van Gompel A, et al. Infectious mononucleosis-like syndromes in febrile travelers returning from the tropics. J Travel Med. 2006 Jul–Aug;13(4):191–7.
3. Freedman DO, Weld LH, Kozarsky PE, Fisk T, Robins R, von Sonnenburg F, et al. Spectrum of disease and relation to place of exposure among ill returned travelers. N Engl J Med. 2006 Jan 12;354(2):119–30.
4. Hochedez P, Canestri A, Guihot A, Brichler S, Bricaire F, Caumes E. Management of travelers with fever and exanthema, notably dengue and chikungunya infections. Am J Trop Med Hyg. 2008 May;78(5):710–3.
5. Jensenius M, Davis X, von Sonnenburg F, Schwartz E, Keystone JS, Leder K, et al. Multicenter GeoSentinel analysis of rickettsial diseases in international travelers, 1996–2008. Emerg Infect Dis. 2009 Nov;15(11):1791–8.
6. Jensenius M, Fournier PE, Raoult D. Rickettsioses and the international traveler. Clin Infect Dis. 2004 Nov 15;39(10):1493–9.
7. Leder K, Tong S, Weld L, Kain KC, Wilder-Smith A, von Sonnenburg F, et al. Illness in travelers visiting friends and relatives: a review of the GeoSentinel Surveillance Network. Clin Infect Dis. 2006 Nov 1;43(9):1185–93.

8. O'Brien D, Tobin S, Brown GV, Torresi J. Fever in returned travelers: review of hospital admissions for a 3-year period. Clin Infect Dis. 2001 Sep 1;33(5):603–9.

9. Ryan ET, Wilson ME, Kain KC. Illness after international travel. N Engl J Med. 2002 Aug 15;347(7):505–16.

10. Wilson ME, Freedman DO. Etiology of travel-related fever. Curr Opin Infect Dis. 2007 Oct;20(5):449–53.

11. Wilson ME, Weld LH, Boggild A, Keystone JS, Kain KC, von Sonnenburg F, et al. Fever in returned travelers: results from the GeoSentinel Surveillance Network. Clin Infect Dis. 2007 Jun 15;44(12):1560–8.

PERSISTENT TRAVELERS' DIARRHEA

Bradley A. Connor

Although most cases of travelers' diarrhea are acute and self-limited, a certain percentage of travelers will develop persistent (>14 days) gastrointestinal symptoms (see Chapter 2, Travelers' Diarrhea). Persistent diarrhea is often associated with enteropathy and consequent malabsorption. This may lead to malnutrition, particularly among young children and the immunosuppressed. The pathogenesis of persistent travelers' diarrhea generally falls into one of the following broad categories: 1) persistent infection or coinfection, 2) chronic underlying gastrointestinal disease unmasked by the enteric infection, or 3) a postinfectious phenomenon.

PERSISTENT INFECTION

Most cases of travelers' diarrhea are the result of bacterial infection and are short-lived and self-limited. Travelers may experience prolonged diarrheal symptoms if they are immunosuppressed, are infected sequentially with diarrheal pathogens, or are infected with protozoan parasites. Parasites as a group are the pathogens most likely to be isolated from patients with persistent diarrhea, and their probability relative to bacterial infections increases with increasing duration of symptoms. Parasites may also be the cause of persistent diarrhea in patients already appropriately treated for a bacterial pathogen.

Giardia is by far the most likely persistent pathogen to be encountered. Suspicion for giardiasis should be particularly high when upper gastrointestinal symptoms predominate. Untreated, symptoms may last for months, even in immunocompetent hosts. The diagnosis can often be made through stool microscopy, antigen detection, or immunofluorescence. However, as *Giardia* infects the proximal small bowel, even multiple stool specimens may fail to detect it, and a duodenal aspirate may be necessary for definitive diagnosis. Given the high prevalence of *Giardia* in persistent travelers' diarrhea, empiric therapy is a reasonable option in the appropriate clinical setting after negative stool microscopy and in lieu of duodenal sampling (Table 5-5). Other intestinal parasites that may cause persistent symptoms include *Cryptosporidium* species, *Entamoeba histolytica*, *Isospora belli*, *Microsporidia*, *Dientamoeba fragilis*, and *Cyclospora cayetanensis*.

Individual bacterial infections rarely cause persistence of symptoms, although persistent diarrhea has been reported in children infected with enteroaggregative or enteropathogenic *Escherichia coli* and among people with diarrhea due to *Clostridium difficile*. C. *difficile*–associated diarrhea may follow treatment of a bacterial pathogen with a fluoroquinolone or other antibiotic, or may even follow malaria chemoprophylaxis. This is especially important to consider in the patient with persistent travelers' diarrhea that seems refractory to multiple courses of empiric antibiotic therapy. The initial work-up of persistent travelers' diarrhea should always include a C. *difficile* stool toxin assay. Treatment is with metronidazole or oral vancomycin, although increasing reports of resistance to both have been noted.

Persistent travelers' diarrhea has also been associated with tropical sprue and Brainerd diarrhea. These syndromes are suspected to result from infectious diseases, but specific pathogens have not been identified. Tropical sprue is associated with deficiencies of vitamins absorbed in the proximal and distal small bowel and most commonly affects long-term travelers to tropical areas. Investigation of an outbreak of Brainerd diarrhea among passengers on a cruise ship to the Galápagos Islands of Ecuador revealed that diarrhea persisted 7 to more than 42 months and did not respond to antimicrobial therapy.

UNDERLYING GASTROINTESTINAL DISEASE

In some cases, persistence of gastrointestinal symptoms relates to chronic underlying gastrointestinal disease or susceptibility unmasked by the enteric infection. Most prominent among these is celiac sprue, a systemic disease manifesting primarily with small bowel changes. In genetically susceptible people, villous atrophy and crypt hyperplasia are seen in response to exposure to antigens found in wheat, leading to malabsorption. The diagnosis is made by obtaining appropriate serologic tests, including tissue transglutaminase antibodies. A biopsy of the small bowel showing villous atrophy confirms the diagnosis. Treatment is with a wheat (gluten)-free diet.

Idiopathic inflammatory bowel disease, both Crohn's disease and ulcerative colitis, may be seen after acute bouts of travelers' diarrhea. One prevailing hypothesis is that an initiating endogenous pathogen triggers inflammatory bowel disease in genetically susceptible people.

In the appropriate clinical setting and age group, it may be necessary to do a more comprehensive search for other underlying causes of chronic diarrhea. Colorectal cancer should be considered, particularly in patients passing occult or gross blood rectally or with the onset of a new iron-deficiency anemia.

POSTINFECTIOUS PHENOMENA

In a certain percentage of patients who present with persistent gastrointestinal symptoms, no specific source will be found.

Patients may experience temporary enteropathy following an acute diarrheal infection, with villous atrophy, decreased absorptive surface area, and disaccharidase deficiencies. This can lead to osmotic diarrhea, particularly when large amounts of lactose, sucrose, sorbitol, or fructose are consumed. Use of antimicrobial medications during the initial days of diarrhea may also lead to alterations in intestinal flora and diarrhea symptoms.

Occasionally, the onset of symptoms of irritable bowel syndrome (IBS) can be traced to an acute bout of gastroenteritis. IBS that develops after acute enteritis has been termed postinfectious (PI)-IBS. In the context of travelers' diarrhea, PI-IBS has been defined as new IBS symptoms by the Rome III criteria:

- ≥3 months of gastrointestinal symptoms, with an onset of symptoms ≥6 months previously.
- Recurrent abdominal pain or discomfort associated with ≥2 of the following features:
  > Improvement with defecation
  > Onset associated with a change in the frequency of stool
  > Onset associated with a change in form (appearance) of stool
- To be labeled PI-IBS, these symptoms should follow an episode of gastroenteritis or travelers' diarrhea if the work-up for microbial pathogens and underlying gastrointestinal disease is negative.

EVALUATION

The hydration and nutritional status of patients with persistent travelers' diarrhea should be assessed. Three or more stool examinations for ova and parasites, including acid-fast stains for *Cryptosporidium*, *Cyclospora*, and *Isospora*; *Giardia* antigen testing; *Clostridium difficile* toxin assay; D-xylose test; tests for stool reducing substances; and duodenal aspirates, may be performed. Fecal lactoferrin testing or microscopy for fecal leukocytes is often present with more severe C. *difficile* colitis and IBS, and noninflammatory diarrhea suggests giardiasis. Patients may also be given empiric treatment for *Giardia* infection. If underlying gastrointestinal disease is suspected, an initial evaluation should include serologic tests for celiac and inflammatory bowel disease. Subsequently, gastrointestinal endoscopy with duodenal aspirate and biopsies may be considered.

MANAGEMENT

Although US travelers are unlikely to become significantly dehydrated or malnourished due to persistent diarrhea, appropriate hydration and nutritional support are of foremost importance. Dietary modifications may help those with malabsorption. If stools are bloody or when disease is caused by *C. difficile*, antidiarrheal medications should not be used in children and should be used cautiously, if at all, in adults. Probiotic medications have been shown to reduce the duration of persistent diarrhea among children in some settings. Antimicrobial medications may be useful in treating persistent diarrhea caused by parasites (Table 5-5). Additional management strategies will depend on the specific cause of persistent diarrhea.

Table 5-5. Treatment of common intestinal protozoan parasites

PARASITE	DISEASE SEVERITY OR INDICATION	DRUG OF CHOICE	ALTERNATIVE DRUGS
Amebiasis (*Entamoeba histolytica*)	Asymptomatic	**Iodoquinol** Adults: 650 mg PO tid × 20 d Pediatric: 30–40 mg/kg/d (max 2 g) PO in 3 doses × 20 d	**Paromomycin** Adults: 25–35 mg/kg/d PO in 3 doses × 7 d Pediatric: 25–35 mg/kg/d PO in 3 doses × 7 d *or* **Diloxanide furoate** Adults: 500 mg PO tid × 10 d Pediatric: 20 mg/kg/d PO in 3 doses × 10 d
	Mild to moderate intestinal disease	1) *Initial:* **Metronidazole** Adults: 500–750 mg PO tid × 7–10 d Pediatric: 35–50 mg/kg/d PO in 3 doses × 7–10 d 2) *Followed by:* **Iodoquinol** Adults: 650 mg PO tid × 20 d Pediatric: 30–40 mg/kg/d (max 2 g) PO in 3 doses × 20 d	1) *Initial:* **Tinidazole** Adults: 2 g PO qd × 5 d Pediatric (age >3 y): 50 mg/kg/d (max 2 g) PO in 1 dose × 3 d 2) *Followed by:* **Paromomycin** Adults: 25–35 mg/kg/d PO in 3 doses × 7 d Pediatric: 25–35 mg/kg/d PO in 3 doses × 7 d
	Severe intestinal and extraintestinal disease	1) *Initial:* **Metronidazole** Adults: 750 mg PO tid × 7–10 d Pediatric: 35–50 mg/kg/d PO in 3 doses × 7–10 d 2) *Followed by:* **Iodoquinol** Adults: 650 mg PO tid × 20 d Pediatric: 30–40 mg/kg/d (max 2 g) PO in 3 doses × 20 d	1) *Initial:* **Tinidazole** Adults: 2 g PO qd × 5 d Pediatric (age >3 y): 50 mg/kg/d (max 2 g) PO in 1 dose × 3 d 2) *Followed by:* **Paromomycin** Adults: 25–35 mg/kg/d PO in 3 doses × 7 d Pediatric: 25–35 mg/kg/d PO in 3 doses × 7 d

continued

TABLE 5-5. TREATMENT OF COMMON INTESTINAL PROTOZOAN PARASITES (continued)

PARASITE	DISEASE SEVERITY OR INDICATION	DRUG OF CHOICE	ALTERNATIVE DRUGS
Cryptosporidiosis (*Cryptosporidium*)	HIV-uninfected (nitazoxanide has not been shown to have efficacy in immunosuppressed people)	**Nitazoxanide** Adults: 500 mg PO bid × 3 d Age 1–3 y: 100 mg PO bid × 3 d Age 4–11 y: 200 mg PO bid × 3 d Age 12–18 y: 500 mg PO q12h × 3 d	
Cyclosporiasis (*Cyclospora cayetanensis*)		**Trimethoprim/ sulfamethoxazole** Adults: TMP 160 mg/SMX 800 mg (1 DS tab) PO bid × 7–10 d Pediatric: TMP 5 mg/kg/d/ SMX 25 mg/kg/d PO in 2 doses × 7–10 d	
Dientamoebiasis (*Dientamoeba fragilis*)		**Iodoquinol** Adults: 650 mg PO tid × 20 d Pediatric: 30–40 mg/kg/d (max 2 g) PO in 3 doses × 20 d	**Paromomycin** Adults: 25–35 mg/kg/d PO in 3 doses × 7 d Pediatric: 25–35 mg/kg/d PO in 3 doses × 7 d *or* **Tetracycline** Adults: 500 mg PO qid × 10 d Pediatric: 40 mg/kg/d (max 2 g) PO in 4 doses × 10 d *or* **Metronidazole** Adults: 500–750 mg PO tid × 10 d Pediatric: 35–50 mg/kg/d PO in 3 doses × 10 d
Giardiasis (*Giardia intestinalis*)		**Metronidazole** Adults: 250 mg PO tid × 5–7 d Pediatric: 15 mg/kg/d PO in 3 doses × 5–7 d *or* **Tinidazole** Adults: 2 g PO once Pediatric: 50 mg/kg PO once (max 2 g) *or* **Nitazoxanide** Adults: 500 mg PO bid × 3 d Age 1–3 y: 100 mg PO q12h × 3 d Age 4–11 y: 200 mg PO q12h × 3 d Age 12–18 y: 500 mg PO q12h × 3 d	**Paromomycin** Adults: 25–35 mg/kg/d PO in 3 doses × 5–10 d Pediatric: 25–35 mg/kg/d PO in 3 doses × 5–10 d *or* **Furazolidone** Adults: 100 mg PO qid × 7–10 d Pediatric: 6 mg/kg/d PO in 4 doses × 7–10 d *or* **Quinacrine** Adults: 100 mg PO tid × 5 d Pediatric: 2 mg/kg/d PO in 3 doses × 5 d (max 300 mg/d)

continued

TABLE 5-5. TREATMENT OF COMMON INTESTINAL PROTOZOAN PARASITES (continued)

PARASITE	DISEASE SEVERITY OR INDICATION	DRUG OF CHOICE	ALTERNATIVE DRUGS
Isosporiasis (*Isospora belli*)		**Trimethoprim/ sulfamethoxazole** Adults: TMP 160 mg/SMX 800 mg (1 DS tab) PO bid × 10 d Pediatric: TMP 5 mg/kg/d/ SMX 25 mg/kg/d PO in 2 doses × 10 d	
Microsporidiosis	Intestinal (*Enterocytozoon bieneusi*, *Encephalitozoon* [*Septata*] *intestinalis*)	Drug of choice for *E. bieneusi*: **Fumagillin** Adults: 20 mg PO tid × 14 d Drug of choice for *E. intestinalis*: **Albendazole** Adults: 400 mg PO bid × 21 d	

BIBLIOGRAPHY

1. Connor BA. Sequelae of traveler's diarrhea: focus on postinfectious irritable bowel syndrome. Clin Infect Dis. 2005 Dec 1;41 Suppl 8:S577–86.
2. Green PH, Jabri B. Coeliac disease. Lancet. 2003 Aug 2;362(9381):383–91.
3. Guerrant RL, Van Gilder T, Steiner TS, Thielman NM, Slutsker L, Tauxe RV, et al. Practice guidelines for the management of infectious diarrhea. Clin Infect Dis. 2001;32:331–50.
4. Jung IS, Kim HS, Park H, Lee SI. The clinical course of postinfectious irritable bowel syndrome: a five-year follow-up study. J Clin Gastroenterol. 2009 Jul;43(6):534–40.
5. Norman FF, Perez-Molina J, Perez de Ayala A, Jimenez BC, Navarro M, Lopez-Velez R. *Clostridium difficile*-associated diarrhea after antibiotic treatment for traveler's diarrhea. Clin Infect Dis. 2008 Apr 1;46(7):1060–3.
6. Osterholm MT, MacDonald KL, White KE, Wells JG, Spika JS, Potter ME, et al. An outbreak of a newly recognized chronic diarrhea syndrome associated with raw milk consumption. JAMA. 1986 Jul 25;256(4):484–90.
7. Porter CK, Tribble DR, Aliaga PA, Halvorson HA, Riddle MS. Infectious gastroenteritis and risk of developing inflammatory bowel disease. Gastroenterology. 2008 Sep;135(3):781–6.
8. Spiller R, Garsed K. Postinfectious irritable bowel syndrome. Gastroenterology. 2009 May;136(6):1979–88.
9. Spiller RC, Jenkins D, Thornley JP, Hebden JM, Wright T, Skinner M, et al. Increased rectal mucosal enteroendocrine cells, T lymphocytes, and increased gut permeability following acute *Campylobacter* enteritis and in post-dysenteric irritable bowel syndrome. Gut. 2000 Dec;47(6):804–11.
10. Taylor DN, Connor BA, Shlim DR. Chronic diarrhea in the returned traveler. Med Clin North Am. 1999 Jul;83(4):1033–52, vii.
11. Walker MM. What is tropical sprue? J Gastroenterol Hepatol. 2003 Aug;18(8):887–90.

SKIN & SOFT TISSUE INFECTIONS IN RETURNED TRAVELERS

Jay S. Keystone

DESCRIPTION

Skin problems are one of the most frequent medical problems in returned travelers. The largest case series of dermatologic problems in returned travelers from the GeoSentinel surveillance network showed that cutaneous larva migrans, insect bites, and bacterial infections were the most frequent skin problems in returned travelers, making up 30% of the 4,742 diagnoses (Table 5-6). In another review of 165 travelers who returned to France with skin problems, cellulitis, scabies,

Table 5-6. Skin lesions in returned travelers, by cause[1]

SKIN LESION	PERCENTAGE (N = 4,742)
Cutaneous larva migrans	9.8
Insect bite	8.2
Skin abscess	7.7
Superinfected insect bite	6.8
Allergic rash	5.5
Rash, unknown origin	5.5
Dog bite	4.3
Superficial fungal infection	4.0
Dengue	3.4
Leishmaniasis	3.3
Myiasis	2.7
Spotted-fever group rickettsiae	1.5
Scabies	1.5

[1] Modified from Lederman ER, Weld LH, Elyazar IR, et al. Dermatologic conditions of the ill returned traveler: an analysis from the GeoSentinel Surveillance Network. Int J Infect Dis. 2008;12(6):593–602.

and pyoderma led the list of skin conditions. These data are biased in that they do not include skin problems that were diagnosed and, in many cases, easily managed during travel or that were self-limited.

Skin problems generally fall into one of the following categories: 1) those associated with fever, usually a rash or secondary bacterial infection (cellulitis, lymphangitis, bacteremia, toxin-mediated) and 2) those not associated with fever. Most skin problems are minor and are not accompanied by fever. Diagnosis of skin problems in returned travelers is based on the following:

- Pattern recognition of the lesions: papular, macular, nodular, linear, or ulcerated
- Location of the lesions: exposed versus unexposed skin surfaces
- Exposure history: freshwater, ocean, insects, animals, or human contact
- Associated symptoms: fever, pain, pruritus

Remember that skin conditions in returned travelers may not have a travel-related cause.

PAPULAR LESIONS

Insect bites, the most common cause of papular lesions, are frequently associated with secondary infection or hypersensitivity reactions. Bed bugs, fleas, and reduviid (triatomine) bugs can all produce papules in groups of 3 ("breakfast, lunch, and dinner"). (For more information about bed bugs, see Box 2-3.) Scabies is a mite that frequently presents with a generalized pruritic, papular rash. Scabies burrows may present as papules or pustules in a short linear pattern on the skin.

Onchocerciasis, also known as river blindness, is caused by the filarial nematode *Onchocerca volvulus*. Generalized pruritus is the rule, often associated with a papular rash. The filariae are transmitted by the bites of day-biting black flies. The main risk occurs in long-stay travelers living in rural sub-Saharan Africa and, rarely, Latin America.

NODULAR OR SUBCUTANEOUS LESIONS, INCLUDING BACTERIAL SKIN INFECTIONS

Bacterial skin infections may occur more frequently after bites and other wounds in the tropics, particularly when good hygiene

cannot be maintained. Organisms responsible are commonly *Staphylococcus aureus* or *Streptococcus pyogenes*. The presentations can include abscess formation, cellulitis, lymphangitis, or ulceration. Furunculosis, or recurrent pyoderma, is the result of colonization of the skin and nasal mucosa with *S. aureus*. Boils may continue to occur weeks or months after a traveler returns.

In addition to pyodermas, cellulitis or erysipelas may complicate excoriated insect bites or any trauma to the skin. Cellulitis and erysipelas manifest as areas of skin erythema, edema, and warmth in the absence of an underlying suppurative focus; unlike cellulitis, erysipelas lesions are raised, there is a clear line of demarcation at the edge of the lesion, and the lesions are more likely to be associated with fever. Cellulitis, on the other hand, is more likely to be associated with lymphangitis. Cellulitis and erysipelas are usually caused by β-hemolytic streptococci; *S. aureus* (including methicillin-resistant staphylococcus) and gram-negative aerobic bacteria may also cause cellulitis. A recent study from France of 60 returned travelers with skin and soft tissue infections found 35% had impetigo and 23% had cutaneous abscesses. Methicillin-susceptible *S. aureus* was detected in 43%, group A *Streptococcus* in 34%, and both in 23%.

Emerging antibiotic resistance among staphylococci and *S. pyogenes* (erythromycin resistance) is problematic, because antimicrobial treatment may be more difficult. After return from travel, antibiotic choice will be determined by symptoms and extent of illness. If a skin problem occurs during travel, the antibiotic choice may depend on whether medical care and follow-up are available, as well as which medications are available. Some travelers may benefit from carrying an antibiotic for self-treatment in these circumstances. Choices are difficult but include trimethoprim-sulfamethoxazole, an extended-spectrum penicillin, a cephalosporin, a broad-spectrum quinolone, and azithromycin. None of these is ideal.

Another common bacterial skin infection in the tropics, due to *S. aureus* or *S. pyogenes*, is impetigo, especially in children. Impetigo is a highly contagious superficial skin infection that generally appears on the arms, legs, or face as "honey-colored" scabs formed from dried serum. The treatment of choice is a topical antibiotic such as mupirocin.

Myiasis presents as a painful, boil-like lesion. It is caused by an infection with the larval stage of the tumbu (*Cordylobia anthropophaga*) or bot fly (*Dermatobia hominis*). The larvae are frequently acquired in Africa and Latin America. The lesions reveal a small, central punctum that allows the larvae to breathe. Several techniques have been described for removal of the larvae; occlusion of the punctum with petroleum jelly is most often used.

Tungiasis is caused by a sand flea (*Tunga penetrans*). The female burrows into the skin, usually the foot, and produces a nodular, pale, subcutaneous lesion with a central dark spot. The lesion expands as the female produces eggs in her uterus. The flea must be extracted surgically.

Loa loa filariasis can rarely occur in long-term travelers living in rural sub-Saharan Africa. It is transmitted by day-biting deer flies. The traveler may present with transient, migratory, subcutaneous, painful, or pruritic swellings produced by the adult nematode migration. Rarely, the worm can be visualized crossing the conjunctiva of the eye or eyelid. Eosinophilia is common. Loa loa can be diagnosed by finding the larval stages (microfilaria) in blood collected during the day. Serologic tests are also available but usually not in commercial laboratories. Infection can be prevented by taking 200 mg of diethylcarbamazine once a week while at risk.

Gnathostomiasis is a nematode infection found primarily in Southeast Asia and less commonly in Africa and Latin America. Infection results from eating undercooked or raw freshwater fish. The traveler experiences transient, migratory, subcutaneous, pruritic, or painful swellings that may occur weeks or even years after exposure. The symptoms are due to worm larva(e) migrating throughout the body, including the central nervous system. Eosinophilia is common, and the diagnosis can be made by serology.

MACULAR LESIONS

By far the most frequent macular lesions seen in returned travelers from warm climates are superficial mycoses, such as tinea versicolor and tinea corporis.

Tinea versicolor, which is due to *Malassezia furfur* (previously *Pityrosporum*

ovale), is characterized by asymptomatic hypopigmented or hyperpigmented oval, slightly scaly patches measuring 1–3 cm, found on the upper chest, neck, and back. Diagnosis is by Wood's lamp or by placing a drop of methylene blue on a slide onto which clear cellulose acetate tape is placed sticky side down, after it has been touched briefly to the skin lesions to pick up superficial scales. Hyphae ("spaghetti") and spores ("meatballs") are readily visible. Treatment with topical or systemic azoles (ketoconazole, fluconazole) or terbinafine is recommended.

Tinea corporis (ringworm) is caused by a number of different superficial fungi. The lesion is often a single lesion with an expanding red, raised ring, with a central area of clearing in the middle. Treatment is several weeks' application of a topical antifungal agent.

Lyme disease, a tickborne infection with *Borrelia burgdorferi*, is common in North America, Europe, and Russia (see Chapter 3, Lyme Disease). The traveler presents with one or more large erythematous patches, with or without central clearing, surrounding a prior tick bite. The patient may not have noted the tick bite.

LINEAR LESIONS

Cutaneous larva migrans is usually the result of infection of the skin with a larva from a dog or cat hookworm (most often *Ancylostoma braziliense*) but can also be caused by infection with other helminth parasites such as *Strongyloides stercoralis* (see Chapter 3, Cutaneous Larva Migrans). Dogs and cats that defecate on beaches appear to be one of the main risks for travelers. Lesions appear on the feet or buttocks most commonly. The traveler presents with an extremely pruritic, serpiginous, linear lesion that migrates within the skin at the rate of 2–4 mm per day. Treatment is with oral albendazole or ivermectin.

Phytophotodermatitis results from spilling lime juice onto the skin in a sunny climate. The result is an exaggerated sunburn that gives rise to a linear, asymptomatic lesion that later develops hyperpigmentation. The hyperpigmentation may take weeks or months to resolve.

Lymphocuticular spread of infection occurs when organisms spread along superficial cutaneous lymphatics, producing a raised, linear, cordlike lesion; nodules or ulcers may also be found. Examples include sporotrichosis, *Mycobacterium marinum* (associated with exposure to water), leishmaniasis, bartonellosis (cat-scratch disease), tularemia, and blastomycosis.

SKIN ULCERS

Ulcerated skin lesions may result from *Staphylococcus* infections or may be the direct result of an unseen spider bite. Often the cause of such an ulcer is not clear. Of particular concern is the ulcer (or nodule) caused by **cutaneous leishmaniasis**, which results from the bite of a sand fly. The main areas of risk are Latin America, the Mediterranean, Middle East, Asia, and parts of Africa. The lesion is a chronic, usually painless ulcer, unless superinfected, with heaped-up margins on exposed skin surfaces. Special diagnostic techniques are necessary to confirm the diagnosis. Both topical and systemic treatments are effective; the species of the infection often determines the treatment modality. If cutaneous leishmaniasis is suspected, clinicians can contact CDC for further advice about diagnosis and treatment (see Chapter 3, Leishmaniasis, Cutaneous for contact information).

MISCELLANEOUS SKIN INFECTIONS
Skin Infections Associated with Water

Soft tissue infections can occur after both freshwater and saltwater exposure, particularly if there is associated trauma. Puncture wounds due to fishhooks and fish spines, lacerations due to inanimate objects during wading and swimming, and bites from fish or other sea creatures may be the source of the trauma leading to waterborne infections. The most common soft tissue infections associated with exposure to water or water-related animals include *M. marinum*, *Aeromonas* spp., *Edwardsiella tarda*, *Erysipelothrix rhusiopathiae*, and *Vibrio vulnificus*. A variety of skin and soft tissue manifestations may occur in association with these infections, including cellulitis, abscess formation, ecthyma gangrenosum, and necrotizing fasciitis. Most *Vibrio* infections occur in men; *V. vulnificus* may be especially severe in those with underlying liver disease. *M. marinum* lesions usually appear as solitary nodules or papules on an extremity, especially on the dorsum of feet and hands that subsequently progress to shallow ulceration and scar formation. Occasionally, "sporotrichoid" spread may occur as the lesions spread proximally along superficial lymphatics.

"Hot tub folliculitis" due to *Pseudomonas aeruginosa* may result from the use of spa pools or whirlpools or exposure to inadequately chlorinated swimming pools and hot tubs. Folliculitis typically develops 8–48 hours after exposure in contaminated water and consists of tender, pruritic papules, papulopustules, or nodules. Most patients have malaise, and some have low-grade fever. The condition is self-limited in 2–12 days; typically no antibiotic therapy is required.

Skin Infections Associated with Bites

Wound infections after dog and cat bites are caused by a variety of microorganisms. *S. aureus*; α-, β-, and γ-hemolytic streptococci; several genera of gram-negative organisms; and a number of anaerobic microorganisms have all been isolated. The prevalence of *Pasteurella multocida* isolates from dog bite wounds is 20%–50%; *P. multocida* is the major pathogen in cat bite wound infections. Management of dog and cat bites includes consideration of rabies prophylaxis, tetanus immunization, and antibiotic prophylaxis. Primary closure of puncture wounds and dog bites to the hand should be avoided. Antibiotic prophylaxis for dog bites is controversial. Since *P. multocida* is a common accompaniment of cat bites, prophylaxis with amoxicillin-clavulanate or a fluoroquinolone for 3–5 days should be considered.

FEVER AND RASH

Fever and rash in returned travelers are most often due to a viral infection. Dengue is the most frequent and perhaps most easily recognizable example.

Dengue fever is caused by 1 of 4 strains of dengue viruses (see Chapter 3, Dengue Fever and Dengue Hemorrhagic Fever). The disease is transmitted by a day-biting *Aedes* mosquito often found in urban areas. The disease is characterized by the abrupt onset of high fever, frontal headache (often accompanied by retroorbital pain), myalgia, and a faint macular rash that becomes evident on the second to fourth day of illness. A petechial rash may be found in classical dengue, as well as dengue hemorrhagic fever. Serologic tests are available to diagnose dengue but often require a convalescent-phase serum sample to confirm. Nonsteroidal anti-inflammatory drugs should be avoided because of the increased risk of capillary leakage.

Chikungunya fever, a virus transmitted by a day-biting *Aedes* mosquito, has recently caused major outbreaks of illness in southeast Africa and South Asia (see Chapter 3, Chikungunya). Chikungunya fever is similar to dengue clinically, including the rash. The major distinguishing feature is that arthritis is common with chikungunya fever and may persist for months, whereas in dengue, arthralgia is the frequent joint problem. Similar to dengue, serologic tests are available for diagnosing chikungunya but often require a convalescent-phase serum sample to confirm. Treatment of the arthritis is with nonsteroidal anti-inflammatory drugs.

South African tick typhus, or African tick-bite fever (*Rickettsia africae*), is the most frequent cause of fever and rash in southern Africa. Transmitted by ticks, the disease is characterized by fever and a papular or vesicular rash associated with localized lymphadenopathy and the presence of an eschar (a mildly painful 1- to 2-cm black necrotic lesion with an erythematous margin). Diagnosis can be suspected clinically and confirmed by serology. Treatment is with doxycycline.

Rocky Mountain spotted fever (RMSF), although uncommon in travelers, is an important cause of fever and rash because of its potential severity and the need for early treatment. This tickborne infection is found in the United States, Mexico, and parts of Central and South America. Most patients with RMSF develop a rash between the third and fifth days of illness. The typical rash of RMSF begins on the ankles and wrists and spreads both centrally and to the palms and soles. The rash commonly begins as a maculopapular eruption and then becomes petechial, although in some patients it begins as petechial. Doxycycline is the treatment of choice.

The category of fever with rash is large, and travel medicine specialists should also consider the following diagnoses: enteroviruses, such as echovirus and coxsackievirus; hepatitis B virus; measles; Epstein-Barr virus; cytomegalovirus; typhus; leptospirosis; and HIV.

BIBLIOGRAPHY

1. Ansart S, Perez L, Jaureguiberry S, Danis M, Bricaire F, Caumes E. Spectrum of dermatoses in 165 travelers returning from the tropics with skin diseases. Am J Trop Med Hyg. 2007 Jan;76(1):184–6.
2. Bernard P. Management of common bacterial infections of the skin. Curr Opin Infect Dis. 2008 Apr;21(2):122–8.
3. Bowers AG. Phytophotodermatitis. Am J Contact Dermat. 1999 Jun;10(2):89–93.
4. Chapman AS, Bakken JS, Folk SM, Paddock CD, Bloch KC, Krusell A, et al. Diagnosis and management of tickborne rickettsial diseases: Rocky Mountain spotted fever, ehrlichioses, and anaplasmosis—United States: a practical guide for physicians and other health-care and public health professionals. MMWR Recomm Rep. 2006 Mar 31;55(RR-4):1–27.
5. Diaz JH. The epidemiology, diagnosis, management, and prevention of ectoparasitic diseases in travelers. J Travel Med. 2006 Mar–Apr;13(2):100–11.
6. Freedman DO, Weld LH, Kozarsky PE, Fisk T, Robins R, von Sonnenburg F, et al. Spectrum of disease and relation to place of exposure among ill returned travelers. N Engl J Med. 2006 Jan 12;354(2):119–30.
7. Heukelbach J, Feldmeier H. Epidemiological and clinical characteristics of hookworm-related cutaneous larva migrans. Lancet Infect Dis. 2008 May;8(5):302–9.
8. Hochedez P, Canestri A, Guihot A, Brichler S, Bricaire F, Caumes E. Management of travelers with fever and exanthema, notably dengue and chikungunya infections. Am J Trop Med Hyg. 2008 May;78(5):710–3.
9. Hochedez P, Canestri A, Lecso M, Valin N, Bricaire F, Caumes E. Skin and soft tissue infections in returning travelers. Am J Trop Med Hyg. 2009 Mar;80(3):431–4.
10. Huang DB, Ostrosky-Zeichner L, Wu JJ, Pang KR, Tyring SK. Therapy of common superficial fungal infections. Dermatol Ther. 2004;17(6):517–22.
11. Klion AD. Filarial infections in travelers and immigrants. Curr Infect Dis Rep. 2008 Mar;10(1):50–7.
12. Lederman ER, Gleeson TD, Driscoll T, Wallace MR. Doxycycline sensitivity of S. *pneumoniae* isolates. Clin Infect Dis. 2003 Apr 15;36(8):1091.
13. Magill AJ. Cutaneous leishmaniasis in the returning traveler. Infect Dis Clin North Am. 2005 Mar;19(1):241–66, x–xi.
14. Medical Letter Inc. Drugs for Parasitic Infections. 2nd ed. New Rochelle, NY: The Medical Letter, Inc; 2010.
15. Menard A, Dos Santos G, Dekumyoy P, Ranque S, Delmont J, Danis M, et al. Imported cutaneous

gnathostomiasis: report of five cases. Trans R Soc Trop Med Hyg. 2003 Mar–Apr;97(2):200–2.

16. Nordlund JJ. Cutaneous ectoparasites. Dermatol Ther. 2009 Nov–Dec;22(6):503–17.

17. Nutman TB, Miller KD, Mulligan M, Reinhardt GN, Currie BJ, Steel C, et al. Diethylcarbamazine prophylaxis for human loiasis. Results of a double-blind study. N Engl J Med. 1988 Sep 22;319(12):752–6.

18. Oostvogel PM, van Doornum GJ, Ferreira R, Vink J, Fenollar F, Raoult D. African tickbite fever in travelers, Swaziland. Emerg Infect Dis. 2007 Feb;13(2):353–5.

19. Tristan A, Bes M, Meugnier H, Lina G, Bozdogan B, Courvalin P, et al. Global distribution of Panton-Valentine leukocidin–positive methicillin-resistant *Staphylococcus aureus*, 2006. Emerg Infect Dis. 2007 Apr;13(4):594–600.

20. Wilson ME, Chen LH. Dermatologic infectious diseases in international travelers. Curr Infect Dis Rep. 2004 Feb;6(1):54–62.

ASYMPTOMATIC POST-TRAVEL SCREENING

Carlos Franco-Paredes

CDC has no official guidelines or recommendations for screening asymptomatic international travelers, except in special populations such as refugees (see Chapter 9, After Arrival in the United States). Cost-effectiveness studies of routine screening in asymptomatic international travelers have not shown a significant benefit to this approach on a population basis. Therefore, a clinic visit or any nondirected laboratory screening for most travelers is not indicated. Exceptions would be for those with known high-risk exposures that are linked to the transmission of certain agents or for people who have lived abroad.

The decision to screen for particular pathogens will depend on the type of travel, itinerary, and exposure history. Travelers who have engaged in casual unprotected sex or have received an injection, a body piercing, or a tattoo may be screened for HIV, hepatitis B and C, and other potential sexually transmitted diseases (such as gonorrhea) with nucleic acid hybridization tests in urine, and for *Chlamydia* infections with nucleic acid amplification tests in urine. When travelers with high-risk factors present with a febrile illness, sometimes testing for hepatitis B DNA, hepatitis C RNA viral load, and HIV RNA viral load is recommended, in order to rule out the possibility of acute hepatitis B or C or an acute HIV syndrome.

Eosinophilia in a returned traveler suggests the possibility of a helminth infection, of which the most important is strongyloidiasis. Travelers with eosinophilia who have been exposed to freshwater in areas endemic for schistosomiasis should be screened for this infection. Travelers exposed to soil should be screened for strongyloidiasis and possibly other intestinal parasites. If left untreated, this infection may last for the lifetime of the host, and in an immunocompromised person, it has the potential to disseminate.

Travelers who received blood products in highly endemic areas for American trypanosomiasis (Chagas disease) should be serologically screened for latent *Trypanosoma cruzi* infection. Asymptomatic international travelers who have been abroad for many months or longer, particularly in developing countries, should be screened for certain diseases by using tests such as hepatitis B serology, HIV serology, syphilis serology, Mantoux intradermal skin test for latent tuberculosis infection (predeparture baseline skin testing should be considered in extended-stay travelers to developing countries or those who will have high-risk exposures), stool examination for ova and parasites, and complete blood count, including a peripheral eosinophil count and red blood cell parameters.

Asymptomatic screening is encouraged in special populations such as refugees and international adoptees. Some of the frequently recommended tests to conduct in these patient groups include the following:

- Hepatitis B serologic panel
- HIV serology
- Syphilis serology
- Complete blood count, including a peripheral eosinophil count and red blood cell parameters

Screening for latent tuberculosis infection can be performed by using one of the following modalities: 1) the Mantoux tuberculin skin test or 2) a blood assay for *Mycobacterium tuberculosis* infection. Currently, the QuantiFERON-TB Gold In-tube Test is approved for screening adults in the United States. Chest radiograph and sputum studies for mycobacterial staining should be performed for those with positive screening results.

CDC has published guidelines for evaluating refugees for intestinal parasites and tissue-invading parasites during domestic medical evaluations. Screening modalities vary according to predeparture presumptive parasitic therapy:

- Screening for parasitic infection among asymptomatic refugees who had no documented

predeparture presumptive antiparasitic therapy should include 2 morning stool samples for ova and parasite examination by the concentration method.
- Screening for parasitic infection among asymptomatic refugees who received single-dose predeparture treatment with albendazole should include the following:
  > An eosinophil count should be performed in every refugee.
  > Refugees from sub-Saharan Africa with persistent eosinophilia should undergo serologic testing for strongyloidiasis and schistosomiasis.
- Screening for parasitic infections in asymptomatic refugees who received high-dose predeparture albendazole (7-day therapy) or ivermectin, with or without praziquantel, should include a follow-up eosinophil count 3–6 months after completion of antiparasitic treatment. Additional treatment is suggested for those identified with residual eosinophilia at the initial evaluation.

Refugee health guidelines are available on the CDC website (www.cdc.gov/immigrant refugeehealth/guidelines/refugee-guidelines. html).

BIBLIOGRAPHY

1. Carroll B, Dow C, Snashall D, Marshall T, Chiodini PL. Post-tropical screening: how useful is it? BMJ. 1993 Aug 28;307(6903):541.
2. CDC. Guidelines for evaluation of refugees for intestinal and tissue-invasive parasitic infections during domestic medical examination. Atlanta:

CDC; 2010 [cited 2008 Nov 26]. Available from: http:// www.cdc.gov/immigrantrefugeehealth/guidelines/ domestic/intestinal-parasites-domestic.html.
3. Stauffer WM, Kamat D, Walker PF. Screening of international immigrants, refugees, and adoptees. Prim Care. 2002 Dec;29(4):879–905.

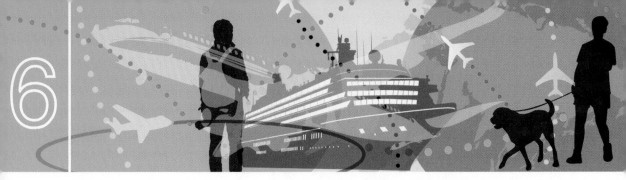

6

Conveyance & Transportation Issues

AIR TRAVEL

Nancy M. Gallagher, Karen J. Marienau, Petra A. Illig, Phyllis E. Kozarsky

Travelers often have concerns about the health risks of flying in airplanes. Those with underlying illness need to be aware that the entire point-to-point travel experience, including buses, trains, taxis, and public waiting areas, can pose challenges. While illness may occur as a direct result of air travel, it is uncommon; the main concerns are:

- Exacerbations of chronic medical problems due to changes in air pressure, humidity, and oxygen concentration
- Relative immobility during flights (risk of thromboembolic disease, see Chapter 2, Deep Vein Thrombosis and Pulmonary Embolism)
- Close proximity to other passengers with certain communicable diseases
- Spraying of airplane cabins with insecticides (disinsection) before landing in certain destinations

EXACERBATION OF CHRONIC DISEASE

During flight, the aircraft cabin pressure is usually maintained at the equivalent of 6,000–8,000 ft (1,829–2,438 m) above sea level. Most healthy travelers will not notice any effects. However, for travelers with cardiopulmonary diseases (especially those who normally require supplemental oxygen), cerebrovascular disease, anemia, or sickle cell disease, conditions in an aircraft can exacerbate underlying medical conditions. Aircraft cabin air is typically dry, usually 10%–20% humidity, which can cause dryness of the mucous membranes of the eyes and airways.

People with chronic illnesses, particularly those whose conditions may be unstable, should be evaluated by a physician to ensure they are fit for air travel. For those who require supplemental in-flight oxygen, the following must be taken into consideration:

- Federal regulations prohibit airlines from allowing passengers to bring their own oxygen aboard; passengers requiring in-flight supplemental oxygen should notify the airline ≥72 hours before departure.
- Information regarding the screening of respiratory equipment (such as oxygen canisters or portable oxygen concentrators) at airports in the United States, and regulations regarding oxygen use on aircraft, can be found at www.tsa.gov/travelers/airtravel.
- Airlines might not offer in-flight supplemental oxygen on all aircraft or flights; some airlines permit only portable oxygen concentrators.
- Travelers must arrange their own oxygen supplies while on the ground, at departure, during layovers, and on arrival. The National Home Oxygen Patients Association provides information to assist patients who require

supplemental oxygen during travel (www. homeoxygen.org/airtrav.html).

BAROTRAUMA DURING FLIGHT

Barotrauma occurs when the pressure inside an air-filled, enclosed body space (such as the middle ear, sinuses, or abdomen) is not the same as air pressure inside the aircraft cabin. It most commonly occurs during rapid changes in environmental pressure, such as during ascent, when cabin pressure rapidly decreases, and during descent, when cabin pressure rapidly increases. Barotrauma most commonly affects the middle ear; it occurs when the eustachian tube is blocked and thus unable to equalize the air pressure in the middle ear with the outside cabin pressure. Middle ear barotrauma is usually not severe or dangerous and can usually be prevented or self-treated. It may rarely cause complications such as a perforated tympanic membrane, dizziness, permanent tinnitus, or hearing loss.

The following suggestions may help avoid potential barotrauma:

- People with ear, nose, and sinus infections or severe congestion may wish to temporarily avoid flying to prevent pain or injury. This is particularly true for infants and toddlers, in whom obstruction occurs more readily.
- Oral pseudoephedrine 30 minutes before flight departure, or a nonsteroidal anti-inflammatory agent, may alleviate symptoms.
- Travelers with seasonal allergies should continue their regular allergy medication.
- Travelers should stay hydrated to help avoid irritation of nasal passages and pharynx and to promote better function of the eustachian tubes.
- Travelers sensitive to abdominal bloating should avoid carbonated beverages and foods that can increase gas production.
- Patients who have had recent surgery, particularly intra-abdominal, neurologic, intra-pulmonary, or intraocular procedures, should consult with their physicians before flying.

VENTILATION AND AIR QUALITY

All commercial jet aircraft built after the late 1980s and a few modified older aircraft recirculate 10%–50% of the air in the cabin mixed with outside air. The recirculated air passes through a series of filters 20–30 times per hour. In most newer-model airplanes, the recycled air passes through high-efficiency particulate air (HEPA) filters, which capture 99.9% of particles (bacteria, fungi, and larger viruses) between 0.1 and 0.3 μm in diameter. Air flow occurs transversely across the plane in limited bands, and air is not forced up and down the length of the plane. As a result, the air cabin environment is not conducive to the spread of most infectious diseases.

IN-FLIGHT MEDICAL EMERGENCIES

Worldwide, more than one billion people travel by commercial aircraft every year, and this number is expected to double in the next 20 years. Increasingly, large aircraft combined with an aging flying population makes the incidence of onboard medical emergencies likely to increase. Approximately 1 in 10,000 to 40,000 passengers has a medical incident during air transport. Of these, approximately 1 in 150,000 requires use of in-flight medical equipment or drugs. The most commonly encountered in-flight medical events, in order of frequency, are the following:

- Vasovagal syncope
- Gastrointestinal events
- Respiratory events
- Cardiac events
- Neurologic events

Deaths aboard commercial aircraft have been estimated at 0.3 per 1 million passengers; approximately two-thirds of these are caused by cardiac problems.

In addition to standard first aid kits, and depending on the size of the aircraft and applicable regulations, enhanced emergency medical kits may include, but are not limited to, the following:

- Automatic external defibrillators
- Intubation equipment (pediatric and adult)
- CPR masks (pediatric and adult)
- Intravenous access equipment and solutions
- Intravenous dextrose
- Antihistamines (oral and injectable)
- First-line cardiac resuscitation drugs (atropine, epinephrine, lidocaine)
- Nitroglycerin
- Bronchodilators
- Analgesics

Although flight attendants receive training in basic first aid procedures, they are generally not certified in emergency medical response. Many airlines use ground-based medical consultants via radio or phone communication to assist volunteer passenger responders and flight attendants in managing medical cases.

The goal of managing in-flight medical emergencies is to stabilize the passenger until appropriate ground-based medical care can safely be reached; it should not be considered a method of maintaining the original flight route in order to reach the scheduled destination. The captain must, therefore, weigh the needs of the ill passenger with other safety considerations such as weather, landing conditions, and terrain. Certain routes, such as transoceanic flights, may severely restrict diversion options, while others may present a number of safe landing choices. In the latter circumstance, consideration should be given to choosing an airport that has timely access to an appropriate medical facility.

IN-FLIGHT TRANSMISSION OF COMMUNICABLE DISEASES

Communicable diseases may be transmitted to other travelers during air travel; therefore, people who are acutely ill, or still within the infectious period for a specific disease, should be discouraged from traveling. Travelers should be reminded to wash their hands frequently and thoroughly (or use an alcohol-based hand cleaner), especially after using the toilet and before preparing or eating food. Travelers should also be reminded to cover their noses and mouths when coughing or sneezing.

If a passenger with a communicable disease is identified as having flown on a particular flight (or flights), passengers who may have been exposed may be contacted by public health authorities, for possible screening or prophylaxis. When necessary, public health authorities will obtain contact information from the airline for potentially exposed travelers so they may be contacted and offered appropriate intervention. To assist in this process, travelers can provide airlines with current contact information.

Tuberculosis

Although the risk of transmission of *Mycobacterium tuberculosis* onboard aircraft is low, international tuberculosis (TB) experts agree that contact investigations for flights >8 hours are warranted when an ill traveler meets World Health Organization (WHO) criteria for being infectious during flight. The concern is most serious when a person may have flown with a highly drug-resistant strain of TB. People known to have infectious TB should not travel by commercial air (or any other commercial means) until they are no longer infectious. State health department TB controllers are valuable resources for advice (http://tbcontrollers.org/?p=10).

Neisseria meningitidis

Meningococcal disease (caused by *Neisseria meningitidis*) can be rapidly fatal; therefore, close contacts need to be quickly identified and provided with prophylactic antimicrobial agents. Antimicrobial prophylaxis should be considered for any of the following:

- Household member traveling with a patient
- Travel companion with very close contact
- Passenger seated directly next to the ill traveler on flights >8 hours

Measles

Most measles cases diagnosed in the United States are imported from countries where measles is endemic. Travelers should ensure they are immune to measles before travel. An ill traveler is considered infectious during a flight of any duration if he or she traveled during the 4 days before rash onset through 4 days after rash onset. Intervention may prevent or mitigate measles in susceptible contacts if MMR vaccine is given within 72 hours of exposure or immune globulin is given within 6 days of exposure.

Influenza and Severe Acute Respiratory Syndrome

Transmission of the influenza virus aboard aircraft has been documented, but data are limited. Transmission is thought to be primarily due to large droplets; therefore, passengers seated closest to the source case are believed to be most at risk for exposure.

The avian influenza virus (H5N1) has infected hundreds of humans since 1997 and is primarily associated with direct contact with infected birds or bird products. No cases have been associated with air travel. The 2009 influenza A (H1N1) pandemic began in April

6

2009, and while air travel played a significant role in its global spread, there are limited data about in-flight transmission. However, data published to date indicate that in-flight transmission did not occur frequently. Severe acute respiratory syndrome (SARS) can be transmitted anywhere people are gathered, including aircraft cabins. The last known case of person-to-person transmission occurred in 2003. See the CDC Travelers' Health website (www.cdc.gov/travel) for more general information and up-to-date, specific guidelines for travelers and the airline industry.

DISINSECTION

To reduce the accidental spread of mosquitoes and other vectors via airline cabins and luggage compartments, a number of countries require disinsection of all inbound flights. WHO and the International Civil Aviation Organization (ICAO) specify 2 approaches for aircraft disinsection:

- Spraying the aircraft cabin with an aerosolized insecticide (usually 2% phenothrin) while passengers are on board

- Treating the aircraft's interior surfaces with a residual insecticide while the aircraft is empty

Some countries use a third method, in which aircraft are sprayed with an aerosolized insecticide while passengers are not on board.

Disinsection is not routinely done on incoming flights to the United States. Although disinsection, when done appropriately, was declared safe by WHO in 1995, there is still much debate about the safety of the agents and methods used. Guidelines for disinsection have been updated for the revised International Health Regulations (www2a.cdc.gov/phlp/docs/58assembly.pdf). Many countries, including the United States, reserve the right to increase the use of disinsection in case of increased threat of vector or disease spread. An updated list of countries that require disinsection and the types of methods used are available at the Department of Transportation website: http://ostpxweb. ost.dot.gov/policy/safetyenergyenv/disinsection.htm.

BIBLIOGRAPHY

1. Aerospace Medical Association Task Force. Medical guidelines for airline travel, 2nd ed. Aviat Space Environ Med. 2003 May;74(5 Suppl):A1–19.
2. Bagshaw M, DeVoll JR, Jennings RT, McCrary BF, Northrup SE, Rayman RB, et al. Medical Guidelines for Airline Passengers. Alexandria, VA: Aerospace Medical Association; 2002. Available from: http://www.asma.org/publications/index.php.
3. Bagshaw M, Nicolls D. Aircraft cabin environment. In: Keystone J, Kozarsky P, Freedman D, Nothdurft H, Connor B, editors. Travel Medicine. 2nd ed. Philadelphia: Mosby; 2008. p. 447–61.
4. CDC. Exposure to patients with meningococcal disease on aircrafts—United States, 1999–2001. MMWR Morb Mortal Wkly Rep. 2001 Jun 15;50(23):485–9.
5. CDC. Multistate measles outbreak associated with an international youth sporting event—Pennsylvania, Michigan, and Texas, August–September 2007. MMWR Morb Mortal Wkly Rep. 2008 Feb 22;57(7):169–73.
6. Delaune EF 3rd, Lucas RH, Illig P. In-flight medical events and aircraft diversions: one airline's experience. Aviat Space Environ Med. 2003 Jan;74(1):62–8.
7. Han K, Zhu X, He F, Liu L, Zhang L, Ma H, et al. Lack of airborne transmission during outbreak of pandemic (H1N1) 2009 among tour group members, China, June 2009. Emerg Infect Dis. 2009 Oct;15(10):1578–81.
8. Harrill WC. Barotrauma of the Middle and Inner Ear. Baylor College of Medicine Grand Rounds, March 23, 1995. Houston: Baylor College of Medicine; 1995. Available from: http://judas.sgul.ac.uk/nelhpc/pcel/cache.php?id=819.
9. Illig P. Passenger health. In: Curdt-Christiansen C, Draeger J, Kriebel J, Antunano M, editors. Principles and Practice of Aviation Medicine. Hackensack, NJ: World Scientific; 2009. p. 667–708.
10. Kenyon TA, Valway SE, Ihle WW, Onorato IM, Castro KG. Transmission of multidrug-resistant Mycobacterium tuberculosis during a long airplane flight. N Engl J Med. 1996 Apr 11;334(15):933–8.
11. Marsden AG. Outbreak of influenza-like illness [corrected] related to air travel. Med J Aust. 2003 Aug 4;179(3):172–3.
12. Mayo Clinic. Airplane ear. Rochester, MN: Mayo Clinic; 2010 [updated Oct 23; cited 2010 Apr 9]. Available from: http://www.mayoclinic.com/health/airplane-ear/DS00472.

13. Mirza S, Richardson H. Otic barotrauma from air travel. J Laryngol Otol. 2005 May;119(5):366–70.

14. Moser MR, Bender TR, Margolis HS, Noble GR, Kendal AP, Ritter DG. An outbreak of influenza aboard a commercial airliner. Am J Epidemiol. 1979 Jul;110(1):1–6.

15. Vogt TM, Guerra MA, Flagg EW, Ksiazek TG, Lowther SA, Arguin PM. Risk of severe acute respiratory syndrome-associated coronavirus transmission aboard commercial aircraft. J Travel Med. 2006 Sep–Oct;13(5):268–72.

16. Wilder-Smith A, Paton NI, Goh KT. Experience of severe acute respiratory syndrome in Singapore: importation of cases, and defense strategies at the airport. J Travel Med. 2003 Sep–Oct;10(5):259–62.

17. World Health Organization. Tuberculosis and Air Travel: Guidelines for Prevention and Control. 3rd ed. Geneva: World Health Organization; 2008 [updated 2008 Jun 24]. Available from: http://www.who.int/tb/publications/2008/WHO_HTM_TB_2008.399_eng.pdf.

CRUISE SHIP TRAVEL

Douglas D. Slaten, Kiren Mitruka

INTRODUCTION

The cruise ship market is the fastest-growing sector of the travel industry. In 2008, the North American cruise industry, which makes up most of the global cruise market, comprised 161 ships carrying more than 13 million passengers to destinations worldwide. Nearly 9 million cruise passengers left from US ports. Florida is the center of US cruise ship travel, accounting for more than half of all US departures. The Caribbean is the top destination, followed by the Mediterranean, Europe, and Alaska. The average length of a cruise is 7 days, although voyages range from a few hours ("voyages to nowhere") to several months for around-the-world cruises. A typical cruise ship carries approximately 2,000 passengers and 800 crew members; however, cruise ship capacities continue to increase and can exceed 5,000 passengers and 2,000 crew. The median age of a cruise ship passenger is 46 years; seniors (≥55 years) represent approximately one-third of passengers. To a certain extent, different cruise lines target different population groups, and longer cruises often attract older passengers.

While most passengers are from the United States or Canada, cruise ships bring together large numbers of people from a variety of communities and backgrounds. Communicable diseases can be introduced onboard by embarking travelers, or acquired during visits to seaports with varying risks of exposure to infectious diseases. The crowded, semi-enclosed environment of the cruise ship facilitates transmission of communicable disease, either person to person or from contaminated food, water, or environmental surfaces. The stress of travel can worsen chronic conditions in specific groups, such as pregnant women and the elderly, who may be more seriously affected by infectious illnesses. Additionally, crew members, who are often from developing countries that may lack routine vaccination programs, can be sources of infection for vaccine-preventable diseases.

HEALTH AND SAFETY REGULATIONS

In 2005, the World Health Organization revised the International Health Regulations, which provide international standards for ship and port sanitation, disease surveillance, and response to infectious diseases. The 2005 revision entered into force in June 2007. The regulations are binding on 194 countries and are intended to help the international community prevent and respond to acute public health risks worldwide (www.who.int/ihr/en).

The Coast Guard enforces safety and security regulations in US waters, and CDC ensures health and sanitation aboard ships with international itineraries arriving at US ports. Federal regulations require such ships to report all shipboard deaths, and certain illnesses suggestive of communicable diseases,

24 hours before arrival at a US seaport. One of CDC's 20 quarantine stations with jurisdiction over the seaport of arrival responds to these reports, providing recommendations to prevent the spread of illness (www.cdc.gov/quarantine/index.html). Since 1975, CDC's Vessel Sanitation Program (VSP) has also helped the cruise ship industry prevent and control gastrointestinal illnesses on cruise ships (www.cdc.gov/nceh/vsp).

CRUISE SHIP MEDICAL CAPABILITIES

Medical facilities on cruise ships can vary widely, depending on a number of ship and traveler characteristics. Generally, shipboard medical clinics are comparable to ambulatory care centers. Although no official agency regulates medical practice aboard cruise ships, consensus-based guidelines have been published, which cruise lines are encouraged to adopt. The Cruise Lines International Association (CLIA) represents 25 major cruise lines, accounting for more than 97% of the North American cruise market (www.cruising.org). CLIA's Medical Facilities Working Group developed industrywide guidelines and recommends cruise ship medical facilities have the capability to:

- Provide emergency medical care for passengers and crew
- Stabilize patients and initiate reasonable diagnostic and therapeutic intervention
- Facilitate the evacuation of seriously ill or injured patients

In 2010, the American College of Emergency Physicians, Section of Cruise Ship and Maritime Medicine, published revised Health Care Guidelines for Cruise Ship Medical Facilities (www.acep.org/practres.aspx?LinkIdentifier=id&id=29980&fid=2184&Mo=No). These guidelines include recommendations for a ship medical center, staffed by physicians and registered nurses on call 24 hours per day. Although the needs of individual ships vary, these guidelines describe desired physician and nurse competencies (including physician board certification in emergency medicine, family practice, or internal medicine), as well as training in drills and preferred shipboard medications and supplies, laboratory and x-ray capabilities, and health equipment.

CRUISE SHIP ILLNESSES AND INJURY

Cruise ship medical clinics deal with a wide variety of illnesses and injuries. Most health-related events are treated or managed onboard. However, medical evacuation and shoreside consultation, particularly for dental problems, are not infrequent. The proportion of reported urgent or emergency conditions is 3%–11%.

Published reviews of cruise ship medical logs have shown that most passenger dispensary visits on cruise ships were due to medical conditions (69%–88%). Respiratory (19%–29%) and gastrointestinal (9%) illnesses were the most frequently reported diagnoses. Injuries accounted for 12%–18% of medical visits.

The most frequently documented cruise ship outbreaks involve respiratory infections (influenza and legionellosis), gastrointestinal infections (norovirus), and vaccine-preventable diseases other than influenza, such as rubella and varicella (chickenpox).

SPECIFIC HEALTH RISKS
Gastrointestinal Illness

VSP conducts twice-annual, unannounced inspections of ships with international itineraries that call on US seaports. In recent years, outbreaks of gastroenteritis (defined as ≥3% of passengers or crew symptomatic) on cruise ships have increased, despite good cruise ship environmental health standards. Most cruise ship gastrointestinal outbreaks are now due to norovirus, which is also the main cause of acute viral gastroenteritis in the United States. Characteristics of norovirus that facilitate outbreaks are low infective dose, easy person-to-person transmissibility, and ability to survive routine cleaning procedures.

Other organisms associated with foodborne and waterborne outbreaks on cruise ships are *Salmonella*, enterotoxigenic *Escherichia coli*, *Shigella*, *Vibrio*, *Staphylococcus aureus*, *Clostridium perfringens*, *Cyclospora*, hepatitis E virus, and *Trichinella*.

Respiratory Illness
Influenza

Since travelers originate from both the Northern and Southern Hemispheres, where the influenza seasons start in October or November and April or May, respectively, shipboard outbreaks of influenza A and B can occur year-round. Outbreaks usually result from the importation of influenza by embarking passengers and crew; infection subsequently spreads person to person.

During the 2009 influenza A (H1N1) pandemic, cruise line medical personnel made case-by-case decisions regarding the boarding of passengers with influenzalike illness. In 2003, the industry instituted similar screening protocols during the outbreak of severe acute respiratory syndrome (SARS) in Asia. Crew members can sustain influenza transmission over successive cruises. Onboard control measures travelers can expect include isolation of ill people, infection control, and antiviral treatment of ill people and contacts.

Legionellosis (Legionnaires' Disease)

Legionnaires' disease is a severe pneumonia caused by inhalation or aspiration of warm, aerosolized water containing *Legionella*. Symptom onset is typically 2–10 days after exposure. There is no person-to-person transmission.

Risk factors for Legionnaires' disease include older age (≥65 years) and underlying medical conditions. Contaminated ships' whirlpool spas and potable water supply systems are the most commonly implicated sources of shipboard *Legionella* outbreaks, although improvements in ship design and standardization of spa and water supply disinfection have reduced the risk of *Legionella* growth and colonization. Most cruise ships can perform *Legionella* urine antigen testing. CDC should be informed of any travel-associated Legionnaires' disease cases by e-mailing travellegionella@cdc.gov.

Vaccine-Preventable Diseases

Although a ship's passenger population is newly introduced at the beginning of each voyage, crew members remain onboard for extended periods. And, although most cruise ship passengers are from countries with routine vaccination programs (mainly the United States and Canada), crew members tend to originate from developing countries, some with low immunization rates. In past cruise ship investigations involving vaccine-preventable diseases, approximately 11% of crew members were found to be acutely infected with or susceptible to rubella, and 13% of crew, mostly from tropical countries,

were susceptible to or acutely infected with varicella.

Crew members should have documented proof of immunity to vaccine-preventable diseases. Passengers should be current on routine vaccinations before travel. Women of childbearing age should be immune to rubella before cruise ship travel.

Vectorborne Diseases

Cruise ship port visits may include countries where vectorborne diseases, such as malaria, dengue, and yellow fever, are endemic. Yellow fever vaccination certificates may be required by some countries for entry. Although cruise lines may schedule arrival and departure times to avoid peak mosquito biting periods, personal protection is still necessary. Preventive measures include the following:

- Remaining in well-screened or air-conditioned areas
- Wearing clothes that cover ankles, legs, and arms
- Using an effective insect repellent (see Chapter 2, Protection against Mosquitoes, Ticks, and Other Insects and Arthropods)
- Antimalarial chemoprophylaxis based on a destination- and activity-specific risk assessment

Other Health Concerns

Stresses of cruise ship travel include varying temperature and weather conditions, as well as unaccustomed changes in diet and physical activity. Foreign travel increases the likelihood of risk-taking behaviors such as alcohol misuse, drug use, and unsafe sex. Deaths on cruise ships are most often due to cardiovascular events. In spite of modern stabilizer systems, seasickness is a common complaint (see Chapter 2, Motion Sickness). Injuries and dental emergencies are frequent occurrences.

PREVENTIVE MEASURES FOR CRUISE SHIP TRAVELERS

Cruise ship travelers often have complex itineraries due to multiple short port visits and potential exposures. Although most of these port visits do not include overnight stays off the cruise ship, many exotic trips have options for travelers to venture off the ship for one or more nights. Cruise ship travelers may be uncertain about which prevention medications, immunizations, and behaviors are appropriate for them and their itineraries. Box 6-1 summarizes recommendations for cruise travelers, and clinicians advising cruise travelers, in pre-travel preparation and healthy behaviors during travel.

After Travel

Travelers who become ill after returning home should inform their health care providers of where they have traveled. Clinicians should report suspected communicable diseases in recently returned cruise ship travelers to public health authorities. Gastrointestinal illnesses related to cruise ship travel should be directed to the CDC VSP: 800-CDC-INFO (800-232-4636) or CDCINFO@cdc.gov. Other suspected communicable illnesses should be reported to the CDC quarantine station with jurisdiction over the cruise ship's port of arrival (www.cdc.gov/quarantine).

BOX 6-1. CRUISE TRAVEL HEALTH PRECAUTIONS

Advice for Clinicians Giving Pre-Travel Cruise Consultations
Risk Assessment and Risk Communication

- Discuss itinerary, including activities at port stops, season, and duration of travel.
- Review traveler's medical and immunization history, allergies, and special health needs.
- Discuss relevant travel-specific health hazards and risk reduction.
- Provide traveler with documentation of his or her medical history, immunizations, and medications.

Immunization and Risk Management

- Provide immunizations that are routine (age-specific), required (yellow fever), and recommended (risk-based).
- Discuss food and water precautions and insect bite prevention.
- Prescribe antimalarial chemoprophylaxis if itinerary includes malaria-endemic areas.
- Older travelers, especially those with a history of heart disease, are advised to carry a baseline EKG with them to facilitate onboard or overseas medical care should it be required.

Medications Based on Risk and Need

- Antimalarials (consider risks at port stops)
- Motion sickness medications for self-treatment (see Chapter 2, Motion Sickness)
- Antibiotics for self-treatment of travelers' diarrhea (see Chapter 2, Travelers' Diarrhea)

Precautions for Cruise Ship Travelers
Pre-Travel

- Consult health care and dental providers before cruise travel.
- Consider additional insurance for overseas health care and medical evacuation.
- Carry prescription medications in their original containers, with a copy of the prescription and accompanying physician's letter.
- Defer travel while acutely ill.

During Travel

- Wash hands frequently, using soap and water or an alcohol-based cleaner.
- Follow safe food and water precautions when eating off the ship at ports of call.
- Use personal protective measures during port visits in malaria- or dengue-endemic areas.
- Use sun protection and maintain good fluid intake.
- Avoid excessive alcohol consumption.
- Avoid contact with ill people.
- If sexually active, practice safe sex.

BIBLIOGRAPHY

1. American College of Emergency Physicians. Health Care Guidelines for Cruise Ship Medical Facilities. Dallas: American College of Emergency Physicians; 2010 [cited 2010 Nov 2]. Available from: http://www.acep.org/practres.aspx?LinkIdentifier=id&id=29980&fid=2184&Mo=No.

2. Bansal V, Fortlage D, Lee JG, Hill LL, Potenza B, Coimbra R. Significant injury in cruise ship passengers a case series. Am J Prev Med. 2007 Sep;33(3):219–21.

3. Carling PC, Bruno-Murtha LA, Griffiths JK. Cruise ship environmental hygiene and the risk of norovirus infection outbreaks: an objective assessment of 56 vessels over 3 years. Clin Infect Dis. 2009 Nov 1;49(9):1312–7.

4. CDC. Quarantine stations: quarantine station contact lists and jurisdictions. Atlanta: CDC; 2010 [cited 2010 Nov 2]. Available from: http://www.cdc.gov/quarantine/QuarantineStations.html.

5. CDC. Rubella among crew members of commercial cruise ships—Florida, 1997. MMWR Morb Mortal Wkly Rep. 1998 Jan 9;46(52–53):1247–50.

6. CDC. Vessel Sanitation Program. Atlanta: CDC; 2010 [updated Oct 28; cited 2010 Apr 19]. Available from: http://www.cdc.gov/nceh/vsp.

7. Cramer EH, Blanton CJ, Blanton LH, Vaughan GH, Jr., Bopp CA, Forney DL. Epidemiology of gastroenteritis on cruise ships, 2001–2004. Am J Prev Med. 2006 Mar;30(3):252–7.

8. Cruise Lines International Association. 2009 CLIA Cruise Market Overview: Statistical Cruise Industry Data Through 2008. Fort Lauderdale, FL: Cruise Lines International Association; 2009 [cited 2010 Apr 5]. Available from: http://www.cruising.org/sites/default/files/pressroom/2009_Market_Overview.pdf.

9. Dahl E. Medical practice during a world cruise: a descriptive epidemiological study of injury and illness among passengers and crew. Int Marit Health. 2005;56(1–4):115–28.

10. Maloney S, Cetron M. Investigation and management of infectious diseases on international conveyances (airplanes and cruise ships). In: DuPont HL, Steffen R, editors. Textbook of Travel Medicine and Health. 2nd ed. Lewiston, NY: BC Decker; 2001. p. 519–30.

11. Minooee A, Rickman LS. Infectious diseases on cruise ships. Clin Infect Dis. 1999 Oct;29(4):737–43.

12. Mitruka K, Wheeler R. Cruise travel. In: Keystone J, Kozarsky P, Freedman D, Nothdurft H, Connor B, editors. Travel Medicine. 2nd ed. Philadelphia: Mosby; 2008. p. 351–60.

13. Mouchtouri V, Black N, Nichols G, Paux T, Riemer T, Rjabinina J, et al. Preparedness for the prevention and control of influenza outbreaks on passenger ships in the EU: the SHIPSAN TRAINET project communication. Euro Surveill. 2009 May 28;14(21):19219.

14. Peake DE, Gray CL, Ludwig MR, Hill CD. Descriptive epidemiology of injury and illness among cruise ship passengers. Ann Emerg Med. 1999 Jan;33(1):67–72.

15. Rowbotham TJ. Legionellosis associated with ships: 1977 to 1997. Commun Dis Public Health. 1998 Sep;1(3):146–51.

16. Said B, Ijaz S, Kafatos G, Booth L, Thomas HL, Walsh A, et al. Hepatitis E outbreak on cruise ship. Emerg Infect Dis. 2009 Nov;15(11):1738–44.

17. Sasso RE, Dale TL. 2010 Cruise Industry Media Update. Cruise Lines International Association; 2009.

18. US Department of Health and Human Services. Title 42, Part 71. Foreign Quarantine. Washington, DC: US Government Printing Office; 2003.

19. Uyeki TM, Zane SB, Bodnar UR, Fielding KL, Buxton JA, Miller JM, et al. Large summertime influenza A outbreak among tourists in Alaska and the Yukon Territory. Clin Infect Dis. 2003 May 1;36(9):1095–102.

20. Vivancos R, Abubakar I, Hunter PR. Foreign travel associated with increased sexual risk-taking, alcohol and drug use among UK university students: a cohort study. Int J STD AIDS. 2010 Jan;21(1):46–51.

21. Wheeler R. Travel health at sea: cruise ship medicine. In: Zuckerman J, editor. Principles and Practices of Travel Medicine. New York: John Wiley and Sons; 2001. p. 275–87.

22. World Health Organization. International Health Regulations. Geneva: World Health Organization; 2005. Available from: http://www.who.int/ihr/en/.

WHAT TO EXPECT WHEN TRAVELING DURING AN INTERNATIONAL OUTBREAK

Todd W. Wilson

OVERVIEW

Outbreaks of communicable disease have occurred throughout history, dramatically shaping the human experience. One of the most recognizable examples of an outbreak with terrible consequences for both human health and culture was the fourteenth-century plague epidemic, or "Black Death," thought to have been caused by *Yersinia pestis*, which killed up to 60% of Europe's population and also spread to Asia and Africa, possibly reducing the global population by 17%.

In recent times, diseases such as Ebola hemorrhagic fever and severe acute respiratory syndrome (SARS) have appeared, seemingly from nowhere, and resulted in high numbers of deaths and illness among those infected. And throughout history—most recently in 2009—new strains of influenza have emerged, circled the globe, and caused social disruption and economic upheaval. These diseases and others like them, which emerge, spread rapidly via travel across international borders, and have significant or initially unknown health effects, have led countries to take public health measures at borders that affect travelers.

Severe Acute Respiratory Syndrome

The 2003 outbreak of SARS has been well chronicled. This newly discovered pathogen was quickly spread by an infected traveler who left Guangdong Province, China, and arrived in Hong Kong, where he infected 10 other people staying in a hotel, leading directly or indirectly to cases in 8 countries. The combined influence of World Health Organization (WHO) travel advisories and media attention to SARS affected traveler behavior to the extent that tourist arrivals in East Asian airports dropped 41% from April 1 to April 21, 2003.

2009 Influenza A (H1N1)

In March 2009, a new strain of influenza A (H1N1) began spreading in Mexico. Within 30 days, cases occurred in US states bordering Mexico. Within 90 days, WHO declared that a pandemic, or global outbreak of H1N1 influenza, was occurring. Analysis of preliminary passenger volume data for the largest airline carriers between Mexico and the United States indicated that during April 27 through May 17, 2010, northbound volume dropped 42%, and southbound volume dropped 57%, as compared to the previous year.

TRAVELER HEALTH SCREENING IS ALWAYS IN PLACE

Modern travel and trade relies on global circumnavigation in less than 24 hours. Therefore, each new outbreak of disease has the potential to significantly affect travelers and the travel industry. When disease threats emerge, countries may take border measures that range from minimal to invasive, regardless of available evidence of the efficacy of those measures. These interventions vary between and within countries, because public health interventions are usually locally driven.

To understand what to expect during an emergency, it is important to know that health screening of travelers is always in place at international ports of entry into most countries. Usually, the form of screening is minimal and routine, since the risk for significant threats to health is low most of the time. When increased health screening occurs, it is usually consistent with the threat of an identified contagious disease with the potential for spread through travel. Below is a list of public health measures used internationally, ranked in order from the least to the most invasive, that may be used to detect or control infection in international travelers, depending on the situation:

- Visual screening—observation of travelers conducted by customs or public health officers at ports of entry, typically without direct interaction with travelers, usually in place at all times
- Traveler health education—health communications intended to educate international travelers about a particular disease and border screening measures in place, including traveler's health alert notices or other printed material handed to travelers upon arrival, announcements or posters in transit areas, public service or social media announcements, and website information
- Travel warning—a notice published by government health authorities advising people to avoid travel to an area where a disease outbreak has been identified
- Passenger locator form—a form used by health officials to gather contact information for travelers believed to have been potentially exposed to an infectious disease during travel, for the purpose of locating or providing information to the travelers
- Traveler's health declaration form—a form often considered a legal, signed document, similar to a customs declaration form, that is used by customs or health officials at ports of entry to gather information related to a traveler's health, prior itinerary, and exposure to infection
- Direct questioning—interview of travelers by customs or health officials to evaluate symptoms and exposure history, to assess the risk of disease exposure or infection
- Temperature check—measurement of a traveler's temperature to identify a fever; can be done remotely by using a thermal imaging camera or through the use of a thermometer
- Detention—holding in custody a traveler suspected of having a communicable disease of concern, to allow further medical screening and examination by public health officials
- Isolation—separating and restricting the movement of an ill person who has a communicable disease of concern from those who are healthy, to minimize disease spread by preventing further transmission
- Quarantine—separating and restricting the movement of people who are well but may have been exposed to a communicable disease, to monitor their health and prevent possible transmission to others, until it is determined that they are not infected

Ultimately, for a given outbreak, the decision on which health measures to use, and how extensively each measure is implemented, will depend on the transmissibility and severity of the disease in question.

WHAT TO EXPECT DURING AN INTERNATIONAL DISEASE OUTBREAK

Whether it is a person's first international trip or that person is a seasoned international traveler, chances are he or she has planned the itinerary carefully to make the trip an enjoyable travel experience. Factoring in some amount of risk and being aware of as many chance variables as possible can help mitigate some of the negative repercussions, should an outbreak of illness occur that impacts travel. The following situations have been observed in nearly all significant international outbreaks of disease during the modern travel era since the 1960s:

- Travel delays—Travel into, out of, or within certain regions may be affected by border health measures or behavior of travelers.
- Inconsistent information—Early in an outbreak, information may change rapidly, be conflicting, or even later be determined to be incorrect, while governments, health officials, and the travel industry work to define the situation and provide reliable information.
- Canceled flights, ship voyages, trains, buses, or routes—Travel cancelations can occur suddenly, especially for air travel, which can be particularly sensitive to shifts in passenger demand and is often unpredictable during outbreaks.
- Voluntary cessation of travel—Travelers may choose to postpone their travel because of official travel warnings, travel advisories, or concerns about their health, border measures, or the possibility of being stranded in a foreign country. Large decreases in travel volume can decrease travel options, and travel schedules may be disrupted, especially to and from the countries most affected by the outbreak.
- Increase in travel—People traveling in affected countries in the early stages of an emerging outbreak may seek unplanned return journeys, as people try to avoid infection or seek health care in their home countries.
- Grounding of flights—In extreme circumstances, flights may be unavailable in a region for a period of time, as occurred in the United States after September 11, 2001, and in the spring of 2010, when clouds of ash resulting from eruptions from Iceland's Eyjafjallajökull volcano stalled air traffic over Europe. Although these instances were emergency disasters and not illness outbreaks, they demonstrate the sensitivity of air travel to health and safety threats.
- Entry or exit screening—The set of border health measures described earlier in this section may be applied, in whole or in part, at international borders, either to prevent the introduction of infection into the country (entry screening) or to prevent infected people from leaving and spreading infection to other countries (exit screening).

Guidelines and practices for what governments ask of travelers on arrival or exit may differ from country to country. Some countries maintain national control over all ports of entry and exit, while in other countries such control is delegated to state, provincial, or local authorities. In either case, requirements and procedures may differ widely and change over time. Flexibility, honesty, and compliance are essential to a successful interaction with public health and other government officials during international travel.

Below is a list of actions travelers might experience upon arrival to or exit from a country during an infectious disease outbreak. This list is not comprehensive or exhaustive. Travelers may be asked or forced to comply with one or more of the following:

- Have their temperatures taken either by thermal imaging camera or oral or ear thermometer
- Provide personal contact information and details about their travel itineraries
- Respond to questions regarding symptoms of illness or exposure to ill people
- Undergo a medical evaluation for infection, including diagnostic testing, such as nasal or throat swabs or blood tests
- Be isolated from other people until they are determined to be noninfectious
- Be hospitalized and given medical treatment if they test positive for or are otherwise diagnosed with an infectious disease of public health concern
- Be quarantined for a specified period of time if they were exposed to someone who is suspected or confirmed to be infected
- Monitor their health during and after travel and report any symptoms they develop to health officials
- Forego communications with family, friends, or traveling companions for a certain period
- Be denied boarding on an airplane, ship, bus, or train, if it is determined they are infectious or may have been exposed to a communicable disease of public health concern

TRAVELER'S RIGHTS AND RESPONSIBILITIES

The United States, acting through the Department of State, takes action to protect US citizens who are abroad via a number of diplomatic channels. However, in the event of an outbreak or epidemic, any country has the right to enact measures to protect its citizens from ill travelers entering its borders or to protect global health from ill travelers exiting the country. These border measures may infringe on the individual rights of any traveler who appears to be infected with or exposed to a disease of public health concern. The ability of the Department of State to intervene in such situations is limited. In effect, if a person chooses to travel abroad, he or she should be aware of the potential for the complete disruption of his or her journey by an outbreak or epidemic of public health significance.

CDC recommends that if a person is planning to travel internationally and feels ill or has symptoms such as fever, rash, or cough, he or she should consult with a medical provider and postpone travel until the illness or symptoms have resolved. Similarly, if a traveler becomes ill during or after international travel, he or she should seek medical attention and postpone further travel until the illness or symptoms have resolved. If an infectious disease is suspected, the traveler should call ahead before arriving at the medical facility, to avoid infecting other patients and staff.

Travelers can consult the embassies of the countries in their travel itineraries for information about health interventions and procedures that may affect their travel, although in some instances, inquiries or embassy websites do not provide correct or up-to-date information. The Department of State website may be helpful (http://travel.state.gov/travel/tips/brochures/brochures_1215.html). Up-to-date information regarding infectious disease risks related to travel may be found at the CDC website (www.cdc.gov/travel). Finally, because of the potential for significant delays and unexpected costs arising from an outbreak of communicable disease, CDC strongly recommends that travelers consider purchasing travel insurance to cover possible trip cancellations, requirements for health care abroad, or possible emergency medical evacuations (see Chapter 2, Travel Health Insurance and Evacuation Insurance).

BIBLIOGRAPHY

1. Barry JM. Observations on past influenza pandemics. Disaster Med Public Health Prep. 2009 Dec;3 Suppl 2:S95–9.
2. Berro A, Gallagher N, Yanni E, Lipman H, Whatley A, Bossak B. World Health Organization (WHO) travel recommendations during the 2003 SARS outbreak: lessons learned for mitigating influenza pandemic and globally emerging infectious diseases. Board 109. International Conference on Emerging Infectious Diseases; 2009 Mar 16–19; Atlanta, Georgia.
3. CDC. Update: outbreak of severe acute respiratory syndrome—worldwide, 2003. MMWR Morb Mortal Wkly Rep. 2003 Mar 28;52(12):241–6, 248.
4. Chan M. World now at the start of 2009 influenza pandemic. Geneva: World Health Organization; 2009 [cited 2010 Apr 26]. Available from: http://www.who.int/mediacentre/news/statements/2009/h1n1_pandemic_phase6_20090611/en/index.html.
5. Christian MD, Poutanen SM, Loutfy MR, Muller MP, Low DE. Severe acute respiratory syndrome. Clin Infect Dis. 2004 May 15;38(10):1420–7.
6. Hays JN. Epidemics and Pandemics: Their Impacts on Human History. Santa Barbara, CA: ABC-CLIO; 2005.
7. Snowden FM. Emerging and reemerging diseases: a historical perspective. Immunol Rev. 2008 Oct;225:9–26.
8. World Health Organization. International Health Regulations. Geneva: World Health Organization; 2005. Available from: http://www.who.int/ihr/en/.
9. World Health Organization. Public health measures taken at international borders during early stages of pandemic influenza A (H1N1) 2009: preliminary results. Wkly Epidemiol Rec. 2010 May 21;85(21):186–95.

DEATH DURING TRAVEL

Clare A. Dykewicz

OBTAINING US DEPARTMENT OF STATE ASSISTANCE

When a US citizen dies outside the United States, the deceased person's family members, domestic partner, or legal representative should notify US consular officials at the Department of State. Consular personnel are available 24 hours a day, 7 days a week, to provide assistance to US citizens for overseas emergencies.

- If a family member, domestic partner, or legal representative is in the foreign country with the deceased US citizen, they should contact the nearest US embassy or consulate for assistance. Contact information for US embassies, consulates, and consular agencies overseas may be found at the Department of State website (www.usembassy.gov).
- If a family member, domestic partner, or legal representative is located in the United States or Canada, he or she should call the Department of State's Office of Overseas Citizens Services in Washington, DC, from 8 AM to 8 PM Eastern Time, Monday through Friday, at 888-407-4747

or 202-501-4444. For emergency assistance after working hours or on weekends and holidays, call the Department of State switchboard at 202-647-4000 and ask to speak with the Overseas Citizens Services Duty Officer.

Emergency services provided by US consular officials can include advising the family, domestic partner, or legal representative about options and costs for disposing of the remains and personal effects of the deceased. Preparing and returning human remains to the United States can be an expensive and lengthy process. The Department of State does not pay for this; these costs are the responsibility of the deceased person's family, domestic partner, or legal representative. Consular officials may also serve as provisional conservators of the deceased person's estate, if no other legal representative is present in the foreign country where the death occurred.

IMPORTATION OF HUMAN REMAINS
General Guidance

People wishing to import human remains, including cremated remains, into the United States must obtain clearance from CDC's Division of Global Migration and Quarantine (CDC/DGMQ). Clearance can be obtained by presenting copies of the foreign death certificate and, if needed, a CDC/DGMQ permit to the CDC Quarantine Station with jurisdiction over the US port of entry of the remains (www.cdc.gov/quarantine/QuarantineStationContactListFull.html).

Remains of a Person Known or Suspected to Have Died from a Quarantinable Communicable Disease

Federal quarantine regulations (42 CFR Part 71) state that the remains of a person who is known or suspected to have died from a quarantinable communicable disease may not be brought into the United States, unless the remains are properly embalmed and placed in a hermetically sealed casket, cremated, or accompanied by a CDC permit to allow importation of human remains, issued by the CDC director.

If a CDC permit is obtained to allow importation of human remains, CDC may impose additional conditions for importation beyond those listed above. Permits for the importation of human remains may be obtained through CDC/DGMQ by calling 866-694-4867 or the CDC Emergency Operations Center at 770-488-7100.

Quarantinable communicable diseases include cholera, diphtheria, infectious tuberculosis, plague, smallpox, yellow fever, viral hemorrhagic fevers (Lassa, Marburg, Ebola, Crimean-Congo, or others not yet isolated or named), severe acute respiratory syndrome, and influenza caused by novel or reemergent influenza viruses that are causing or have the potential to cause a pandemic.

A copy of the foreign death certificate and the CDC/DGMQ permit must accompany the human remains at all times during shipment. The foreign death certificate must state the cause of death and be translated into English.

The US mortician handling the importation and disposition of the remains is also subject to the regulations of state and local health authorities for interstate and intrastate shipment. After disposition of the remains, the US mortician must submit a letter to CDC/DGMQ certifying that the human remains were imported, handled, and disposed of according to the terms of the CDC permit.

Remains of a Person Who Died of a Nonquarantinable Communicable Disease

Federal regulations also give CDC authority to restrict the importation of the remains of a person who died of a nonquarantinable communicable disease, when necessary to prevent the spread of communicable disease.

Remains of a Person Who Died of a Noncommunicable Disease

CDC places no restrictions on the importation of the remains of a person who died of a noncommunicable disease, although other federal, state, or local regulations may apply.

EXPORTATION OF HUMAN REMAINS

CDC places no restrictions on the exportation of human remains outside the United States, although other federal, state, and local regulations may apply. Exporters of human remains and travelers taking human remains out of the United States should be aware that the importation requirements of the destination country must be met. Information regarding these requirements may be obtained from the appropriate foreign embassy or consulate.

BIBLIOGRAPHY

1. CDC. Quarantine Stations: Quarantine Station Contact Lists and Jurisdictions. Atlanta: CDC; 2010 [cited 2010 Nov 2]. Available from: http://www.cdc.gov/quarantine/QuarantineStations.html.
2. Federal Register. Executive order 13295 of April 4, 2003—revised list of quarantinable communicable diseases. Washington, DC: Federal Register; 2003. p. 17255.
3. US Department of Health and Human Services. Title 42. Public Health. Chapter 1. Public Health Service, Department of Health and Human Services. Part 71. Foreign Quarantine. US Government Printing Office; 2001.
4. US Department of State. International Travel Information: Country Specific Information. Washington, DC: US Department of State. Available from: http://travel.state.gov/travel/cis_pa_tw/cis/cis_4965.html.
5. US Department of State. Death or Injury of an American Citizen Abroad. Washington, DC: US Department of State. Available from: http://travel.state.gov/travel/tips/emergencies/emergencies_3878.html.
6. US Department of State. Emergencies and Crises. Washington, DC: US Department of State. Available from: http://travel.state.gov/travel/tips/emergencies/emergencies_1212.html.
7. US Department of State. Emergency Abroad Getting Help. Washington, DC: US Department of State. Available from: http://www.travel.state.gov/travel/tips/emergencies/emergencies_1205.html.

TAKING ANIMALS & ANIMAL PRODUCTS ACROSS INTERNATIONAL BORDERS

G. Gale Galland, Robert J. Mullan, Heather Bair-Brake

CDC restricts the importation of animals and products, such as trophies and vectors, that may pose an infectious disease threat to humans. These restrictions apply to some pets, such as dogs and cats, as well as turtles, nonhuman primates, African rodents, civets, bats, and animal products capable of causing human disease (see www.cdc.gov/animalimportation/index.html). Animals taken out of the United States are subject, upon return, to the same regulations as those entering for the first time.

In addition to CDC, the Department of Agriculture (USDA) and the Fish and Wildlife Service (FWS) have jurisdiction over the importation of some animals. States may also have additional restrictions on the importation of animals.

ANIMAL HEALTH CERTIFICATES

CDC regulations do not require general health certificates for animals (including dogs or cats) entering the United States. However, health certificates may be required for entry of animals into some states and may be required by airlines in order to transport animals. Before departure, travelers should check with the public health veterinarian in their destination state, and with the airline, for any certificate requirements.

DOGS

Dogs are subject to inspection and may be denied entry into the United States if they have evidence of an infectious disease that can be transmitted to humans or if they have not been vaccinated against rabies. If a dog appears to be ill, further examination by a licensed veterinarian, at the owner's expense, may be required before it is released for official entry into the United States.

Rabies vaccination is required for all dogs entering the United States from a country where rabies is present. Unless a dog is being imported from a country considered "rabies-free" by the World Health Organization (Table 3-13), it must be accompanied by a current, valid rabies vaccination certificate that includes the following information:

- The breed, sex, age, color, markings, and other identifying information for the dog
- Date of rabies vaccination

- Signature of a licensed veterinarian
- Date of expiration of vaccination
  > Rabies certificates have expiration dates that range from 1 to 3 years from the date of vaccination, depending on the type of vaccine given

Dogs must be at least 3 months old before getting a rabies vaccine for the first time. Since it takes 30 days for the vaccine to take effect, dogs must have had their first rabies vaccination ≥30 days prior to arrival.

- If dogs arrive in the United States unvaccinated, CDC requires that they receive a rabies vaccine within 4–10 days of arrival and that they be confined for the 30-day period until the vaccination takes effect.
- If dogs arrive that have received their first rabies vaccine <30 days prior to arrival, CDC requires that the dogs be confined for the remainder of the 30-day period.
- Older dogs that have had prior rabies vaccination may be given a rabies vaccine up to the day of travel.

Dogs that do not meet CDC's rabies vaccination requirement may enter the United States only if the importer or owner completes a legal document called a *confinement agreement*. A copy of the confinement agreement (CDC Form 75.37) can be found on the CDC website at www.cdc.gov/animalimportation/dogs.html. By signing a confinement agreement, the importer or owner promises to confine the animal until it is fully vaccinated against rabies. Confinement agreements must be completed for:

- Dogs not accompanied by a current, valid rabies certificate.
- Dogs younger than 4 months of age.
- Dogs that received their first rabies vaccination <30 days prior to arrival in the United States.

Confinement is defined as isolation away from people and other animals, except for contact necessary for the dog's care. Conditions of the confinement agreement are as follows:

- The dog must be kept confined at a place of the owner's choosing, including the owner's home, until a rabies vaccination has been obtained and/or until 30 days have passed since vaccination.
- If the dog is allowed out of its enclosure, the owner must muzzle the dog and use a leash.
- The dog may not be sold or transferred from the responsibility of the importer during the confinement period.

Routine rabies vaccination of dogs is recommended in the United States and required by most state and local health authorities. Check with state authorities at the final destination to determine any state requirements for rabies vaccination. State-specific information is found at http://www.aphis.usda.gov/import_export/animals/animal_import/animal_imports_states.shtml. All pet dogs arriving in the state of Hawaii and the territory of Guam, even from the US mainland, are subject to locally imposed quarantine requirements. For more information about Hawaii, consult http://hawaii.gov/hdoa/ai/aqs/info or call 808-483-7151. For more information about Guam, see www.guamcourts.org/CompilerofLaws/GAR/09GAR/09GAR001-1.pdf or call 671-475-1426.

CATS

Cats are subject to inspection at US ports of entry and must appear healthy on arrival. If a cat appears to be ill, further examination by a licensed veterinarian, at the owner's expense, may be required before entry is permitted. Cats are not required to have proof of rabies vaccination for importation into the United States. States may require rabies vaccination for cats, however, so check with state and local health authorities at the final destination to determine any state requirements for rabies vaccination. All pet cats arriving in the state of Hawaii and the territory of Guam, even from the US mainland, are subject to locally imposed quarantine requirements. For more information about Hawaii, consult http://hawaii.gov/hdoa/ai/aqs/info or call 808-483-7151. For more information about Guam, see www.guamcourts.org/CompilerofLaws/GAR/09GAR/09GAR001-1.pdf or call 671-475-1426.

OTHER ANIMALS, ANIMAL PRODUCTS, AND VECTORS

Nonhuman Primates (Monkeys, Apes)

Nonhuman primates can transmit a variety of serious diseases to humans, including Ebola and tuberculosis. Nonhuman primate entry into the United States is restricted (see www.cdc.gov/animalimportation/monkeys.html). Nonhuman primates may only be imported into the United States by a CDC-registered importer and only for scientific, educational, or exhibition purposes. Nonhuman primates may not be imported as pets. All nonhuman primates are considered endangered or threatened and require additional FWS permits for importation. Nonhuman primates that leave the United States may only return through a registered importer, and only if they are imported for science, education, or exhibition.

Turtles

Turtles can transmit salmonella to humans, and because turtles are often kept as pets, restrictions apply to their importation. More information is available at www.cdc.gov/animalimportation/turtles.html. A person may import no more than 6 viable turtle eggs or live turtles with a carapace (shell) length of <4 in (10 cm). More turtles may be imported with CDC permission but only for science, education, or exhibition. CDC has no restrictions on the importation of live turtles with a carapace length >4 in. Check with USDA or FWS regarding additional requirements to import turtles.

African Rodents and Civets

To reduce the risk of introducing monkeypox and the severe acute respiratory syndrome (SARS) coronavirus, live African rodents and civets, as well as potentially infectious products made from these animals, may not be imported into the United States (see www.cdc.gov/ncidod/monkeypox/embargoqa.htm or www.cdc.gov/ncidod/sars/civetembargo.htm). Exceptions may be made for animals imported for science, education, or exhibition purposes, with permission from CDC.

Bats

Bats are reservoirs of many viruses that can infect humans, including rabies virus, Nipah virus, and SARS coronavirus. To reduce the risk of introducing these viruses, the importation of all live bats requires a CDC permit. Because they may be endangered species, bats also require additional permits issued by FWS. The applications for a CDC import permit for bats can be found at www.cdc.gov/animalimportation/bats.html.

Other Animals, Trophies, Animal Products, and Vectors

Certain live animals, hosts, or vectors of human disease, including insects, biological materials, tissues, and other unprocessed animal products, may pose an infectious disease risk to humans and be restricted from entry. For example, goatskin souvenirs (such as goatskin drums) from Haiti have been associated with human anthrax cases, and CDC restricts their entry into the United States. Potentially infectious nonhuman primate trophies may be imported if they are treated to render them noninfectious or if accompanied by a permit issued by CDC. In some circumstances, restricted items may be admitted with a permit from CDC for science, education, or exhibition (see www.cdc.gov/od/eaipp). USWFS and USDA may also have requirements for animal products and trophies.

Travelers planning to import horses, ruminants, swine, poultry or other birds, or dogs used for handling livestock should contact USDA's Animal Plant Health Inspection Service at 301-734-8364 or visit www.aphis.usda.gov to learn about additional requirements.

Travelers planning to import fish, reptiles, spiders, wild birds, rabbits, bears, wild members of the cat family, or other wild or endangered animals should contact FWS at 800-358-1949 or visit www.fws.gov/international/DMA_DSA/CITES/CITES_home.html.

For additional CDC information regarding animal and animal product importations, travelers should call 404-639-3441 or visit www.cdc.gov/animalimportation/index.html.

TRAVELING ABROAD WITH A PET

Travelers planning to take a companion animal to a foreign country should be advised to meet the entry requirements of the destination country and transportation guidelines of the airline. To obtain this information, travelers should contact the country's embassy in Washington, DC, or the nearest consulate (see www.state.gov/s/cpr/rls/fco/).

BIBLIOGRAPHY

1. CDC. Human rabies prevention—United States, 1999. Recommendations of the Advisory Committee on Immunization Practices (ACIP). MMWR Recomm Rep. 1999 Jan 8;48(RR-1):1–21.

2. CDC. Multistate outbreak of monkeypox—Illinois, Indiana, and Wisconsin, 2003. MMWR Morb Mortal Wkly Rep. 2003 Jun 13;52(23):537–40.

3. DeMarcus TA, Tipple MA, Ostrowski SR. US policy for disease control among imported nonhuman primates. J Infect Dis. 1999 Feb;179 Suppl 1:S281–2.

4. Dobson AP. What links bats to emerging infectious diseases? Science. 2005 Oct 28;310(5748):628–9.

5. Editorial: bongo-drum disease. Lancet. 1974 Jun 8;1(7867):1152.

6. National Association of State Public Health Veterinarians, Inc. Compendium of animal rabies prevention and control, 2009. MMWR Recomm Rep. 2009;58(RR-1):1–15.

7. Stam F, Romkens TE, Hekker TA, Smulders YM. Turtle-associated human salmonellosis. Clin Infect Dis. 2003 Dec 1;37(11):e167–9.

8. Wu D, Tu C, Xin C, Xuan H, Meng Q, Liu Y, et al. Civets are equally susceptible to experimental infection by two different severe acute respiratory syndrome coronavirus isolates. J Virol. 2005 Feb;79(4):2620–5.

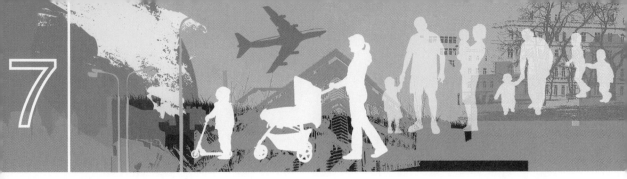

7

International Travel with Infants & Children

TRAVELING SAFELY WITH INFANTS & CHILDREN

Nicholas Weinberg, Michelle Weinberg, Susan A. Maloney

OVERVIEW

The number of children who travel or live outside their home countries has increased dramatically. An estimated 1.9 million children travel internationally each year. Although data about the incidence of pediatric illnesses associated with international travel are limited, the risks that children face while traveling are likely similar to the risks that their parents face. The most commonly reported health problems among children are:

- Diarrheal illnesses
- Dermatologic conditions
- Systemic febrile illnesses, especially malaria
- Respiratory disorders

Motor vehicle and water-related accidents are also major health problems for child travelers. In assessing a child who is planning international travel, clinicians should:

- Review routine childhood and travel-related vaccinations. The pre-travel visit is an opportunity to ensure that children are up to date on routine vaccinations.
- Assess all travel-related activities.
- Provide preventive counseling and interventions tailored to specific risks, including special travel preparations and treatment that may be required for children with underlying conditions, chronic diseases, or immunocompromising conditions.
- Give special consideration to the risks of children who are visiting friends and relatives in developing countries. These conditions may include increased risk of malaria, intestinal parasites, and tuberculosis.
- Consider counseling adults and older children to take a course in basic first aid before travel.

DIARRHEA

Diarrhea and associated gastrointestinal illness are among the most common travel-related problems affecting children. Infants and children with diarrhea can become dehydrated more quickly than adults. The etiology of travelers' diarrhea (TD) in children is similar to that in adults (see Chapter 2, Travelers' Diarrhea).

Prevention

For infants, breastfeeding is the best way to reduce the risk of foodborne and waterborne illness. Infant formulas available abroad may not be the same as in the United States; if parents are feeding their child formula, they should consider whether they need to bring formula from home.

Water served to young children, including water used to prepare infant formula, should be disinfected (see Chapter 2, Water Disinfection for Travelers). In some parts of the world, bottled water may also harbor germs and should be disinfected before consumption.

Similarly, food precautions should be followed diligently. Foods served to children should be thoroughly cooked and eaten while still hot; fruits eaten raw should be peeled immediately before consumption. Additionally, caution should be used with fresh dairy products, which may not be pasteurized and may be diluted with untreated water. For short trips, parents may want to bring a supply of safe snacks from home for times when the children are hungry and the available food may not be appealing or safe. See the section in Chapter 2, Food and Water Precautions for more information.

Scrupulous attention should be paid to handwashing and cleaning bottles, pacifiers, teething rings, and toys that fall to the floor or are handled by others; water used to clean these items should be potable. Parents should be particularly careful to wash hands well after diaper changes, especially for infants with diarrhea, to avoid spreading infection to themselves and other family members. When proper handwashing facilities are not available, an alcohol-based hand cleaner can be used as a disinfecting agent. However, because alcohol-based hand cleaners are not effective against certain types of germs, hands should be washed with soap and water as soon as possible. Additionally, alcohol does not remove organic material; visibly soiled hands should be washed with soap and water.

Management

Adults traveling with children should be counseled about the signs and symptoms of dehydration and the proper use of oral rehydration salts (ORS). Medical attention may be required for an infant or young child with diarrhea who has:

- Signs of moderate to severe dehydration (Table 7-1)
- Bloody diarrhea

- Temperature >101.5°F (38.6°C)
- Persistent vomiting (unable to maintain oral hydration)

The biggest threat to the infant with diarrhea and vomiting is dehydration. Fever or increased ambient temperature increases fluid loss and speeds dehydration. Parents should be advised that dehydration is best prevented and treated by use of ORS, in addition to the infant's usual food (see Table 2-5). ORS should be provided to the infant by bottle, cup, oral syringe (often available in pharmacies), or spoon while medical attention is obtained. Low-osmolarity ORS is the most effective in preventing dehydration, although other formulations are available and may be used if they are more acceptable to young children. Homemade sugar-salt solutions are not recommended. Adults traveling with children should be counseled that sports drinks, which are designed to replace water and electrolytes lost through sweat, do not contain the same proportions of electrolytes as the solution recommended by the World Health Organization for rehydration during diarrheal illness. However, if ORS is not readily available, children should be offered whatever palatable liquid they will take until ORS is obtained.

ORS Use and Availability

ORS packets are available at stores or pharmacies in almost all developing countries. ORS is prepared by adding one packet to boiled or treated water. Travelers should be advised to check packet instructions carefully to ensure that the salts are added to the correct volume of water. ORS solution should be consumed or discarded within 12 hours if held at room temperature or 24 hours if kept refrigerated.

A dehydrated child will usually drink ORS avidly; travelers should be advised to give it to the child as long as the dehydration persists. As dehydration lessens, the salty-tasting ORS solution may be refused, and another liquid can be offered. An infant or child who has been vomiting will usually keep ORS down if it is offered by spoon or oral syringe in small sips; these small amounts must be offered frequently, however, so the child can receive an adequate volume of ORS. Older children will often drink well by sipping through a straw. Severely dehydrated children, however, often

Table 7-1. Assessment of dehydration in infants

SIGN	SEVERITY		
	MILD	MODERATE	SEVERE
General condition	Thirsty, restless, agitated	Thirsty, restless, irritable	Withdrawn, somnolent, or comatose; rapid, deep breathing
Pulse	Normal	Rapid, weak	Rapid, weak
Anterior fontanelle	Normal	Sunken	Very sunken
Eyes	Normal	Sunken	Very sunken
Tears	Present	Absent	Absent
Mucous membranes	Slightly dry	Dry	Dry
Skin turgor	Normal	Decreased	Decreased with tenting
Urine	Normal	Reduced, concentrated	None for several hours
Weight loss	4%–5%	6%–9%	≥10%

will be unable to drink adequately. Severe dehydration is a medical emergency that usually requires administration of fluids by intravenous or intraosseous routes.

Children weighing <22 lb (10 kg) who have mild to moderate dehydration should be administered 2–4 oz (60–120 mL) ORS for each diarrheal stool or vomiting episode. Children who weigh ≥22 lb (10 kg) should receive 4–8 oz (120–240 mL) of ORS for each diarrheal stool or vomiting episode.

ORS packets are available in the United States from Jianas Brothers Packaging Company (816-421-2880). ORS packets may also be available at stores that sell outdoor recreation and camping supplies. In addition, Cera Products (410-309-1000 or 888-237-2598; www.ceraproductsinc.com) markets a rice-based, rather than glucose-based, product.

Dietary Modification

Breastfed infants should continue nursing on demand. Formula-fed infants should continue their usual formula during rehydration. They should receive a volume that is sufficient to satisfy energy and nutrient requirements. Lactose-free or lactose-reduced formulas are usually unnecessary. Diluting formula may slow resolution of diarrhea and is not recommended. Older infants and children receiving semisolid or solid foods should continue to receive their usual diet during the illness. Recommended foods include starches, cereals, yogurt, fruits, and vegetables. Foods that are high in simple sugars, such as soft drinks, undiluted apple juice, gelatins, and presweetened cereals, can exacerbate diarrhea by osmotic effects and should be avoided. In addition, foods high in fat may not be tolerated because of their tendency to delay gastric emptying.

The practice of withholding food for 24 hours or more is not recommended. Early feeding can decrease changes in intestinal permeability caused by infection, reduce illness duration, and improve nutritional outcome. Highly specific diets (such as the BRAT [bananas, rice, applesauce, and toast] diet) have been commonly recommended; however, similar to juice-based and clear fluid diets, such severely restrictive diets have no scientific basis and should be avoided.

Antibiotics

Chemoprophylaxis is not generally used in children. Few data are available regarding empiric treatment of TD in children. The antimicrobial options for empiric treatment of TD in children are limited. In practice, when an antibiotic is indicated for moderate to severe diarrhea, some clinicians prescribe azithromycin as a single dose (10 mg/kg) for 3 days. Physicians can prescribe unreconstituted azithromycin powder before travel, with instructions from the pharmacist as to how to mix it into an oral suspension if it becomes necessary to use it.

Although fluoroquinolones are frequently used for the empiric treatment of TD in adults, they are not approved by the Food and Drug Administration for this purpose among children aged <18 years because of cartilage damage seen in animal studies. The American Academy of Pediatrics suggests that fluoroquinolones be considered for the treatment of children with severe infections caused by multidrug-resistant strains of *Shigella* species, *Salmonella* species, *Vibrio cholerae*, or *Campylobacter jejuni*. Routine use of fluoroquinolones for chemoprophylaxis or empiric treatment for TD among children is not recommended.

MALARIA

Malaria is among the most serious and life-threatening diseases that can be acquired by pediatric international travelers. Children who are visiting friends and relatives are at particularly high risk for acquiring malaria if they do not receive chemoprophylaxis. Children with malaria can rapidly develop a high level of parasitemia. They are at increased risk for severe complications of malaria,

including shock, seizures, coma, and death. Initial symptoms of malaria in children may mimic many other common causes of pediatric febrile illness and therefore may result in delayed diagnosis and treatment. Clinicians should counsel adults traveling with children in malarious areas to use the appropriate preventive measures, be aware of the signs and symptoms of malaria, and seek prompt medical attention if they develop.

Antimalarial Drugs

Pediatric doses for malaria chemoprophylaxis are provided in Table 3-11. Pediatric doses of medications used for treatment are included in Table 3-9. All dosing should be calculated on the basis of body weight. Medications used for infants and young children are the same as those recommended for adults, except under the following circumstances:

- Doxycycline should not be given to children aged <8 years because of the risk of teeth staining.
- Atovaquone-proguanil should not be used for prophylaxis in children weighing <5 kg (11 lb) because of lack of data on safety and efficacy.

Chloroquine, mefloquine, and atovaquone-proguanil have a bitter taste. Before departure, pharmacists can be asked to pulverize tablets and prepare gelatin capsules with calculated pediatric doses. Mixing the powder in a small amount of food or drink can facilitate the administration of antimalarial drugs to infants and children. Additionally, any compounding pharmacy can alter the flavoring of malaria medication tablets so that they are more willingly ingested by children. Assistance with finding a compounding pharmacy is available on the International Academy of Compounding Pharmacists' website (www.iacprx.org). Because overdose of antimalarial drugs, particularly chloroquine, can be fatal, medication should be stored in childproof containers and kept out of the reach of infants and children.

Personal Protection Measures

Children should sleep in rooms with air conditioning and screened windows, or under bed nets, when available. Mosquito netting should be used over infant carriers. Children can reduce skin exposed to mosquitoes by wearing long pants and long sleeves while outdoors in areas where malaria is transmitted. Clothing and mosquito nets can be treated with insect repellents such as permethrin, a repellent and insecticide that repels and kills ticks, mosquitoes, and other arthropods. Permethrin remains effective through multiple washings. Clothing and bed nets should be retreated according to the product label. Permethrin should not be applied to the skin. Although permethrin provides longer duration protection, recommended repellents that can be applied to skin (DEET [N,N-diethyl-m-toluamide], picaridin, oil of lemon eucalyptus [OLE] or PMD, and IR3535) can also be used on clothing and mosquito nets. See Chapter 2, Protection against Mosquitoes, Ticks, and Other Insects and Arthropods for more details about these protective measures.

Repellent Use

CDC recommends the use of DEET, picaridin, OLE or PMD, and IR3535, which are repellents containing active ingredients registered with the US Environmental Protection Agency, according to the product labels. Most repellents can be used on children aged >2 months, with the following considerations:

- Products containing OLE specify that they should not be used on children aged <3 years.
- Repellent products must state any age restriction. If none is stated, the Environmental Protection Agency has not required a restriction on the use of the product.
- Many repellents contain DEET as the active ingredient. The concentration of DEET varies considerably among products. The duration of protection varies with the DEET concentration: higher concentrations protect longer. Products with DEET concentration above 50% do not offer a marked increase in protection time. The American Academy of Pediatrics recommends:
  > ≤30% DEET should be used on children aged >2 months.
  > Repellents with DEET should not be used on infants aged <2 months.

Repellents can be applied to exposed skin and clothing; however, they should not be applied under clothing. Repellents should never be used over cuts, wounds, or irritated skin. Young children should not be allowed to handle the product. When using repellent on a child, an adult should apply it to his or her own hands and then rub them on the child, with the following considerations:

- Avoid the child's eyes and mouth, and apply sparingly around the ears.
- Do not apply repellent to children's hands, since children tend to put their hands in their mouths.
- Do not apply repellent under clothing.
- Heavy application and saturation are generally unnecessary for effectiveness. If biting insects do not respond to a thin film of repellent, then apply a bit more.
- After returning indoors, wash treated skin with soap and water or bathe. This is particularly important when repellents are used repeatedly in a day or on consecutive days.

Products that contain repellents and sunscreen are generally not recommended, because instructions for use are different and the need to reapply sunscreen is usually more frequent than with repellent alone. In general, apply sunscreen first, then apply repellent. Mosquito coils should be used with caution in the presence of children to avoid burns and inadvertent ingestion.

For more information about repellent use, see Chapter 2, Protection against Mosquitoes, Ticks, and Other Insects and Arthropods.

INFECTION AND INFESTATION FROM SOIL CONTACT

Children are more likely than adults to have contact with soil or sand, and therefore, they may be exposed to diseases caused by infectious stages of parasites present in soil, including ascariasis, hookworm infestation, cutaneous or visceral larva migrans, trichuriasis, and strongyloidiasis. Children and infants should wear protective footwear and play on a sheet or towel rather than directly on the ground. Clothing should not be dried on the ground. When traveling in countries with a tropical climate, clothing or diapers dried in the open air should be ironed before use to prevent infestation with fly larvae.

ANIMAL BITES AND RABIES

Worldwide, rabies is more common in children than adults. In addition to the potential for increased contact with animals, children are also more likely to be bitten on the head or neck, leading to more severe injuries. Children and their families should be counseled to avoid all stray or unfamiliar animals and to inform adults of any contact or bites. Bats throughout the world are considered to have the potential to transmit rabies virus. Mammal-associated injuries should be washed thoroughly with water and soap (and povidone iodine if available), and the child should be evaluated promptly to assess the need for rabies post-exposure prophylaxis. Because of the potential unavailability of rabies vaccine and rabies immune globulin in certain destinations, families should seriously consider purchasing medical evacuation insurance.

AIR TRAVEL

Although air travel is safe for healthy newborns, infants, and children, a few issues should be considered in preparation for travel. Children with chronic heart or lung problems may be at risk for hypoxia during flight, and a physician should be consulted before travel. Making sure that children can be safely restrained during a flight is a safety consideration. Severe turbulence or crash can create enough momentum that a parent cannot hold onto a child:

- Children should be placed in a rear-facing Federal Aviation Authority-approved child-safety seat until they are aged ≥1 year and weigh ≥20 lb.
- Children aged ≥1 year and 20–40 lb should use a forward-facing Federal Aviation Authority-approved child-safety seat.
- Children who weigh >40 lb can be secured in the aircraft seat belt.

Ear pain can be troublesome for infants and children during descent. Pressure in the middle ear can be equalized by swallowing or chewing:

- Infants should nurse or suck on a bottle.
- Older children can try chewing gum.
- Antihistamines and decongestants have not been shown to be of benefit.

There is no evidence that air travel exacerbates the symptoms or complications associated with otitis media. Travel to different time zones, "jet lag," and schedule disruptions can disturb sleep patterns in infants and children, as well as adults.

ACCIDENTS
Vehicle-Related

Vehicle-related accidents are the leading cause of death in children who travel. While traveling in automobiles and other vehicles, children weighing ≤40 lb should be restrained in age-appropriate car seats or booster seats, as described above. These seats often must be carried from home, since availability of well-maintained and approved seats may be limited abroad. In general, children are safest traveling in the rear seat; no one should ever travel in the bed of a pickup truck. Families should be counseled that in many developing countries, cars may lack front or rear seatbelts.

Drowning and Water-Related Illness and Injuries

Drowning is the second leading cause of death in young travelers. Children may not be familiar with hazards in the ocean or in rivers. Swimming pools may not have protective fencing to keep toddlers from falling into the pool. Close supervision of children around water is essential. Appropriate water safety devices such as life vests may not be available abroad, and families should consider bringing these from home. Protective footwear is important to avoid injury in many marine environments. Schistosomiasis is a risk to children and adults in endemic areas. While in schistosomiasis-endemic areas (see Map 3-14), children should not swim in fresh, unchlorinated water such as lakes or ponds.

Accommodations

Conditions at hotels and other lodging may not be as safe as those in the United States, and accommodations should be carefully inspected for exposed wiring, pest poisons, paint chips, or inadequate stairway or balcony railings.

ALTITUDE

Children are as susceptible to altitude illness as adults. Young children who cannot talk can show nonspecific symptoms, such as loss of appetite and irritability. They may present with unexplained fussiness and change in sleep and activity patterns. Older children may complain of headache or shortness of breath. If a child demonstrates unexplained symptoms after an ascent, it may be necessary to descend to see if they improve. Acetazolamide is not approved for pediatric use for altitude illness, but it is generally safe in children when used for other indications.

SUN EXPOSURE

Sun exposure, and particularly sunburn before age 15 years, is strongly associated with melanoma and other forms of skin cancer (see Chapter 2, Sunburn). Exposure to UV light is highest near the equator, at high altitudes, during midday (10 AM–4 PM), and where light is reflected off water or snow. Sunscreens are generally recommended for use in children aged >6 months. Sunscreens (or sun blocks), either physical (such as titanium or zinc oxides) or chemical (SPF ≥15 and providing protection from both UVA and UVB), should be applied as directed and reapplied, as needed, after sweating and water exposure. Babies aged <6 months require extra protection from the sun because of their thinner and more sensitive skin; severe sunburn for this age group is considered a medical emergency. Babies should be kept in the shade and wear clothing that covers the entire body. A minimal amount of sunscreen can be applied to small exposed areas, including the infant's face and hands.

Sun-blocking shirts are available that are made for swimming and preclude having to rub sunscreen over the entire trunk. Hats and sunglasses also reduce sun injury to skin and eyes. If both sunscreen and a DEET-containing insect repellent are applied, the sun protection factor (SPF) of the sunscreen may be diminished by one-third, and covering clothing should be worn or time in the sun decreased accordingly.

OTHER GENERAL CONSIDERATIONS
Travel Stress
Changes in schedule, activities, and environment can be stressful for children. Including children in planning for the trip and bringing along familiar toys or other objects can decrease these stresses. For children with chronic illnesses, decisions regarding timing and itinerary should be made in consultation with the child's health care providers.

Insurance
As for any traveler, insurance coverage for illnesses and accidents while abroad should be verified before departure. Consideration should be given to purchasing special travel insurance for airlifting or air ambulance to an area with adequate medical care.

Identification
In case family members become separated, each infant or child should carry identifying information and contact numbers in his or her own clothing or pockets. Because of concerns about illegal transport of children across international borders, if only one parent is traveling with the child, he or she may need to carry relevant custody papers or a notarized permission letter from the other parent.

BIBLIOGRAPHY

1. American Academy of Pediatrics. A parent's guide to insect repellants. 2005. Available from: http://www.arlingtonpediatrics.com/A%20Parent's%20Guide%20to%20Insect%20Repellents.pdf.
2. Committee on Infectious Disease, American Academy of Pediatrics. The use of systemic fluoroquinolones. Pediatrics. 2006;118(3):1287–92.
3. DuPont HL, Ericsson CD, Farthing MJ, Gorbach S, Pickering LK, Rombo L, et al. Expert review of the evidence base for prevention of travelers' diarrhea. J Travel Med. 2009 May–Jun;16(3):149–60.
4. Hagmann S, Neugebauer R, Schwartz E, Perret C, Castelli F, Barnett ED, et al. Illness in children after international travel: analysis from the GeoSentinel Surveillance Network. Pediatrics. 2010 May;125(5):e1072–80.
5. King CK, Glass R, Bresee JS, Duggan C. Managing acute gastroenteritis among children: oral rehydration, maintenance, and nutritional therapy. MMWR Recomm Rep. 2003 Nov 21;52(RR-16):1–16.
6. Murphy ME, Montemarano AD, Debboun M, Gupta R. The effect of sunscreen on the efficacy of insect repellent: a clinical trial. J Am Acad Dermatol. 2000 Aug;43(2 Pt 1):219–22.

VACCINE RECOMMENDATIONS FOR INFANTS & CHILDREN

Sheila M. Mackell

Vaccinating children for travel requires careful evaluation. Whenever possible, children should complete the routine immunizations of childhood on a normal schedule. However, travel at an earlier age may require accelerated schedules. **Not all travel-related vaccines are effective in infants, and some are specifically contraindicated.**

The recommended childhood and adolescent immunization schedules are depicted in Tables 7-2 and 7-3. Table 7-4 depicts the catch-up schedule for children and adolescents who start their vaccination schedule late or who are >1 month behind. This table also describes the recommended minimum intervals between doses for children who need to be vaccinated on an accelerated schedule, which may be necessary before international travel. Proof of yellow fever vaccination is required for entry into certain countries.

MODIFYING THE IMMUNIZATION SCHEDULE FOR INADEQUATELY IMMUNIZED INFANTS AND YOUNGER CHILDREN BEFORE INTERNATIONAL TRAVEL

Several factors influence recommendations for the age at which a vaccine is administered, including age-specific risks of the disease and its complications, the ability of people of a given age to develop an adequate immune response to the vaccine, and potential interference with the immune response by passively transferred maternal antibody.

The routine immunization recommendations and schedules for infants and children in the United States do not provide specific guidelines for those traveling internationally before the age when specific vaccines and toxoids are routinely recommended. Recommended age limitations are based on potential adverse events (yellow fever), lack of efficacy data or inadequate immune response (polysaccharide vaccines and influenza), maternal antibody interference (measles,

mumps, rubella), or lack of safety data. In deciding when to travel with a young infant or child, parents should be advised that the earliest opportunity to receive routinely recommended immunizations in the United States (except for the dose of hepatitis B vaccine at birth) is at age 6 weeks.

Routine Infant and Childhood Vaccinations

Hepatitis B Vaccine

Hepatitis B virus (HBV) is a cause of acute and chronic hepatitis, cirrhosis, and hepatocellular carcinoma. There are more than 350 million chronically infected people worldwide. The risk of chronic infection is highest when infection occurs in infancy or childhood and declines with age. Infants and children who have not previously been vaccinated and who are traveling to areas where HBV is intermediately or highly endemic are at risk if they are directly exposed to blood (or body fluids containing blood) from the local population. HBV transmission could occur in children if they receive blood transfusions not screened for HBV surface antigen (HBsAg), are exposed to unsterilized medical or dental equipment, or have continuous close contact with local residents who have open skin lesions (impetigo, scabies, or scratched insect bites).

Hepatitis B vaccine is recommended for all infants in the United States, with the first dose administered soon after birth and before hospital discharge. Infants and children who will travel should receive 3 doses of HBV vaccine before traveling:

- The interval between doses 1 and 2 should be ≥4 weeks.
- The interval between doses 2 and 3 should be ≥8 weeks.
- The interval between doses 1 and 3 should be ≥16 weeks.
- The third dose should not be given before the infant is at least 24 weeks of age.

Table 7-2. Recommended immunization schedule for ages 0–6 years—United States, 2011

For those who fall behind or start late, see the catch-up schedule.

Vaccine ▼	Birth	1 month	2 months	4 months	6 months	12 months	15 months	18 months	19–23 months	2–3 years	4–6 years
Hepatitis B[1]	HepB	HepB				HepB					
Rotavirus[2]			RV	RV	RV[2]						
Diphtheria, Tetanus, Pertussis[3]			DTaP	DTaP	DTaP	see footnote[3]	DTaP				DTaP
Haemophilus influenzae type b[4]			Hib	Hib	Hib[4]	Hib					
Pneumococcal[5]			PCV	PCV	PCV	PCV				PPSV	PPSV
Inactivated Poliovirus[6]			IPV	IPV	IPV						IPV
Influenza[7]					Influenza (Yearly)						
Measles, Mumps, Rubella[8]						MMR		see footnote[8]			MMR
Varicella[9]						Varicella		see footnote[9]			Varicella
Hepatitis A[10]						HepA (2 doses)				HepA Series	HepA Series
Meningococcal[11]										MCV4	MCV4

Legend:

■ Range of recommended ages for all children

■ Range of recommended ages for certain high-risk groups

This schedule includes recommendations in effect as of December 21, 2010. Any dose not administered at the recommended age should be administered at a subsequent visit, when indicated and feasible. The use of a combination vaccine generally is preferred over separate injections of its equivalent component vaccines. Considerations should include provider assessment, patient preference, and the potential for adverse events. Providers should consult the relevant Advisory Committee on Immunization Practices statement for detailed recommendations: www.cdc.gov/vaccines/pubs/acip-list.htm. Clinically significant adverse events that follow immunization should be reported to the Vaccine Adverse Event Reporting System (VAERS) at http://vaers.hhs.gov or by telephone, 800-822-7967.

1. **Hepatitis B vaccine (HepB).** (Minimum age: birth)
   At birth:
   - Administer monovalent HepB to all newborns before hospital discharge.
   - If mother is hepatitis B surface antigen (HBsAg)-positive, administer HepB and 0.5 mL of hepatitis B immune globulin (HBIG) within 12 hours of birth.
   - If mother's HBsAg status is unknown, administer HepB within 12 hours of birth. Determine mother's HBsAg status as soon as possible and, if HBsAg-positive, administer HBIG (no later than age 1 week).

Doses following the birth dose:

- The second dose should be administered at age 1 or 2 months. Monovalent HepB should be used for doses administered before age 6 weeks.
- Infants born to HBsAg-positive mothers should be tested for HBsAg and antibody to HBsAg 1 to 2 months after completion of at least 3 doses of the HepB series, at age 9 through 18 months (generally at the next well-child visit).
- Administration of 4 doses of HepB to infants is permissible when a combination vaccine containing HepB is administered after the birth dose.
- Infants who did not receive a birth dose should receive 3 doses of HepB on a schedule of 0, 1, and 6 months.
- The final (3rd or 4th) dose in the HepB series should be administered no earlier than age 24 weeks.

2. **Rotavirus vaccine (RV).** [Minimum age: 6 weeks]
- Administer the first dose at age 6 through 14 weeks (maximum age: 14 weeks 6 days). Vaccination should not be initiated for infants aged 15 weeks 0 days or older.
- The maximum age for the final dose in the series is 8 months 0 days.
- If Rotarix is administered at ages 2 and 4 months, a dose at 6 months is not indicated.

3. **Diphtheria and tetanus toxoids and acellular pertussis vaccine (DTaP).** [Minimum age: 6 weeks]
- The fourth dose may be administered as early as age 12 months, provided at least 6 months have elapsed since the third dose.

4. *Haemophilus influenzae* **type b conjugate vaccine (Hib).** [Minimum age: 6 weeks]
- If PRP-OMP (PedvaxHIB or Comvax [HepB-Hib]) is administered at ages 2 and 4 months, a dose at age 6 months is not indicated.
- Hiberix should not be used for doses at ages 2, 4, or 6 months for the primary series but can be used as the final dose in children aged 12 months through 4 years.

5. **Pneumococcal vaccine.** [Minimum age: 6 weeks for pneumococcal conjugate vaccine [PCV]; 2 years for pneumococcal polysaccharide vaccine [PPSV]]
- Administer 1 dose of PCV to all healthy children aged 24 through 59 months who are not completely vaccinated for their age.
- A PCV series begun with 7-valent PCV (PCV7) should be completed with 13-valent PCV (PCV13).
- A single supplemental dose of PCV13 is recommended for all children aged 14 through 59 months who have received an age-appropriate series of PCV7.
- A single supplemental dose of PCV13 is recommended for all children aged 60 through 71 months with underlying medical conditions who have received an age-appropriate series of PCV7.
- The supplemental dose of PCV13 should be administered at least 8 weeks after the previous dose of PCV7. See *MMWR* 2010;59[No.RR-11].
- Administer PPSV at least 8 weeks after last dose of PCV to children aged 2 years or older with certain underlying medical conditions, including a cochlear implant.

6. **Inactivated poliovirus vaccine (IPV).** [Minimum age: 6 weeks]
- If 4 or more doses are administered prior to age 4 years an additional dose should be administered at age 4 through 6 years.
- The final dose in the series should be administered on or after the fourth birthday and at least 6 months following the previous dose.

7. **Influenza vaccine (seasonal).** [Minimum age: 6 months for trivalent inactivated influenza vaccine [TIV]; 2 years for live, attenuated influenza vaccine [LAIV]]
- For healthy children aged 2 years and older (i.e., those who do not have underlying medical conditions that predispose them to influenza complications), either LAIV or TIV may be used, except LAIV should not be given to children aged 2 through 4 years who have had wheezing in the past 12 months.
- Administer 2 doses (separated by at least 4 weeks) to children aged 6 months through 8 years who are receiving seasonal influenza vaccine for the first time or who were vaccinated for the first time during the previous influenza season but only received 1 dose.
- Children aged 6 months through 8 years who received no doses of monovalent 2009 H1N1 vaccine should receive 2 doses of 2010-2011 seasonal influenza vaccine. See *MMWR* 2010;59[No.RR-8]:33-34.

8. **Measles, mumps, and rubella vaccine (MMR).** [Minimum age: 12 months]
- The second dose may be administered before age 4 years, provided at least 4 weeks have elapsed since the first dose.

9. **Varicella vaccine.** [Minimum age: 12 months]
- The second dose may be administered before age 4 years, provided at least 3 months have elapsed since the first dose.
- For children aged 12 months through 12 years the recommended minimum interval between doses is 3 months. However, if the second dose was administered at least 4 weeks after the first dose, it can be accepted as valid.

10. **Hepatitis A vaccine (HepA).** [Minimum age: 12 months]
- Administer 2 doses at least 6 months apart.
- HepA is recommended for children aged older than 23 months who live in areas where vaccination programs target older children, who are at increased risk for infection, or for whom immunity against hepatitis A is desired.

11. **Meningococcal conjugate vaccine, quadrivalent (MCV4).** [Minimum age: 2 years]
- Administer 2 doses of MCV4 at least 8 weeks apart to children aged 2 through 10 years with persistent complement component deficiency and anatomic or functional asplenia, and 1 dose every 5 years thereafter.
- Persons with human immunodeficiency virus (HIV) infection who are vaccinated with MCV4 should receive 2 doses at least 8 weeks apart.
- Administer 1 dose of MCV4 to children aged 2 through 10 years who travel to countries with highly endemic or epidemic disease and during outbreaks caused by a vaccine serogroup.
- Administer MCV4 to children at continued risk for meningococcal disease who were previously vaccinated with MCV4 or meningococcal polysaccharide vaccine after 3 years if the first dose was administered at age 2 through 6 years.

The Recommended Immunization Schedules for Persons Aged 0 Through 18 Years are approved by the Advisory Committee on Immunization Practices (www.cdc.gov/vaccines/pubs/ACIP-list. html), the American Academy of Pediatrics (www.aap.org), and the American Academy of Family Physicians (www.aafp.org).

Table 7-3. Recommended immunization schedule for ages 7–18 years—United States, 2011

For those who fall behind or start late, see the schedule below and the catch-up schedule.

Vaccine ▼ Age ▶	7–10 years	11–12 years	13–18 years
Tetanus, Diphtheria, Pertussis[1]		Tdap	Tdap
Human Papillomavirus[2]	see footnote[2]	HPV (3 doses) (females)	HPV series
Meningococcal[3]	MCV4	MCV4	MCV4
Influenza[4]	Influenza (Yearly)		
Pneumococcal[5]	Pneumococcal		
Hepatitis A[6]	HepA Series		
Hepatitis B[7]	HepB Series		
Inactivated Poliovirus[8]	IPV Series		
Measles, Mumps, Rubella[9]	MMR Series		
Varicella[10]	Varicella Series		

Range of recommended ages for all children

Range of recommended ages for catch-up immunization

Range of recommended ages for certain high-risk groups

This schedule includes recommendations in effect as of December 21, 2010. Any dose not administered at the recommended age should be administered at a subsequent visit, when indicated and feasible. The use of a combination vaccine generally is preferred over separate injections of its equivalent component vaccines. Considerations should include provider assessment, patient preference, and the potential for adverse events. Providers should consult the relevant Advisory Committee on Immunization Practices statement for detailed recommendations: www.cdc.gov/vaccines/pubs/acip-list.htm. Clinically significant adverse events that follow immunization should be reported to the Vaccine Adverse Event Reporting System (VAERS) at www.vaers.hhs.gov or by telephone, 800-822-7967.

1. **Tetanus and diphtheria toxoids and acellular pertussis vaccine (Tdap).** (Minimum age: 10 years for Boostrix and 11 years for Adacel)
   - Persons aged 11 through 18 years who have not received Tdap should receive a dose followed by Td booster doses every 10 years thereafter.
   - Persons aged 7 through 10 years who are not fully immunized against pertussis (including those never vaccinated or with unknown pertussis vaccination status) should receive a single dose of Tdap. Refer to the catch-up schedule if additional doses of tetanus and diphtheria toxoid–containing vaccine are needed.
   - Tdap can be administered regardless of the interval since the last tetanus and diphtheria toxoid–containing vaccine.

2. **Human papillomavirus vaccine (HPV). (Minimum age: 9 years)**
   - Quadrivalent HPV vaccine (HPV4) or bivalent HPV vaccine (HPV2) is recommended for the prevention of cervical precancers and cancers in females.
   - HPV4 is recommended for prevention of cervical precancers, cancers, and genital warts in females.
   - HPV4 may be administered in a 3-dose series to males aged 9 through 18 years to reduce their likelihood of genital warts.
   - Administer the second dose 1 to 2 months after the first dose and the third dose 6 months after the first dose (at least 24 weeks after the first dose).

3. **Meningococcal conjugate vaccine, quadrivalent (MCV4). (Minimum age: 2 years)**
   - Administer MCV4 at age 11 through 12 years with a booster dose at age 16 years.
   - Administer 1 dose at age 13 through 18 years if not previously vaccinated.
   - Persons who received their first dose at age 13 through 15 years should receive a booster dose at age 16 through 18 years.
   - Administer 1 dose to previously unvaccinated college freshmen living in a dormitory.
   - Administer 2 doses at least 8 weeks apart to children aged 2 through 10 years with persistent complement component deficiency and anatomic or functional asplenia, and 1 dose every 5 years thereafter.
   - Persons with HIV infection who are vaccinated with MCV4 should receive 2 doses at least 8 weeks apart.
   - Administer 1 dose of MCV4 to children aged 2 through 10 years who travel to countries with highly endemic or epidemic disease and during outbreaks caused by a vaccine serogroup.
   - Administer MCV4 to children at continued risk for meningococcal disease who were previously vaccinated with MCV4 or meningococcal polysaccharide vaccine after 3 years (if first dose administered at age 2 through 6 years) or after 5 years (if first dose administered at age 7 years or older).

4. **Influenza vaccine (seasonal).**
   - For healthy nonpregnant persons aged 7 through 18 years (i.e., those who do not have underlying medical conditions that predispose them to influenza complications), either LAIV or TIV may be used.
   - Administer 2 doses (separated by at least 4 weeks) to children aged 6 months through 8 years who are receiving seasonal influenza vaccine for the first time or who were vaccinated for the first time during the previous influenza season but only received 1 dose. Children 6 months through 8 years of age who received no doses of monovalent 2009 H1N1 vaccine should receive 2 doses of 2010–2011 seasonal influenza vaccine. See MMWR 2010;59[No. RR-8]:33-34.

5. **Pneumococcal vaccines.**
   - A single dose of 13-valent pneumococcal conjugate vaccine (PCV13) may be administered to children aged 6 through 18 years who have functional or anatomic asplenia, HIV infection or other immunocompromising condition, cochlear implant or CSF leak. See MMWR 2010;59[No. RR-11].
   - The dose of PCV13 should be administered at least 8 weeks after the previous dose of PCV7.
   - Administer pneumococcal polysaccharide vaccine at least 8 weeks after the last dose of PCV to children aged 2 years or older with certain underlying medical conditions, including a cochlear implant. A single revaccination should be administered after 5 years to children with functional or anatomic asplenia or an immunocompromising condition.

6. **Hepatitis A vaccine (HepA).**
   - Administer 2 doses at least 6 months apart.
   - HepA is recommended for children aged older than 23 months who live in areas where vaccination programs target older children, or who are at increased risk for infection, or for whom immunity against hepatitis A is desired.

7. **Hepatitis B vaccine (HepB).**
   - Administer the 3-dose series to those not previously vaccinated. For those with incomplete vaccination, follow the catch-up schedule.
   - A 2-dose series (separated by at least 4 months) of adult formulation Recombivax HB is licensed for children aged 11 through 15 years.

8. **Inactivated poliovirus vaccine (IPV).**
   - The final dose in the series should be administered on or after the fourth birthday and at least 6 months following the previous dose.
   - If both OPV and IPV were administered as part of a series, a total of 4 doses should be administered, regardless of the child's current age.

9. **Measles, mumps, and rubella vaccine (MMR).**
   - The minimum interval between the 2 doses of MMR is 4 weeks.

10. **Varicella vaccine.**
   - For persons aged 7 through 18 years without evidence of immunity (see MMWR 2007;56[No. RR-4]), administer 2 doses if not previously vaccinated or the second dose if only 1 dose has been administered.
   - For persons aged 7 through 12 years, the recommended minimum interval between doses is 3 months. However, if the second dose was administered at least 4 weeks after the first dose, it can be accepted as valid.
   - For persons aged 13 years and older, the minimum interval between doses is 4 weeks.

The Recommended Immunization Schedules for Persons Aged 0 Through 18 Years are approved by the Advisory Committee on Immunization Practices (www.cdc.gov/vaccines/recs/acip), the American Academy of Pediatrics (www.aap.org), and the American Academy of Family Physicians (www.aafp.org).

Table 7-4. Recommended childhood catch-up immunization schedule—United States, 2011. Children and adolescents who start late or who are more than 1 month behind.

The table below provides catch-up schedules and minimum intervals between doses for children whose vaccinations have been delayed. A vaccine series does not need to be restarted, regardless of the time that has elapsed between doses. Use the section appropriate for the child's age.

VACCINE	MINIMUM AGE FOR DOSE 1	MINIMUM INTERVAL BETWEEN DOSES			
		DOSE 1 TO DOSE 2	DOSE 2 TO DOSE 3	DOSE 3 TO DOSE 4	DOSE 4 TO DOSE 5
Persons Aged 4 Months Through 6 Years					
Hepatitis B[1]	Birth	**4 weeks**	**8 weeks** (and at least 16 weeks after first dose)		
Rotavirus[2]	6 weeks	**4 weeks**	**4 weeks[2]**		
Diphtheria, Tetanus, Pertussis[3]	6 weeks	**4 weeks**	**4 weeks**	**6 months**	**6 months[3]**
Haemophilus influenzae type b[4]	6 weeks	**4 weeks** if first dose administered at younger than age 12 months **8 weeks (as final dose)** if first dose administered at age 12–14 months **No further doses needed** if first dose administered at age 15 months or older	**4 weeks[4]** if current age is younger than 12 months **8 weeks (as final dose[4]** if current age is 12 months or older and first dose administered at younger than age 12 months and second dose administered at younger than 15 months **No further doses needed** if previous dose administered at age 15 months or older	**8 weeks (as final dose)** This dose only necessary for children aged 12 months through 59 months who received 3 doses before age 12 months	

continued

Pneumococcal[5]	6 weeks	**4 weeks** if first dose administered at younger than age 12 months **8 weeks (as final dose for healthy children)** if first dose administered at age 12 months or older or current age 24 through 59 months **No further doses needed** for healthy children if first dose administered at age 24 months or older	**4 weeks** if current age is younger than 12 months **8 weeks (as final dose for healthy children)** if current age is 12 months or older **No further doses needed** for healthy children if previous dose administered at age 24 months or older	**8 weeks (as final dose)** This dose only necessary for children aged 12 months through 59 months who received 3 doses before age 12 months or for children at high risk who received 3 doses at any age
Inactivated Poliovirus[6]	6 weeks	**4 weeks**	**4 weeks**	**6 months[6]**
Measles, Mumps, Rubella[7]	12 months	**4 weeks**		
Varicella[8]	12 months	**3 months**		
Hepatitis A[9]	12 months	**6 months**		
Persons Aged 7 Through 18 Years				
Tetanus, Diphtheria/ Tetanus, Diphtheria, Pertussis[10]	7 years[10]	**4 weeks** if first dose administered at younger than age 12 months **6 months** if first dose administered at 12 months or older	**6 months** if first dose administered at younger than age 12 months	

7

TABLE 7-4. RECOMMENDED CHILDHOOD CATCH-UP IMMUNIZATION SCHEDULE—UNITED STATES, 2011. CHILDREN AND ADOLESCENTS WHO START LATE OR WHO ARE MORE THAN 1 MONTH BEHIND. (continued)

VACCINE	MINIMUM AGE FOR DOSE 1	MINIMUM INTERVAL BETWEEN DOSES			
		DOSE 1 TO DOSE 2	DOSE 2 TO DOSE 3	DOSE 3 TO DOSE 4	DOSE 4 TO DOSE 5
Human Papillomavirus[11]	9 years	Routine dosing intervals are recommended (females)[11]			
Hepatitis A[9]	12 months	6 months			
Hepatitis B[1]	Birth	4 weeks	8 weeks (and at least 16 weeks after first dose)		
Inactivated Poliovirus[6]	6 weeks	4 weeks	4 weeks[6]	6 months[6]	
Measles, Mumps, Rubella[7]	12 months	4 weeks			
Varicella[8]	12 months	3 months if person is younger than age 13 years / 4 weeks if person is aged 13 years or older			

1. **Hepatitis B vaccine (HepB).**
   - Administer the 3-dose series to those not previously vaccinated.
   - The minimum age for the third dose of HepB is 24 weeks.
   - A 2-dose series (separated by at least 4 months) of adult formulation Recombivax HB is licensed for children aged 11 through 15 years.

2. **Rotavirus vaccine (RV).**
   - The maximum age for the first dose is 14 weeks 6 days. Vaccination should not be initiated for infants aged 15 weeks 0 days or older.
   - The maximum age for the final dose in the series is 8 months 0 days.
   - If Rotarix was administered for the first and second doses, a third dose is not indicated.

3. **Diphtheria and tetanus toxoids and acellular pertussis vaccine (DTaP).**
   - The fifth dose is not necessary if the fourth dose was administered at age 4 years or older.

4. **Haemophilus influenzae type b conjugate vaccine (Hib).**
   - 1 dose of Hib vaccine should be considered for unvaccinated persons aged 5 years or older who have sickle cell disease, leukemia, or HIV infection, or who have had a splenectomy.
   - If the first 2 doses were PRP-OMP (PedvaxHIB or Comvax), and administered at age 11 months or younger, the third (and final) dose should be administered at age 12 through 15 months and at least 8 weeks after the second dose.
   - If the first dose was administered at age 7 through 11 months, administer the second dose at least 4 weeks later and a final dose at age 12 through 15 months.

5. **Pneumococcal vaccine.**
   - Administer 1 dose of 13-valent pneumococcal conjugate vaccine (PCV13) to all healthy children aged 24 through 59 months with any incomplete PCV schedule (PCV7 or PCV13).
   - For children aged 24 through 71 months with underlying medical conditions, administer 1 dose of PCV13 if 3 doses of PCV were received previously or administer 2 doses of PCV13 at least 8 weeks apart if fewer than 3 doses of PCV were received previously.
   - A single dose of PCV13 is recommended for certain children with underlying medical conditions through 18 years of age. See age-specific schedules for details.
   - Administer pneumococcal polysaccharide vaccine (PPSV) to children aged 2 years or older with certain underlying medical conditions, including a cochlear implant, at least 8 weeks after the last dose of PCV. A single revaccination should be administered after 5 years to children with functional or anatomic asplenia or an immunocompromising condition. See *MMWR* 2010;59(No. RR-11).

6. **Inactivated poliovirus vaccine (IPV).**
   - The final dose in the series should be administered on or after the fourth birthday and at least 6 months following the previous dose.
   - A fourth dose is not necessary if the third dose was administered at age 4 years or older and at least 6 months following the previous dose.

   In the first 6 months of life, minimum age and minimum intervals are only recommended if the person is at risk for imminent exposure to circulating poliovirus (i.e., travel to a polio-endemic region or during an outbreak).

7. **Measles, mumps, and rubella vaccine (MMR).**
   - Administer the second dose routinely at age 4 through 6 years. The minimum interval between the 2 doses of MMR is 4 weeks.

8. **Varicella vaccine.**
   - Administer the second dose routinely at age 4 through 6 years.
   - If the second dose was administered at least 4 weeks after the first dose, it can be accepted as valid.

9. **Hepatitis A vaccine (HepA).**
   - HepA is recommended for children aged older than age 23 months who live in areas where vaccination programs target older children, or who are at increased risk for infection, or for whom immunity against hepatitis A is desired.

10. **Tetanus and diphtheria toxoids (Td) and tetanus and diphtheria toxoids and acellular pertussis vaccine (Tdap).**
    - Doses of DTaP are counted as part of the Td/Tdap series.
    - Tdap should be substituted for a single dose of Td in the catch-up series for children aged 7 through 10 years or as a booster for children aged 11 through 18 years; use Td for other doses.

11. **Human papillomavirus vaccine (HPV).**
    - Administer the series to females at age 13 through 18 years if not previously vaccinated or have not completed the vaccine series.
    - Quadrivalent HPV vaccine (HPV4) may be administered in a 3-dose series to males aged 9 through 18 years to reduce their likelihood of genital warts.
    - Use recommended routine dosing intervals for series catch-up (i.e., the second and third doses should be administered at 1 to 2 and 6 months after the first dose). The minimum interval between the first and second doses is 4 weeks. The minimum interval between the second and third doses is 12 weeks, and the third dose should be administered at least 24 weeks after the first dose.

Information about reporting reactions after immunization is available online at www.vaers.hhs. gov or by telephone, 800-822-7967. Suspected cases of vaccine-preventable diseases should be reported to the state or local health department. Additional information, including precautions and contraindications for immunization, is available from the National Center for Immunization and Respiratory Diseases at www.cdc.gov/vaccines or telephone, 800-CDC-INFO (800-232-4636).

Adolescents not previously vaccinated with hepatitis B vaccine should be vaccinated at age 11–12 years:

- For adolescents, the usual schedule is 2 doses separated by ≥4 weeks, followed by a third dose 4–6 months after the second dose.
- A 2-dose series is licensed for adolescents aged 11–15 years, and doses can be separated by 4–6 months.

Diphtheria and Tetanus Toxoid and Pertussis Vaccine

Diphtheria, tetanus, and pertussis each occur worldwide and are endemic in countries with low immunization levels. Infants and children leaving the United States should be immunized before traveling. Optimum protection against diphtheria, tetanus, and pertussis is achieved with at least 3 but preferably 4 doses of diphtheria and tetanus toxoids and acellular pertussis vaccine (DTaP). Two doses of DTaP received at intervals ≥4 weeks apart can provide some protection; however, a single dose offers little protective benefit. Parents should be informed that infants and children who have not received ≥3 doses of DTaP might not be fully protected against pertussis.

The usual primary series includes 4 doses given at ages 2, 4, 6, and 15–18 months. A fifth (booster) dose is recommended when the child is aged 4–6 years. The fifth dose is not necessary, if the fourth dose in the primary series was given after the child's fourth birthday.

The schedule can be accelerated as soon as the infant is 6 weeks of age, with the second and third doses given 4 weeks after each preceding dose. The fourth dose should not be given before the infant is 12 months of age and should be separated from the third dose by ≥6 months. The fifth (booster) dose should not be given before the child is 4 years of age.

Haemophilus influenzae Type b Conjugate Vaccine

Haemophilus influenzae type b (Hib) is an endemic disease worldwide that can cause fatal meningitis, epiglottitis, and other invasive diseases. Infants and children should have optimal protection before traveling. Routine Hib vaccination beginning at age 2 months is recommended for all US children.

The first dose may be given when an infant is as young as 6 weeks of age. Children aged <6 weeks should not be given Hib vaccine, because it may induce immune tolerance to subsequent vaccines.

A primary series consists of 2 or 3 doses (depending on the type of vaccine used) with a minimum interval of 4 weeks between doses. A booster dose is recommended when the infant is aged ≥12 months and at least 8 weeks have passed since the previous dose. If Hib vaccination is started when the infant or child is aged ≥7 months, fewer doses are required.

A shortage of Hib vaccine supply in the United States in 2008 and 2009 may have resulted in deferral of the booster dose at 12–15 months. Clinicians need to review a child's earlier vaccination history with Hib and update if indicated.

Considerations for travel by age include the following:

- If previously unvaccinated, infants aged <15 months should receive at least 2 vaccine doses before travel. An interval as short as 4 weeks between these 2–3 doses is acceptable.
- Unvaccinated infants and children aged 15–59 months should receive a single dose of Hib vaccine.
- Children aged >59 months, adolescents, and adults do not need to be vaccinated unless a specific condition exists, such as functional or anatomic asplenia, immunodeficiency, immunosuppression, or HIV infection.

If different brands of vaccine are administered, a total of 3 doses of Hib conjugate vaccine completes the primary series. After completion of the primary infant vaccination series, any of the licensed Hib conjugate vaccines may be used for the booster dose when the infant is aged 12–15 months.

Polio Vaccine

Although polio has been eliminated in the United States, poliovirus continues to circulate in other parts of the world. In the United States, all infants and children should receive 4 doses of inactivated poliovirus vaccine (IPV) at ages 2, 4, 6–18 months, and 4–6 years. If accelerated protection is needed, the minimum interval between doses is 4 weeks. The minimum age for the fourth dose is 4 years. If a child has received 4 doses of poliovirus

7

vaccine before the fourth birthday, a fifth dose is recommended. The interval between the next-to-last and last dose should be ≥6 months. Infants and children who had initiated the poliovirus vaccination series with 1 or more doses of oral poliovirus vaccine (OPV) should receive IPV to complete the series.

Rotavirus Vaccine

Rotavirus is the most common cause of severe gastroenteritis in infants and young children worldwide. In developing countries, rotavirus gastroenteritis is responsible for approximately 500,000 deaths per year among children aged <5 years. Routine rotavirus vaccination beginning at age 2 months is recommended for all US infants.

Two rotavirus vaccines, RotaTeq (RV5) and Rotarix (RV1), are licensed for use in US infants. RV5 is administered orally in a 3-dose series at ages 2, 4, and 6 months. RV1 is administered orally in a 2-dose series at ages 2 and 4 months. The minimum age for the first dose of rotavirus vaccine is 6 weeks; the maximum age for the first dose is 14 weeks, 6 days. Vaccination should not be initiated for infants aged 15 weeks 0 days or older because of insufficient data on the safety of the first dose of rotavirus vaccine in older infants. The minimum interval between doses of rotavirus vaccine is 4 weeks. All doses should be administered before age 8 months 0 days.

Measles, Mumps, and Rubella Vaccine (MMR)

Measles is an endemic disease in many countries, and outbreaks occur even in developed countries. International travelers are at increased risk for measles exposure. Infants and children should be protected against measles, and the immunization series should be completed before traveling, if possible. While the risk for serious disease from either mumps or rubella is low, these diseases circulate in many parts of the world, and vaccination is recommended.

The Advisory Committee for Immunization Practices (ACIP) generally recommends combination vaccines over single-component vaccines. ACIP recommends that MMR vaccine be administered when any of the individual components is indicated as part of the routine immunization schedule. However, the risk of seizures after vaccination is increased if MMRV is used for the first dose in the series between the ages of 12 and 47 months. So for this dose, MMR and varicella administered separately are preferred over MMRV. The combination product MMRV is generally recommended for the second dose of the series, or for the first dose if it is given to someone aged 47 months through 12 years. Monovalent measles, monovalent mumps, monovalent rubella, and combination measles-rubella vaccines are not currently available in the United States. MMRV vaccine is licensed for children aged 12 months to 12 years and may be used in place of MMR vaccine, if vaccination for measles, mumps, rubella, and varicella is needed.

Two doses of MMR are routinely recommended for all children, usually at age 12 months and again at age 4–6 years. The second dose of MMR can be given as soon as 28 days after the first dose.

Children traveling abroad should be vaccinated at an earlier age than children remaining in the United States. Before departure, children aged 6–11 months should receive the first dose of MMR vaccine, and children aged ≥12 months should have received 2 doses of MMR vaccine before departure. Infants vaccinated before age 12 months must be revaccinated on or after their first birthday with 2 doses of MMR vaccine, separated by at least 28 days.

Varicella Vaccine

Varicella (chickenpox) is an endemic disease throughout the world. Two doses of varicella vaccine are recommended for all susceptible children and adolescents. The first dose is recommended at age 12–15 months. The second dose is routinely recommended at age 4–6 years but can be given earlier, provided that ≥3 months have passed since the first dose.

Efforts should be made to ensure varicella immunity before age 13 years, because varicella disease can be more severe among older children and adults. Children aged ≥13 should receive 2 doses of varicella vaccine 4–8 weeks apart.

Vaccination is not necessary for children with a history of documented chickenpox. When a prior history of chickenpox is uncertain, the vaccine should be given.

Meningococcal Vaccine

Meningococcal disease, caused by the bacterium *Neisseria meningitidis*, is associated with high morbidity and mortality. Epidemics occur in sub-Saharan Africa during the dry season, December through June (see Map 3-13), and CDC recommends that travelers be vaccinated before traveling to this region. Meningococcal vaccination is a requirement to enter Saudi Arabia when traveling to Mecca during the annual Hajj. Health requirements and recommendations for US travelers planning to travel to Saudi Arabia for Hajj are available on the CDC Travelers' Health website after these recommendations are determined each fall (www.cdc.gov/travel).

Three vaccines are available in the United States that protect against 4 serogroups of *N. meningitidis* (A, C, Y, and W-135): 2 meningococcal conjugate vaccines (MenACWY) and 1 meningococcal polysaccharide vaccine (MPSV4). The 2 conjugate vaccines are differentiated by their protein conjugate. Both vaccines are licensed for people aged 2–55 years.

CDC recommends routine vaccination of people with MenACWY at age 11 or 12 years, with a booster dose at age 16 years. For adolescents who receive the first dose at age 13–15 years, a one-time booster dose should be administered, preferably at age 16–18 years. People who receive their first dose of MenACWY at or after age 16 years do not need a booster dose, unless they remain at continued risk for meningococcal disease.

Meningococcal vaccine is also recommended for people aged 2–10 years and ≥19 years who travel to or reside in areas where *N. meningitidis* is hyperendemic or epidemic. A conjugate product is preferred where licensed for a person's age group, and providers should take care to use a meningococcal vaccine that is licensed for a particular age. MPSV4 (licensed for people aged ≥2 years) can be used when neither MenACWY vaccine is available.

Age considerations:

- The serogroup A polysaccharide in MPSV4 induces an antibody response in some children as young as 3 months. Thus, vaccinating infants traveling to high-risk areas can provide some degree of protection.
- For children vaccinated with either MPSV4 or MenACWY at age <7 years, revaccination with MenACWY in 3 years is recommended, if the children remain at high risk for infection, and every 5 years thereafter, if they remain at continued risk.
- For children vaccinated with either MPSV4 or MenACWY at age ≥7 years, revaccination with MenACWY is recommended in 5 years, if they remain at high risk, and every 5 years thereafter, if they remain at continued risk.

Pneumococcal Vaccines

Streptococcus pneumoniae is a leading cause of illness and death worldwide. In the United States, 2 vaccines are available to prevent pneumococcal disease: the 13-valent pneumococcal conjugate vaccine (PCV13) is recommended for routine use in children aged ≤5 years, and the pneumococcal polysaccharide vaccine (PPSV23) is recommended for children and adults aged ≥2 years who have certain underlying medical conditions, and for all adults aged ≥65 years. Before March 2010, the 7-valent vaccine (PCV7) was used. Licensure of PCV13 with its improved serotype protection has prompted its use in place of PCV7 on the same schedule.

All infants should be vaccinated with PCV13. Infant vaccination provides the earliest protection, and children aged <2 years have high rates of pneumococcal disease. The primary series for PCV13 includes 3 doses given at ages 2, 4, and 6 months, with a fourth (booster) dose at age 12–15 months. Children who have been completely vaccinated with PCV7 should receive a single dose of PCV13 between the ages of 14 and 59 months to afford extra seroprotection to the additional components of the new vaccine. For children at risk of invasive *S. pneumoniae* disease, this supplemental dose is recommended through age 71 months. PCV13 should be given ≥8 weeks after the last dose of PCV7 or PPSV23.

Children aged ≥2 years who are at high risk for pneumococcal disease (such as those with sickle cell disease, asplenia, HIV, chronic illness, or immunocompromising conditions) should receive a dose of PPSV23 ≥2 months after their last dose of PCV7 or PCV13. A second dose of PPSV23 is recommended 5 years after the first dose of PPSV23 for people aged ≥2 years who are immunocompromised, have sickle cell disease, or have functional or anatomic asplenia.

7

All healthy children aged 24–59 months who have not completed any recommended schedule for PCV7 should receive 1 dose of PCV13. All children with underlying medical conditions through age 71 months who have received 3 doses should receive 1 dose of PCV13. This includes those who have previously received PPSV23. All children with underlying medical conditions aged 24–59 months who have received <3 doses and have not received any doses after age 12 months should receive 2 doses of PCV13 at least 8 weeks apart. The PCV13 vaccine is not routinely recommended for people aged >5 years, but providers are permitted to give a dose to children aged 6–18 years if they are at high risk of invasive *S. pneumoniae* disease.

Influenza Vaccine

Influenza viruses circulate predominantly in the winter months in temperate regions (typically November–April in the Northern Hemisphere and April–September in the Southern Hemisphere) but can occur year-round in tropical climates. Annual influenza vaccination of all people aged ≥6 months is recommended by ACIP as the most effective measure for preventing influenza and its associated complications. Prevention of influenza is particularly important for people who are (or live with those who are) at increased risk for influenza-related complications, such as children aged <5 years (particularly infants aged <6 months who are not eligible for influenza vaccination), people with medical conditions (such as immunosuppression, diabetes, asthma, pregnancy, and neurologic disorders) and children and adolescents who are receiving long-term aspirin therapy.

Two types of influenza vaccines are available for use in the United States: trivalent inactivated vaccine (TIV), administered by intramuscular injection; and live, attenuated influenza vaccine (LAIV), administered by nasal spray. LAIV is approved for use only in healthy people aged 2–49 years who are not pregnant. LAIV may result in an increase in asthma or reactive airway disease in children aged <5 years; therefore, LAIV should not be administered to children aged <2 years or to children aged 2–4 years who have a history of wheezing in the past year or who had a diagnosis of asthma.

Children receiving TIV should be administered an age-appropriate dose (0.25 mL for those aged 6–35 months and 0.5 mL for those aged ≥36 months). One dose of influenza vaccine per season is recommended for most people. Children aged <9 years who are receiving influenza vaccine for the first time or who received only 1 dose the previous season (if it was their first vaccination season) should receive 2 doses (separated by a 4-week interval). Only 1 dose per year is needed in previously unvaccinated children aged ≥9 years. More specific information about these influenza vaccine recommendations can be found on the CDC website (www.cdc.gov/flu).

Hepatitis A Vaccine or Immune Globulin for Hepatitis A

Hepatitis A virus (HAV) is endemic in most parts of the world, and infants and children traveling to these areas are at increased risk for acquiring HAV infection. Although HAV is often not severe in infants and children aged <5 years, infected children may transmit the infection to older children and adults, who are at higher risk for severe disease.

Hepatitis A vaccine

Hepatitis A vaccine is a routine immunization of childhood in the United States. It is recommended for all children at age 1 year (12–23 months). Vaccination should be ensured for all susceptible children traveling to areas where there is an intermediate or high risk of HAV infection. The hepatitis A vaccine is not approved for children aged <1 year. The HAV vaccine series consists of 2 doses ≥6 months apart. One dose of monovalent hepatitis A vaccine administered at any time before departure can provide adequate protection for most healthy children. The second dose is necessary for long-term protection.

Immune globulin

Children aged <1 year who are traveling to high-risk areas can receive immune globulin (IG). For optimal protection, children aged ≥1 year who are immunocompromised or have chronic medical conditions and who are planning to depart to a high-risk area in <2 weeks should receive the initial dose of vaccine, along with IG (0.02 mL/kg intramuscularly) at a separate anatomic injection site.

IG does not interfere with the response to yellow fever vaccine but can interfere with the response to other live injected vaccines (such as MMR and varicella vaccines). Administration of MMR should be delayed for ≥3 months and varicella for >5 months after administration of IG. IG should not be administered for 2 weeks after measles-, mumps-, rubella-, and varicella-containing vaccines. If IG is given during this time, the child should be revaccinated with the live vaccine ≥3 months after administration of IG. When travel plans do not allow adequate time to administer live vaccines and IG before travel, the severity of the diseases and their epidemiology at the destination will help determine the most appropriate course of preparation.

Human Papillomavirus Vaccine

Human papillomavirus (HPV) infection can be prevented with 2 licensed vaccines. One vaccine, HPV4, protects against HPV types 6, 11, 16, and 18; the other, HPV2, protects against types 16 and 18. Both protect against cervical cancer, and HPV4 also protects against genital warts. HPV vaccination is recommended for girls aged 11–12 years with catch-up vaccination recommended through 26 years. HPV2 is licensed for girls/women aged 10–25 years and HPV4 is licensed for girls and women aged 9-26 years. HPV4 is also licensed for use in boys and men aged 9–26 years. The schedule for both vaccines is 3 doses at 0, 1–2, and 6 months. The minimum interval between dose 1 and dose 2 is 4 weeks. Dose 3 should be given ≥12 weeks after dose 2.

Other Vaccines
Yellow Fever Vaccine

Yellow fever, a disease transmitted by mosquitoes, is endemic in certain areas of Africa and South America (see Maps 3-18 and 3-19). Proof of yellow fever vaccination is required for entry into some countries (see Chapter 3, Yellow Fever and Malaria Information, by Country). Infants and children aged ≥9 months can be vaccinated if they travel to countries within the yellow fever-endemic zone.

Infants are at high risk for developing encephalitis from yellow fever vaccine, a live virus vaccine. Vaccination of infants should be considered on an individual basis. Although the incidence of these adverse events has not been clearly defined, 14 of 18 reported cases of postvaccination encephalitis were in infants aged <4 months. One fatal case confirmed by viral isolation was in a 3-year-old child.

Travelers with infants <9 months of age should be advised against traveling to areas within the yellow fever-endemic zone. ACIP recommends that yellow fever vaccine *never* be given to infants aged <6 months. Infants ages 6–8 months should be vaccinated only if they must travel to areas of ongoing epidemic yellow fever and if a high level of protection against mosquito bites is not possible (see Chapter 3, Yellow Fever). Physicians considering vaccinating infants 6–8 months of age may contact their respective state health departments or CDC at 800-232-4636.

Typhoid Vaccine

Typhoid fever is caused by the bacterium *Salmonella enterica* serotype Typhi. Vaccination is recommended for travelers to areas where there is a recognized risk of exposure to S. Typhi.

Two typhoid vaccines are available: a Vi capsular polysaccharide vaccine (ViCPS) administered intramuscularly and an oral, live, attenuated vaccine (Ty21a). Both vaccines induce a protective response in 50%–80% of recipients. The ViCPS vaccine can be administered to children who are aged ≥2 years, with a booster dose 2 years later, if continued protection is needed. The Ty21a vaccine, which consists of a series of 4 capsules (1 taken every other day) can be administered to children aged ≥6 years. A booster series for Ty21a should be taken every 5 years, if indicated. The capsule cannot be opened for administration but must be swallowed whole. All 4 doses should be taken ≥1 week before potential exposure.

Japanese Encephalitis Vaccine

Japanese encephalitis (JE) virus is transmitted by mosquitoes and is endemic throughout Asia. The risk can be seasonal in temperate climates and year-round in more tropical climates. The risk to short-term travelers and those who confine their travel to urban centers is low. Travelers who plan to travel for ≥1 month or take up residence in an endemic area should be vaccinated against JE. The decision to vaccinate a child should follow the more detailed recommendations in Chapter 3, Japanese Encephalitis.

JE vaccine (licensed for children aged 1–16 years [JE-Vax]) is administered as a series of 3 injections on days 0, 7, and 30. Children aged 1–2 years receive 0.5 mL of vaccine per dose; those aged ≥3 years receive 1.0 mL of vaccine per dose. No data are available on vaccine efficacy for infants aged <1 year. For children who remain at risk, a booster can be given after 2 years.

JE-Vax carries a risk of hypersensitivity reactions that range from 10 to 180 cases per 100,000 vaccinees. Hypersensitivity reactions can be delayed for 1–2 weeks after receipt of the vaccine. Children receiving the vaccine series should be observed for 30 minutes after immunization, and the series should be completed ≥10 days before departure.

JE-Vax is no longer manufactured and all remaining doses expired in May 2011. A new JE vaccine (IC51, trade name Ixiaro) was licensed by the Food and Drug Administration on March 30, 2009, for use in the United Stated for travelers aged ≥17 years of age. The IC51 vaccine is not approved for use in children aged <17 years of age. Pediatric clinical trials are being conducted to enable licensure of Ixiaro for use in children.

Rabies Vaccine

Rabies virus causes an acute viral encephalitis that is virtually 100% fatal. Traveling children may be at increased risk of rabies exposure, mainly from street dogs in developing countries. Bat bites carry a potential risk of rabies throughout the world. There are 2 strategies to prevent rabies in humans:

- Avoiding bite or scratch exposures.
- A 3-shot preexposure immunization series, on days 0, 7, and 21 or 28. In the event of a subsequent possible rabies virus exposure, the child will require 2 more doses of rabies vaccine on days 0 and 3. The decision whether to obtain preexposure immunization for children should follow the recommendations in Chapter 3, Rabies.

For children who have not received preexposure immunization and may have been exposed to rabies, a weight-based dose of human rabies immune globulin and a series of 4 rabies vaccine injections are required on days 0, 3, 7, and 14.

BIBLIOGRAPHY

1. Broder KR, Cortese MM, Iskander JK, Kretsinger K, Slade BA, Brown KH, et al. Preventing tetanus, diphtheria, and pertussis among adolescents: use of tetanus toxoid, reduced diphtheria toxoid and acellular pertussis vaccines—recommendations of the Advisory Committee on Immunization Practices (ACIP). MMWR Recomm Rep. 2006 Mar 24;55(RR-3):1–34.

2. CDC. Epidemiology and prevention of vaccine-preventable diseases. 9th ed. Atkinson W, Hamborsky J, McIntyre L, Wolfe S, editors. Washington, DC: Public Health Foundation; 2006.

3. CDC. Licensure of a 13-valent pneumococcal conjugate vaccine (PCV13) and recommendations for use among children—Advisory Committee on Immunization Practices (ACIP), 2010. MMWR Morb Mortal Wkly Rep. 2010 Mar 12;59(9):258–61.

4. CDC. Notice to readers: recommendation from the Advisory Committee on Immunization Practices (ACIP) for use of quadrivalent meningococcal conjugate vaccine (MCV4) in children aged 2–10 years at increased risk for invasive meningococcal disease. MMWR Morb Mortal Wkly Rep. 2007;56(48):1265–6.

5. CDC. Revised recommendations of the Advisory Committee on Immunization Practices to vaccinate all persons aged 11–18 years with meningococcal conjugate vaccine. MMWR Morb Mortal Wkly Rep. 2007 Aug 10;56(31):794–5.

6. CDC. Update: recommendations from the Advisory Committee on Immunization Practices (ACIP) regarding administration of combination MMRV vaccine. MMWR Morb Mortal Wkly Rep. 2008 Mar 14;57(10):258–60.

7. CDC. Updated recommendations for use of meningococcal conjugate vaccines—Advisory Committee on Immunization Practices (ACIP), 2010. MMWR Morb Mortal Wkly Rep. 2011 Jan 28;60(3):72–6.

8. CDC. Updated recommendations of the Advisory Committee on Immunization Practices (ACIP) regarding routine poliovirus vaccination. MMWR Morb Mortal Wkly Rep. 2009 Aug 7;58(30):829–30.

9. Cetron MS, Marfin AA, Julian KG, Gubler DJ, Sharp DJ, Barwick RS, et al. Yellow fever vaccine. Recommendations of the Advisory Committee on Immunization Practices (ACIP), 2002. MMWR Recomm Rep. 2002 Nov 8;51(RR-17):1–11.

10. Cortese MM, Parashar UD. Prevention of rotavirus gastroenteritis among infants and children: recommendations of the Advisory Committee on

Immunization Practices (ACIP). MMWR Recomm Rep. 2009 Feb 6;58(RR-2):1–25.

11. Fiore AE, Shay DK, Broder K, Iskander JK, Uyeki TM, Mootrey G, et al. Prevention and control of seasonal influenza with vaccines: recommendations of the Advisory Committee on Immunization Practices (ACIP), 2009. MMWR Recomm Rep. 2009 Jul 31;58(RR-8):1–52.

12. Fiore AE, Wasley A, Bell BP. Prevention of hepatitis A through active or passive immunization: recommendations of the Advisory Committee on Immunization Practices (ACIP). MMWR Recomm Rep. 2006 May 19;55(RR-7):1–23.

13. Fischer M, Lindsey N, Staples JE, Hills S. Japanese encephalitis vaccines: recommendations of the Advisory Committee on Immunization Practices (ACIP). MMWR Recomm Rep. 2010 Mar 12;59(RR-1):1–27.

14. Mast EE, Margolis HS, Fiore AE, Brink EW, Goldstein ST, Wang SA, et al. A comprehensive immunization strategy to eliminate transmission of hepatitis B virus infection in the United States: recommendations of the Advisory Committee on Immunization Practices (ACIP) part 1: immunization of infants, children, and adolescents. MMWR Recomm Rep. 2005 Dec 23;54(RR-16):1–31.

15. Rupprecht CE, Briggs D, Brown CM, Franka R, Katz SL, Kerr HD, et al. Use of a reduced (4-dose) vaccine schedule for postexposure prophylaxis to prevent human rabies: recommendations of the advisory committee on immunization practices. MMWR Recomm Rep. 2010 Mar 19;59(RR-2):1–9.

TRAVEL & BREASTFEEDING

Katherine Shealy, Jessica Allen

The medical preparation of a traveler who is breastfeeding differs only slightly than that of other travelers and depends in part on whether the mother and child will be separated or together during travel. Most travelers should be advised to continue breastfeeding throughout travel. Before departure, mothers may wish to carry with them a written list of local breastfeeding resources at their destination. Clinicians may be able to help breastfeeding mothers find out about available breastfeeding support experts at their destination through sources that may include:

- International Board-Certified Lactation Consultants (IBCLCs)—health professionals in approximately 50 countries who specialize in the clinical management of breastfeeding (http://gotwww.net/ilca or www.iblce.org).
- La Leche League Leaders (LLLLs)—trained and accredited volunteer mothers in approximately 60 countries who provide mother-to-mother breastfeeding support and help (www.llli.org).

Mothers who plan to use a breast pump while traveling should have a back-up option available, including written instructions for hand expression; for more detailed instructions about hand expression, see www.workand pump.com/handexpression.htm.

IMMUNIZATIONS AND MEDICATIONS

In almost all situations, clinicians can and should select immunizations and medications that are compatible with breastfeeding. In most circumstances, it is inappropriate to counsel mothers to wean in order to be vaccinated or to withhold vaccination due to breastfeeding status.

Breastfeeding and lactation do not affect maternal or infant dosage guidelines for any immunization or medication; children always require their own immunization or medication, regardless of maternal dose. In the absence of documented risk to the breastfeeding child of a particular maternal medication, known risks of stopping breastfeeding generally outweigh a theoretical risk of exposure via breastfeeding.

Immunizations

Breastfeeding mothers and children should be vaccinated according to routine, recommended schedules; only preventive vaccinia (smallpox) vaccine is contraindicated for use in breastfeeding mothers. Administration of most live and inactivated vaccines does not affect breastfeeding, breast milk, or the process of lactation.

Special Consideration: Yellow Fever Vaccination

Whether this vaccine is excreted in human milk is unknown. However, at least 2 cases of yellow fever vaccine-associated neurologic disease have been documented in infants, presumably associated with breastfeeding transmission of yellow fever vaccine virus. No testing has been done to detect the yellow fever vaccine virus in breast milk, so it can only be said that the vaccine virus was transmitted through breastfeeding, but it has not been definitively determined that transmission occurred via the breast milk. Therefore, breastfeeding is a precaution to yellow fever vaccination, and women should be cautioned to avoid this vaccination while breastfeeding. Since risk exists and there are many gaps in knowledge, breastfeeding mothers should be discouraged from traveling to yellow fever–endemic areas. However, if travel to a yellow fever–endemic area cannot be avoided or postponed, then the mother should be vaccinated.

Medications

The American Academy of Pediatrics (AAP) 2001 Policy Statement: The Transfer of Drugs and Other Chemicals into Human Milk provides an overview of the compatibility or effects on breastfeeding of approximately 250 drugs. The pharmaceutical reference guide, Medications and Mothers' Milk, is updated every 2 years and provides a comprehensive review of the compatibility or effects on breastfeeding of approximately 1,000 drugs, including generic and trade names, AAP recommendations, risk categories, pharmacologic properties, interactions with other drugs, suitable alternatives, theoretic and relative child dose, pediatric half-life, and many other pediatric concerns.

Special Consideration: Antimalarial Medications

Since chloroquine and mefloquine may be safely prescribed to infants, both are considered safe to prescribe to mothers who are breastfeeding. Most experts consider short-term use of doxycycline compatible with breastfeeding. Primaquine may be used for breastfeeding mothers and children with normal glucose-6-phosphate dehydrogenase (G6PD) levels. Breastfeeding mothers should not use atovaquone-proguanil when the breastfeeding infant weighs <5 kg (about 11 lb).

AIR TRAVEL

X-rays used in airport screenings have no effect on breastfeeding, breast milk, or the process of lactation. Airlines typically consider breast pumps as personal items to be carried onboard, similar to laptop computers, handbags, and diaper bags.

Before departure, mothers who will be traveling by air and expect to have expressed milk with them during travel need to carefully plan how they will transport their milk. Airport security regulations for passengers carrying expressed milk vary internationally and are subject to change. In the United States, the Transportation Security Administration (TSA) recognizes expressed milk in the category of liquid medications that may be carried on, regardless of whether the breastfeeding child is traveling, as long as it is declared before screening. TSA recommends that travelers carrying expressed milk have with them a printed copy of the TSA website page www.tsa.gov/travelers/airtravel/children/formula.shtm to help prevent inadvertent problems at security checkpoints.

Travelers carrying expressed milk in checked luggage should refer to cooler pack storage guidelines in "Proper Handling and Storage of Human Milk" on CDC's website at www.cdc.gov/breastfeeding/recommendations/handling_breastmilk.htm to protect milk during travel. Expressed milk is not considered a biohazard. International Air Transport Authority regulations for shipping category B biological substances (UN 3373) do not apply to expressed milk; it is considered a food for individual use. Travelers shipping frozen milk should follow guidelines for shipping other frozen foods and liquids. Expressed milk does not need to be declared at US Customs upon return to the United States.

TRAVELING WITH A BREASTFEEDING CHILD

Breastfeeding provides unique benefits to mothers and children traveling together.

Health clinicians should explain clearly to breastfeeding mothers the value of continuing breastfeeding during travel. Exclusive breast-milk feeding (only breast milk, no other food or drink) protects infants from exposure to contamination and pathogens via foods or liquids. Additionally, feeding only at the breast protects infants from exposure to contamination from containers (bottles, cups, utensils).

Breastfeeding infants require no water supplementation, even in extreme heat environments. Breastfeeding protects children from eustachian tube pain and collapse during air travel, especially during ascent and descent, by allowing them to stabilize and gradually equalize internal and external air pressure, which cannot be replicated by sucking on a bottle or pacifier.

Clinicians should offer information to breastfeeding mothers so that they are better able to continue breastfeeding during travel. Frequent, unrestricted breastfeeding opportunities ensure the mother's milk supply remains ample and the child's nutrition and hydration are ideal. Safe use of a fabric infant carrier helps maintain breastfeeding by increasing breastfeeding opportunities and skin-to-skin contact with the child, while also protecting the child from environmental hazards and easing the burden of carrying a heavy child. Mothers who are concerned about breastfeeding away from home may breastfeed modestly with the child in a fabric carrier. In many countries around the world, breastfeeding in public places is more widely practiced than in the United States. US federal legislation protects mothers' and children's right to breastfeed on federal property, which includes US Customs and embassies overseas.

Special Consideration: Travelers' Diarrhea

Exclusive breastfeeding protects infants against travelers' diarrhea. Breastfeeding is ideal rehydration therapy. Children who are suspected of having travelers' diarrhea should breastfeed more frequently. Children in this situation should not be offered other fluids or foods that replace breastfeeding. Breastfeeding mothers with travelers' diarrhea should continue breastfeeding and increase their own fluid intake. The organisms that cause travelers' diarrhea do not pass through breast milk. Breastfeeding mothers should not use bismuth subsalicylate compounds, because they may transfer salicylate to the child. Compatible alternatives are kaolin-pectin and loperamide. Use of oral rehydration salts is fully compatible with breastfeeding.

TRAVELING WITHOUT A BREASTFEEDING CHILD

A breastfeeding mother traveling without her breastfeeding infant or child may wish to express and store a supply of milk to be fed to the infant or child during her absence. Building a supply to be fed in her absence takes time and patience and is most successful when begun gradually, many weeks in advance of the mother's departure. Infants who have never consumed milk from a bottle or cup need opportunities to practice this skill with another caregiver before the mother's departure.

A mother's milk supply can diminish if she does not express milk while away from her nursing child, but this does not need to be a reason to stop breastfeeding. Clinicians should help mothers determine the best course for breastfeeding based on a variety of factors, including the amount of time she has to prepare for her trip, her flexibility of time while traveling, her options for expressing and storing expressed milk while traveling, the duration of her travel, and her destination. A mother who returns to her nursing infant or child can continue breastfeeding and, if necessary, supplement as needed until her milk supply returns to its prior level. Often, after returning from travel, a nursing infant or child will help bring her milk supply to its prior level. However, nursing infants or children who are separated from their mother for an extended time may have difficulty transitioning back to breastfeeding.

BIBLIOGRAPHY

1. American Academy of Pediatrics Committee on Drugs. Transfer of drugs and other chemicals into human milk. Pediatrics. 2001 Sep;108(3):776–89.

2. CDC. Update: universal precautions for prevention of transmission of human immunodeficiency virus, hepatitis B virus, and other bloodborne pathogens in health-care

settings. MMWR Morb Mortal Wkly Rep. 1988 Jun 24;37(24):377–82, 87–8.

3. Cetron MS, Marfin AA, Julian KG, Gubler DJ, Sharp DJ, Barwick RS, et al. Yellow fever vaccine. Recommendations of the Advisory Committee on Immunization Practices (ACIP), 2002. MMWR Recomm Rep. 2002 Nov 8;51(RR-17):1–11.

4. Eglash A, Chantry, C, Howard, C. ABM clinical protocol #8: human milk storage information for home use for full-term infants. The Academy of Breastfeeding Medicine Protocol Committee; 2010. Available from: http://www.bfmed.org/Media/Files/Protocols/Protocol%208%20-%20English.pdf.

5. Gartner LM, Morton J, Lawrence RA, Naylor AJ, O'Hare D, Schanler RJ, et al. Breastfeeding and the use of human milk. Pediatrics. 2005 Feb;115(2):496–506.

6. Hale TW. Medications and mothers' milk 2008. 13th ed. Amarillo, TX: Pharmasoft Medical Publishing; 2008.

7. Kroger AT, Atkinson WL, Marcuse EK, Pickering LK. General recommendations on immunization: recommendations of the Advisory Committee on Immunization Practices (ACIP). MMWR Recomm Rep. 2006 Dec 1;55(RR-15):1–48.

8. Lawrence RA. Breastfeeding: a guide for the medical profession. 4th ed. New York: Mosby-Yearbook; 1994.

9. Sachdev HP, Krishna J, Puri RK, Satyanarayana L, Kumar S. Water supplementation in exclusively breastfed infants during summer in the tropics. Lancet. 1991 Apr 20;337(8747):929–33.

10. Staples JE, Gershman M, Fischer M. Yellow fever vaccine: recommendations of the Advisory Committee on Immunization Practices (ACIP). MMWR Recomm Rep. 2010 Jul 30;59(RR-7):1–27.

INTERNATIONAL ADOPTION
Cynthia R. Howard, Chandy C. John

OVERVIEW

The number of internationally adopted children that arrive in the United States was an average of about 21,400 each year from 2003 through 2007, but dropped to an average of about 15,000 in 2008 and 2009. These children accounted for 1.3% of all legal immigrants and approximately 15% of all legal pediatric immigrants in 2009. The demography of international adoption is in constant flux, and the epidemiology of diseases in these children shifts as a consequence. In 2009, the most common countries of origin for internationally adopted children were, in order, China, Ethiopia, Russia, South Korea, Guatemala, Ukraine, Vietnam, Haiti, India, and Kazakhstan (Map 7-1). In 2009, 25% of internationally adopted children were aged <1 year, 51% were aged 1–4 years, and 23% were aged ≥5 years; 56% were girls.

Families traveling to unite with their adoptive child, siblings who wait at home for the child's arrival, extended family, and child care providers all are at risk for acquiring infectious diseases secondary to travel or contact with the newly arrived child. International adoptees are usually underimmunized and are at increased risk for infections such as measles and hepatitis A because of crowded living conditions, malnutrition, lack of clean water, and exposure to endemic diseases that are not common in the United States. The absence of medical history, unavailability of biological family history, questionable reliability of immunization records, variation in preadoption living standards, varying disease epidemiology in countries of origin, and increased risk for developmental delays are challenges in providing care.

TRAVEL PREPARATION FOR ADOPTIVE PARENTS AND THEIR FAMILIES

A pre-travel visit is strongly recommended for prospective adoptive parents. In preparation, the travel health provider must know the disease risks in the adoptive child's country of origin and the medical and social history of the adoptee (if available), as well as which family members will be traveling, their immunization and medical histories, the season of travel, and length of stay in the country.

Family members who remain at home, including extended family, should be current on their routine immunizations, as

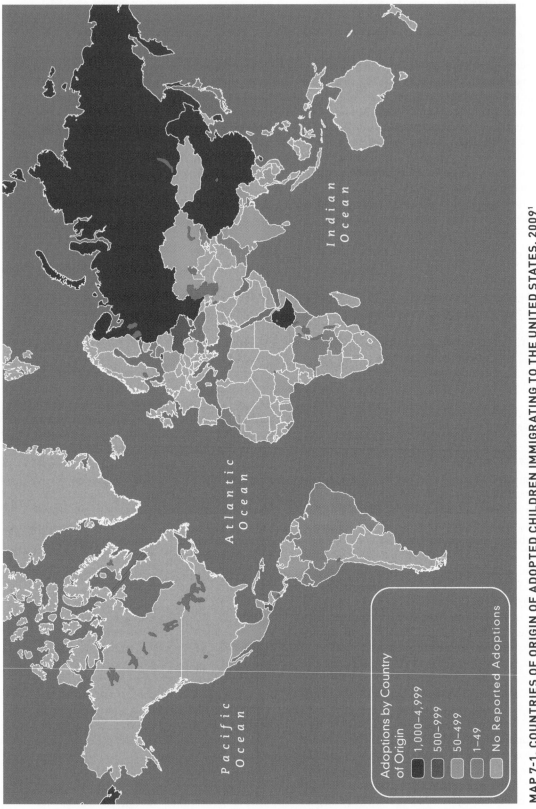

MAP 7-1. COUNTRIES OF ORIGIN OF ADOPTED CHILDREN IMMIGRATING TO THE UNITED STATES, 2009[1]

Adoptions by Country of Origin

- 1,000–4,999
- 500–999
- 50–499
- 1–49
- No Reported Adoptions

Pacific Ocean

Atlantic Ocean

Indian Ocean

[1] Data from: US Department of Homeland Security. Yearbook of Immigration Statistics: 2009. Washington, DC: US Department of Homeland Security, Office of Immigration Statistics; 2010.

recommended by the Advisory Committee on Immunization Practices (ACIP). Protection against measles, hepatitis A, and hepatitis B must be ensured for everyone who will be in the household or providing child care for the adopted child. Measles immunity or 2 doses of MMR should be documented for all people born in or after 1957. Most adult family members will also require immunization with hepatitis A virus (HAV) and hepatitis B virus (HBV) vaccines. ACIP recommends that unprotected family members and close contacts of the adopted child be immunized against HAV before the child's arrival. Adults aged 19–64 who have not previously received the diphtheria, tetanus, and acellular pertussis (Tdap) vaccine should receive a single dose of Tdap to protect against *Bordetella pertussis* in addition to tetanus and diphtheria. Adults aged ≥65 years who have or who anticipate having close contact with an infant aged <12 months and who have not previously received Tdap should receive a single dose of Tdap to protect against pertussis and reduce the likelihood of transmission; all other adults ≥65 years who have not previously received Tdap may be given a single dose of Tdap instead of Td. A one-time inactivated polio booster is also recommended for adults.

Prospective adoptive parents should receive advice on travel safety, food safety, immunization, malaria prophylaxis, diarrhea prevention and treatment, and other travel-related health issues, as outlined elsewhere in this book. In addition, any child traveling with adoptive parents should receive appropriate health care counseling, immunizations, and travel preparation advice. Instructions on car seats, injury prevention, food safety, and air travel apply equally to the adoptive child, so the travel health provider should also be familiar with and provide information on these child-specific issues.

OVERSEAS MEDICAL EXAMINATION OF THE ADOPTED CHILD

All immigrants, including infants and children adopted internationally by US citizens, must undergo a medical examination in their country of origin, performed by a physician designated by the Department of State. The medical examination is used primarily to detect certain serious contagious diseases that may make the immigrant ineligible for a visa. Prospective adoptive parents should not rely on this medical examination to detect all possible disabilities and illnesses. Laboratory results from the country of origin may be unreliable.

The medical examination consists of a brief physical examination and a medical history. A chest radiograph examination for tuberculosis (TB) and a blood test for syphilis are required for immigrants aged ≥15 years. Immigration applicants aged <15 years are tested only if there is reason to suspect any of these diseases. However, children aged 2–14 years who are coming from countries with an estimated TB incidence of ≥20 cases per 100,000 population per year must have a tuberculin skin test or interferon-γ release assay (IGRA) before arrival in the United States. TB incidence exceeds this rate in all of the top 10 countries from which children were adopted internationally in 2009.

Additional information about the medical examination and the vaccination exemption form for internationally adopted children is available on the Department of State website at http://adoption.state.gov/about/how/health.html and http://travel.state.gov/pdf/DS-1981.pdf, respectively.

FOLLOW-UP MEDICAL EXAMINATION AFTER ARRIVAL IN THE UNITED STATES

The adopted child should have a medical examination within 2 weeks of arrival in the United States, or earlier if the child has fever, anorexia, diarrhea, or vomiting. Items to consider during medical examination of an adopted child include the following:

- Temperature (fever requires further investigation)
- General appearance: alert, interactive, referring to parents, consoled by parents, smiling
- Anthropometric measurements: height/age, weight/age, weight/height, head circumference/age
- Facial features: length of palpebral fissures, philtrum, upper lip (fetal alcohol syndrome: short palpebral fissures, thin upper lip, indistinct philtrum)
- Hair: texture, color
- Eyes: jaundice, pallor, strabismus, visual acuity screen
- Ears: hearing screen
- Mouth: palate, teeth

- Neck: thyroid (enlargement secondary to hypothyroidism, iodine deficiency)
- Heart: murmurs
- Abdomen: liver or spleen enlargement
- Skin: Mongolian spots, scars, Bacillus Calmette-Guérin (BCG) scar
- Lymph nodes: enlargement suggestive of TB

In addition, all children should receive a complete neurodevelopmental examination by a clinician with experience in child development. Further evaluation will depend on the country of origin, the age of the child, previous living conditions, number of transitions, nutritional status, developmental status, and the adoptive family's specific questions. Concerns raised during the preadoption medical review may dictate further investigation.

SCREENING FOR INFECTIOUS AND NONINFECTIOUS DISEASES

The current panel of tests for infectious diseases recommended by the American Academy of Pediatrics (AAP) for screening internationally adopted children is as follows:

- HBV serologic testing (repeat at 6 months if negative or if child is aged <12 months at initial testing)
- Syphilis serologic testing
- HIV 1 and 2 serologic testing
- Complete blood cell count with differential and red blood cell indices
- Stool examination for ova and parasites (3 specimens)
- Stool examination for *Giardia intestinalis* and *Cryptosporidium* antigen (1 specimen)
- Tuberculin skin test (TST) or IGRA (repeat at 6 months if negative)

Additional screening tests that may be useful, depending on the child's country of origin or specific risk factors, are HAV serology, hepatitis C virus (HCV) serology, Chagas disease serology, malaria smears, and *Helicobacter pylori* antigen screening of stool if there is persistent abdominal pain or refractory anemia.

Gastrointestinal Parasites

Gastrointestinal parasites have been found in up to 51% of internationally adopted children. *G. intestinalis* is the most common parasite identified. The highest rates of infection have been reported from Russia, Eastern Europe,

and China. Three stool samples collected in the early morning, 2–3 days apart, and placed in an appropriate container that contains preservative are recommended for ova and parasite analysis. Only one of these samples needs to be analyzed for *Giardia* antigen and *Cryptosporidium* antigen. Although theoretically possible, transmission of intestinal parasites from internationally adopted children to family and school contacts has not been reported. Stool samples should be cultured for enteric bacterial pathogens for any child with diarrhea.

Hepatitis A

HAV serology is useful in identifying the infant or child from a HAV-endemic area who may be asymptomatic but is acutely infected and shedding virus. In 2007 and early 2008, multiple cases of hepatitis A secondary to exposure to a newly arrived internationally adopted child were reported in the United States. Some of these cases involved extended family members who were not living in the household. Identification of acutely infected toddlers new to the United States is necessary to prevent further transmission. In addition, identifying children who have natural immunity and do not need the HAV vaccine is cost-effective.

Hepatitis B

HBV surface antigen (HBsAg) has been reported in 1%–5% of newly arrived adoptees. Because of widespread use of the HBV vaccine, the prevalence of HBV infection has decreased. Children found to be positive for HBsAg should be retested for confirmation. Results of a positive HBsAg test should be reported to the state health department. HBV is highly transmissible within the household. All members of households adopting children with chronic HBV infection must be immunized and should have follow-up antibody titers to determine whether levels consistent with immunity have been achieved. Children with chronic HBV infection should receive additional tests for HBV E antigen, hepatitis D virus antibody, and liver function; they should also have a consultation with a pediatric gastroenterologist. Repeat screening at 6 months after arrival should be done on all children who initially test negative for HBV surface antibody.

7

Hepatitis C

Routine screening for HCV is not recommended. However, AAP suggests that providers consider HCV serologic screening for children from Russia, Eastern Europe, Egypt, and China. HCV screening for children from other areas may be indicated depending on presence of symptoms consistent with hepatitis and on histories of prevalence in the country of origin, receipt of blood products, and maternal drug use.

Syphilis

Screening for *Treponema pallidum* is recommended for all internationally adopted children. Initial screening may be done with either a nontreponemal or treponemal test, but any positive result must be confirmed by using the opposite test. Care must be taken in interpreting either test method. Treponemal tests remain positive for life in most cases even after successful treatment and are specific for treponemal diseases, which includes syphilis and other diseases (such as yaws, pinta, and bejel) that are seen in tropical countries. If syphilis cannot be satisfactorily excluded, a full evaluation for disease must be undertaken and antitreponemal treatment given.

HIV

Clinical symptoms of malnutrition, long-term institutionalization, and acquired immunodeficiency may overlap, but positive HIV antibodies in children aged <18 months may reflect maternal antibody and not infection. Assaying for HIV DNA with PCR will confirm the diagnosis of HIV in the infant or child. Some experts recommend PCR for any infant aged <6 months on arrival. If PCR testing is done, 2 negative assays administered 1 month apart, at least one of which is done after the age of 6 months, are necessary to exclude infection. Some experts recommend repeating the screen for HIV antibodies 6 months after arrival.

Chagas Disease

Chagas disease is endemic throughout much of Mexico, Central America, and South America. Risk of Chagas disease varies by region within endemic countries. Although the risk of Chagas disease is likely low in adopted children from endemic countries,

treatment of infected children is very effective. If a child comes from a country with endemic Chagas disease, testing for Chagas disease should be considered. Serologic testing when the child is aged >1 year will avoid possible false-positive results due to maternal antibody.

Malaria

Thick and thin malaria smears should be obtained immediately for any newly arrived child from a malaria-endemic area who has a fever. The child with fever should have 3 sets of malaria smears ≥12 hours apart before the diagnosis can be excluded.

Tuberculosis

Internationally adopted children are at 4–6 times the risk for TB than are their US-born peers. The TST of purified protein derivative is indicated for all children, regardless of their BCG status. TST results must be interpreted carefully for internationally adopted children; guidelines may be found in the bibliography. For children aged >5 years, IGRAs (such as QuantiFERON-TB Gold) are considered an acceptable screening alternative to the TST. A chest radiograph and complete physical examination to assess for pulmonary and extrapulmonary TB are indicated for all children with positive TST results. Hilar lymphadenopathy is a more sensitive finding for TB in young children than are pulmonary infiltrates or cavitation. A repeat TST 3–6 months after arrival is recommended for children who initially tested negative. Children who had a positive TST result but have no evidence of active disease should be treated with isoniazid for 9 months. If active disease is found, every effort should be made to isolate the organism and determine sensitivities, particularly if the child is from a region of the world with a high rate of multidrug-resistant TB, such as Russia, Eastern Europe, and Asia.

Eosinophilia

Children with eosinophil counts >450 cells/mm³ may warrant further evaluation. One option for children who appear well is to repeat a complete blood count with differential 4 weeks after the initial test. If eosinophilia persists, further investigations should be based on the child's country of origin and might include evaluation for *Strongyloides* stercoralis, *Toxocara canis*, *Schistosoma* species, *Ancylostoma* species, *Trichinella spiralis*, intestinal parasites that can migrate through tissues, and filarial worms.

Noninfectious Diseases

Several screening tests for noninfectious diseases should be performed in all or select internationally adopted children. These tests include thyroid-stimulating hormone, iron, iron saturation and binding capacity, lead, hemoglobin electrophoresis, glucose-6-phosphate dehydrogenase, metabolic screen, vitamin D screen, and calcium. In certain circumstances, neurological and psychological testing may also be considered.

IMMUNIZATIONS

The US Immigration and Nationality Act requires that any person seeking an immigrant visa for permanent residency must show proof of having received the ACIP-recommended vaccines (Tables 7-2 and 7-3) before immigration. This applies to all immigrant infants and children entering the United States, but internationally adopted children aged <10 years are exempt from the overseas immunization requirements. Adoptive parents are required to sign a waiver indicating their intention to comply with the immunization requirements within 30 days of the infant's or child's arrival in the United States.

Most children throughout the developing world receive BCG, oral polio, measles, diphtheria, tetanus, and pertussis vaccines per the original immunization schedule of the United Nations Expanded Programme of Immunizations (begun in 1974). In many developing countries, HBV and *Haemophilus influenzae* type B vaccines have become more widely available. Upon arrival in the United States, >90% of newly arrived internationally adopted children need catch-up immunizations to meet ACIP guidelines. Varicella, pneumococcal conjugate, rubella, mumps, and *Haemophilus influenzae* type b vaccines are often not available in developing countries.

Reliability of vaccine records appears to differ by, and even within, country of origin. Providers can choose 1 of 2 approaches for vaccination of internationally adopted children. The first is to reimmunize regardless of immunization record. The second, applicable to children aged ≥6 months, is to test antibody titers to the vaccines reportedly administered and reimmunize only for those to which the child has no protective titers. Immunity to *B. pertussis* is an exception; antibody titers do not correlate with immune status to *B. pertussis*. However, protective antibody levels to diphtheria and tetanus imply protective antibody levels to *B. pertussis*.

Most experts recommend serologic testing for infants and children aged ≥6 months. MMR is not given in most countries of origin. Measles vaccine is administered as a single antigen. Unless the child has had mumps and rubella, administration of the MMR vaccine is recommended over serologic testing. Varicella testing for children coming from tropical countries is not recommended before age 12 years, unless there is a history of disease. In the tropics, varicella is a disease of adolescents and adults.

Immunizations should be given according to the current ACIP schedule for catch-up vaccination. If the infant is <6 months old and there is uncertainty regarding immunization status or validity of immunization record, the child should be reimmunized according to the ACIP schedule.

BIBLIOGRAPHY

1. American Academy of Pediatrics. Medical evaluation of internationally adopted children for infectious diseases. In: Pickering LK, Baker CJ, Kimberlin DW, Long SS, editors. Red Book: 2009 Report of the Committee on Infectious Diseases. 28th ed. Elk Grove Village, IL; 2009. p. 183.
2. CDC. CDC immigration requirements: technical instructions for tuberculosis screening and treatment: using cultures and directly observed therapy. 2009 [cited 2010 Nov 17]. Available from: http://www.cdc. gov/immigrantrefugeehealth/pdf/tuberculosis-ti-2009. pdf.
3. CDC. Recommended adult immunization schedule—United States. MMWR Morb Mortal Wkly Rep. 2010;59(1):1–4.
4. CDC. Recommended immunization schedules for persons aged 0 through 18 years—United States, 2010. MMWR Morb Mortal Wkly Rep. 2010;58(51, 52):1–4.
5. CDC. Updated recommendations for use of tetanus toxoid, reduced diphtheria toxoid and acellular

pertussis (Tdap) vaccine from the Advisory Committee on Immunization Practices, 2010. MMWR Morb Mortal Wkly Rep. 2011 Jan 14;60(1):13–5.

6. CDC. Updated recommendations from the Advisory Committee on Immunization Practices (ACIP) for use of hepatitis A vaccine in close contacts of newly arriving international adoptees. MMWR Morb Mortal Wkly Rep. 2009 Sep 18;58(36):1006–7.

7. Chen LH, Barnett ED, Wilson ME. Preventing infectious diseases during and after international adoption. Ann Intern Med. 2003 Sep 2;139(5 Pt 1):371–8.

8. Hostetter MK, Iverson S, Dole K, Johnson D. Unsuspected infectious diseases and other medical diagnoses in the evaluation of internationally adopted children. Pediatrics. 1989 Apr;83(4):559–64.

9. Lee PJ. Vaccines for travel and international adoption. Pediatr Infect Dis J. 2008 Apr;27(4):351–4.

10. Mandalakas AM, Kirchner HL, Iverson S, Chesney M, Spencer MJ, Sidler A, et al. Predictors of *Mycobacterium tuberculosis* infection in international adoptees. Pediatrics. 2007 Sep;120(3):e610–6.

11. Mazurek GH, Jereb J, Vernon A, LoBue P, Goldberg S, Castro K. Updated guidelines for using interferon gamma release assays to detect *Mycobacterium tuberculosis* infection—United States, 2010. MMWR Recomm Rep. 2010 Jun 25;59(RR-5):1–25.

12. Mazzulli T. Laboratory diagnosis of infection due to viruses, *Chlamydia*, *Chlamydophila*, and *Mycoplasma*. In: Long SS, Pickering LK, Prober CG, editors. Principles and Practice of Pediatric Infectious Diseases. 3rd ed. China: Churchill Livingstone; 2008.

13. Miller LC. International adoption: infectious diseases issues. Clin Infect Dis. 2005 Jan 15;40(2):286–93.

14. Schulte JM, Maloney S, Aronson J, San Gabriel P, Zhou J, Saiman L. Evaluating acceptability and completeness of overseas immunization records of internationally adopted children. Pediatrics. 2002 Feb;109(2):E22.

15. Stauffer WM, Kamat D, Walker PF. Screening of international immigrants, refugees, and adoptees. Prim Care. 2002 Dec;29(4):879–905.

16. US Department of Homeland Security. Yearbook of Immigration Statistics: 2007. Washington, DC: US Department of Homeland Security, Office of Immigration Statistics; 2008.

7

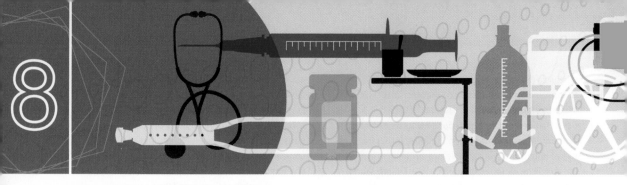

Advising Travelers with Specific Needs

IMMUNOCOMPROMISED TRAVELERS
Elaine C. Jong, David O. Freedman

APPROACH TO THE IMMUNOCOMPROMISED TRAVELER

The pre-travel preparation of travelers with immune suppression due to any medical condition, drug, or treatment must address several categories of concern:

- Is the traveler's underlying medical condition stable? The travel health provider may need to contact the traveler's primary and specialty care providers (with the patient's permission) to discuss the traveler's fitness to travel, give specific medical advice for the proposed itinerary, and verify the drugs and doses composing the usual maintenance regimen.
- Do the conditions, medications, and treatments of the traveler constitute contraindications to or decrease the effectiveness of any of the disease-prevention measures recommended for the proposed trip? Depending on the destination, these measures include but are not limited to immunizations and drugs used for malaria chemoprophylaxis and management of travelers' diarrhea.
- Could any of the disease-prevention measures recommended for the proposed trip destabilize the underlying medical condition, directly or through drug interactions?
- Are there specific health hazards at the destination that would exacerbate the underlying

condition or be more severe in an immunocompromised traveler? If so, can specific interventions be recommended to mitigate these risks?

The traveler's immune status is particularly relevant to immunizations. Overall considerations for vaccine recommendations, such as destination and the likely risk of exposure to disease, are the same for immunocompromised travelers as for other travelers, although the consequences of not administering an indicated vaccine may be more severe. In some complex cases when travelers cannot tolerate recommended immunizations or prophylaxis, the traveler should consider changing the itinerary, altering the activities planned during travel, or deferring the trip. For purposes of clinical assessment and approach to immunizations, immunocompromised travelers fall into 1 of 4 groups, based on mechanism and level of immune suppression. Vaccine recommendations for different categories of immunocompromised adults are shown in Table 8-1.

MEDICAL CONDITIONS WITHOUT SIGNIFICANT IMMUNOLOGIC COMPROMISE

With regard to travel immunizations, travelers whose health status places them in one of the following groups are not considered significantly immunocompromised and should be prepared as any other traveler, although the nature of the previous or underlying disease needs to be kept in mind.

1. Travelers receiving corticosteroid therapy under any of the following circumstances:
   > Short- or long-term daily or alternate-day therapy with <20 mg of prednisone or equivalent.
   > Long-term, alternate-day treatment with short-acting preparations.
   > Maintenance physiologic doses (replacement therapy).
   > Steroid inhalers.
   > Topical steroids (skin, ears, or eyes).
   > Intraarticular, bursal, or tendon injection of steroids.
   > If >1 month has passed since high-dose steroids ($\geq$20 mg per day of prednisone or equivalent for >2 weeks) have been used. However, after short-term (<2 weeks) therapy with daily or alternate-day dosing of $\geq$20 mg of prednisone or equivalent, some experts will wait 2 weeks before administering measles vaccine.
2. HIV patients with >500/mm^3 CD4 T lymphocytes.
3. Travelers with a history of cancer who received their last chemotherapy treatment $\geq$3 months previously and whose malignancy is in remission.
   > These recommendations refer primarily to corticosteroids; it remains unknown how long other drugs should be discontinued for optimal immunization.
   > When patients are on immunosuppressive medications (including tumor necrosis factor [TNF] blockers) for conditions other than hematologic malignancies and cancer, some clinicians suggest waiting only 1 month since a last dose of such medications before immunization.
4. Bone marrow transplant recipients who are >2 years posttransplant, not on immunosuppressive drugs, and without graft-versus-host disease.
5. Travelers with autoimmune disease (such as systemic lupus erythematosus, inflammatory bowel disease, rheumatoid arthritis, or multiple sclerosis [MS]) who are not being treated with immunosuppressive drugs, although definitive data are lacking. Decisions should be made on an individual basis by the clinician and traveler.
6. CDC advises following its usual guidelines for use of vaccines in MS patients who lack prior immunity and who are not experiencing an exacerbation of disease. This advice concurs with that of the National Multiple Sclerosis Society (www.nationalmssociety.org).

MEDICAL CONDITIONS AND TREATMENTS ASSOCIATED WITH LIMITED IMMUNE DEFICITS
Asymptomatic HIV Infection
Asymptomatic HIV-infected people with CD4 cell counts of 200–500/mm^3 are considered to have limited immune deficits. CD4 counts increased by antiretroviral drugs, rather than nadir counts, should be used to categorize HIV-infected people. The exact time at which reconstituted lymphocytes are fully functional is not well defined. To achieve a maximal vaccine response with minimal risk, many clinicians advise a delay of 3 months after reconstitution, if possible, before immunizations are administered. While seroconversion rates and geometric mean titers of antibody in response to vaccines may be less than those measured in healthy controls, most vaccines can elicit seroprotective levels of antibody in most HIV-infected patients in this category.

Transient increases in HIV viral load, which return quickly to baseline, have been observed after administration of several different vaccines to HIV-infected people. The clinical significance of these increases is not known, but they do not preclude the use of any vaccine.

Multiple Sclerosis
The Multiple Sclerosis Council for Clinical Practice Guidelines, published in 2001, contain the clinical practice guidance on "Immunizations and Multiple Sclerosis." The expert panel that developed this guidance used CDC recommendations as their foundation. Updated comments are posted on the National Multiple Sclerosis Society website (www.nationalmssociety.org). People with MS who are having a serious relapse (exacerbation) interfering with the activities of daily living should defer immunization until 4–6 weeks after onset of the relapse.

Table 8-1. Immunization of immunocompromised adults

	HIV INFECTION, CD4 CELLS ≥200/mm³	SEVERE IMMUNO-SUPPRESSION (HIV/AIDS), CD4 CELLS <200/mm³	SEVERE IMMUNOSUPPRESSION (NOT HIV-RELATED)	ASPLENIA	RENAL FAILURE	CHRONIC LIVER DISEASE, DIABETES
Live Vaccines						
Bacillus Calmette-Guérin (BCG)	X	X	X	U	U	U
Influenza, live attenuated (LAIV)	X	X	X	U	X	X
Measles-mumps-rubella (MMR)[1]	R	W	X	U	U	U
Typhoid, Ty21a	X	X	X	U	U	U
Varicella (adults)[2]	U	X	X	U	U	U
Yellow fever[3]	W	X	X	U	W	W
Inactivated Vaccines						
Haemophilus influenzae type b (Hib)	C[4]	C[4]	R	R	U	U
Hepatitis A	U[5]	U[5]	U	U[5]	U[5]	U[5]
Hepatitis B	U[5,6]	U[5,6]	U[6]	U[6]	R[7]	U[6]

Vaccine						
Influenza (inactivated)	R	R	R	R	R	R
Japanese encephalitis	U	U	U	U	U	U
Meningococcal polysaccharide or conjugate	U	U	R	U	C	C
Pneumococcal polysaccharide	R	R	R	R	R	R
Polio (IPV)	U	U	U	U	U	U
Rabies	U	U	R	U	R	R
Td or Tdap	R	R	R	R	R	R
Typhoid, Vi	U	U	U	U	U	U

Abbreviations: C, Consider; R, Recommended for all in this patient category; U, Use as indicated for normal hosts; W, Warning; X, Contraindicated.

[1] MMR vaccination should be considered for all symptomatic HIV-infected patients with CD4 counts >200/mm³ without evidence of measles immunity. Immune globulin may be administered for short-term protection of those facing high risk of measles and for whom MMR vaccine is contraindicated.

[2] Varicella vaccine should not be administered to people who have cellular immunodeficiencies, but people with impaired humoral immunity (including congenital or acquired hypoglobulinemia or dysglobulinemia) may be vaccinated. Immunocompromised hosts should receive 2 doses of vaccine spaced at 3-month intervals.

[3] See detail in the text.

[4] Decision should be based on consideration of the individual patient's risk of Hib disease and the effectiveness of the vaccine for that person. In some settings, the incidence of Hib disease may be higher among HIV-infected adults than among HIV-uninfected adults, and the disease can be severe in these patients.

[5] Routinely indicated for all men who have sex with men, people with multiple sexual partners, hemophiliacs, patients with chronic hepatitis, and injection drug users.

[6] Test for antibodies to hepatitis B virus surface antigen serum titer after vaccination, and revaccinate if initial antibody response is absent or suboptimal (<10 mIU/mL). HIV-infected nonresponders may react to a subsequent vaccine course if CD4 cell counts rise to 500/mm³ after institution of highly active antiretroviral therapy. See text for discussion of other immunocompromised groups.

[7] Use special double-dose vaccine formulation. Test for antibodies to hepatitis B virus surface antigen after vaccination and revaccinate if initial antibody response is absent or suboptimal (<10 mIU/mL).

Inactivated vaccines are generally considered safe for people with MS. Administration of tetanus, hepatitis B, or influenza vaccines does not appear to increase the short-term risk of relapses in people with MS. However, published studies are lacking on the safety and efficacy of other vaccines (such as those against pneumonia, meningitis, typhoid, polio, hepatitis A, human papilloma virus, and pertussis). Inactivated vaccines are theoretically safe for people being treated with an interferon medication, glatiramer acetate, mitoxantrone, or natalizumab, although efficacy data are lacking.

In the past, many practicing neurologists have strongly advised their MS patients against the use of live-virus vaccines at any time. Live-virus vaccines should not be given to people during therapy with immunosuppressants, such as mitoxantrone, azathioprine, methotrexate, or cyclophosphamide, or during chronic corticosteroid therapy. However, a few published studies suggest that measles, rubella, and varicella vaccines may be safe in people with MS if administered several weeks in advance of, or several weeks after, immunosuppressive therapy. Yellow fever vaccine and smallpox vaccine have not been studied in people with MS and should not be given unless there is a compelling reason to do so (such as unavoidable direct exposure) and there has been a consultation with the patient's neurologist.

Other Chronic Conditions

Chronic medical conditions that may be associated with varying degrees of immune deficit include asplenia, chronic renal disease, chronic liver disease (including hepatitis C), diabetes mellitus, and complement deficiencies. Because no information is available regarding possible increased adverse events or decreased vaccine efficacy following administration of live, attenuated viral or bacterial antigen vaccines to patients with these diseases, caution should be used if considering the administration of live vaccines to such patients. Factors to consider in assessing the general level of immune competence of these patients include disease severity, duration, clinical stability, complications, and comorbidities.

A blunted response to hepatitis B vaccine has been reported in patients with chronic liver disease; a decreased response to hepatitis B vaccine has also been observed in patients with diabetes. Additional doses of hepatitis B vaccine beyond the primary 3-dose series may be necessary. Double-dose hepatitis B vaccine preparations are used to promote optimal immunization of people with chronic renal failure and other patients with absent or suboptimal response to standard hepatitis B vaccine doses. Adjuvanted hepatitis B candidate vaccines undergoing clinical trials appear to be more effective for immunization of liver transplant patients and patients with renal insufficiency.

Asplenic patients are susceptible to overwhelming sepsis with encapsulated bacterial pathogens. Although response to vaccines may be less than in people with a functioning spleen, many clinical guidelines recommend immunization against meningococcal, pneumococcal, and *Haemophilus influenzae* disease in these patients, regardless of travel plans.

- Limited data show that vaccine response in people who have had a splenectomy was more impaired if splenectomy was performed because of hematologic malignancy rather than for splenic trauma.
- The meningococcal A/C/Y/W-135 conjugate vaccine is indicated for both pediatric and adult populations at risk.
- Although the polysaccharide-protein conjugate vaccines against disease due to *Streptococcus pneumoniae* (PCV13) and *H. influenzae* type b (Hib conjugate vaccine) infections appear to elicit an increased immune response and duration of protection in vaccine recipients, there are few published clinical studies and there are no approved indications for use of these vaccines in adults at this time.

People with terminal complement deficiencies appear to have increased susceptibility to meningococcal infections and should be immunized against meningococcal disease.

Severe Immune Compromise (Non-HIV)

Severely immunocompromised people include those who have active leukemia or lymphoma, generalized malignancy, aplastic anemia, graft-versus-host disease, or congenital immunodeficiency; others in this category include people who have received recent radiation therapy, people who have had solid-organ or bone marrow transplants, within 2 years of transplantation, or transplant recipients who are still taking immunosuppressive drugs.

People with chronic lymphocytic leukemia have poor humoral immunity, even early in the disease course, and rarely respond to vaccines. Complete revaccination with standard childhood vaccines should begin 12 months after bone marrow transplantation. However, measles, mumps, and rubella (MMR) vaccine should be administered 24 months after transplant if the recipient is presumed to be immunocompetent. Influenza vaccine should be administered 6 months after transplant and annually thereafter.

For solid-organ transplants, the risk of infection is highest in the first year after transplant, so travel to high-risk destinations should be postponed until after that time. Vaccine doses received while concurrently receiving immunosuppressive therapy or during the 2 weeks before starting therapy are not considered valid. At least 3 months after therapy is discontinued, patients should be revaccinated with all vaccines that are still indicated. People taking any of the following categories of medications are considered severely immunocompromised:

- **High-dose corticosteroids**—Most clinicians consider a dose of either >2 mg/kg of body weight or ≥20 mg per day of prednisone or equivalent in people who weigh >10 kg, when administered for ≥2 weeks, as sufficiently immunosuppressive to raise concern about the safety of vaccination with live-virus vaccines. Furthermore, the immune response to vaccines may be impaired. Clinicians should wait ≥1 month after discontinuation of high-dose systemic corticosteroid therapy before administering a live-virus vaccine.
- **Alkylating agents** (such as cyclophosphamide)
- **Antimetabolites** (such as azathioprine, 6-mercaptopurine)
- **Transplant-related immunosuppressive drugs** (such as cyclosporine, tacrolimus, sirolimus, mycophenolate mofetil, and mitoxantrone)
- **Cancer chemotherapeutic agents**, excluding tamoxifen but including low-dose methotrexate weekly regimens, are classified as severely immunosuppressive, as evidenced by increased rates of opportunistic infections and blunting of responses to certain vaccines

among patient groups. Limited studies show that methotrexate monotherapy had no effect on the response to influenza vaccine, but it did impair the response to pneumococcal vaccine.

- **TNF blockers** such as etanercept, rituximab, adalimumab, and infliximab blunt the immune response to certain vaccines and certain chronic infections. When used alone or in combination regimens with methotrexate to treat rheumatoid disease, TNF blockers were associated with an impaired response to influenza vaccine and to pneumococcal vaccine as well.
  > Despite measurable impairment of the immune response, postvaccination antibody titers were often sufficient to provide protection for most people; therefore, treatment with TNF blockers does not preclude immunization against influenza and pneumococcal disease.
  > Although the potential benefits of live-viral and live-bacterial vaccines in patients receiving TNF blockers need to be weighed carefully against potential risks, most clinicians would be reluctant to use vaccines such as yellow fever in this situation, as the safety of using live vaccines is unknown for these agents.

Severe Immune Compromise Due to Symptomatic HIV/AIDS

Knowledge of the HIV-infected traveler's current CD4 T-lymphocyte count is necessary for pre-travel consultation. HIV-infected people with CD4 cell counts <200/mm³, history of an AIDS-defining illness, or clinical manifestations of symptomatic HIV are considered to have severe immunosuppression (see Chapter 3, HIV and AIDS) and should not receive live attenuated viral or bacterial vaccines because of the risk that the vaccine could cause serious systemic disease. The response to inactivated vaccines also will be suboptimal; thus, vaccine doses received by HIV-infected people while CD4 cell counts are <200/mm³ should be ignored, and the person should be revaccinated ≥3 months after immune reconstitution with antiretroviral therapy.

In newly diagnosed, treatment-naïve patients with CD4 cell counts <200/mm³, travel should be delayed pending reconstitution of CD4 cell counts with antiretroviral therapy. This delay will minimize risk of infection and avoid immune reconstitution illness during the travel.

Household Contacts

Household contacts of severely immunocompromised patients may be given live-virus vaccines such as yellow fever, MMR, or varicella vaccines but should not be given the live attenuated influenza vaccine.

SPECIAL CONSIDERATIONS FOR IMMUNOCOMPROMISED TRAVELERS
Yellow Fever Vaccine

Travelers with severe immune compromise should be strongly discouraged from travel to destinations that present a true risk for yellow fever (YF). If travel to an area where YF vaccine is recommended (see Maps 3-18 and 3-19) is unavoidable and the vaccine is not given, these travelers should be carefully instructed in methods to avoid mosquito bites and be provided with a vaccination medical waiver (see Chapter 3, Yellow Fever).

Patients with limited immune deficits or asymptomatic HIV going to YF-endemic areas may be offered YF vaccine and monitored closely for possible adverse effects. As vaccine response may be suboptimal, such vaccinees are candidates for serologic testing 1 month after vaccination. For information about serologic testing, contact your state health department or CDC's Division of Vector-Borne Diseases at 970-221-6400. Data from clinical and epidemiologic studies are insufficient at this time to evaluate the actual risk of severe adverse effects associated with YF vaccine among recipients with limited immune deficits.

If international travel requirements, and not true exposure risk, are the only reasons to vaccinate a traveler with asymptomatic HIV-infection or a limited immune deficit, the physician should provide a waiver letter. Travelers should be warned that vaccination waiver documents may not be accepted by some countries; if the waiver is rejected, the option of deportation might be preferable to receipt of YF vaccine at the destination.

Malaria Chemoprophylaxis

Immunocompromised travelers to malaria-endemic areas should be prescribed appropriate drugs for malaria chemoprophylaxis and receive counseling about mosquito bite avoidance—the same as for immunocompetent travelers (see Chapter 3, Malaria). However, special concerns for immunocompromised travelers include any of the following possibilities:

- Drugs used for malaria chemoprophylaxis may interact with drugs in the traveler's maintenance regimen.
- The underlying medical condition will predispose the immunocompromised traveler to more serious disease from malaria infection.
- A malaria infection and the drugs used to treat the malaria infection may exacerbate the underlying disease.

The severity of malaria is increased in HIV-infected people: malaria infection increases HIV viral load and thus may exacerbate disease progression. There is a lack of published data on the safety and efficacy of CDC-recommended antimalarial regimens in the HIV-infected traveler taking highly active antiretroviral therapy (HAART) while traveling to malaria-endemic areas. Table 8-2 gives some examples of potential interactions between drugs used for malaria chemoprophylaxis and those used in HAART regimens:

- Tetracyclines have no clinically significant interactions expected with the protease inhibitors and nonnucleoside reverse transcriptase inhibitors, so doxycycline might be a reasonable recommendation for malaria chemoprophylaxis in a traveler on HAART going to a malaria-endemic area.
- Atovaquone-proguanil might be a reasonable malaria chemoprophylaxis choice for a traveler whose HAART regimen includes nelfinavir (protease inhibitor) and nevirapine (nonnucleoside reverse transcriptase inhibitor). Atovaquone is not expected to have any significant interaction with common nucleoside reverse transcriptase inhibitors, although no data are available for proguanil.
- New classes of antiretroviral drugs include entry inhibitors and integrase inhibitors, and little data are available. Since new drugs and drug combinations for HIV treatment are under continuous development, clinicians are encouraged to review the most current information regarding possible drug interactions. An interactive web-based resource for checking on drug interactions involving HAART drugs is found at the University of Liverpool website (www.hiv-druginteractions.org).

Artemisinin combination therapy, consisting of 6 oral doses of artemether-lumefantrine taken over 3 days, is one of the recommended

8

Table 8-2. Potential interactions between malaria drugs and HIV drugs[1,2]

DRUG	PROTEASE INHIBITORS	NRTIs	NNRTIs
Mefloquine	Potential interaction with all protease inhibitors	No available data	Decreased levels of mefloquine with efavirenz or nevirapine
Atovaquone-proguanil	Atovaquone: potential interactions with indinavir, ritonavir, lopinavir, atazanavir, darunavir, tipranavir	Atovaquone: no clinically significant interaction expected	Atovaquone: potential interaction with efavirenz
	Proguanil: potential interactions with ritonavir and lopinavir	Proguanil: no available data	Proguanil: potential interaction with efavirenz
Doxycycline	No clinically significant interactions expected	No available data	No clinically significant interactions expected
Chloroquine	Potential interaction with ritonavir only	No available data	No clinically significant interactions expected
Primaquine	No clear data	No available data	No available data

Abbreviations: NRTI, nucleoside reverse transcriptase inhibitor; NNRTI, nonnucleoside reverse transcriptase inhibitor.
[1] Adapted from Table 2 in Bhadelia N, Klotman M, Caplivski D. The HIV-positive traveler. Am J Med. 2007 Jul;120(7):574–80, and information available at www.hiv-druginteractions.org.
[2] All potential interactions within an HIV drug class are noted in the table. There are no drug combinations with absolute contraindications to coadministration.

treatments for uncomplicated malaria due to *Plasmodium falciparum*. For severe malaria infections, intravenous artesunate is available in the United States through an investigational new drug protocol by CDC (see Chapter 3, Malaria). Limited data have raised concerns that parasite clearance of *P. falciparum* after therapy with artemisinins may be delayed in malaria patients coinfected with HIV compared with those who are HIV seronegative, raising the possibility that the host's immunity affects the efficacy of antimalarial drug treatment. The use of quinidine (and by implication quinine) in patients taking nelfinavir or ritonavir is contraindicated because of potential cumulative cardiotoxicity. However, if a patient has severe and complicated malaria, there may be no choice. In these circumstances, as in others, quinidine should be used only with close monitoring. In addition,

careful monitoring should accompany quinidine therapy in patients taking amprenavir, delavirdine, or the lopinavir-ritonavir combination. Although the clinical significance, if any, is not known, several protease inhibitors have been shown in laboratory testing to inhibit the growth of malaria parasites.

Some clinical case reports suggest that asplenic people may be at higher risk of acquisition and complications of malaria, so asplenic travelers to malaria areas should be counseled to adhere conscientiously to the malaria chemoprophylaxis regimen prescribed for them.

Enteric Infections

Many foodborne and waterborne infections, such as those caused by *Salmonella*, *Campylobacter*, *Giardia*, and *Cryptosporidium*, can be severe or become chronic in immunocompromised people. Enteroaggregative

Escherichia coli is an emerging enteric pathogen causing persistent diarrhea among children, adults, and HIV-infected people.

Safe food and beverage precautions should be followed by all travelers, but travelers' diarrhea can occur despite strict adherence. Selection of antimicrobials to be used for self-treatment of travelers' diarrhea may require special consideration of potential drug interactions among patients already taking medications for chronic medical conditions. Fluoroquinolones and rifaximin are active against several enteric pathogens and are not known to have significant interactions with HAART drugs. However, macrolide antibiotics may have significant interactions with HAART drugs (Table 8-3). Emerging therapies for diarrhea in HIV/AIDS patients may involve probiotics such as *Lactobacillus rhamnosus* GR-1, *L. reuteri* RC-14, and others.

Waterborne infections might result from swallowing water during recreational activities. To reduce the risk for cryptosporidiosis and giardiasis, patients should avoid swallowing water during swimming and should not swim in water that might be contaminated (with sewage or animal waste, for example).

Attention to hand hygiene, including frequent and thorough handwashing, is the best prevention against gastroenteritis. Hands should be washed after contact with public surfaces and also after any contact with animals or their living areas.

Reducing Risk for Other Diseases

Geographically focal infections that pose an increased risk of severe outcome for immunocompromised people include visceral leishmaniasis and several fungal infections acquired by inhalation (such as *Penicillium marneffei* infection in Southeast Asia and coccidioidomycosis in the Americas). Many developing areas have high rates of tuberculosis (TB), and establishing the TB status of immunocompromised travelers going to such destinations may be helpful in the evaluation of any subsequent travel-associated illness. Depending on the traveler's degree of immune suppression, the baseline TB status may be assessed by obtaining a tuberculin skin test, chest radiograph, or *Mycobacterium tuberculosis* antigen-specific interferon-γ assay.

Patients with advanced HIV and transplant recipients frequently take either primary or secondary prophylaxis for one or more opportunistic infections (such as pneumocystis, mycobacteria, and toxoplasma). Complete adherence to all indicated regimens should be confirmed before travel (see Chapter 3, HIV and AIDS).

Table 8-3. Potential interactions between antibiotics for travelers' diarrhea and HIV drugs[1]

DRUG	PROTEASE INHIBITORS	NRTIs	NNRTIs
Fluoroquinolones	No clinically significant interactions	No clinically significant interactions	No clinically significant interactions
Macrolides	Possible increased levels of clarithromycin with ritonavir, atazanavir, and lopinavir	Decreased levels of zidovudine with clarithromycin; no data available for azithromycin	Possible interactions with clarithromycin, efavirenz, and nevirapine
Rifaximin	No available data	No available data	No available data

Abbreviations: NRTI, nucleoside reverse transcriptase inhibitor; NNRTI, nonnucleoside reverse transcriptase inhibitor.
[1] Adapted from Table 2 in Bhadelia N, Klotman M, Caplivski D. The HIV-positive traveler. Am J Med. 2007 Jul;120(7):574–80.

BIBLIOGRAPHY

1. Amenta M, Dalle Nogare ER, Colomba C, Prestileo TS, Di Lorenzo F, Fundaro S, et al. Intestinal protozoa in HIV-infected patients: effect of rifaximin in *Cryptosporidium parvum* and *Blastocystis hominis* infections. J Chemother. 1999 Oct;11(5):391–5.

2. Anukam KC, Osazuwa EO, Osadolor HB, Bruce AW, Reid G. Yogurt containing probiotic *Lactobacillus rhamnosus* GR-1 and *L. reuteri* RC-14 helps resolve moderate diarrhea and increases CD4 count in HIV/AIDS patients. J Clin Gastroenterol. 2008 Mar;42(3):239–43.

3. Beran J. Safety and immunogenicity of a new hepatitis B vaccine for the protection of patients with renal insufficiency including pre-haemodialysis and haemodialysis patients. Expert Opin Biol Ther. 2008 Feb;8(2):235–47.

4. Bhadelia N, Klotman M, Caplivski D. The HIV-positive traveler. Am J Med. 2007 Jul;120(7):574–80.

5. Boerbooms AM, Kerstens PJ, van Loenhout JW, Mulder J, van de Putte LB. Infections during low-dose methotrexate treatment in rheumatoid arthritis. Semin Arthritis Rheum. 1995 Jun;24(6):411–21.

6. Brezinschek HP, Hofstaetter T, Leeb BF, Haindl P, Graninger WB. Immunization of patients with rheumatoid arthritis with antitumor necrosis factor alpha therapy and methotrexate. Curr Opin Rheumatol. 2008 May;20(3):295–9.

7. Brinkman DM, Jol-van der Zijde CM, ten Dam MM, te Boekhorst PA, ten Cate R, Wulffraat NM, et al. Resetting the adaptive immune system after autologous stem cell transplantation: lessons from responses to vaccines. J Clin Immunol. 2007 Nov;27(6):647–58.

8. CDC. Recommendations of the Advisory Committee on Immunization Practices (ACIP): use of vaccines and immune globulins for persons with altered immunocompetence. MMWR Recomm Rep. 1993 Apr 9;42(RR-4):1–18.

9. CDC. Vaccination of persons with primary and secondary immune deficiencies. Washington, DC: Public Health Foundation; 2009. Available from: http://www.cdc.gov/vaccines/pubs/pinkbook/downloads/appendices/A/immuno-table.pdf.

10. Cohen C, Karstaedt A, Frean J, Thomas J, Govender N, Prentice E, et al. Increased prevalence of severe malaria in HIV-infected adults in South Africa. Clin Infect Dis. 2005 Dec 1;41(11):1631–7.

11. De Sousa dos Santos S, Lopes MH, Simonsen V, Caiaffa Filho HH. *Haemophilus influenzae* type b immunization in adults infected with the human immunodeficiency virus. AIDS Res Hum Retroviruses. 2004 May;20(5):493–6.

12. Douvin C, Simon D, Charles MA, Deforges L, Bierling P, Lehner V, et al. Hepatitis B vaccination in diabetic patients. Randomized trial comparing recombinant vaccines containing and not containing pre-S2 antigen. Diabetes Care. 1997 Feb;20(2):148–51.

13. Duchini A, Goss JA, Karpen S, Pockros PJ. Vaccinations for adult solid-organ transplant recipients: current recommendations and protocols. Clin Microbiol Rev. 2003 Jul;16(3):357–64.

14. Eigenberger K, Sillaber C, Greitbauer M, Herkner H, Wolf H, Graninger W, et al. Antibody responses to pneumococcal and hemophilus vaccinations in splenectomized patients with hematological malignancies or trauma. Wien Klin Wochenschr. 2007;119(7-8):228–34.

15. Fomin I, Caspi D, Levy V, Varsano N, Shalev Y, Paran D, et al. Vaccination against influenza in rheumatoid arthritis: the effect of disease modifying drugs, including TNF alpha blockers. Ann Rheum Dis. 2006 Feb;65(2):191–4.

16. Furst DE, Breedveld FC, Kalden JR, Smolen JS, Burmester GR, Bijlsma JW, et al. Updated consensus statement on biological agents, specifically tumour necrosis factor {alpha} (TNF{alpha}) blocking agents and interleukin-1 receptor antagonist (IL-1ra), for the treatment of rheumatic diseases, 2005. Ann Rheum Dis. 2005 Nov;64 Suppl 4:iv2-14.

17. Geretti AM, Doyle T. Immunization for HIV-positive individuals. Curr Opin Infect Dis. 2010 Feb;23(1):32–8.

18. Huang DB, Mohanty A, DuPont HL, Okhuysen PC, Chiang T. A review of an emerging enteric pathogen: enteroaggregative *Escherichia coli*. J Med Microbiol. 2006 Oct;55(Pt 10):1303–11.

19. Kamya MR, Gasasira AF, Yeka A, Bakyaita N, Nsobya SL, Francis D, et al. Effect of HIV-1 infection on antimalarial treatment outcomes in Uganda: a population-based study. J Infect Dis. 2006 Jan 1;193(1):9–15.

20. Kapetanovic MC, Saxne T, Sjoholm A, Truedsson L, Jonsson G, Geborek P. Influence of methotrexate, TNF blockers and prednisolone on antibody responses to pneumococcal polysaccharide vaccine in patients with rheumatoid arthritis. Rheumatology (Oxford). 2006 Jan;45(1):106–11.

21. Kaplan JE, Masur H, Holmes KK. Guidelines for preventing opportunistic infections among HIV-infected persons—2002. Recommendations of the US Public Health Service and the Infectious Diseases Society of America. MMWR Recomm Rep. 2002 Jun 14;51(RR-8):1–52.

22. Kofidis T, Pethig K, Ruther G, Simon AR, Strueber M, Leyh R, et al. Traveling after heart transplantation. Clin Transplant. 2002 Aug;16(4):280–4.

23. Laurence JC. Hepatitis A and B immunizations of individuals infected with human immunodeficiency virus. Am J Med. 2005 Oct;118 Suppl 10A:75S–83S.

24. Matulis G, Juni P, Villiger PM, Gadola SD. Detection of latent tuberculosis in immunosuppressed patients with autoimmune diseases: performance of a *Mycobacterium tuberculosis* antigen-specific interferon gamma assay. Ann Rheum Dis. 2008 Jan;67(1):84–90.

25. Mishra LC, Bhattacharya A, Sharma M, Bhasin VK. HIV protease inhibitors, indinavir or nelfinavir, augment antimalarial action of artemisinin in vitro. Am J Trop Med Hyg. 2010 Jan;82(1):148–50.

26. Nevens F, Zuckerman JN, Burroughs AK, Jung MC, Bayas JM, Kallinowski B, et al. Immunogenicity and safety of an experimental adjuvanted hepatitis B candidate vaccine in liver transplant patients. Liver Transpl. 2006 Oct;12(10):1489–95.

27. Skinner-Adams TS, McCarthy JS, Gardiner DL, Andrews KT. HIV and malaria co-infection: interactions and consequences of chemotherapy. Trends Parasitol. 2008 Jun;24(6):264–71.

TRAVELERS WITH CHRONIC ILLNESSES
Deborah Nicolls Barbeau

GENERAL TRAVEL PREPARATION: PRACTICAL CONSIDERATIONS

Although traveling abroad can be relaxing and rewarding, the physical demands of travel can be stressful, particularly for travelers with underlying chronic illnesses. With adequate preparation, however, those with chronic illnesses can have safe and enjoyable trips. The following is a list of recommendations for patients with chronic illnesses:

- Ensure that any chronic illnesses are stable. Patients with underlying illness should see their physicians to ensure that the management of their illness is optimized.
- Recommend seeking pre-travel consultation early, at least 4–6 weeks before departure, to ensure adequate time to respond to immunizations and, in some circumstances, to try medications before travel (see the Immunocompromised Travelers section earlier in this chapter).
- Provide a physician's letter. The letter should be on office letterhead stationery, outlining existing medical conditions, medications prescribed (including generic names), and any equipment required to manage the condition.
- Advise travelers to pack medications in their original containers in carry-on luggage and to carry a copy of their prescriptions. Ensure sufficient quantities of medications for the entire trip, plus extra in case of unexpected delays. When crossing time zones, medications should be taken based on elapsed time, not time of day.
- Educate regarding drug interactions. Medications used to treat chronic medical illnesses (such as warfarin) may interact with medications prescribed for self-treatment of travelers' diarrhea or malaria chemoprophylaxis. Discuss all medications used, either daily or on an as-needed basis.
- Recommend consideration of supplemental insurance. Consideration should be given for 3 types of insurance policies: 1) trip cancellation in the event of illness; 2) supplemental insurance so that money paid for health care abroad may be reimbursed, since most medical insurance policies do not cover health care in other countries; and 3) medical evacuation insurance (see Chapter 2, Travel Health Insurance and Evacuation Insurance).
- Help devise a health plan. This plan should give instructions for managing minor problems or exacerbations of underlying illnesses and should include information about medical facilities available in the destination country (see Chapter 2, Obtaining Health Care Abroad for the Ill Traveler).
- Recommend that the traveler wear a medical alert bracelet or carry medical information on his or her person (various brands of jewelry or tags, even electronic, are available).
- Always advise the traveler about packing a health kit (see Chapter 2, Travel Health Kits).

SPECIFIC CHRONIC MEDICAL ILLNESSES

Issues related to specific chronic medical illnesses are addressed in Table 8-4. These recommendations should be used in conjunction with the other recommendations given

Table 8-4. Special considerations for travelers with chronic medical illnesses

CONDITION	ABSOLUTE AND RELATIVE CONTRAINDICATIONS TO AIRLINE TRAVEL	PRE-TRAVEL CONSIDERATIONS	IMMUNIZATION CONSIDERATIONS	MISCELLANEOUS
Cardiovascular diseases	Uncomplicated MI within 2–3 weeks Complicated MI within 6 weeks Unstable angina CHF, severe, decompensated Uncontrolled hypertension CABG within 10–14 days CVA within 2 weeks Uncontrolled arrhythmia Eisenmenger syndrome Severe symptomatic valvular heart disease	Supplemental oxygen Plan for self-management of dehydration and volume overload; may include adjusting medications Bring copy of recent EKG Bring pacemaker or AICD card DVT precautions	Influenza Pneumococcal Consider hepatitis B	Have sublingual nitroglycerine available in carry-on bag Mefloquine not recommended for people with cardiac conduction abnormalities, particularly for those with ventricular arrhythmias Self-monitoring and management of INR should be tailored to the individual patient by the anticoagulant primary provider
Pulmonary diseases	Severe, labile asthma Recent hospitalization for asthma Active respiratory infection Pneumothorax within 2–3 weeks Pleural effusion within 14 days High supplemental oxygen requirements at baseline Major chest surgery within 10–14 days	Supplemental oxygen Discuss with airline need for other equipment on plane (such as nebulizer) Plan for self-management of exacerbations (including COPD, asthma) DVT precautions	Influenza Pneumococcal Consider hepatitis B	Consider carrying short course of antibiotics and steroids, as appropriate, for exacerbations Consider advising an inhaler available in carry-on bag, even if not routinely used

continued

TABLE 8-4. SPECIAL CONSIDERATIONS FOR TRAVELERS WITH CHRONIC MEDICAL ILLNESSES (continued)

CONDITION	ABSOLUTE AND RELATIVE CONTRAINDICATIONS TO AIRLINE TRAVEL	PRE-TRAVEL CONSIDERATIONS	IMMUNIZATION CONSIDERATIONS	MISCELLANEOUS
Gastrointestinal diseases	Surgery, including laparoscopic, within 10–14 days Gastrointestinal bleed within 24 hours Colonoscopy within 24 hours Partial bowel obstruction Chronic liver disease (especially cirrhosis or heavy alcohol use)	Emphasize food and water precautions Consider prescribing prophylactic antibiotic for TD Recommend avoiding undercooked seafood, if cirrhosis or heavy alcohol use (*Vibrio vulnificus*)	Influenza Pneumococcal Hepatitis A Hepatitis B	May experience increased colostomy output during air travel H₂ blockers and PPIs increase susceptibility to TD Use mefloquine with caution in any chronic liver disease For YF vaccine, see the Immunocompromised Travelers section earlier in this chapter
Renal failure and chronic renal insufficiency	None	Emphasize food and water precautions Plan for self-management of dehydration, which can worsen renal function Arrange dialysis abroad, if needed Adjust medications for CrCl	Influenza Pneumococcal Hepatitis B	Know HIV, hepatitis C, and hepatitis B status Atovaquone-proguanil contraindicated when CrCl <30 mL/min Kidney Foundation and Global Dialysis websites can help with finding dialysis centers; check for JCI accreditation For YF vaccine, see the Immunocompromised Travelers section earlier in this chapter
Diabetes mellitus	None	Plan for self-management of dehydration, diabetic foot, and pressure sores Insulin adjustments	Influenza Pneumococcal Consider hepatitis B	Keep insulin and all glucose meter supplies in carry-on bag Bring food and supplies needed to manage hypoglycemia during travel

8

		Should check FSBG at 4- to 6-hour intervals during air travel Discuss changes in insulin regimen or oral agent with diabetes specialist Provide physician's letter stating need for all equipment, including syringes, glucose meter, and supplies		Check feet daily for pressure sores For YF vaccine, see the Immunocompromised Travelers section earlier in this chapter
Severe allergic reactions	None	Plan for managing allergic reaction while traveling and consider bringing short course of steroids for possible allergic reactions Should carry injectable epinephrine and antihistamines (H$_1$ and H$_2$ blockers)—always have on person		Many airlines already have policies in place for dealing with peanut allergies Make sure to carry injectable epinephrine in case of severe reaction while in flight
Autoimmune and rheumatologic diseases	None	Should have a baseline TST or IGRA before starting TNF blockers.	Immunosuppressive medications and TNF blockers may alter response to immunizations Live attenuated vaccines may be contraindicated	Particular emphasis should be placed on food and water precautions and hand hygiene

Abbreviations: AICD, automatic implantable cardioverter defibrillators; CABG, coronary artery bypass graft; CHF, congestive heart failure; COPD, chronic obstructive pulmonary disease; CrCl, creatinine clearance; CVA, cerebrovascular accident; DVT, deep vein thrombosis; EKG, electrocardiogram; FSBG, fingerstick blood glucose; IGRA, interferon-γ release assay; INR, international normalized ratio; JCI, Joint Commission International; MI, myocardial infarction; PPIs, proton-pump inhibitors; TD, travelers' diarrhea; TNF, tumor necrosis factor; TST, tuberculin skin test; YF, yellow fever.

throughout this book. Additional resources for information include:

- American Diabetes Association (www.diabetes.org)
- American Heart Association (www.heart.org)
- American Lung Association (www.lungusa.org)
- Anticoagulation Forum (www.acforum.org)
- Crohn's and Colitis Foundation of America (www.ccfa.org)
- Global Dialysis (www.globaldialysis.com)
- International Self-Monitoring Association of Oral Anticoagulated Patients (www.ismaap.org)

- National Kidney Foundation (www.kidney.org)
- US Department of State (www.state.gov)

Also, many health care facilities outside the United States are accredited by Joint Commission International, an affiliate of the Joint Commission, which is the largest accreditor of US-based health care organizations. A list of accredited international facilities is available at their website (www.jointcommissioninternational.org).

If travelers or their health care providers have concerns about fitness for air travel, the medical unit affiliated with the specific airline is also a valuable source for information.

BIBLIOGRAPHY

1. Aerospace Medical Association. Medical Guidelines for Airline Travel. Alexandria, VA: Aerospace Medical Association; 2003 [cited 18 Nov 2010]. Available from: http://www.asma.org/pdf/publications/medguid.pdf.
2. Bassetti M, Nicco E, Delfino E, Viscoli C. Disseminated *Salmonella paratyphi* infection in a rheumatoid arthritis patient treated with infliximab. Clin Microbiol Infect. 2010 Jan;16(1):84–5.
3. Chandran M, Edelman SV. Have insulin, will fly: diabetes management during air travel and time zone adjustment strategies. Clin Diabetes. 2003;21(2):82–5.
4. McCarthy AE. Travelers with pre-existing disease. In: Keystone JS, Kozarsky PE, Freedman DO, Nothdurft HD, Connor BA, editors. Travel Medicine. 2nd ed. Philadelphia: Mosby; 2008. p. 249–55.
5. Ringwald J, Strobel J, Eckstein R. Travel and oral anticoagulation. J Travel Med. 2009 Jul–Aug;16(4):276–83.
6. Schwartz M. Travel and oral anticoagulants. J Travel Med. 2009 Sep–Oct;16(5):369–70.
7. Simons FE. Anaphylaxis. J Allergy Clin Immunol. 2008 Feb;121(2 Suppl):S402–7.

8

PREGNANT TRAVELERS
Madeline Y. Sutton

OVERVIEW

Since as many as 50% of pregnancies are unplanned, women of reproductive age should consider maintaining current immunizations during routine check-ups in case an unplanned pregnancy coincides with a need to travel. Because of the decreased risk to the unborn child, preconceptional immunizations are preferred to vaccination during pregnancy. A woman should defer pregnancy for ≥28 days after receiving live vaccines (such as measles-mumps-rubella or yellow fever) because of a theoretical risk of transmission to the fetus. However, small studies of women who received these vaccines unintentionally during pregnancy have not found a definitive link between the vaccines and poor pregnancy outcomes. Therefore, pregnancy termination is not recommended after an inadvertent exposure.

According to the American College of Obstetrics and Gynecology, the safest time for a pregnant woman to travel is during the second trimester, when she usually feels best and is in least danger of spontaneous abortion or premature labor. A woman in the third trimester should be advised to defer overseas travel because of concerns about access to medical care in case of problems such as hypertension, phlebitis, or premature labor. Pregnant women should be advised to consult with their health care providers before making any travel decisions. Collaboration between travel health experts and obstetricians is helpful in weighing benefits and risks based on destination and recommended preventive and treatment measures. Table 8-5 lists relative contraindications to international travel during pregnancy. In general, pregnant women with serious underlying illnesses should be advised not to travel to developing countries.

PREPARATION FOR TRAVEL DURING PREGNANCY

Once a pregnant woman has decided to travel, a number of issues need to be considered before her departure:

- An intrauterine pregnancy should be confirmed by a clinician and ectopic pregnancy excluded before beginning any travel.
- General health insurance policies may or may not provide coverage of pregnancy-related problems while abroad. Pregnant travelers should inquire about what their health insurance policies cover and, if needed, obtain a supplemental policy for their trip. Many supplemental travel insurance policies and prepaid medical evacuation insurance policies do not cover pregnancy-related problems, so this issue should be clarified before obtaining a policy.
- Check medical facilities at the destination. For a woman in the last trimester, medical facilities should be able to manage complications of pregnancy, toxemia, cesarean sections, and premature or ill neonates.
- Determine beforehand whether prenatal care will be required while abroad and who will provide it. The pregnant traveler should make sure she does not miss prenatal visits requiring specific timing.
- Determine beforehand whether blood is routinely screened for HIV and hepatitis B and C at the destination. Pregnant travelers should consider the safety of blood transfusions, if needed, when making plans for international travel. The pregnant traveler should also be advised to know her blood type, and Rh-negative pregnant women should receive anti-D immune globulin (a plasma-derived

product) prophylactically at about 28 weeks' gestation. The immune globulin dose should be repeated after delivery if the infant is Rh positive.
- Determine if the traveler risks influenza on this trip, and recommend influenza vaccine accordingly.
- Determine whether the prevalence of tuberculosis (TB) is high in the destination region and whether the planned itinerary will put the traveler at risk for TB. If exposure to TB is determined to be a risk, the pregnant traveler should receive skin testing before and after travel (see Chapter 3, Tuberculosis).

GENERAL RECOMMENDATIONS FOR TRAVEL DURING PREGNANCY

A pregnant woman should be advised to travel with at least one companion; she should also be advised that, during her pregnancy, her level of comfort may be adversely affected by traveling. Table 8-6 lists the most serious risks that pregnant women face during international travel.

Typical problems of pregnant travelers are the same as those experienced by any pregnant woman: fatigue, heartburn, indigestion, constipation, vaginal discharge, leg cramps, increased frequency of urination, and hemorrhoids. During travel, pregnant women can take preventive measures, including avoiding gas-producing food or drinks before scheduled flights (entrapped gases can expand at higher altitudes) and periodically moving the legs (to decrease venous stasis). Pregnant women should always use seatbelts while seated, as air turbulence is not predictable and may cause significant trauma.

Signs and symptoms that indicate the need for immediate medical attention are vaginal bleeding, passing tissue or clots, abdominal pain or cramps, contractions, ruptured membranes, excessive leg swelling or pain, headaches, or visual problems.

AIR TRAVEL DURING PREGNANCY

Commercial air travel poses no special risks to a healthy pregnant woman or her fetus. The American College of Obstetricians and Gynecologists states that women with healthy, single pregnancies can fly safely up to 36 weeks' gestation.

Table 8-5. Potential contraindications to international travel during pregnancy

OBSTETRIC RISK FACTORS	GENERAL MEDICAL RISK FACTORS	TRAVEL TO POTENTIALLY HAZARDOUS DESTINATIONS
• History of miscarriage • Incompetent cervix • History of ectopic pregnancy (current ectopic pregnancy should be ruled out before travel) • History of premature labor or premature rupture of membranes • History of or existing placental abnormalities • Threatened abortion or vaginal bleeding during current pregnancy • Multiple gestation in current pregnancy • Fetal growth abnormalities • History of toxemia, hypertension, or diabetes with any pregnancy • Primigravida at age ≥35 years or ≤15 years	• History of thromboembolic disease • Pulmonary hypertension • Severe asthma or other chronic lung disease • Valvular heart disease (if NYHA class III or IV heart failure) • Cardiomyopathy • Hypertension • Diabetes • Renal insufficiency • Severe anemia or hemoglobinopathy • Chronic organ system dysfunction requiring frequent medical interventions	• High altitudes • Areas endemic for or experiencing ongoing outbreaks of life-threatening foodborne or insectborne infections • Areas where chloroquine-resistant *Plasmodium falciparum* malaria is endemic • Areas where live virus vaccines are required or recommended

Abbreviation: NYHA, New York Heart Association.

Table 8-6. Greatest risks for pregnant travelers

Motor vehicle accidents	• Safety belts should be worn whenever possible. • Fasten seatbelts at the pelvic area, not across the lower abdomen. Lap and shoulder restraints are best. • In most accidents, the fetus recovers quickly from the safety belt pressure. However, consult a physician even for mild trauma.
Hepatitis E	• Hepatitis E is not vaccine preventable and is especially dangerous in pregnant women. • As with other enteric infections, pregnant women should be advised that the best preventive measures are to avoid potentially contaminated water and food.
Scuba diving	• Scuba diving should be avoided in pregnancy because of the risk of decompression syndrome in the fetus.

The lowered cabin pressure (kept at the equivalent of 5,000–8,000 ft [about 1,500–2,400 m]) has minimal effect on fetal oxygenation because of the favorable fetal hemoglobin-oxygen dynamics. If supplemental oxygen is required during flight because of preexisting medical conditions, arrangements for oxygen need to be made in advance. Severe anemia, sickle-cell disease or trait, or history of thrombophlebitis are relative contraindications to flying. Pregnant women with placental abnormalities or risks for premature labor should avoid air travel.

Airline Policies and Airport Security

Each airline has policies regarding pregnancy and flying; it is always safest to check with the airline when booking reservations, because some will require medical forms to be completed. Domestic travel is usually permitted until the pregnant traveler is in week 36 of gestation, and international travel may be permitted until weeks 32–35, depending on the airline. A pregnant woman should be advised to carry documentation stating the expected day of delivery, contact information for her obstetric provider, and her blood type. For pregnant flight attendants and pilots, work-related air travel is restricted by most airlines by 20 weeks' gestation.

To date, airport security radiation exposure is minimal for pregnant women and has not been linked to an increase in adverse outcomes for unborn children. However, because of early reports of a possible association of radiation exposure during pregnancy with subsequent increased risk of childhood leukemia and cancer, a pregnant passenger may request a hand or wand search rather than being exposed to the radiation of the airport security machines.

General Tips

- An aisle seat at the bulkhead will provide the most space and comfort, but a seat over the wing in the midplane region will give the smoothest ride.
- A pregnant woman should be advised to walk every half hour during a smooth flight and flex and extend her ankles frequently to prevent phlebitis.
- Dehydration can lead to decreased placental blood flow and hemoconcentration, increasing risk of thrombosis. Thus, pregnant women should drink plenty of fluids during flights.

TRAVEL TO HIGH ALTITUDES DURING PREGNANCY

There have been no documented reports of adverse pregnancy outcomes related to high-altitude exposure during pregnancy. High-altitude destinations, however, often are remote from medical care in an emergency, and any decision to trek or climb to high altitudes while pregnant should take into account the uncertainties of being in a remote environment while pregnant and the unknown possible effects of high altitude on the fetus. Conservative advice for pregnant women is to avoid altitudes >12,000 ft (3,658 m).

FOODBORNE AND WATERBORNE ILLNESS DURING PREGNANCY

Pregnant women should be advised of the following:

- Adhere strictly to food and water precautions in developing countries, because the consequences of foodborne and waterborne illness may be more severe than diarrhea and may have serious sequelae (such as toxoplasmosis or listeriosis).
- Boil suspect drinking water to avoid long-term use of iodine-containing purification systems. Iodine tablets can probably be used for travel up to several weeks, but congenital goiters have been reported in association with administration of iodine-containing drugs during pregnancy.
- Oral rehydration (boiled or bottled water) is the mainstay of therapy for travelers' diarrhea.
- Bismuth subsalicylate compounds are contraindicated because of the theoretical risks of fetal bleeding from salicylates and teratogenicity from the bismuth.
- The combination of kaolin and pectin may be used, and loperamide should be used only when necessary.
- The antibiotic treatment of travelers' diarrhea during pregnancy can be complicated. Azithromycin or an oral third-generation cephalosporin may be the best option for treatment, if an antibiotic is needed.

MALARIA DURING PREGNANCY

Advise pregnant women to avoid travel to malaria-endemic areas if possible. Women who choose to go to areas with malaria can reduce their risk of acquiring malaria by taking appropriate malaria chemoprophylaxis and following insect precautions (see Chapter 2, Protection against Mosquitoes, Ticks, and Other Insects and Arthropods and Chapter 3, Malaria). Pregnant women should use insect repellents as recommended for adults sparingly, but as needed. Pyrethrum-containing house sprays may also be used indoors, if insects are a problem.

Antimalarial Medications

For pregnant women who travel to areas with chloroquine-sensitive *Plasmodium falciparum* malaria, chloroquine can be taken for malaria chemoprophylaxis, since it has been used for decades with no documented increase in birth defects. For pregnant women who travel to areas with chloroquine-resistant *P. falciparum*, mefloquine should be recommended for chemoprophylaxis. Evidence suggests that mefloquine prophylaxis causes no significant increase in spontaneous abortions or congenital malformations when taken during the first trimester.

Because there is no evidence that chloroquine and mefloquine are associated with congenital defects when used for prophylaxis, CDC does not recommend that women planning pregnancy wait a specific period of time after their use before becoming pregnant.

However, if women or their health care providers wish to decrease the amount of antimalarial drug in the body before conception, Table 8-7 provides information on the half-lives of selected antimalarial drugs. After 2, 4, and 6 half-lives, approximately 25%, 6%, and 2%, respectively, of the drug remain in the body.

Doxycycline and primaquine are contraindicated for malaria prophylaxis during pregnancy, because both may cause adverse effects on the fetus. Atovaquone-proguanil is not recommended for use by pregnant women to prevent malaria because of the lack of safety studies during pregnancy.

Treatment and Management

Malaria must be treated as a medical emergency in any pregnant traveler. A woman who has traveled to an area that has chloroquine-resistant strains of *P. falciparum* should be treated as if she has illness caused by chloroquine-resistant organisms. The management of malaria in a pregnant woman should include frequent blood glucose determinations and careful fluid monitoring (being careful not to give too much intravenous fluid).

Table 8-7. Half-lives of selected antimalarial drugs

DRUG	HALF LIFE
Atovaquone	2–3 days
Chloroquine	Can extend 6–60 days
Doxycycline	12–24 hours
Mefloquine	2–3 weeks
Primaquine	4–7 hours
Proguanil	14–21 hours
Pyrimethamine	3–4 days
Sulfadoxine	6–9 days

IMMUNIZATIONS FOR PREGNANT TRAVELERS

Risk to a developing fetus from vaccination of the mother during pregnancy is primarily theoretical. No evidence exists of risk from vaccinating pregnant women with inactivated virus, bacterial vaccines, or toxoids. The benefits of vaccinating pregnant women usually outweigh potential risks when the likelihood of disease exposure is high, infection would pose a risk to the mother or fetus, and the vaccine is unlikely to cause harm.

Table 8-8 is intended for women who may require immunizations during pregnancy. Pregnant travelers may visit areas of the world where diseases eliminated by routine vaccination in the United States are still endemic, and therefore may require immunizations before travel.

TRAVEL HEALTH KITS FOR PREGNANT WOMEN

Additions and substitutions to the usual travel health kit (see Chapter 2, Travel Health Kits) need to be made during pregnancy. Talcum powder, a thermometer, oral rehydration salt packets, prenatal vitamins, a topical antifungal agent for vaginal yeast, acetaminophen, and a sunscreen with a high SPF should be included. Women in the third trimester may be advised to carry a blood-pressure cuff and urine dipsticks and be trained to use this equipment to check for hypertension, proteinuria, and glucosuria, any of which would require prompt medical attention. Antimalarial and antidiarrheal self-treatment medications should be evaluated individually, depending on the traveler's itinerary and her health history. Medications should only be used after consultation with a physician.

Table 8-8. Vaccination during pregnancy

VACCINE/ IMMUNOBIOLOGIC	TYPE	USE
Immune globulins, pooled or hyperimmune	Immune globulin or specific globulin preparations	If indicated for preexposure or postexposure use; no known risk to fetus
Vaccination of Pregnant Women is Recommended		
Hepatitis B	Recombinant or plasma-derived	Recommended for women at risk of infection
Influenza[1]	Inactivated whole virus or subunit	All people >6 months, including women who will be or are pregnant during the flu season (September–March), regardless of trimester, and women at high risk for pulmonary complications, regardless of trimester
Tetanus-diphtheria (Td)	Toxoid	If indicated, such as lack of primary series or no booster within past 10 years

continued

TABLE 8-8. VACCINATION DURING PREGNANCY (continued)

VACCINE/ IMMUNOBIOLOGIC	TYPE	USE
Tetanus-diphtheria-pertussis (Tdap)	Toxoid, acellular	Not contraindicated, but no data are available on safety, immunogenicity, and outcomes of pregnancy. ACIP recommends Td when tetanus and diphtheria protection are required but Tdap to add protection against pertussis in some situations. Second or third trimester is preferred.
Hepatitis A	Inactivated virus	No data are available on safety in pregnancy. Because hepatitis A vaccine is produced from inactivated hepatitis A virus, the theoretical risk of vaccination should be weighed against the risk of disease. Consider immune globulin rather than vaccine.

Pregnancy is a Precaution, and Under Normal Circumstances, Vaccination Should Be Deferred; Vaccine Should Only Be Given when Benefits Outweigh Risks

Japanese encephalitis	Inactivated virus	No data are available on safety in pregnancy. Pregnant women who must travel to an area where the risk is high should be vaccinated when the theoretical risks are outweighed by the risk of disease.
Meningococcal meningitis	Polysaccharide	Meningococcal conjugate vaccine (MenACWY) is preferred for adults; however, no data are available on safety and immunogenicity in pregnant women. Meningococcal polysaccharide vaccine (MPSV4) can be administered during pregnancy if the woman is entering an epidemic area. Indications for prophylaxis are not altered by pregnancy; vaccine is recommended in unusual outbreak situations.
Pneumococcal	Polysaccharide	The safety of pneumococcal (PPV23) vaccine during the first trimester of pregnancy has not been evaluated, although no adverse events have been reported after inadvertent vaccination during pregnancy. Women with chronic diseases, smokers, and immunosuppressed women should consider vaccination.
Polio, inactivated	Inactivated virus	Indicated for susceptible pregnant women traveling in endemic areas or in other high-risk situations.
Rabies	Inactivated virus	Indications for postexposure prophylaxis not altered by pregnancy. If risk for exposure to rabies is substantial, preexposure prophylaxis may also be indicated.

continued

8

TABLE 8-8. VACCINATION DURING PREGNANCY (continued)

VACCINE/ IMMUNOBIOLOGIC	TYPE	USE
Typhoid (ViCPS)	Polysaccharide	If indicated for travel to endemic areas
Typhoid (Ty21a)	Live bacterial	No data are available on safety in pregnancy; theoretical risk exists, because it is a live-attenuated vaccine.
Yellow fever	Live attenuated	The safety of YF vaccination in pregnancy has not been studied in a large prospective trial. If travel is unavoidable and the risks for YFV exposure outweigh the vaccination risks, a pregnant woman should be vaccinated. If the risks for vaccination outweigh the risks for YFV exposure, a pregnant woman should be issued a medical waiver to fulfill health regulations. If a pregnant woman is vaccinated, her infant should be monitored after birth for evidence of congenital infection and other possible adverse effects resulting from YF vaccination. Pregnancy may interfere with the immune response to YF vaccine; therefore, serologic testing to document a protective immune response to the vaccine should be considered (see Chapter 3, Yellow Fever for more details).

Pregnancy is a Contraindication to Vaccination; Vaccine Should Not Be Administered to Pregnant Women

Tuberculosis (BCG)	Attenuated mycobacterial	Contraindicated due to theoretical risk of disseminated disease. Skin testing for tuberculosis exposure before and after travel is preferable when the risk of possible exposure is high.
Measles-mumps-rubella	Live attenuated virus	Contraindicated. Vaccination of susceptible women should be part of postpartum care. Unvaccinated women should delay travel to countries where measles is endemic until after delivery. Unvaccinated pregnant women with a documented exposure to measles should receive immune globulin within 6 days to prevent illness.
Human papillomavirus	Recombinant quadrivalent	Contraindicated. The vaccine has not been causally associated with adverse outcomes of pregnancy; however, additional information is needed for further recommendations. Pregnancy testing is not needed before vaccination.

continued

TABLE 8-8. VACCINATION DURING PREGNANCY (continued)

VACCINE/ IMMUNOBIOLOGIC	TYPE	USE
Varicella	Live attenuated virus	Contraindicated. Vaccination of susceptible women should be considered postpartum. Unvaccinated pregnant women should consider postponing travel until after delivery, when the vaccine can be given safely.
Influenza[1]	Live attenuated virus, including intranasal preparations	Contraindicated during pregnancy; postpartum and breastfeeding mothers may receive live attenuated virus vaccines.

Abbreviations: ACIP, Advisory Committee on Immunization Practices; BCG, Bacillus Calmette-Guérin; YF, yellow fever; YFV, yellow fever virus.

[1] Starting with the 2010–11 influenza season, most influenza vaccines will offer protection against both seasonal and H1N1 influenza virus strains.

BIBLIOGRAPHY

1. ACOG Committee on Obstertic Practice. Committee opinion: number 264, December 2001. Air travel during pregnancy. Obstet Gynecol. 2001 Dec;98(6):1187–8.
2. American College of Obstetricians and Gynecologists. ACOG Committee Opinion. Immunization during pregnancy. Obstet Gynecol. 2003 Jan;101(1):207–12.
3. Barish RJ. In-flight radiation exposure during pregnancy. Obstet Gynecol. 2004 Jun;103(6):1326–30.
4. Bia FJ. Medical considerations for the pregnant traveler. Infect Dis Clin North Am. 1992 Jun;6(2):371–88.
5. Bilukha OO, Rosenstein N. Prevention and control of meningococcal disease. Recommendations of the Advisory Committee on Immunization Practices (ACIP). MMWR Recomm Rep. 2005 May 27;54(RR-7):1–21.
6. Boice JD, Miller RW. Childhood and adult cancer after intrauterine exposure to ionizing radiation. Teratology. 1999 Apr;59(4):227–33.
7. CDC. Guidelines for vaccinating pregnant women, Advisory Committee on Immunization Practices. Atlanta: CDC; 1998 [updated 2007 May; cited 2010 Oct 26]. Available from: http://www.cdc.gov/vaccines/pubs/downloads/b_preg_guide.pdf.
8. CDC. Guiding principles for development of ACIP recommendations for vaccination during pregnancy and breastfeeding. MMWR Morb Mortal Wkly Rep. 2008 May 30;57(21):580.
9. CDC. Human rabies prevention—United States, 1999. Recommendations of the Advisory Committee on Immunization Practices (ACIP). MMWR Recomm Rep. 1999 Jan 8;48(RR-1):1–21.
10. CDC. Revised ACIP recommendation for avoiding pregnancy after receiving a rubella-containing vaccine. MMWR Morb Mortal Wkly Rep. 2001 Dec 14;50(49):1117.
11. CDC. Typhoid immunization: recommendations of the Advisory Committee on Immunization Practices (ACIP). MMWR Morb Mortal Wkly Rep. 1994;43(RR-14):1–7.
12. Cetron MS, Marfin AA, Julian KG, Gubler DJ, Sharp DJ, Barwick RS, et al. Yellow fever vaccine. Recommendations of the Advisory Committee on Immunization Practices (ACIP), 2002. MMWR Recomm Rep. 2002 Nov 8;51(RR-17):1–11.
13. Fiore AE, Shay DK, Broder K, Iskander JK, Uyeki TM, Mootrey G, et al. Prevention and control of influenza: recommendations of the Advisory Committee on Immunization Practices (ACIP), 2008. MMWR Recomm Rep. 2008 Aug 8;57(RR-7):1–60.
14. Fiore AE, Uyeki TM, Broder K, Finelli L, Euler GL, Singleton JA, et al. Prevention and control of influenza with vaccines: recommendations of the Advisory Committee on Immunization Practices (ACIP), 2010. MMWR Recomm Rep. 2010 Aug 6;59(RR-8):1–62.
15. GlaxoSmithKline. Malarone (atovaquone and proguanil hydrochloride) tablets and pediatric tablets prescribing information. Research Triangle Park, NC: GlaxoSmithKline; 2009. Available from: http://us.gsk.com/products/assets/us_malarone.pdf.
16. Marin M, Guris D, Chaves SS, Schmid S, Seward JF. Prevention of varicella: recommendations of the Advisory Committee on Immunization Practices (ACIP). MMWR Recomm Rep. 2007 Jun 22;56(RR-4):1–40.

17. Mast EE, Margolis HS, Fiore AE, Brink EW, Goldstein ST, Wang SA, et al. A comprehensive immunization strategy to eliminate transmission of hepatitis B virus infection in the United States: recommendations of the Advisory Committee on Immunization Practices (ACIP). Part 1: immunization of infants, children, and adolescents. MMWR Recomm Rep. 2005 Dec 23;54(RR-16):1–31.

18. Watson JC, Hadler SC, Dykewicz CA, Reef S, Phillips L. Measles, mumps, and rubella—vaccine use and strategies for elimination of measles, rubella, and congenital rubella syndrome and control of mumps: recommendations of the Advisory Committee on Immunization Practices (ACIP). MMWR Recomm Rep. 1998 May 22;47(RR-8):1–57.

TRAVELERS WITH DISABILITIES

Emad A. Yanni, Amanda Cantor

OVERVIEW

Travelers with disabilities are defined as travelers whose mobility is reduced because of a physical incapacity (sensory or locomotor), an intellectual deficiency, age, illness, or another cause, and who may require special attention and adaptation of the transportation services that are available to all passengers. The medical preparation of a traveler with a stable, ongoing disability does not differ from that of any other traveler. The following recommendations are key to ensuring safe, accessible travel:

- Assess each international itinerary on an individual basis, in consultation with specialized travel agencies or tour operators.
- Consult travel health providers for additional recommendations.
- Use print and internet resources.

AIR TRAVEL

Regulations and Codes

Carriers may not refuse transportation on the basis of disability. By law, US air carriers must comply with highly detailed regulations that affect people with disabilities. These do not cover foreign carriers serving the United States.

All US and non-US carriers are required to file annual reports of disability-related complaints with the Department of Transportation (DOT). The DOT maintains a toll-free hotline (800-778-4838, available 7 AM–11 PM, Eastern Time) to provide real-time assistance in facilitating compliance with DOT rules and to suggest customer-service solutions to the airlines.

The Transportation Security Administration (TSA) has established a program for screening travelers with disabilities and their equipment, mobility aids, and devices. TSA permits prescriptions, liquid medications, and other liquids needed by people with disabilities and medical conditions. International Air Transport Association (IATA) member airlines voluntarily adhere to codes of practice that are similar to US legislation based on guidance from the International Civil Aviation Organization. However, smaller airlines overseas may not be IATA members.

Airlines are obliged to accept a declaration by a passenger that he or she is self-reliant. Medical certificates can be required only in specific situations (for example, if a person intends to travel with a possible communicable disease, will require a stretcher or oxygen, or if unusual behavior is anticipated that may affect the operation of the flight).

Assistance and Accommodations

When a traveler with a disability requests assistance, the airline is obliged to provide access to the aircraft door (preferably by a level entry bridge), an aisle wheelchair, and a seat with removable armrests. Aircraft with fewer than 30 seats are generally exempt. Airline personnel are not required to transfer passengers from wheelchair to wheelchair, wheelchair to aircraft seat, or wheelchair to lavatory seat. Travelers with disabilities who cannot transfer themselves should travel with a companion or attendant, but carriers may not, without reason, require a person with a disability to travel with an attendant.

Only wide-body aircraft with 2 aisles are required to have fully accessible lavatories, although any aircraft with more than 60 seats must have an onboard wheelchair, and personnel must help move the wheelchair from a seat to the lavatory area. Airline personnel are not obliged to assist with feeding, visiting the lavatory, or dispensing medication to travelers.

Airlines may not require advance notice of a passenger with a disability; however, they may require up to 48 hours' advance notice and 1-hour advance check-in for certain accommodations that require preparation time, such as the following:

- Medical oxygen for use on board the aircraft, if the service is available on the flight
- Carriage of an incubator, if the service is available on the flight
- Hook-up for a respirator to the aircraft electrical power supply, if the service is available on the flight
- Accommodation for a passenger who must travel in a stretcher, if the service is available on the flight
- Transportation of an electric wheelchair on a flight scheduled on an aircraft with fewer than 60 seats
- Provision by the airline of hazardous material packaging for a battery used in a wheelchair or other assistive devices
- Accommodation for a group of 10 or more people with disabilities who make a reservation and travel as a group
- Provision of an onboard wheelchair to be used on an aircraft that does not have an accessible lavatory

Assessment and Preparation

With high incidence of cardiopulmonary disease and millions of people traveling by air, many people are at risk for significant hypoxia and respiratory symptoms while flying. Generally, patients with an oxygen saturation by pulse oximetry >95% do not require supplemental oxygen, and those with a saturation <92% will require it during air travel. The hypoxia altitude simulation test can identify those patients (with an oxygen saturation by pulse oximetry between 92% and 95%) who may benefit from oxygen supplementation during air travel, decreasing their risk for significant cardiopulmonary effects of induced hypoxia at higher altitudes.

Internationally standardized codes for classifying disabled passengers and their needs are available in all computerized reservations systems. Passengers with disabilities should use travel agents experienced in the use of the disability coding; it is critical that appropriate codes and interairline messages are sequentially entered for all flights. The delivering carrier is always responsible for a traveler with disabilities until a subsequent carrier physically accepts responsibility for that passenger.

SERVICE ANIMALS

Service animals are not exempt from compliance with quarantine regulations and so may not be allowed to travel to all international destinations. They are also subject to US animal import regulations on return (see Chapter 6, Taking Animals and Animal Products across International Borders). However, carriers must permit guide dogs or other service animals with appropriate identification to accompany a person with a disability on a flight. Carriers must permit a service animal to accompany a traveler with a disability to any seat in which the person sits, unless the animal obstructs an aisle or other area that must remain clear to facilitate an emergency evacuation, in which case the passenger will be assigned another seat.

CRUISE SHIPS

US companies or entities conducting programs or tours on cruise ships have obligations regarding access for travelers with disabilities, even if the ship itself is of foreign registry (see Chapter 6, Cruise Ship Travel). However, all travelers with disabilities should check with individual cruise lines regarding availability of requested or needed items before booking. Cruises are available that cater to travelers with special needs, such as dialysis patients.

USEFUL LINKS

- MossRehab ResourceNet (www.mossresource net.org/travel.htm)
- Department of Transportation, Aviation Consumer Protection Division
  > New Horizons Information for the Air Traveler with a Disability (http://

airconsumer.ost.dot.gov/publications/horizons.htm#NewEnvironment)
> Nondiscrimination on the Basis of Disability in Air Travel: 14 CFR Part 382, Federal Rules (http://airconsumer.ost.dot.gov/rules/rules.htm)
- American Council of the Blind—lists cruises, books, useful telephone numbers, and links to products for purchase (www.acb.org/resources/travel.html)
- Access-Able—resource for mature travelers and those with special needs (www.access-able.com)
- Transportation Security Administration—travelers with disabilities and medical conditions (www.tsa.gov/travelers/airtravel/specialneeds)
- Society for Accessible Travel and Hospitality (www.sath.org)
- Aerospace Medical Association—medical guidelines for airline travel (www.asma.org/publications/medicalguideline.php)
- Mobility International USA (www.miusa.org)
> Preparing for Departure (www.miusa.org/ncde/goingabroad/survivalsteps/preparingtodepart)
> Equipment and Tools that Make Traveling with a Disability Easy (www.miusa.org/ncde/tipsheets/tools)

BIBLIOGRAPHY

1. Bucks C. A World of Options: a Guide to International Exchange, Community Service and Travel for Persons with Disabilities. 3rd ed. Eugene, OR: ILR Press; 1997.
2. Convention on International Civil Aviation. ICAO-recommended practices relating to persons with disabilities. International Civil Aviation Organization. Available from: http://www.icao.int/icao/en/atb/sgm/disabilities.htm.
3. Dine CJ, Kreider ME. Hypoxia altitude simulation test. Chest. 2008 Apr;133(4):1002–5.

IMMIGRANTS RETURNING HOME TO VISIT FRIENDS & RELATIVES (VFRs)

Jay S. Keystone

DEFINITION OF VFR

A traveler categorized as a VFR is an immigrant, ethnically and racially distinct from the majority population of the country of residence (a higher-income country), who returns to his or her home country (lower-income country) to visit friends or relatives. Included in the VFR category are family members, such as the spouse or children, who were born in the country of residence. Some experts have recently recommended that the term VFR refer to all those visiting friends and relatives regardless of the traveler's country of origin; however, this more recently proposed definition may be too broad and not take into consideration cultural, economic, and attitudinal issues, and thus we use the more classic definition.

DISPROPORTIONATE INFECTIOUS DISEASE RISKS IN VFRs

Altered migration patterns to North America in the past 30 years have resulted in many immigrants originating from Asia, Southeast Asia, and Latin America instead of Europe. Although 12% of the US population is foreign born, in 2008, 34% of those from the United States traveling overseas listed VFR as a reason for travel. VFRs experience a higher incidence of travel-related infectious diseases, such as malaria, typhoid fever, tuberculosis, hepatitis A, and sexually transmitted diseases, than do other groups of international travelers, for a number of reasons:

- Lack of awareness of risk
- ≤30% have a pre-travel health care encounter

- Financial barriers to pre-travel health care
- Clinics are not geographically convenient
- Cultural and language barriers with health care providers
- Lack of trust in the medical system
- Last-minute travel plans and longer trips
- Travel to higher-risk destinations, such as staying in homes and living the local lifestyle that often includes lack of food and water precautions and use of bed nets
- Belief that they are immune (VFR health beliefs likely contribute to lower rates of vaccination against hepatitis A and typhoid and infrequent use of malaria chemoprophylaxis, compared with other international travelers.)

Malaria

In 2008, 65% of imported malaria cases in US civilians occurred among VFRs. Data from GeoSentinel show VFRs are 8 times more likely to acquire malaria than are tourist travelers. Reports from the United Kingdom have shown that VFR travelers to West Africa were 10 times more likely to develop malaria than were tourists. Many VFRs assume they are immune; however, in most VFRs, especially those who left their countries of origin years previously, immunity has waned and is no longer protective. In recent years, a number of VFRs have died of malaria on their return to North America.

Other Infections

In the United States, 66% of typhoid cases occur in VFRs, mostly from South Asia and Latin America; 90% of paratyphoid A cases are imported from South Asia as well. Most typhoid isolates showed lower sensitivity to fluoroquinolones.

VFR children aged <15 years are at highest risk for hepatitis A, and many are symptomatic. In a British study, most cases were acquired in south Asia. Other diseases, such as tuberculosis, hepatitis A and B, cholera, and measles occur more commonly in VFRs after travel.

PRE-TRAVEL HEALTH COUNSELING FOR VFRs

Table 8-9 summarizes VFR health risks and prevention recommendations. It is important to increase awareness among travelers regarding their unique risks for travel-related infections and the barriers to travel health services. If possible, clinics should incorporate culturally sensitive educational materials, provide language translators, and provide handouts in multiple languages (see www. tropical.umn.edu/TTM/VFR/index.htm).

Vaccinations

Travel immunization recommendations and requirements for VFRs are the same as those for US-born travelers. It is crucial, however, to first try to establish whether the immigrant traveler has had routine immunizations (such as measles and tetanus) or has a history of the diseases. Adult travelers, in the absence of documentation of immunizations, may be considered to be nonimmune, and age-appropriate vaccinations (or serologic studies to check for antibody status) should be provided, with 2 important caveats:

- Immunity to hepatitis A should not be assumed; many young adults and adolescents from developing countries are still susceptible. Pre-travel serologic testing for both hepatitis A and B may be worthwhile.
- Consider varicella immunization for immigrants from South and Southeast Asia and Latin America. These travelers may be more susceptible, because infection occurs at an older age in tropical than in temperate regions. Also, rates of death and complications from varicella disease are higher in adults than in children.

Malaria Prevention

VFR travelers to endemic areas should not only be encouraged to take prophylactic medications, but also be reminded of the benefits of barrier methods of prevention, such as bed nets and insect repellents, particularly for children (see Chapter 2, Protection against Mosquitoes, Ticks, and Other Insects and Arthropods). VFRs should be advised that drugs such as chloroquine and pyrimethamine, as well as proguanil monotherapy, are no longer effective in most areas, especially in sub-Saharan Africa. These medications are often readily available and inexpensive in their home countries but are not efficacious.

VFRs should also be encouraged to purchase their medications before traveling to ensure good drug quality. Studies in Africa and Southeast Asia show that one-third to half of antimalarial drugs purchased locally were counterfeit or substandard; a recently published study from Laos showed that 88% of oral artesunate sold in pharmacies was of poor quality.

Table 8-9. Diseases for which VFR travelers are at increased risk, proposed reasons for risk variance, and recommendations to reduce risks specific to travelers visiting friends and relatives[1]

SPECIFIC DISEASES	REASON FOR RISK VARIANCE[2]	RECOMMENDATIONS TO STRESS WITH VFR TRAVELERS
Foodborne and waterborne illness	Social and cultural pressure (eat the meal served by hosts)	Frequent handwashing Avoid high-risk foods (dairy products, undercooked foods) Simplify treatment regimens (single dose, such as azithromycin, 1,000 mg, or ciprofloxacin, 500 mg) Discuss food preparation
Fish-related toxins and infections	Eating high-risk foods Less pre-travel advice	Avoidance counseling about specific foods (such as raw freshwater fish)
Malaria	Longer stays Higher-risk destinations Less pre-travel advice leading to less use of chemoprophylaxis and fewer personal protection measures Belief that already immune	Education on malaria, mosquito avoidance, and the need for chemoprophylaxis Consider cost of chemoprophylaxis Use of insecticide-treated bed nets
Tuberculosis (particularly multidrug-resistant)	Increased close contact with local population Increased contact with HIV-coinfected people	Check PPD 2–3 months after return if history of negative Mantoux text and long stay (>3 months) Educate about tuberculosis signs, symptoms, and avoidance
Bloodborne and sexually transmitted diseases	More likely to seek substandard, local care Cultural practices (tattoos, female genital mutilation) Longer stays and increased chance of blood transfusion Higher likelihood of sexual encounters with local population	Discuss high-risk behaviors, including tattoos, piercings, dental work, sexual encounters Encourage purchase of condoms before travel Consider providing syringes, needles, and intravenous catheters for long-term travel
Schistosomiasis and geohelminths	Limited access to piped-in water in rural areas for bathing and washing clothes	Avoid freshwater exposure Use liposomal DEET preparation with freshwater exposures[3] Discourage children from playing in dirt Use ground cover Use protective footwear
Respiratory problems	Increased close exposure to fires, smoking, or pollution	Prepare for asthma exacerbations by considering stand-by bronchodilators and steroids

continued

TABLE 8-9. DISEASES FOR WHICH VFR TRAVELERS ARE AT INCREASED RISK, PROPOSED REASONS FOR RISK VARIANCE, AND RECOMMENDATIONS TO REDUCE RISKS SPECIFIC TO TRAVELERS VISITING FRIENDS AND RELATIVES[1] (continued)

SPECIFIC DISEASES	REASON FOR RISK VARIANCE[2]	RECOMMENDATIONS TO STRESS WITH VFR TRAVELERS
Zoonotic diseases (such as rickettsial, leptospirosis, viral fevers, leishmaniasis, anthrax)	Rural destinations Staying with family where animals are kept Increased exposure to insects Increased exposure to mice and rats Sleeping on floors	Avoid animals Wash hands Wear protective clothing Check for ticks daily Avoid thatched roofs and mud walls in Latin America Avoid sleeping at floor level
Envenomations (snakes, spiders, scorpions)	Sleeping on floors	Avoid sleeping at floor level Use footwear out-of-doors at night
Toxin ingestion (medication adverse events, heavy metal ingestion)	Purchase of local medications Use of traditional therapies Use of contaminated products (such as pottery with lead glaze) Eating contaminated freshwater fish	Anticipate and purchase medications before travel Counsel avoidance of known traditional medications (such as Hmong bark tea with aspirin) and high-risk items (such as large reef fish)
Yellow fever and Japanese encephalitis (risk is decreased in adults)	Unclear, partial immunity from previous exposure or vaccination	Avoid mosquitoes by taking protective measures and receiving vaccination when appropriate
Dengue fever (especially risk of DHF and DSS)	DHF and DSS occur on repeat exposure to a different serotype of dengue; VFRs more likely to have had previous exposure	Avoid mosquitoes by taking protective measures

Abbreviations: DEET, *N,N*-diethyl-*m*-toluamide; DHF, dengue hemorrhagic fever; DSS, dengue shock syndrome; VFR, visiting friends and relatives.
[1] Adapted from: Bacaner N, Stauffer B, Boulware DR, Walker PF, Keystone JS. Travel medicine considerations for North American immigrants visiting friends and relatives. JAMA. 2004;291(23):2856–64.
[2] Hypothesis unless referenced to support assertions
[3] In animal models, DEET (liposomal preparations) prevents *Schistosoma* cercariae from penetrating the skin.

BIBLIOGRAPHY

1. Angell SY, Cetron MS. Health disparities among travelers visiting friends and relatives abroad. Ann Intern Med. 2005 Jan 4;142(1):67–72.
2. Arguin PM. A definition that includes first and second generation immigrants returning to their countries of origin to visit friends and relatives still makes sense to me. J Travel Med. 2010 May–Jun;17(3):147–9.
3. Bacaner N, Stauffer B, Boulware DR, Walker PF, Keystone JS. Travel medicine considerations for North American immigrants visiting friends and relatives. JAMA. 2004 Jun 16;291(23):2856–64.
4. Barnett ED, Christiansen D, Figueira M. Seroprevalence of measles, rubella, and varicella in refugees. Clin Infect Dis. 2002 Aug 15;35(4):403–8.
5. Barnett ED, MacPherson DW, Stauffer WM, Loutan L, Hatz CF, Matteelli A, et al. The visiting friends or

relatives traveler in the 21st century: time for a new definition. J Travel Med. 2010 May–Jun;17(3):163–70.
6. Bate R, Coticelli P, Tren R, Attaran A. Antimalarial drug quality in the most severely malarious parts of Africa—a six country study. PLoS One. 2008;3(5):e2132.
7. dos Santos CC, Anvar A, Keystone JS, Kain KC. Survey of use of malaria prevention measures by Canadians visiting India. CMAJ. 1999 Jan 26;160(2):195–200.
8. Greenaway C, Dongier P, Boivin JF, Tapiero B, Miller M, Schwartzman K. Susceptibility to measles, mumps, and rubella in newly arrived adult immigrants and refugees. Ann Intern Med. 2007 Jan 2;146(1):20–4.
9. Gupta SK, Medalla F, Omondi MW, Whichard JM, Fields PI, Gerner-Smidt P, et al. Laboratory-based surveillance of paratyphoid fever in the United

States: travel and antimicrobial resistance. Clin Infect Dis. 2008 Jun 1;46(11):1656–63.

10. Jacobsen KH, Koopman JS. Declining hepatitis A seroprevalence: a global review and analysis. Epidemiol Infect. 2004 Dec;132(6):1005–22.

11. Leder K, Tong S, Weld L, Kain KC, Wilder-Smith A, von Sonnenburg F, et al. Illness in travelers visiting friends and relatives: a review of the GeoSentinel Surveillance Network. Clin Infect Dis. 2006 Nov 1;43(9):1185–93.

12. Lee BW. Review of varicella zoster seroepidemiology in India and Southeast Asia. Trop Med Int Health. 1998 Nov;3(11):886–90.

13. Lynch MF, Blanton EM, Bulens S, Polyak C, Vojdani J, Stevenson J, et al. Typhoid fever in the United States, 1999–2006. JAMA. 2009 Aug 26;302(8):859–65.

14. Mandal BK, Mukherjee PP, Murphy C, Mukherjee R, Naik T. Adult susceptibility to varicella in the tropics is a rural phenomenon due to the lack of previous exposure. J Infect Dis. 1998 Nov;178 Suppl 1:S52–4.

15. Pavli A, Maltezou HC. Malaria and travellers visiting friends and relatives. Travel Med Infect Dis. 2010 May;8(3):161–8.

16. Schilthuis HJ, Goossens I, Ligthelm RJ, de Vlas SJ, Varkevisser C, Richardus JH. Factors determining use of pre-travel preventive health services by West African immigrants in The Netherlands. Trop Med Int Health. 2007 Aug;12(8):990–8.

17. US Census Bureau. The foreign-born population in 2004. Washington, DC: US Census Bureau; 2004 [cited 2007 Jul 17]. Available from: http://www.census.gov/population/pop-profile/dynamic/ForeignBorn.pdf.

18. US Department of Commerce. Profile of US resident travelers visiting overseas destinations: 2008 outbound. Washington, DC: International Trade Administration, Manufacturing and Services, Office of Travel and Tourism Industries; 2008 [cited 2010 Jun 25]. Available from: http://www.tinet.ita.doc.gov/outreachpages/download_data_table/2008_Outbound_Profile.pdf.

19. US Department of Homeland Security. US legal permanent residents: 2005. Washington, DC: Office of Immigration Statistics; 2006 [cited 2006 Jul 17]. Available from: http://www.dhs.gov/xlibrary/assets/statistics/publications/USLegalPermEst_5.pdf.

ADVICE FOR AIR CREWS
Phyllis E. Kozarsky

OVERVIEW

As airlines expand their reach and air crews are asked to travel to more exotic destinations, these travelers need to prepare ahead of time for the exposures they may encounter. To some degree, air crews are similar to all travelers to such destinations, but the differences require some modifications of travel health guidance for several reasons:

- Layovers are short, often <24 hours.
- Travel is frequent.
- Travel to new destinations may be on short notice.
- Despite short travel times, air crews may be more adventuresome and thus have more risk than typical package tourists.
- Air crews may perceive themselves to be low risk because of their generally healthy status and because their exposure time in-country is short.

Given these factors, it is worth noting some guidelines for this special group. In general, American carriers traveling to destinations in the developing world try to inform their air crews about health issues they may face. However, airlines do not necessarily have available on their staff occupational health or other providers who are experts in travel medicine, and the airlines may not be aware of special risks at their destinations. Air crews and clinicians seeing such travelers should, therefore, encourage airlines to avail themselves of professionals who are knowledgeable in the field and who can help determine recommendations for the various destinations served.

Pilots typically know some of the medications and classes of medications that are not permitted while flying, so clinicians should always discuss medication options. Medications with central nervous system adverse events should not be prescribed, and a trial should be taken between trips of any medication that could have side effects that may interfere with flying. Pilots and flight attendants should also be aware that certain foods and beverages containing trace amounts of products could cause a drug screen to turn positive. They should also consider the effects of drinking too much water (possibly causing hyponatremia) on health and drug tests. If questions arise, an aeromedical examiner should be consulted who will know the Federal Aviation Administration rules for what medications can and cannot be taken by pilots. These physicians are responsible for certifying that pilots are fit to fly, and they examine pilots on a regular basis.

Although any travel health provider can see and advise flight crews, it is important to ask the crew member what the airline may require, in addition to what is required or recommended to maintain the person's health while traveling. If in doubt, the travel health provider should contact the airline medical director or occupational health department for guidance. For example, some air crews primarily fly domestic routes or routes to Western Europe or Japan, so would not fly to a region of yellow fever risk in their normal daily work. However, an airline may require that crew members without contraindications be vaccinated against yellow fever, so that the airline has flexibility to shift crews and be able to address any urgent need.

GENERAL HEALTH MEASURES

Although pilots are required to have periodic physician visits to ensure they are fit to fly, these may not address some issues that may affect them when they travel internationally, particularly to destinations in the developing world. Flight attendants and others should also consider asking their health care providers about these recommendations:

- Administering a periodic tuberculin skin test, if traveling frequently to destinations where the prevalence of tuberculosis is much higher than in the United States, where the incidence of antimicrobial resistance is higher, and where the crew member will be in close contact with crowds (www.who.int/tb/challenges/mdr/en/).

- Checking at each visit to make sure that routine immunizations are up to date (see below).
- Immunizing against seasonal influenza every year when the vaccine becomes available, and immunizing against any outbreak influenza strain, should a special vaccine be available.

In addition, all medications for chronic conditions should be carried in extra quantities, as they may not be available at some locations, and even if available and less costly, may be counterfeit (see Chapter 2, Perspectives: Counterfeit Drugs). The business of manufacturing counterfeit medications in developing countries is huge and growing; it is impossible to tell from the packaging or pills if they are counterfeit. Some counterfeit drugs contain little or no active ingredient, and others contain toxic contaminants.

Vaccinations

Because of the frequency of travel to international destinations, air crews may be exposed to various diseases that are not common in the United States. For example, measles can be a life-threatening illness for adults and is more common in most of the world, including Europe, because of lack of mandatory childhood immunization against the disease in many countries. International flight crews should consider a travel health visit to ensure as complete protection as possible. Some may have short notice before traveling to new destinations; thus, travelers should be asked about this possibility during their visit, so that vaccinations for an upcoming trip—that may not be imminent—may be given, or a series may be started early. Providers should educate travelers about health risks in the various destinations; whether certain vaccinations are administered will depend on the traveler's tolerance for risk.

Routine Vaccinations

All travelers should make sure they are up to date with routine vaccinations (see the separate sections on these diseases in Chapter 3):

- **Measles**—A person born in the United States before 1957 is assumed to be immune to measles. If born after, it is important to have documentation of having had the disease or having had 2 vaccine doses against measles. Measles vaccine is typically given as MMR (measles-mumps-rubella).

- **Varicella**—Strongly recommended for travelers with no history of chickenpox
- **Polio**—A single booster is recommended as an adult. Although transmission of the polio virus is not a problem in the Western Hemisphere, it remains a risk in some countries in sub-Saharan Africa and in Asia.
- **Diphtheria-tetanus-pertussis**—Administered at 10-year intervals (a single booster of the triple combination, and thereafter Td) for complete protection
- **Hepatitis B**—Administered to all children and adolescents in the United States, it is advisable for frequent travelers because of unpredictability of exposure.
- **Hepatitis A**—Administered to all children in the United States, it is advisable for all travelers.
- **Others**—Any age-related (such as varicella-zoster) or health maintenance-related (such as pneumococcal) vaccinations should be considered.

Special Vaccinations for Travel

Although there are no established guidelines or recommendations for the use of travel vaccinations in pilots and other air crews, it may be reasonable to offer meningococcal, Japanese encephalitis, yellow fever, and typhoid vaccine to this special population because of their frequent, short-stay, and at times unpredictable travel and destinations. As well, they are generally a group who travels frequently beyond work, so they should always be asked during a consultation whether they plan other travel itineraries that can be addressed at the same time.

Malaria Chemoprophylaxis

Crew members are typically informed by their airline as to which destinations harbor malaria. Some European and Asian air carriers have longer experience flying to destinations where malaria is endemic, and these airlines have various policies with respect to its prevention. Although there may be malaria transmission in some areas of destination countries, sometimes there is none in the capitals or the larger urban areas to which the major American carriers fly (such as in China or the Philippines). This is generally not the case in sub-Saharan Africa, where there can be substantial exposure during a short 24-hour layover (however, in

Kenya, there is no malaria risk in Nairobi). Although there may be little risk at the hotels in the destination, risk may be increased at the international airports and during unpredictable delays in transit. Even during short single stops (for example, in West Africa en route to South Africa) there is some risk when the aircraft doors are open. Little published data are available on the risk of malaria for flight crews with short layovers, but some information suggests that it is less than that for tourists.

Flight crew members should be educated about the risk of malaria at their destinations and have an individual risk assessment for preventive measures. For destinations where the prevalence of malaria is high (countries in West Africa, for example), crew members should take prophylaxis for layovers. For other destinations where crews are thought to be at low risk based on local intensity of transmission, accommodations, and personal behaviors, they may be advised to use insect repellents and no chemoprophylaxis. Flight crews should always:

- Educate themselves as much as possible about malaria.
- Understand the importance of personal protective measures such as repellents, and use them properly.
- Take chemoprophylaxis if recommended by their doctor.
- Know that if fever or chills occur after exposure, it is a medical emergency.
- Know how they can get medical assistance at their destinations or at home in the event of symptoms or signs of malaria.

There are several options for malaria chemoprophylaxis, depending on the destination city. The combination of country-specific recommendations that can be accessed either in this text (see Chapter 3, Yellow Fever and Malaria Information, by Country) or on the CDC Travelers' Health website (www.cdc.gov/travel) should help with this decision, along with the individual assessment. Chemoprophylaxis recommendations for pilots and air crew include the following:

- **Mefloquine**—The current product label for mefloquine contains a caution against using mefloquine for malaria prophylaxis in pilots.

- **Chloroquine**—There are no contraindications for use of chloroquine in pilots or air crew. Chloroquine may not be the preferred option for many because of the need to continue taking the drug for 4 weeks after the last exposure, thus requiring more than 4 weeks of drug administration for even a single night of exposure. In addition, in many areas malaria is resistant to chloroquine.
- **Atovaquone-proguanil**—There are no contraindications for use of atovaquone-proguanil in pilots or air crew members. In addition, because of the short-stay nature of their travel, use of atovaquone-proguanil as chemoprophylaxis may be preferred because of the need to take the drug for only 7 days after leaving an area of exposure risk.
- **Doxycycline**—There are no contraindications for use of doxycycline in pilots or air crew. Doxycycline may not be the preferred option for many because of the need to continue taking the drug for 28 days after the last exposure, thus requiring >4 weeks of drug administration for even a single night of exposure.
- **Primaquine**—There are no contraindications for use of primaquine in pilots or air crew. Like atovaquone-proguanil, use of primaquine as chemoprophylaxis may be attractive because of the need to take the drug for only 7 days after leaving an area of exposure risk. A blood test for the enzyme glucose-6-phosphate

dehydrogenase is required before prescribing. CDC recommends primaquine for prevention of malaria in areas with mainly *Plasmodium vivax*.

Food and Water Precautions and Travelers' Diarrhea

Pilots and air crew members should follow the same safe food and water precautions and prevention and management of travelers' diarrhea as other travelers (see Chapter 2, Travelers' Diarrhea). They should also be well versed in the recognition and self-treatment of travelers' diarrhea to avoid unnecessary illness that would affect their job performance.

Bloodborne Infections and Sexually Transmitted Diseases

Although these risks and preventions are addressed in more detail in other sections, it is worth reiterating that frequent travelers have an increased likelihood of engaging in casual and unprotected sex. It is common to think that people from Western countries would have the same risk of HIV and STDs; however, travelers have far higher rates of such infections. Dental procedures and activities such as acupuncture, tattooing, and piercing also are ill-advised during travel to developing countries.

BIBLIOGRAPHY

1. Bagshaw M, Nicolls DS. Aircraft cabin environment. In: Keystone JS, Kozarsky PE, Freedman DO, Nothdurft HD, Connor BA, editors. Travel Medicine. Philadelphia: Mosby; 2008. p. 447–61.
2. Byrne N. Urban malaria risk in sub-Saharan Africa: where is the evidence? Travel Med Infect Dis. 2007 Mar;5(2):135–7.
3. Byrne NJ, Behrens RH. Airline crews' risk for malaria on layovers in urban sub-Saharan Africa: risk assessment and appropriate prevention policy. J Travel Med. 2004 Nov–Dec;11(6):359–63.

HUMANITARIAN AID WORKERS
Brian D. Gushulak

OVERVIEW
Through organizations and agencies or individual activities, many thousands of people are involved in the delivery of humanitarian aid in diverse locations every year. After large-scale events such as the Haitian

earthquake of January 2010, the number of those traveling to provide humanitarian aid and assistance can increase significantly. Maintaining the health of humanitarian workers is important to ensure that they are able to deliver care to those in need.

In common with other travelers, people who travel to provide humanitarian aid or disaster relief must first address their personal health and welfare before, during, and after travel. This includes knowledge and preparation for all the usual elements associated with travel to the area. In addition, aid workers can experience specific risks and situations related to the provision of humanitarian care, such as:

- Exposure to the environment that precipitated or sustains a crisis or event, such as a natural disaster or conflict
- Working long hours under adverse or extreme conditions, often in close contact with the affected population
- Damaged or absent infrastructure, including availability of food, water, lodging, transportation, and health services
- Reduced levels of security and protection
- Stress, ethical, and moral challenges related to the event and the resource capacities of the situation

Humanitarian service can damage personal health. Studies involving long-term humanitarian workers have noted that >35% report that their personal health status deteriorated during the mission. Accidents and violence are documented risks for humanitarian workers and cause more deaths than disease and natural causes. Recent estimates place the risk of violence-related deaths, medical evacuations, and hospitalizations at approximately 6 per 10,000 aid worker person-years. Conditions and outcomes vary by location, nature of the humanitarian event, and time spent in the field.

A recent study of Red Cross workers noted a 10% ratio of injury or accident and an exposure to violence of 16%. That study also showed that >40% found the experience more stressful than expected. An earlier study of deaths among Peace Corps volunteers noted that unintentional injuries were the cause of nearly 70% of deaths, followed by homicide

at 17%. Illness was responsible for 14% of the Peace Corps fatalities.

However, risks to humanitarian workers are not uniformly distributed across the spectrum of humanitarian aid. For example, in 2009 a survey of violence against humanitarian workers found that a small number of insecure locations (Afghanistan, Darfur [Sudan], and Somalia) accounted for >60% of these events.

PRE-TRAVEL CONSIDERATIONS
Evaluation and Pre-Travel Medical Care
Giving careful attention to pre-travel evaluation, both medical and psychological, in addition to educating travelers can reduce the likelihood of illness and the need for repatriation. Comprehensive medical examinations can prepare travelers by helping identify previously unrecognized disease and allowing for treatment before travel. Careful evaluation of risk factors (family history, history of alcohol or substance abuse, sexually transmitted diseases, and psychiatric illness) may direct additional evaluation and identify previously unrecognized psychological problems or chronic conditions. Identifying alcohol or substance dependence, depression, or other psychiatric illness is important, as these conditions may be exacerbated by the stress of the mission and are often the reason for emergency repatriation.

Those who will be providing medical care as part of their humanitarian activities should be evaluated in terms of occupational risk and the need for preventive or post-exposure interventions. Humanitarian aid workers destined to areas of active conflict or limited police presence may benefit from specialized security briefings, either provided by the employing agency or private sources. Medical facilities may be compromised by the disaster or overwhelmed in responding to it. Therefore, volunteers with underlying conditions or pregnant women should be counseled against travel and encouraged to support the response in other ways.

Regardless of the area of the world in which the aid worker will be deployed, certain basics should be addressed in the pre-travel encounter, including routine vaccinations, malaria prophylaxis (if appropriate), food and water precautions, self-treatment for travelers' diarrhea, risks from insect bites, and injury prevention.

Counseling and Advice

Predeployment education and training are essential, as personal illness or injury burdens the community the worker has come to support. Injuries and motor vehicle accidents are a common risk for travelers anywhere in the world; thus, travelers should be sensitive to their surroundings and carefully select the type of transportation and hour of travel, if possible. In disaster and emergency situations, the traveler should also be aware of physical hazards such as debris, unstable structures, downed power lines, environmental hazards, and extremes of temperature.

Travelers to conflict areas should be aware of landmines and other potential hazards associated with unexploded ordnance. In situations associated with damage or destruction to local services and facilities, humanitarian workers should expect limited accommodation, logistics, and personal support. Humanitarian workers destined for low-resource areas or situations may benefit from pre-travel training and counseling regarding the moral complexities of providing service in these environments.

Preparation

Health Items

The traveler should be advised to prepare a travel health kit that is more extensive than the typical kit and should also be familiar with basic first aid to self-treat any injury until medical attention can be obtained. Aid workers may need to disinfect their own water and may want to carry high-energy, nonperishable food items for emergency use. Humanitarian workers should research the available resources in the destination to tailor how extensive their packed supplies should be. In addition to a basic travel health kit (see Chapter 2, Travel Health Kits), humanitarian aid workers should consider bringing the following items:

Toiletries

- Toothbrush/toothpaste
- Skin moisturizer
- Soap, shampoo
- Lip balm
- If corrective lenses are used:
  > Extra pair of prescription glasses in a protective case and a copy of the prescription
  > Eyeglasses cleaning supplies and repair kit
  > Extra contact lenses and lens cleaner
- Razor, extra blades[1]
- Nail clippers[1]
- Toilet paper
- Menstrual supplies
- Sewing kit
- Laundry detergent
- Small clothesline/pins

Clothing

- Comfortable, lightweight clothing
- Long pants
- Long-sleeved shirts
- Hat
- Boots
- Shower shoes
- Rain gear
- Bandana/handkerchief
- Towel (highly absorbent travel towel if possible)
- Gloves (leather gloves if physical labor will be performed; rubber gloves if handling blood or body fluids)

Activities of daily living

- Sunglasses
- Waterproof watch
- Flashlight
- Spare batteries
- Travel plug adapters for electronics
- Knife, such as a Swiss Army knife or Leatherman[1]
- If traveling to an area where food and water may be contaminated:
  > Bottled water or water filters/purification system/water purification tablets
  > Nonperishable food items
- If traveling to malaria-endemic areas:
  > Personal bed net (insecticide impregnated)

Safety and security

- Money belt
- Cash
- Cellular telephone, equipped to work internationally, or satellite telephone (with charger)

[1] Pack these items in checked baggage, since they may be considered sharp objects and confiscated by airport or airline security if packed in carry-on bags.

- Candles, matches, and lighter in a zip-top bag
- Extra zip-top bags
- Safety goggles

Personal Items

Because of the loss of life, serious injuries, missing and separated families, and destruction often associated with disasters, relief workers should recognize that situations they encounter may be extremely stressful. Keeping a personal item nearby, such as a family photo, favorite music, or religious material, can offer comfort in such situations. Checking in with family members and close friends from time to time is another means of support. Satellite telephones are small, can work almost anywhere in the world, and can be rented for less than $10 per day.

Important Documents

In uncertain circumstances, extra passport-style photos may be required for certain types of visas or for additional work permits. Travelers should bring photocopies of important documents, such as passports and credit cards, as well as copies of their medical or nursing license, if applicable. Medical information, such as immunization records and blood type, is also helpful to have. The traveler should carry these copies and also leave a copy with someone back home. In addition, they should carry contact information for the person who should be notified in an emergency.

Registration with Embassies

Travelers should register before departure with the US embassy in the destination country, so that the local consulate is aware of their presence, and they may be accounted for and included in evacuation plans. They should also consider supplemental health insurance to cover medical care and evacuation should they become ill or injured. See the Department of State website for additional information (https://travelregistration.state.gov/ibrs/ui).

POST-TRAVEL CONSIDERATIONS

Returning aid workers should be advised to seek medical care if they sustained injuries during their travel or become ill on return. To ensure proper evaluation, they should advise their providers of the nature of their recent travel.

Depending upon the length of time away or their activities (such as working in health care), returning aid workers may benefit from a complete medical review. Homecoming has also been identified as a risk period for difficulties in psychological adjustment, and appropriate treatment or counseling should be sought. Workers who witnessed or were involved in situations of mass casualties, deaths, or serious injuries or who have been victims of violence (assault, kidnapping, or serious accident) should be considered for referral for critical incident counseling.

Studies have indicated that >30% of aid workers report depression shortly after returning home. The adjustment process can be assisted by a skilled debriefing. Generally, humanitarian workers are able to adapt to the acute and chronic stressors of their work and demonstrate considerable resilience, but they will also benefit from proper rest and support to help them fully adjust back into the home environment.

BIBLIOGRAPHY

1. Callahan MV, Hamer DH. On the medical edge: preparation of expatriates, refugee and disaster relief workers, and Peace Corps volunteers. Infect Dis Clin North Am. 2005 Mar;19(1):85–101.
2. Campbell S. Responding to international disasters. Nurs Stand. 2005 Feb 2–8;19(21):33–6.
3. CDC. Coping with a traumatic event: information for the public. Atlanta: CDC; 2005 [cited 2008 Apr 12]. Available from: http://www.bt.cdc.gov/masscasualties/copingpub.asp.
4. Coppola DP. Introduction to International Disaster Management. Amsterdam: Butterworth Heinemann; 2006.
5. Gamble K, Lovell D, Lankester T, Keystone JS. Aid workers, expatriates and travel. In: Zuckerman J, editor. Principles and Practice of Travel Medicine. Hoboken, NJ: Wiley; 2001. p. 448–66.
6. Jung P, Banks RH. Tuberculosis risk in US Peace Corps Volunteers, 1996 to 2005. J Travel Med. 2008 Mar–Apr;15(2):87–94.

7. McFarlane CA. Risk associated with the psychological adjustment of humanitarian aid workers. The Australasian Journal of Disaster and Trauma Studies [serial on the Internet]. 2004 [cited 2008 Oct 2]. Available from: http://www.massey.ac.nz/~trauma/issues/2004-1/mcfarlane.htm.

8. Mitchell AM, Sakraida TJ, Kameg K. Critical incident stress debriefing: implications for best practice. Disaster Manag Response. 2003 Apr–Jun;1(2):46–51.

9. Nurthen NM, Jung P. Fatalities in the Peace Corps: a retrospective study, 1984 to 2003. J Travel Med. 2008 Mar–Apr;15(2):95–101.

10. Pearn J. Pre-deployment education and training for refugee emergencies: health and safety aspects. J Refug Stud. 1997;10:495–502.

11. Peytremann I, Baduraux M, O'Donovan S, Loutan L. Medical evacuations and fatalities of United Nations High Commissioner for Refugees field employees. J Travel Med. 2001 May–Jun;8(3):117–21.

12. Sheik M, Gutierrez MI, Bolton P, Spiegel P, Thieren M, Burnham G. Deaths among humanitarian workers. BMJ. 2000 Jul 15;321(7254):166–8.

LONG-TERM TRAVELERS & EXPATRIATES

Anne E. McCarthy

UNIQUE CONSIDERATIONS FOR LONG-TERM TRAVEL

A prolonged stay of ≥6 months in low- and middle-income countries, whether for tourism or employment purposes, increases the risk of travel-related and travel-unrelated illness. The risk includes both infectious diseases and trauma, due in part to the cumulative risk over months to years of potential exposure.

The most commonly reported health problems in long-term travelers include diarrheal diseases, respiratory illness, and skin conditions. Infectious diseases, although important causes of illness, are not common causes of travel-related death, even in long-term travelers. A Canadian study of international travel-related deaths documented rare occurrences due to vaccine-preventable or exotic disease. Similarly, a US study found that those residing abroad were more likely to sustain fatal injuries, particularly due to motor vehicle crashes and drowning, suggesting that these travelers should be educated about road and water safety. A recent review of more than 4,000 long-term travelers seen in GeoSentinel clinics after travel showed increased cases of chronic diarrhea and gastrointestinal complaints, vectorborne diseases including malaria and cutaneous leishmaniasis, fatigue, eosinophilia, and schistosomiasis.

The authors stressed the importance of vector and contact-transmitted diseases, as well as psychological problems.

Those spending prolonged periods abroad are likely to eventually relax preventive measures, resulting in increased risk of acquiring vectorborne, foodborne, and waterborne diseases. This risk will increase the chance of requiring local medical care, which may have limited resources (personnel and therapeutic) and suboptimal therapy (such as counterfeit or poor-quality medications). Approximately 3% of more than 4,000 UK diplomats living overseas during 1995 required medical evacuation, most (70%) of which were because of unsuitable medical facilities in the host country.

PRE-TRAVEL CARE

Providing pre-travel care for long-term travelers includes prevention strategies, as well as therapy for illness that may be inevitable with time. Before departure, all long-term travelers should undergo an extensive medical and dental examination to exclude underlying disease. The pre-travel consultation for long-term and expatriate travelers should include consideration of vaccine-preventable and other diseases and discussion about acquiring medical care while abroad, as well as appropriate medical care and evacuation insurance. The need for eventual medical care should be anticipated, and strategies to reduce the risk of counterfeit or ineffective medication should be discussed.

With prolonged travel, there may be more than just the immediate destination to consider, since over time there may be travel to surrounding regions and possibly repeated short-term exposures that translate into significant cumulative risk. Expatriates often live in areas or cities with low or negligible infectious risks but take frequent recreational or business trips to destinations with increased risk.

VACCINE-PREVENTABLE INFECTIOUS DISEASES

Routine vaccines, including influenza vaccination, should be updated. In addition, a number of travel-related vaccines warrant consideration:

- Hepatitis A and typhoid vaccines are appropriate given the cumulative risk, although the traveler should be aware that the latter does not provide full protection.
- Hepatitis B vaccine is increasingly provided in the United States; however, many adults may not have protection. They may be at substantial risk, as demonstrated by a survey of mostly short-term travelers, showing that 15% of 400 travelers had potential blood and body fluid exposure.
- Meningococcal disease is more likely in travelers with prolonged exposure to local populations in endemic or epidemic areas; quadrivalent vaccine should be considered for those at risk.
- According to the Advisory Committee on Immunization Practices recommendations, Japanese encephalitis (JE) vaccine is recommended for travelers to endemic areas who stay ≥1 month during the JEV transmission season. JE vaccine is also recommended for travelers to rural areas whose activities may increase the risk of JE virus exposure.
- Rabies prevention is of increased importance with prolonged residence in endemic countries. Foreign residents in Nepal reported an exposure risk of 5.7 per 1,000 people per year, compared with 1.9 per 1,000 people per year for tourists. Rabies prevention strategies are complicated by the cost and availability

of preexposure vaccine and by the potential lack of availability of safe or effective postexposure prophylaxis, particularly rabies immune globulin, in some countries. In one survey, only 38% of 293 missionary personnel stationed abroad had received preexposure prophylaxis. More concerning was that just 8% of 38 potential exposures received appropriate postexposure care.

INFECTIOUS DISEASES NOT PREVENTED BY VACCINES
Malaria

Standard strategies appropriate for malaria prevention in short-term travel may need to be modified and adapted for those with long-term malaria risk. These travelers or expatriates often do not optimize personal protection measures for bite avoidance (insect repellents and insecticide-treated nets and clothing) on a daily basis. They may not adhere to continuous prophylaxis regimens or not want to take medications long term. A retrospective cohort analysis study conducted by reviewing pharmacy records and by interviews in person of chemoprophylaxis adherence in 183 expatriate households in coastal Nigeria showed that only 127 (69%) collected their prophylaxis regularly, and overall, only 39% of households were compliant. Many cited concerns about the real and perceived risks for adverse drug reactions, particularly with long-term use.

There are no consensus guidelines on the prevention of malaria in long-term travelers. Many different malaria prevention strategies have been recommended, such as initial prophylaxis followed by discontinuation or intermittent use at times of higher risk (seasonal chemoprophylaxis). If long-term travelers choose not to take chemoprophylaxis, they should have good access to medical care and seek medical attention when sick for the best quality diagnosis and treatment (see Chapter 3, Malaria).

Long-term travelers:
- Must be aware of their risk
- Should use appropriate malaria prevention interventions, which may include chemoprophylaxis and the use of repellents, window screens, and insecticide-treated bed nets
- Should be educated on malaria symptoms and the need to seek early medical attention for a febrile illness

Other Diseases

Diarrhea and gastrointestinal diseases are common in long-term travelers residing in the tropics, and these people should be educated about the management of acute diarrhea, including rehydration, the use of antimotility agents, and empiric antimicrobial therapy. Prolonged diarrhea is more suggestive of a protozoal etiology.

HIV and sexually transmitted disease risks have increased in travelers and expatriates. Furthermore, the consistent use of condoms in expatriates is low (approximately 20%). Long-term travelers should be educated about the risk of HIV and sexually transmitted diseases in their destination. The potential for occupational exposure to HIV is important to consider in health care workers; postexposure prophylaxis with highly active antiretroviral therapy and risk avoidance should be included in the pre-travel consultation (see Chapter 2, Occupational Exposure to HIV).

Transfusion is an important risk for hepatitis C infection in expatriates. The risk of hepatitis E, spread by the fecal-oral route, is highest in Asia, although it has been transmitted in many different tropical locations. Pregnant women are at highest risk of fulminant disease. Other infections vary with location and include schistosomiasis, which may be prevented by not swimming or wading in fresh water. Tuberculosis risk eventually equates to that of the local population, increasing with length of stay and contact with the local population.

BIBLIOGRAPHY

1. Arguin PM, Krebs JW, Mandel E, Guzi T, Childs JE. Survey of rabies preexposure and postexposure prophylaxis among missionary personnel stationed outside the United States. J Travel Med. 2000 Jan;7(1):10–4.

2. Banta JE, Jungblut E. Health problems encountered by the Peace Corps overseas. Am J Public Health Nations Health. 1966 Dec;56(12):2121–5.

3. Berg J, Visser LG. Expatriate chemoprophylaxis use and compliance: past, present and future from an occupational health perspective. J Travel Med. 2007 Sep–Oct;14(5):357–8.

4. Chen LH, Wilson ME, Davis X, Loutan L, Schwartz E, Keystone J, et al. Illness in long-term travelers visiting GeoSentinel clinics. Emerg Infect Dis. 2009 Nov;15(11):1773–82.

5. Chen LH, Wilson ME, Schlagenhauf P. Prevention of malaria in long-term travelers. JAMA. 2006 Nov 8;296(18):2234–44.

6. Cobelens FG, van Deutekom H, Draayer-Jansen IW, Schepp-Beelen AC, van Gerven PJ, van Kessel RP, et al. Risk of infection with Mycobacterium tuberculosis in travellers to areas of high tuberculosis endemicity. Lancet. 2000 Aug 5;356(9228):461–5.

7. Cockburn R, Newton PN, Agyarko EK, Akunyili D, White NJ. The global threat of counterfeit drugs: why industry and governments must communicate the dangers. PLoS Med. 2005 Apr;2(4):e100.

8. Correia JD, Shafer RT, Patel V, Kain KC, Tessier D, MacPherson D, et al. Blood and body fluid exposure as a health risk for international travelers. J Travel Med. 2001 Sep–Oct;8(5):263–6.

9. Freeman RJ, Mancuso JD, Riddle MS, Keep LW. Systematic review and meta-analysis of TST conversion risk in deployed military and long-term civilian travelers. J Travel Med. 2010 Jul;17(4):233–42.

10. Guse CE, Cortes LM, Hargarten SW, Hennes HM. Fatal injuries of US citizens abroad. J Travel Med. 2007 Sep–Oct;14(5):279–87.

11. Hillel O, Potasman I. Correlation between adherence to precautions issued by the WHO and diarrhea among long-term travelers to India. J Travel Med. 2005 Sep–Oct;12(5):243–7.

12. Leutscher PD, Bagley SW. Health-related challenges in United States Peace Corps volunteers serving for two years in Madagascar. J Travel Med. 2003 Sep–Oct;10(5):263–7.

13. MacPherson DW, Gushulak BD, Sandhu J. Death and international travel—the Canadian experience: 1996 to 2004. J Travel Med. 2007 Mar–Apr;14(2):77–84.

14. Pandey P, Shlim DR, Cave W, Springer MF. Risk of possible exposure to rabies among tourists and foreign residents in Nepal. J Travel Med. 2002 May–Jun;9(3):127–31.

15. Patel D, Easmon CJ, Dow C, Snashall DC, Seed PT. Medical repatriation of British diplomats resident overseas. J Travel Med. 2000 Mar–Apr;7(2):64–9.

16. Toovey S, Moerman F, van Gompel A. Special infectious disease risks of expatriates and long-term travelers in tropical countries. Part I: malaria. J Travel Med. 2007 Jan–Feb;14(1):42–9.

17. Toovey S, Moerman F, van Gompel A. Special infectious disease risks of expatriates and long-term travelers in tropical countries. Part II: infections other than malaria. J Travel Med. 2007 Jan–Feb;14(1):50–60.

SPECIAL CONSIDERATIONS FOR US MILITARY DEPLOYMENTS

Alan J. Magill, Steven B. Cersovsky, Robert F. DeFraites*

OVERVIEW

The US military, as a matter of policy, follows most of the recommendations in the CDC Yellow Book. However, there are unique situations that apply only to the US military, and some policies or recommendations differ from what is recommended in the Yellow Book for civilian travel. Active-duty military physicians generally manage pre-deployment medicine, but civilian physicians may interact with people who are on reserve status, home on leave, recently discharged from active duty, or veterans. Pre-deployment and post-deployment information, policies, and guidelines for clinicians, service members and their families, and veterans can be found on the Deployment Health Clinical Center website (www.pdhealth.mil). The purpose of this section is to inform US military medical corps officers, who routinely consult the Yellow Book, about these differences and also make civilian clinicians, who frequently see military personnel, aware of these differences.

In many countries, one of the largest traveling populations is their military personnel. The military should be considered a special population with demographics, destinations, and needs different from civilian travelers. This section focuses on the unique aspects of using pre-travel vaccines and malaria chemoprophylaxis in the military population. The specific examples will be from the US military, but the concepts may be applicable to other militaries, as well. In 2010, approximately 1.5 million US military members were on active duty and approximately 1.0 million were in the reserve forces.

Several characteristics of the military force differ from those of the civilian population (Table 8-10). The active duty military is younger, in better health, and predominately male.

FORCE HEALTH PROTECTION

Force Health Protection (FHP) is an important concept in military medicine. FHP is broadly defined as a strategy that applies preventive health techniques and emerging technologies to environmental surveillance and combat medicine to protect all service members before, during, and after deployment. Delivery of vaccines and the appropriate use of malaria chemoprophylaxis agents are 2 aspects of FHP.

Medical countermeasures for FHP are the responsibility of the unit commander, with advice from the unit medical officer. When pre-deployment vaccines or malaria chemoprophylaxis are indicated, the commander includes such requirements in the mission plan. Service members are then required to receive the interventions under medical supervision. People who have a medical contraindication to a vaccine or drug receive alternative agents, when they are available. The unit medical officer documents which military personnel have not received standard preventive measures, so these people may receive additional monitoring or treatment if they become ill.

FHP policy positions in the Department of Defense (DoD) are issued as directives and instructions. All directives and instructions can be found online at Policy and Program for Immunizations to Protect the Health of Service Members and Military Beneficiaries is found in directive 6205.O2E (September 19, 2006) (www.dtic.mil/whs/directives/corres/pdf/620502p.pdf). Although policy may be made at higher levels in Washington, DC, the final decision to use vaccines or malaria chemoprophylaxis under FHP is made by commanders in the field, guided by their medical staff.

8

---

* The views and opinions expressed in this section are those of the authors and do not represent the official views of the US Department of Defense, The US Army, the Armed Forces Health Surveillance Center, or the Walter Reed Army Institute of Research.

Table 8-10. Differences between military populations and civilian traveling populations

CHARACTERISTIC	TRAVEL MEDICINE	MILITARY MEDICINE
Primary focus	Individual	Unit
Goal	Optimizing advice and interventions for individual travelers	Ensuring mission success; optimizing advice and interventions for each person is difficult
Adherence	Strongly encouraged but travelers are free to choose	Required; vaccines and malaria chemoprophylaxis are part of Force Health Protection (FHP)
Education	One-on-one encounters	Unit education
Population	Not prescreened; travel health providers see all ages and people with preexisting medical conditions	Prescreened; people with significant medical problems are not allowed to join the military or be deployed
Special populations	Infants, children, pregnant women, elderly people, people with renal or hepatic impairment	Not part of military population or deployments
Disease comorbidity	Similar to civilian population	Limited, generally healthy
Gender	50% male, 50% female	85% male
Unusual activities	Adventure activities, such as trekking, climbing, scuba diving, spelunking	Housed in barracks or other group settings, Aviators, Special Forces, operating complex weapons systems, hostile and extreme environments, stress of combat operations, night operations and use of night-vision goggles
Duration of use	Mostly short term, 2–3 weeks	The US military often uses chemoprophylaxis for longer periods of time than do short-term travelers. Many deployments, to Afghanistan for example, are for 1 year or longer.

ROUTINE AND TRAVEL-RELATED IMMUNIZATIONS

DoD policy states that the recommendations for immunization from CDC and the Advisory Committee for Immunization Practices shall generally be followed, consistent with requirements and guidance of the Food and Drug Administration (FDA) and with consideration for the unique needs of military settings and exposure risks. The Military Vaccine Agency (MILVAX) supports all 5 branches of the US Armed Services to enhance

ADVISING TRAVELERS WITH SPECIFIC NEEDS

military medical readiness by coordinating DoD immunization (vaccination) programs worldwide. A valuable source of service-specific information on immunizations for all branches of the US military is found at the MILVAX website (www.vaccines.mil/default.aspx).

In particular, the quick reference section of the MILVAX website (www.vaccines.mil/default.aspx?cnt=resource/qr) provides an easily accessible and complete source of information with product specifics and policy documents that both military and civilian providers will find useful. DoD and service-specific policies for vaccines and geographic-specific vaccine recommendations can be also be downloaded from this site.

GEOGRAPHIC AREAS OF RESPONSIBILITY

The US military issues FHP recommendations based on geographic areas of responsibility (AOR) (www.vaccines.mil/default.aspx?cnt=resource/qr). Command and control over US military personnel in each AOR are under a unified combatant command, which is a joint (all branches of the US military) command that provides recommendations for all service members being deployed to that AOR. For example, Afghanistan is in the Central Command (CENTCOM) AOR. All people on orders to deploy or travel to Afghanistan should receive the vaccines listed in the above web page under the CENTCOM tab of the vaccine recommendations page, unless there is a medical contraindication.

MALARIA CHEMOPROPHYLAXIS

Preventing malaria in military units deployed to endemic areas is an essential objective of FHP. Malaria can be prevented through 1) education and training, 2) appropriate use of personal protection measures that include individual bed nets, permethrin-impregnated uniforms, and insect repellents, and 3) use of chemoprophylaxis where indicated.

Malaria cases seen in returning US military personnel reflect the current deployments around the world. In 2010, the highest risk was in Afghanistan, with exposures to chloroquine-resistant *Plasmodium falciparum* and *P. vivax* malaria. There is also significant risk from frequent training and development missions to sub-Saharan Africa.

Several features of malaria chemoprophylaxis under FHP that are unique to the US military are derived from the activities and stressors of military deployments. When anti-malarial drugs are used for chemoprophylaxis as part of FHP, the military can only use FDA-approved chemoprophylaxis agents in accordance with the specific FDA-approved indications. Off-label use of drugs is not allowed when given under FHP. If off-label indications are felt to be in the best interest of the person or unit, trained and knowledgeable clinicians must provide one-on-one medical evaluations, document in the medical record the rationale for such use, and provide a by-name prescription for the drug or vaccine to each person.

In September 2009, the Assistant Secretary of Defense (Health Affairs) issued a policy memorandum on the use of mefloquine in malaria chemoprophylaxis throughout the DoD. In chloroquine-resistant areas in which doxycycline and mefloquine are equally efficacious in preventing malaria, doxycycline is the drug of choice for malarial chemoprophylaxis. Those personnel with a history of neurobehavioral disorders who cannot take doxycycline should be prescribed atovaquone-proguanil for travel to chloroquine-resistant areas.

The rationale for recommending doxycycline over mefloquine is as follows:

- With the increasing recognition of possible neuropsychiatric side effects of mefloquine in some people, new relative contraindications have been added to the product label since 2003. In addition, each person prescribed mefloquine must be given an FDA-approved medication guide. Complying with this guidance requires a one-on-one encounter with a knowledgeable provider, which can be difficult with large deployments.
- Neuropsychiatric side effects may confound the diagnosis and management of post-traumatic stress disorder and traumatic brain injury, which makes the continued routine use of mefloquine less desirable.

The US military routinely uses primaquine for presumptive antirelapse treatment (PART) in returning military populations to prevent the late relapse of *P. vivax* malaria or *P. ovale* malaria as a matter of policy. PART is also referred to as "terminal prophylaxis." In PART,

Table 8-11. Differences between CDC recommendations and US military's use of malaria chemoprophylaxis

	CDC RECOMMENDATION	US MILITARY POLICY
Choice of malaria chemoprophylaxis agent	Chemoprophylaxis guidelines do not recommend one drug versus another, but rather emphasize the goal of individualizing the recommendation for the individual traveler on the basis of past experience, itinerary, possible drug interaction, potential side effects, costs, and medical contraindications such as drug allergies.	Individualizing advice and recommendations for large military deployments is rarely logistically possible or feasible. Recognizing this reality, in September 2009, the US military adopted a new policy on the use of malaria chemoprophylaxis in the US military. Doxycycline is now the drug of choice to prevent malaria in deployed US military forces.
Chloroquine	Chemoprophylaxis option only in areas with chloroquine-sensitive malaria	Chemoprophylaxis option only in areas with chloroquine-sensitive malaria
Doxycycline	An option for chemoprophylaxis in all areas	Recommended first-line chemoprophylaxis in all areas
Mefloquine	An option for chemoprophylaxis in all areas	Mefloquine is not recommended as a primary option. It should be used only in those whose travel requires malaria chemoprophylaxis, who cannot take either doxycycline or atovaquone-proguanil, and who meet all requirements of the current FDA-approved product label.
Atovaquone-proguanil	An option for chemoprophylaxis in all areas	Atovaquone-proguanil is recommended for those who are intolerant of or who have contraindications to doxycycline.
Primaquine chemoprophylaxis	CDC recommends the use of primaquine as primary chemoprophylaxis in geographic areas with mainly *P. vivax* malaria.	There is no FDA-approved indication for the use of primaquine to prevent malaria. Therefore, the US military cannot use primaquine as a chemoprophylaxis agent under current FHP guidelines.
PART	Primaquine at 30 mg (base) for 14 days	There is no FDA-approved indication for the use of primaquine at the higher dose of 30 mg (base) for 14 days. Therefore, the US military must use primaquine in the PART indication at 15 mg (base) for 14 days under current FHP guidelines. If the CDC-recommended (higher) dose is used, it must be given as an individual medical care intervention and not as FHP

Abbreviations: FDA, Food and Drug Administration; FHP, Force Health Protection; PART, presumptive antirelapse treatment.

primaquine is given to otherwise healthy people on their return from an endemic area. Primaquine is used for this indication much more frequently in the military than in most civilian travelers.

The FDA-approved regimen for PART is 15 mg (base) given daily for 14 days. This regimen was approved in 1952 and has not been revisited since. In the intervening decades, an overwhelming amount of data has accumulated to show that the total dose of primaquine to eliminate the dormant hypnozoite stages responsible for late relapses is dependent on the infecting *P. vivax* strain, and therefore, the optimal human dose should be based on weight and adjusted for the infecting *P. vivax* strain.

In 2003, CDC recommended 30 mg (base) of primaquine daily for 14 days based on available evidence, but the FDA-approved regimen remains the lower dose. Adherence to the daily 14-day regimen is poor unless primaquine is given under directly observed therapy, which is rarely done. As a result of noncompliance and subtherapeutic dosing with the 15 mg (base) for 14 days regimen, periodic outbreaks of relapsed *P. vivax* malaria occur in returning military personnel.

Current policy is for all US military personnel to be screened for glucose-6-phosphate dehydrogenase (G6PD) deficiency on entry into military service. However, some people, such as reservists, may have deployed without testing, or clinicians may not be able to confirm results for all people in a unit requiring PART. Clinicians should be aware that hemolytic reactions to primaquine may occur in those with unrecognized G6PD deficiency.

Under FHP, people are required to take their chemoprophylaxis agents as prescribed to maintain mission readiness. Individual soldiers do not have the right to refuse an order given under FHP. There is great variability in practice as to how seriously individual commanders enforce these policies, however, and continued outbreaks of malaria occur in military populations because of poor compliance.

Differences between civilian and US military use of chemoprophylaxis drugs are summarized in Table 8-11.

UNIQUE NEEDS FOR THE MILITARY

US military personnel may encounter threats, such as biological warfare agents, that are not usually considered for civilian travelers. Vaccines, immunoglobulins, drug prophylaxis, and drug treatment regimens can be given under FHP but only in accordance with FDA-licensed products and regimens and for FDA-approved indications.

Products not approved by the FDA are given to soldiers only with voluntary informed consent under an institutional review board–approved protocol and in accordance with a current and FDA-approved investigational new drug application.

Only under exceptional circumstances would products not approved by the FDA be given to soldiers without informed consent. This circumstance is governed by emergency use authorization procedures. Section 564 of the Federal Food, Drug, and Cosmetic Act (21 USC 360bbb-3), as amended by the Project BioShield Act of 2004 (Public Law 108-276), permits the FDA commissioner to authorize the use of an unapproved medical product or an unapproved use of an approved medical product during a declared emergency involving a heightened risk of attack on the public or US military forces, or when there is a significant potential to affect national security.

BIBLIOGRAPHY

1. Carr ME Jr, Fandre MN, Oduwa FO. Glucose-6-phosphate dehydrogenase deficiency in 2 returning Operation Iraqi Freedom soldiers who developed hemolytic anemia while receiving primaquine prophylaxis for malaria. Mil Med. 2005 Apr;170(4):273–6.

2. Food and Drug Administration. Emergency use authorization of medical products. Rockville, MD: Food and Drug Administration; 2007 [updated 2010 Mar 1; cited 2010 Oct 26]. Available from: http://www.fda.gov/RegulatoryInformation/Guidances/ucm125127.htm.

3. Kotwal RS, Wenzel RB, Sterling RA, Porter WD, Jordan NN, Petruccelli BP. An outbreak of malaria in US Army Rangers returning from Afghanistan. JAMA. 2005 Jan 12;293(2):212–6.

4. Llanos JK. The reporting and recording of unspecified malaria in the military, 1998–2007. US Army Med Dep J. 2009 Apr–Jun:42–5.

5. Office of the Assistant Secretary of Defense. Policy memorandum on the use of mefloquine (Lariam) in malaria prophylaxis. Washington, DC: TRICARE Management Activity; 2009.

6. US Department of Defense. Department of Defense directive, force health protection (FHP): 6200.04. Washington, DC: US Department of Defense; 2004. Available from: http://www.dtic.mil/whs/directives/corres/pdf/620004p.pdf

7. US Department of Defense. Force health protection. Falls Church, VA: TRICARE Management; 2001 [updated 2001 Aug 30; cited 2010 Oct 26]. Available from: http://www.ha.osd.mil/forcehealth/about/main.html.

8. US Department of Defense. Unified combatant commands. Washington, DC: US Department of Defense. Available from: http://www.defense.gov/OrgChart/office.aspx?id=45.

9. Whitman TJ, Coyne PE, Magill AJ, Blazes DL, Green MD, Milhous WK, et al. An outbreak of *Plasmodium falciparum* malaria in US Marines deployed to Liberia. Am J Trop Med Hyg. 2010 Aug;83(2):258–65.

STUDY ABROAD

Gary Rhodes, Tricia A. Schwartz, Jodi Ebner

OVERVIEW

Study-abroad programs are designed to allow students to travel outside the United States to obtain academic credit or to take part in community service projects, research, or internships sponsored through their college or university. Students may also travel to participate in athletics, adventure, and volunteer or mission groups.

The number of US study-abroad students has increased significantly in the past 10 years. In 1997, fewer than 100,000 students studied abroad; however, in 2008, more than 250,000 students received academic credit through study-abroad programs. Students study in countries all over the world. In 1998–99, approximately 62% of study-abroad students traveled to Europe. By 2007–08, this number had dropped to 56%. Substantial numbers of students now study in developing countries, where health concerns and challenges compared with those in the United States differ more widely than those in Europe. Table 8-12 shows the host regions of US study-abroad students from 1999–2000 through 2008–2009.

ELEMENTS OF STUDY-ABROAD PROGRAMS

Study-abroad programs are implemented in various ways. Some programs are administered overseas by an international university, with no US staff support onsite. Other US colleges and universities obtain legal status where the program is offered and bring faculty and staff from the United States to run the program.

Institutional administrative structures vary as well. Some universities have more than 20 study-abroad staff with an administrator to focus on health and safety issues. Some large colleges and universities have a travel health clinic for students to visit. Other institutions have no full-time study-abroad office or staff or support from a health clinic. Some study-abroad programs require health insurance that integrates comprehensive medical care, 24-hour assistance, emergency evacuation, and repatriation. Other institutions may recommend that students obtain health insurance for study abroad but may provide limited or no information about available options.

The pre-travel consultation for students planning to study abroad should provide background on health issues in the host country, including country health information and information on how to obtain medical care.

PREDEPARTURE PLANNING

Study-abroad program advisors should work with medical professionals to provide the following to students:

- Cautions about alcohol and drug abuse
- Information about physiologic and psychological consequences they may encounter as a result of changes in their routine
- General instructions for emergency medical situations

Table 8-12. US study-abroad students, percentage by host region[1]

HOST REGION	1999–00	2000–01	2001–02	2002–03	2003–04	2004–05	2005–06	2006–07	2007–08	2008–09
Africa	2.8%	2.9%	2.9%	2.8%	3.0%	3.5%	3.8%	4.2%	4.5%	5.3%
Asia	6.2%	6.0%	6.8%	5.6%	6.9%	8.0%	9.3%	10.3%	11.1%	11.4%
Europe[2]	62.4%	63.1%	62.6%	62.9%	60.9%	60.3%	58.3%	57.4%	56.3%	54.5%
Latin America	14.0%	14.5%	14.5%	15.3%	15.2%	14.4%	15.2%	15.0%	15.3%	15.4%
Middle East	2.9%	1.1%	0.8%	0.4%	0.5%	1.0%	1.2%	1.1%	1.3%	1.4%
North America	0.9%	0.7%	0.8%	0.7%	0.6%	0.5%	0.5%	0.6%	0.4%	0.5%
Oceania	5.0%	6.0%	6.8%	7.3%	7.4%	6.7%	6.3%	5.7%	5.3%	5.5%
Multiple destinations	5.8%	5.6%	4.9%	5.1%	5.5%	5.6%	5.5%	5.6%	5.7%	6.0%
Total number	**143,590**	**154,168**	**160,920**	**174,629**	**191,321**	**205,983**	**223,534**	**241,791**	**262,416**	**260,327**

[1] Data from: Open Doors. US study abroad: host regions 1999/00–2009/10. New York: Institute of International Education; 2010. Available from: http://www.iie.org/en/Research-and-Publications/Open-Doors/Data/US-Study-Abroad/Host-Regions/1999-2009.
[2] Cyprus and Turkey were previously classified in the Middle East category but were moved to the Europe category in 2004–05.

- General advice on nutrition and dietary deficiencies
- Advice for students with disabilities
- Gender-specific health information
- Full health and accident insurance policy coverage information and identification
- Region-specific health information

The information in the Humanitarian Aid Workers section earlier in this chapter can be useful for students participating in study abroad, internships, or research in the developing world.

Before departure, advisors and professionals should encourage students to learn about the destination. Students should understand the health and safety issues of the countries they will visit. This includes reading about the cultural and political climate of those countries. The Department of State's travel website (http://travel.state.gov/travel) provides information about travel abroad, primarily focusing on topics of passports, visas, safety, security, and resources for US citizens during international travel. For some countries, the department posts travel alerts or travel warnings to describe situations such as security risks, political or civil unrest, armed conflicts, natural disasters, and terrorist attacks. Travel warnings are issued when the Department of State recommends against travel to a certain country. The Department of State also hosts a website specifically for students (http://studentsabroad.state.gov/). The CDC Travelers' Health website (www.cdc.gov/travel) contains advice for travelers on the most current health recommendations for international destinations.

Students may need to get vaccines to protect themselves from infectious diseases endemic in the areas they will visit. All travelers should visit a travel health provider, ideally 4–6 weeks before departure, to allow enough time to get recommended vaccines and prescriptions. Even if travel is imminent, students should still visit their travel health provider before departure. The quality of dental and medical care may be different in host countries or more expensive than similar care would be in the United States. Students should receive thorough medical and dental examinations, especially those who are going abroad for several months. Students should be encouraged to bring a well-stocked travel health kit as a first line of defense (see Chapter 2, Travel Health Kits).

HEALTH AND SAFETY WHILE ABROAD
Food and Water Safety
Being mindful with food and water selection can minimize the risk of diarrhea and other illnesses. Specific food and water recommendations depend on the destination country; however, some useful tips to help students regarding food and water safety are the following:

- Find out if water is safe to drink.
- Purify unsafe water before drinking or drink only bottled water, making sure that the bottles are sealed when purchased. Use only purified or bottled water for brushing teeth. For more information, see Chapter 2, Water Disinfection for Travelers.
- Avoid ice in drinks, since it can also be unsafe, depending on the water used to make it.
- Poor refrigeration, undercooked meat, and food purchased from street vendors could pose problems related to food contamination.
- See Chapter 2, Food and Water Precautions for more information.

Adherence to Host Country Laws and Codes of Conduct
Administrators should make students aware of the rules and regulations of the study-abroad program sponsor and the local laws and customs of the countries visited. Students must abide by the legal system of their host country.

Mental and Physical Health
The Association of International Educators' publication "Best Practices in Addressing Mental Health Issues Affecting Education Abroad Participants" encourages study-abroad programs "to sensitively offer support that connects the student to professional help before a problem reaches a crisis state or seriously derails the student's academic and career plans." Likewise, students must consider their own mental and physical health issues when applying for a study-abroad program. Program administrators need to be made aware of all necessary health information to assist students with any special needs or advise on common risks. Dealing with stressful situations abroad may be difficult

for students away from their known support system, which may lead to mental and physical issues.

Prescriptions

A signed prescription for all medications needed while abroad should be obtained. Some prescriptions may need to be translated if they are to be filled abroad. It is preferable to have all prescriptions filled before departure, reducing the need to purchase medication overseas and decreasing potential exposure to counterfeit medications (see Chapter 2, Perspectives: Counterfeit Drugs).

Emergency Contacts

Students can print and fill out an emergency card that includes important contact numbers and personal information. Students should leave copies of it with their US-based emergency contacts and emergency contacts abroad; students should also keep a copy with them at all times (http://studentsabroad.com/emergencycard.asp). Additionally, students should keep program staff and an emergency contact at home well informed of their whereabouts and activities and provide them with copies of their important travel documents (passport, visa, plane tickets, traveler's checks, and prescriptions).

Transportation

Accidents involving in-country travel are a major cause of injury to students abroad. It is imperative for students to understand what safe modes of travel are available at their destination.

Alcohol and Drugs

The use and abuse of alcohol and drugs abroad can increase the risk of accident and injury.

Many students are not given adequate alcohol and drug health and safety training before going abroad, but this is a population that may be at risk for heavy drinking. Violating drug laws abroad may result in serious consequences. In some countries, being found guilty of violating drug laws can result in consequences as serious as death. Therefore, study-abroad administrators should conduct a proper orientation with medical and other professionals about the risks associated with drinking and abusing drugs abroad.

RESOURCES

The Association of International Educators has published a set of good practices titled "Responsible Study Abroad: Good Practices for Health and Safety" for study-abroad sponsors to work with their overseas partners to develop plans and procedures for implementing good practices for students, especially with health and safety issues (www.nafsa.org/uploadedFiles/responsible_study_abroad_2.pdf?n=4131). As study abroad becomes more common among K–12 students, the Council on Standards for International Educational Travel has developed standards for exchange programs for US high school students going abroad (http://csiet.org/about/standards.html).

The Center for Global Education has developed the SAFETI (Safety Abroad First–Educational Travel Information) Clearinghouse to disseminate resources to support study-abroad program development and implementation, emphasizing health and safety issues and resources for US colleges and universities supporting study abroad (http://globaled.us/safeti). Part of this resource includes the SAFETI Program Audit Checklist (http://globaled.us/safeti/auditchklst.html).

BIBLIOGRAPHY

1. CDC. Travelers' Health. Atlanta: CDC; 2010 [cited 2010 Oct 29]. Available from: http://wwwnc.cdc.gov/travel/.

2. Center for Global Education. Emergency card. Los Angeles: Center for Global Education. Available from: http://studentsabroad.com/emergencycard.asp.

3. Center for Global Education. SAFETI adaptation of Peace Corps resources. Los Angeles: Center for Global Education; 2009 [cited 2010 Oct 29]. Available from: http://globaled.us/peacecorps/index.html.

4. Center for Global Education. SAFETI clearinghouse. Los Angeles: Center for Global Education; 2005 [cited 2010 Oct 29]. Available from: http://globaled.us/safeti/.

5. Center for Global Education. SAFETI on-line newsletter. Los Angeles: Center for Global Education; 2005 [cited 2010 Oct 29]. Available from: http://globaled.us/safeti/newsletter.html.

6. Center for Global Education. SAFETI program audit checklist. Los Angeles: Center for Global Education;

2005 [cited 2010 Oct 29]. Available from: http://globaled.us/safeti/auditchklst.html.

7. Center for Global Education. Study Abroad Student Handbook. Center for Global Education; 2010. Available from: http://studentsabroad.com/.

8. Council on Standards for International Educational Travel. CSIET standards. Alexandria [cited 2010 Oct 29]. Available from: http://csiet.org/about/standards.html.

9. Gore J, Green J. Issues and advising responsibilities. NAFSA's Guide to Education Abroad for Advisors and Administrators. 3rd ed. Washington, DC: NAFSA Association of International Educators; 2005. p. 261.

10. Interorganizational Task Force on Safety and Responsibility in Study Abroad. Responsible study abroad: good practices for health and safety. Washington, DC: NAFSA: Association of International Educators; 2001 [cited 2010 Oct 29]. Available from: http://www.nafsa.org/knowledge_community_network.sec/education_abroad_1/developing_and_managing/practice_resources_36/policies/guidelines_for_health/.

11. Lindeman B. Best Practices in Addressing Mental Health Issues Affecting Education Abroad Participants 2008. Available from: http://www.nafsa.org/knowledge_community_network.sec/education_abroad_1/developing_and_managing/practice_resources_36/onsite/best_practices_in_addressing/.

12. Open Doors. Americans study abroad in increasing numbers. New York: Institute of International Education; 2009 [cited 2010 Oct 29]. Available from: http://www.iie.org/en/Who-We-Are/News-and-Events/Press-Center/Press-Releases/2009/2009-11-16-Americans-Study-Abroad-Increasing.

13. Open Doors. US study abroad: host regions 1999/00–2009/10. New York: Institute of International Education; 2010 [cited 2010 Nov 30]. Available from: http://www.iie.org/en/Research-and-Publications/Open-Doors/Data/US-Study-Abroad/Host-Regions/1999-2009.

14. Pedersen ER, LaBrie JW, Hummer JF. Perceived behavioral alcohol norms predict drinking for college students while studying abroad. J Stud Alcohol Drugs. 2009;70(6):924–8.

15. Sobel R. The association for safe international road travel. Los Angeles: Center for Global Education; 1999. Available from: http://globaled.us/safeti/newsletter_for_ge.html.

16. The Forum on Education Abroad. Code of ethics for education abroad. Carlisle, PA: Dickinson College; 2008. Available from: http://www.forumea.org/documents/ForumonEducationAbroadCodeofEthics.pdf.

17. US Department of State. Country specific information. Washington, DC: US Department of State; 2010 [cited 2010 Oct 29]. Available from: http://travel.state.gov/travel/cis_pa_tw/cis/cis_4965.html.

18. US Department of State. International travel. Washington, DC: US Department of State; 2010 [cited 2010 Oct 29]. Available from: http://travel.state.gov/travel/travel_1744.html.

TRAVEL TO MASS GATHERINGS

C. Virginia Lee, Nancy M. Gallagher, Gary W. Brunette

OVERVIEW

Every year, millions of people travel internationally to engage in mass gatherings ranging from major sports events to fairs, festivals, concerts, or even political rallies. These mass gatherings may pose special risks for travelers, because large numbers of people in small areas can facilitate the spread of infectious diseases or increase the risk of injury. These issues should be considered when providing pre-travel consultations.

A mass gathering is usually defined as more than a specified number of people (which may be as few as 1,000 people, although 25,000 people is most commonly used) at a specific location for a specific purpose for a defined period of time. The World Health Organization defines a mass gathering as "an event [where] the number of people attending is sufficient to strain the planning and response resources of the community, state, or nation hosting the event." While mass gatherings can be spontaneous events, such as a funeral for a head of state or a form of political expression, such as a rally or march, most are planned events. Some mass gatherings occur regularly at different locations (such as the Olympic Games or the Soccer World Cup), and others recur in the same location (such as the Hajj or Wimbledon).

Mass gatherings can be characterized by purpose, location, participants, and duration. The reason for the gathering will often set a predictable tone for the event. Rock concerts are expected to be loud and boisterous, and segments of the crowd will engage in more risky behaviors. On the other hand, a religious event, such as a papal visit, would have other predictable characteristics. The purpose often influences the characteristics of the participants (age, origin, culture, homogeneity). For example, religious and family oriented events tend to have participants at the extremes of age, who may have increased susceptibility to certain diseases.

The location will determine the climate and weather and will give some indication of social and political stability in that area. There will be diseases endemic to that area, and there may be specific disease outbreaks occurring that could affect the health of visitors. Geography (particularly altitude) and climate can predispose visitors to problems such as altitude sickness, heat-related illnesses, and dehydration. The actual venue can be fixed (stadium, open space) or mobile (procession, pilgrimage). Some gatherings are indoors or in protected spaces that can shield against the elements, while others are completely exposed. The health infrastructure at the event and in the area will determine the ability to respond to both anticipated and unanticipated incidents. Facilities for food, water, and sanitation can affect the health of attendees. Often these facilities are temporary, recently erected, and may not meet the needs of the population.

The density of the crowd influences the potential risks, such as problems with crowd control, disease transmission, and injury. Large crowds can quickly overwhelm facilities. Crowd characteristics, such as age, mood, and availability of drugs or alcohol, will influence whether violence is a risk. Densely packed crowds are more likely to be violent. Events with large numbers of international participants tend have increased risk of infectious disease outbreaks. This is in part related to varying endemic diseases in host and home countries and different levels of vaccinations in those locations. The longer an event lasts, the more likely that stresses to facilities, organizers, and participants will be observed.

The most common health problems reported at mass gatherings are injuries, respiratory and cardiac issues, heat-related illness, alcohol or drug effects, and gastrointestinal illnesses. These problems can typically be addressed by either on-site clinics or nearby health facilities. However, circumstances leading to mass casualties have occurred at many different types of events.

Although communicable diseases are an understandable concern for organizers of large gatherings, they have historically not been a significant cause of adverse health events. For example, infectious diseases contributed to <1% of health care visits during the 1996 Atlanta Olympic Games and the 2000 Sydney Olympic Games. On the other hand, meningococcal meningitis transmission during the Hajj not only caused illness but also resulted in changes in requirements for Hajj pilgrims (see Chapter 4, Hajj Pilgrimage, Saudi Arabia). In addition, illnesses such as influenza may be difficult to definitively attribute to attendance at an event.

GUIDANCE FOR INTERNATIONAL TRAVELERS TO MASS GATHERINGS

All travelers to international mass gatherings should be evaluated by a travel health provider, ideally 4–6 weeks before travel, to assess the level of risk faced by the traveler and to take steps to manage the risk. Travelers should take precautions to mitigate risks associated with mass gatherings:

- Be aware of the most likely health risks associated with the event they are attending and what they can do to stay healthy and safe.
- Avoid gatherings where drug and alcohol use could contribute to dangerous behavior, where political or religious fervor may contribute to violence, or where inadequate facilities may contribute to an unhealthy environment.
- Avoid densely congested areas with limited egress.
- Be aware of emergency precautions and the location of exit routes and medical facilities.

Knowledge of the country or region being visited is essential. This can be obtained from destination pages on the CDC Travelers' Health website (wwwnc.cdc.gov/travel/destinations/list.aspx), which provides destination-specific information and will also often post specific guidance for major events. The Department of State website (http://travel.state.gov/travel/travel_1744.html) may provide additional information about countries or specific events.

For all international travel, travelers should practice healthy and safe behaviors, including:

- Safe food and water habits
- Prevention of insect bites
- Avoidance of animals, especially dogs
- Hygiene and regular handwashing
- Safe driving

BIBLIOGRAPHY

1. Emergency Management Australia. Safe and Healthy Mass Gatherings: a Health, Medical and Safety Planning Manual for Public Events. Commonwealth of Australia; 1999.
2. Fapore D, Lurie P, Moll M, Weltman A, Rankin J. Public health aspects of the rainbow family of living light annual gathering—Allegheny National Forest, Pennsylvania, 1999. MMWR Morb Mortal Wkly Rep. 2000;49(15):324–6.
3. Kaiser R, Coulombier D. Epidemic intelligence during mass gatherings. Euro Surveill. 2006;11(12):E061221.3.
4. Lombardo JS, Sniegoski CA, Loschen WA, Westercamp M, Wade M, Dearth S, et al. Public health surveillance for mass gatherings. Johns Hopkins APL Technical Digest. 2008;27(4):1–9.
5. Milsten AM, Maguire BJ, Bissell RA, Seaman KG. Mass-gathering medical care: a review of the literature. Prehosp Disaster Med. 2002 Jul–Sep;17(3):151–62.
6. World Health Organization. Communicable disease alert and response for mass gatherings: key considerations. Geneva: World Health Organization; 2008. Available from: http://www.who.int/csr/Mass_gatherings2.pdf.

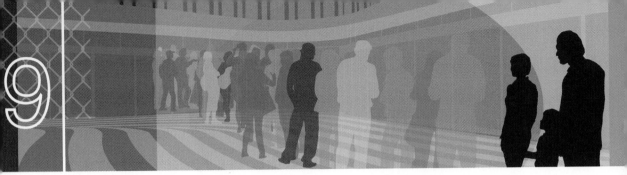

Health Considerations for Newly Arrived Immigrants & Refugees

INTRODUCTION
Christine Dubray, Mary P. Naughton, Luis S. Ortega

According to the Department of Homeland Security, approximately 75,000 refugees were admitted into the United States in 2009 (Figure 9-1). In addition, 1.1 million immigrants obtained legal permanent status, of whom 670,000 were already living in the United States and 460,000 came directly from overseas. Approximately 163 million nonimmigrant visitors are admitted to the United States annually. Of these, 127 million are Canadian and Mexican commuters who are not required to submit an arrival-departure record (I-94 form), and 36 million are nonimmigrant visitors who are required to submit an I-94 form.

A medical examination is mandatory for refugees and immigrant applicants, whether living overseas or in the United States. CDC's Division of Global Migration and Quarantine (DGMQ) provides the Department of State and the Citizenship and Immigration Services with technical instructions for conducting the medical examinations.

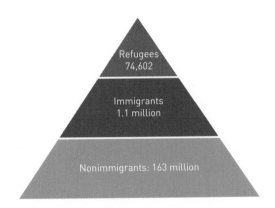

FIGURE 9-1. ANNUAL ESTIMATE OF MIGRANTS ENTERING THE UNITED STATES[1]

BIBLIOGRAPHY
1. US Department of Homeland Security. 2009 Yearbook of Immigrant Statistics. Washington, DC: US Department of Homeland Security; 2010 [cited 2010 Aug]. Available from: http://www.dhs.gov/xlibrary/assets/statistics/yearbook/2009/ois_yb_2009.pdf.

[1] Modified from the 2009 Yearbook of Immigrant Statistics, Office of Immigration Statistics, US Department of Homeland Security. Figure not to scale.

BEFORE ARRIVAL IN THE UNITED STATES: PANEL PHYSICIANS & THE OVERSEAS MEDICAL EXAMINATION

Christine Dubray, Mary P. Naughton, Luis S. Ortega

PANEL PHYSICIANS

The Immigration and Nationality Act (INA), which relates to the immigration, temporary admission, naturalization, and removal of foreigners, mandates that all immigrants and refugees migrating to the United States undergo an overseas medical screening examination performed by panel physicians. A panel physician is a medically trained, licensed, and experienced medical doctor practicing overseas who is appointed by the local US embassy or consulate. More than 760 panel physicians perform overseas predeparture medical examinations in accordance with requirements, referred to as technical instructions, provided by CDC (www.cdc. gov/immigrantrefugeehealth/exams/ti/panel/ technical-instructions-panel-physicians. html).

In 2008, CDC amended the regulations that govern the required overseas medical examination for immigrants and refugees. In addition to the communicable diseases specified in the INA, the following disease categories were added: 1) quarantinable diseases designated by presidential executive order and 2) diseases that meet the criteria of public health emergency of international concern, which require notification to the World Health Organization under the revised International Health Regulations (2005). CDC also amended the provisions that describe the scope of the medical examination by incorporating a more flexible, risk-based approach based on medical and epidemiologic factors. This approach will determine which diseases are included in the medical screening and testing of immigrants and refugees in areas of the world that are experiencing outbreaks of specific diseases. In addition, CDC updated the screening requirements for tuberculosis (TB) to be consistent with current medical knowledge and practice. These changes will reduce the health risk to the United States from emerging diseases, without imposing undue burden on either the immigrants and refugees or the US health care system.

MEDICAL EXAMINATION

The mandated medical examination focuses primarily on detecting diseases determined to be inadmissible conditions for the purposes of visa eligibility and on preventing the importation of diseases of public health importance. These medical conditions include infectious diseases such as TB, Hansen disease, and sexually transmitted diseases; mental disorders associated with harmful behavior; and substance abuse or addiction (www.cdc.gov/ immigrantrefugeehealth/exams/ti/panel/ technical-instructions-panel-physicians. html). As of January 4, 2010, testing for HIV is no longer a required part of the US immigration medical screening process, and HIV infection is no longer an inadmissible condition that prevents non-US citizens from entering the United States (www.cdc.gov/ immigrantrefugeehealth/laws-regs/hiv-ban-removal/final-rule.html).

The visit to the panel physician also provides an opportunity to give preventive medical interventions, such as updating vaccines and administering presumptive therapy for parasitic or other infectious diseases that may be affecting a specific refugee population at the time of migration, including nematode infections, malaria, and specific vaccine-preventable diseases.

CLASSIFICATION OF APPLICANTS

To determine the inadmissibility of an applicant, medical conditions are categorized as class A or B. Class A conditions are defined as those that preclude an immigrant or refugee from entering the United States. Class B conditions are defined as physical or mental

9

abnormalities, diseases, or disabilities serious enough or permanent in nature, as to amount to a substantial departure from normal well-being. Follow-up evaluation soon after US arrival is recommended for immigrants or refugees with class B TB. If an immigrant or refugee has an inadmissible condition, a visa may still be issued after the illness has been adequately treated or after a waiver of the visa ineligibility has been approved by the Citizenship and Immigration Services (www. uscis.gov).

PROOF OF VACCINATION

In 1996, a subsection was added to the INA requiring that people seeking immigrant visas for permanent residency show proof of receipt of at least 1 dose of all vaccination series recommended by the Advisory Committee on Immunization Practices (ACIP) (www.cdc.gov/vaccines/recs/acip). As of December 14, 2009, CDC adopted revised vaccination criteria to determine which vaccines recommended by ACIP should be required for immigrant visa applicants. These criteria allow CDC the flexibility to adapt vaccination requirements based on public health needs (www.cdc.gov/immigrantrefugeehealth/laws-regs/vaccination-immigration/revised-vaccination-criteria-immigration.html). The new vaccination criteria state that the vaccine must:

- be age-appropriate
- protect against a disease that has the potential to cause an outbreak
- protect against a disease that has been eliminated or is in the process of being eliminated in the United States.

These regulations apply to all adult immigrants and most immigrant children. However, internationally adopted children who are aged <10 years may obtain a waiver of exemption from the immunization requirements. Adoptive parents are required to sign a waiver indicating their intention to comply with the immunization requirements within

30 days of the infant's or child's arrival in the United States. Refugees are not required to meet the INA immunization requirements at the time of entry into the United States but must show proof of vaccination at the time they apply for permanent US residence, typically 1 year after arrival.

Updated instructions regarding vaccination requirements are available on the CDC website (http://www.cdc.gov/immigrantrefugeehealth/exams/ti/panel/vaccination-panel-technical-instructions.html).

TECHNICAL INSTRUCTIONS

CDC is responsible for providing technical instructions to the panel physicians performing the overseas medical screening examination. The testing modalities recommended for the medical examination include a medical history, physical examination, and diagnostic tests (see Table 9-1). CDC also monitors the quality of the overseas medical examination process through its Quality Assessment Program.

Additionally, CDC notifies state or local health departments of all arriving refugees, immigrants with class A conditions (with waiver), and immigrants with class B TB who are resettling in their jurisdiction and need follow-up evaluation and possible treatment. Department of State forms are collected at US ports of entry at the time of arrival. These forms summarize the results of the overseas medical examination and include classification of health conditions. This information is transmitted to state or local health departments electronically through CDC's Electronic Disease Notification System.

State and local health departments are asked to report to CDC the results of these US follow-up evaluations and any significant public health conditions identified among recently arrived immigrants and refugees, as a way to better understand epidemiologic patterns of disease in recently arrived immigrants and refugees, and to monitor the quality of overseas medical examination.

Table 9-1. Testing for required overseas medical screening examination

HEALTH CONDITION	TESTING
TB	Chest radiograph, followed by AFB smears and sputum cultures if chest radiograph suggests TB
Syphilis	Serology
Other sexually transmitted diseases	Physical examination, laboratory testing
Hansen disease	Physical examination, laboratory testing
Mental disorders with associated harmful behavior	History, mental health evaluation
Drug abuse or addiction	History, physical examination
Vaccinations	History and vaccination records, serology

Abbreviations: AFB, acid-fast bacilli; TB, tuberculosis.

BIBLIOGRAPHY

1. CDC. Technical instructions for panel physicians. Atlanta: CDC; 2010 [updated 2010 May 28; cited 2010 Apr12]. Available from: http://www.cdc.gov/immigrantrefugeehealth/exams/ti/panel/technical-instructions-panel-physicians.html.

2. Maloney S, Ortega L, Cetron M. Overseas medical screening for immigrants and refugees. In: Walker PF, Barnett ED, editors. Immigrant Medicine. Philadelphia: Saunders; 2007.

3. Office of Immigration Statistics. US Legal permanent residents: 2009. Washington, DC: US Department of Homeland Security; 2010 [cited 2010 Oct 29]. Available from: http://www.dhs.gov/xlibrary/assets/statistics/publications/lpr_fr_2009.pdf.

4. US Department of Homeland Security. Immigration and Nationality Act. Washington, DC: US Department of Homeland Security; 1952 [cited 2010 Nov 22]. Available from: http://www.uscis.gov/portal/site/uscis/menuitem.f6da51a2342135be7e9d7a10e0dc91a0/?vgnextoid=fa7e539dc4bed010VgnVCM1000000ecd190aRCRD&vgnextchannel=fa7e539dc4bed010VgnVCM1000000ecd190aRCRD&CH=act.

5. US Department of Homeland Security. Title 8 of Code of Federal Regulations (CFR). Washington DC: US Department of Homeland Security; 1938 [cited 2010 Nov 22]. Available from: http://www.uscis.gov/portal/site/uscis/menuitem.f6da51a2342135be7e9d7a10e0dc91a0/?vgnextoid=fa7e539dc4bed010VgnVCM1000000ecd190aRCRD&vgnextchannel=fa7e539dc4bed010VgnVCM1000000ecd190aRCRD&CH=8cfr.

ARRIVAL IN THE UNITED STATES: PROCESS, HEALTH STATUS, & SCREENING OF REFUGEES & IMMIGRANTS

Patricia F. Walker, William M. Stauffer, Elizabeth D. Barnett

There is great diversity among immigrant populations arriving in the United States each year, with a concomitant wide spectrum of health needs. Some immigrants arrive with infectious diseases of personal or public health significance; others with untreated chronic conditions such as vitamin deficiencies, diabetes, or hypertension; and many with both infectious and chronic disease issues. Two of these groups, refugees and internationally adopted children, have more health information available than other groups, so much of the published screening recommendations is based on studies of these groups.

State health departments are notified by CDC about refugee new arrivals. A secure electronic system, the Electronic Disease Notification System, alerts states of refugee arrivals that have class A conditions (with waiver) and class B conditions. Class A conditions are defined as those that preclude an immigrant or refugee from entering the United States. Class B conditions are defined as physical or mental abnormalities, diseases, or disabilities that are permanent or serious enough to amount to a substantial departure from normal well-being.

Newly arrived refugees are encouraged to receive stateside evaluation and treatment, conducted at state or local health departments, as well as private clinics and community health centers. Ideally, these examinations are done within 3 months of US arrival. Because there is no required nationwide process for postarrival health assessments, the timing and thoroughness of postarrival refugee health evaluations vary from state to state. For nonrefugee immigrants, no formal mechanism or funding source is available for medical screening; therefore, immigrants, with the exception of international adoptees, do not routinely receive any postarrival medical screening services. Many clinicians are unfamiliar with screening recommendations and diseases endemic to immigrants' countries of origin and are unprepared to deal with language, social, and cultural barriers in caring for new arrivals. In addition, refugees and immigrants often have other demands related to their new environment that may compete with their perception of need for health evaluations and treatment. To address the special health challenges of refugees, the Office of Refugee Resettlement (ORR), Department of Health and Human Services, provides guidance, resources, and oversight for medical assistance, initial medical screening, and physical and mental health technical assistance and consultation for refugees (www.acf.hhs.gov/programs/orr). CDC, in collaboration with ORR and other partners, has developed guidelines to assist states and clinicians in providing medical screening services to refugees. These guidelines, found at www.cdc.gov/immigrantrefugeehealth/guidelines/refugee-guidelines.html, include screening for malaria, intestinal parasites, and blood lead levels, as well as a general outline for the history and physical examination.

MEDICAL SCREENING FOR NEWLY ARRIVED REFUGEES

After arrival in the United States, it is recommended but not required that all refugees receive medical screening. In addition, this visit provides an opportunity to provide preventive services, such as immunizations and initiation of treatment for latent tuberculosis (TB) and individual counseling (such as nutritional and mental health), and to establish ongoing primary care. Recommendations for this initial medical evaluation should ideally be tailored to the specific population and based on such factors as receipt of predeparture presumptive therapy (malaria and intestinal parasites), ethnicity, and epidemiologic risks in the country of origin, as well as the country or countries of first asylum. Refugees may be able to qualify for the federally funded, state-administered Refugee Medical Assistance program for their medical care needs. Refugees may be eligible for the program for up to 8 months from the date of their arrival and can apply for the program in their state of residence during that time. For more information, clinicians and refugees can contact their state health departments and also access more information through the Office of Refugee Resettlement (US Department of Health and Human Services), which supports this program (www.acf.hhs.gov/programs/orr/programs/cma.htm).

DOMESTIC HEALTH ASSESSMENT

Many refugees and immigrants originate from countries with a high prevalence of tropical and other infectious diseases, which may be a threat to individual or public health. In addition, untreated chronic health conditions are common. Infectious diseases with long latency periods can be particularly challenging, including TB, hepatitis B, and certain intestinal nematodes, such as *Schistosoma* spp. and *Strongyloides stercoralis*.

All migrants who are medically screened should have a detailed history and physical examination. Medical screening for new arrivals should include basic components outlined in Box 9-1. Many refugees will not have had age-appropriate cancer screening, such as a Papanicolaou test, mammography, and colon cancer screening, and these needs should be addressed at early follow-up visits. Clinicians should be aware of cancers with a higher prevalence in many immigrant populations, such as cervical, liver, stomach, and nasopharyngeal cancer. HIV testing has recently been removed from requirements for US admission, which has implications for providers seeing patients from higher-prevalence countries. Culturally sensitive counseling regarding HIV testing is critical.

In addition to CDC's postarrival domestic medical screening guidelines for refugees, other published resources are available to the clinician to obtain expert opinion regarding appropriate medical screening in refugees. Most recently, the Public Health Authority of Canada has produced consensus documents on the evidence base for screening newly arriving refugees to Canada. The Migrant Health Resources section of this chapter includes a list of clinical resources for providers and organizations.

BOX 9-1. RECOMMENDED COMPONENTS OF DOMESTIC HEALTH ASSESSMENTS[1]

- Review all available records, chest radiograph (ask for overseas records)
- Complete history and physical examination
- Vision and hearing screening
- Dental evaluation
- Mental health screening
- Tuberculosis
- Laboratory testing (hepatitis B for those arriving from countries with prevalence rates more than 2%, hematologic testing, urinalysis, lead, and HIV testing, when clinically appropriate)
- Presumptive treatment of malaria
- Evaluation for intestinal parasites (ova and parasites [2–3 times], serology for schistosomiasis and strongyloidiasis in certain groups)
- Presumptive treatment for schistosomiasis in groups at risk
- Evaluation and update of immunizations as needed

[1] Formal refugee health guidelines are available from www.cdc.gov/immigrantrefugeehealth/guidelines/refugee-guidelines.html.

MEDICAL SCREENING FOR INTERNATIONAL ADOPTEES

There are many similarities in health conditions on arrival between international adoptees and refugees. However, an important distinction is that international adoptees frequently enter into households and communities that are naive to many infections common in resource-poor settings. On the other hand, refugees generally remain within their own cultural group for some time after arrival and have limited interactions with the wider community. This distinction is particularly pertinent for conditions that may continue to be infectious for weeks to months after arrival (such as hepatitis A or *Giardia*). The American Academy of Pediatrics offers guidance for clinicians who will be serving this population after their arrival in the United States in the Red Book, which may be accessed at http://aapredbook.aappublications.org. For more information, see Chapter 7, International Adoption.

CONCLUSION

Limited health interventions are provided to immigrants and refugees before their entry into the United States. Points of contact during the migration process, such as overseas examination, transit stops (such as quarantine stations), and postarrival medical visits offer opportunities to intervene to improve the health status of the person, as well as to minimize any public health risk.

BIBLIOGRAPHY

1. Avery R. Immigrant women's health: infectious diseases. Part 1: clinical assessment, tuberculosis, hepatitis, and malaria. West J Med. 2001 Sep;175(3):208–11.

2. Barnett E. Immunizations for immigrants. In: Walker P, Barnett E, editors. Immigrant Medicine. Philadelphia: Elsevier; 2007. p. 151–70.

3. Barnett ED. Immunizations and infectious disease screening for internationally adopted children. Pediatr Clin North Am. 2005 Oct;52(5):1287–309, vi.

4. Barnett ED. Infectious disease screening for refugees resettled in the United States. Clin Infect Dis. 2004 Sep 15;39(6):833–41.

5. CDC. Final rule removing HIV infection from US immigration screening. Atlanta: CDC; 2010 [updated 2010 Apr 2; cited 2010 Oct 29]. Available from: http://www.cdc.gov/immigrantrefugeehealth/laws-regs/hiv-ban-removal/final-rule.html.

6. CDC. Revised vaccination criteria for US immigration. Atlanta: CDC; 2010 [updated January 19, 2010]. Available from: http://www.cdc.gov/immigrantrefugeehealth/laws-regs/vaccination-immigration/fact-sheet.html.

7. Chen LH, Barnett ED, Wilson ME. Preventing infectious diseases during and after international adoption. Ann Intern Med. 2003 Sep 2;139(5 Pt 1):371–8.

8. Ivey SL, Faust S. Immigrant women's health: screening and immunization. West J Med. 2001 Jul;175(1):62–5.

9. Miller LC. International adoption: infectious diseases issues. Clin Infect Dis. 2005 Jan 15;40(2):286–93.

10. Posey DL, Blackburn BG, Weinberg M, Flagg EW, Ortega L, Wilson M, et al. High prevalence and presumptive treatment of schistosomiasis and strongyloidiasis among African refugees. Clin Infect Dis. 2007 Nov 15;45(10):1310–5.

11. Pottie K, Tugwell P, Feightner J, Welch V, Greenaway C, Swinkels H, et al. Summary of clinical preventive care recommendations for newly arriving immigrants and refugees to Canada. CMAJ. 2010 Jul 26.

12. Seybolt L, Barnett ED, Stauffer W. US Medical screening for immigrants and refugees: clinical issues. In: Walker PF, Barnett ED, editors. Immigrant Medicine. Philadelphia: Saunders; 2007. p. 135–50.

13. Stauffer WM, Kamat D, Walker PF. Screening of international immigrants, refugees, and adoptees. Prim Care. 2002 Dec;29(4):879–905.

14. Stauffer WM, Maroushek S, Kamat D. Medical screening of immigrant children. Clin Pediatr (Phila). 2003 Nov–Dec;42(9):763–73.

MIGRANT HEALTH RESOURCES

William M. Stauffer

Historically, the Yellow Book has addressed travel health issues for US residents visiting countries outside the United States. In this increasingly mobile world, the discipline of travel medicine is evolving to recognize non-traditional groups who cross international boundaries into and out of the United States. One such group includes people who originate in other countries and migrate to the United States, either temporarily or permanently. Recognized migrants to the United States include immigrants (documented and undocumented), refugees, asylum seekers, and adoptees. In addition, students and corporate workers are frequent visitors to the United States. Many clinics serving the traditional travel population also function as contact points with the US medical system for these populations, particularly for immigrants and refugees. This section provides resources to assist clinicians and organizations that serve these populations to access up-to-date patient-care guidelines, online education materials, and print resources.

CLINICAL REFERENCES
Organizational Guidelines
- **Centers for Disease Control and Prevention:** predeparture and postarrival presumptive treatment and medical screening guidelines for refugees relocating to the United States available at www.cdc.gov/immigrantrefugee health/exams/medical-examination.html
- **American Academy of Pediatrics:** online Red Book guidance on medical screening and vaccination issues in adoptees, refugees, and immigrants at http://aapredbook.aappublica tions.org
- **Canadian Collaboration for Immigrant and Refugee Health:** clinical preventive guidelines for primary care for newly arriving immigrants and refugees at www.ccirh.uottawa.ca

Websites
- **Centers for Disease Control and Prevention**
  > Division of Global Migration and Quarantine: information on immigrants and refugees who are resettling in the United States plus resources at www.cdc. gov/immigrantrefugeehealth/index.html
  > Division of Parasitic Diseases and Malaria: clinical and public policy information on parasitic diseases at www.cdc.gov/parasites and www.cdc.gov/malaria/
  > Travelers' Health: health information for international travelers at www.cdc.gov/ travel
  > International Emergency and Refugee Health Branch: health information pertaining to complex humanitarian emergencies at www. cdc.gov/globalhealth/ierh
- **Minnesota Department of Health:** multiple resources for clinicians in refugee health at www.health.state.mn.us/divs/idepc/refugee/ hcp/index.html
- **Healthy Roads Media:** health education materials, including video, in a variety of languages at http://healthyroadsmedia.org
- **EthnoMed:** information about cultural beliefs, medical issues, and other related issues pertinent to the health care of recent immigrants at http://ethnomed.org/ethnomed
- **Health Information Translations:** set of common hospital signs with multiple translations at www.healthinfotranslations.com
- **Medical Leadership Council on Cultural Proficiency:** database of patient information resources in a variety of languages and organizations providing services in languages other than English at www.medicalleadership.org/resources/ patient_education.shtml
- **Refugee Health Information Network:** multilingual information for clinicians, refugees, and asylum seekers in print, audio, and video formats at www.rhin.org
- **US Committee for Refugees and Immigrants:** toolkits on multiple health issues for clinicians, immigrants, and communities in multiple languages at www.refugees.org/resources/ for-refugees-immigrants/health
- **US Citizenship and Immigration Services:** information regarding adjustment of status at www.uscis.gov

Reference Books
Textbooks with a Focus on Migrant Health
- **Immigrant Medicine.** Walker PF, Barnett ED, editors. Philadelphia: Saunders; 2007.
- **Migration Medicine and Health: Principles and Practice.** Gushulak BD, MacPherson D, editors. Hamilton, ON: BC Decker; 2006.
- **Travel Medicine and Migrant Health.** Lockie C, Walker E, Calvert L, Cossar J, Knill-Jones R, Raeside F, editors. Edinburgh: Churchill Livingstone; 2000.
- **Refugee and Immigrant Health. A Handbook for Health Professionals.** Kemp C, Rasbridge LA, editors. New York: Cambridge University Press; 2004.

Textbooks with a Focus on Tropical Diseases
- **Atlas of Tropical Medicine and Parasitology. 6th ed.** Peters W, Pasvol G, editors. Mosby; 2006.
- **Douglas and Bennett's Principles & Practice of Infectious Diseases. 5th ed.** Mandell GL, Bennett JE, Dolin R, editors. Philadelphia: Churchill Livingstone; 2000.
- **Hunter's Tropical Medicine and Emerging Infectious Diseases. 8th ed.** Hunter GW, Strickland GT, Magill AJ, editors. Philadelphia: WB Saunders Company; 2000.
- **Manson's Tropical Diseases. 22nd ed.** Cook GC, Zumla AI, editors. Edinburgh, UK: Saunders Ltd; 2008.
- **Tropical Infectious Diseases. 2nd ed.** Guerrant RL, Walker DH, Weller PF, editors. Philadelphia: Churchill Livingstone; 2006.

GENERAL RESOURCES
Reading Lists
- **Global Health Education Consortium's Global Health Bibliography:** bibliography of selected citations for use by students and faculty in global health at http://globalhealthedu.org/resources/Pages/GlobalHealthBibliography.aspx
- **University of Minnesota reading list on refugee and immigrant health:** comprehensive reading list for people interested in refugee and immigrant health at www.globalhealth.umn.edu/residenttraining/reading/home.html

Educational Opportunities
- **University of Minnesota/CDC ASTMH-accredited course in global health:** focus on immigrant and refugee health at www.global-health.umn.edu/globalhealthcourse/home.html (in-person course) and www.global-health.umn.edu/onlinetrainingglobalhealth/home.html (online course)
- **ASTMH-accredited courses in tropical and travel medicine:** list of ASTMH-accredited tropical and travel medicine courses at www.astmh.org/Approved_Diploma_Courses/2867.htm

Non-CDC Organizations
- **US Department of Health and Human Services**
  > Office of Refugee Resettlement: www.acf.hhs.gov/programs/orr
  > Office of Global Health Affairs: www.globalhealth.gov
- **United Nations High Commissioner for Refugees:** www.unhcr.org/cgi-bin/texis/vtx/home
- **World Health Organization refugee page:** www.who.int/topics/refugees/en
- **American Society of Tropical Medicine and Hygiene:** www.astmh.org
- **International Organization for Migration:** www.iom.int
- **International Society of Travel Medicine Health of Migrants and Refugees Committee:** www.istm.org/WebForms/Members/MemberActivities/VolunteerActivities/interest_groups/migrants.aspx
- **Global Health Education Consortium:** http://globalhealtheducation.org
- **Global Health Council:** www.globalhealth.org

Other Resources
- **Pre-travel handouts for non-English-speaking patients** (multiple topics in over 15 languages): www.tropical.umn.edu/TTM/VFR/index.htm
- **The Providers' Guide to Quality and Culture:** http://erc.msh.org/mainpage.cfm?file=1.0.htm&module=provider&language=English

Appendices

APPENDIX A: PROMOTING QUALITY IN THE PRACTICE OF TRAVEL MEDICINE

Stephen M. Ostroff

Travel medicine is a young area of medical practice, but even as the field continues to mature based on a growing body of scientific and medical information, there remains no recognized specialty or subspecialty of travel medicine anywhere in the world, including the United States. Clinicians offering travel medicine services are not "board certified" in travel medicine. Instead, travel medicine physicians generally have credentials in other disciplines, usually infectious diseases, internal medicine, family practice, or general practice. The same applies to nurses, pharmacists, and other allied health professionals. Clinics in the United States that offer travel medicine services are also not specifically credentialed for this purpose.

Given these circumstances, how can travelers maximize the likelihood their provider will deliver quality travel-related medical care and that the advice, preventive measures, and treatment services they are given fall within accepted standards? Similarly, how can providers assure patients they have sufficient knowledge of the subject matter relevant to travel medicine?

Research into the quality of travel health care is limited, but several studies suggest that travelers who visit a clinician with training in travel medicine are more likely to receive appropriate pre- and post-travel advice and care than if they see other clinicians for such services. Similarly, 2006 guidelines on travel medicine published by the Infectious Diseases Society of America (Box A-1) recommend that pre- and post-travel care be obtained from a clinician with expertise in travel medicine. This is especially relevant for travelers going to exotic destinations, engaging in adventure travel, or who have special needs or medical problems.

Below is a partial list of resources for clinicians who wish to enhance their knowledge of travel medicine. People seeking travel-related medical services may want to inquire about whether their provider or clinic participates in these organizations or activities.

INTERNATIONAL SOCIETY OF TRAVEL MEDICINE (ISTM)

Founded in 1991, ISTM (www.istm.org) is the preeminent multinational organization dealing exclusively with travel medicine. ISTM has more than 2,500 members worldwide, slightly fewer than half of whom are located in the United States.

ISTM activities include the following:

- *Journal of Travel Medicine*
- An active listserv where members share information and can ask questions
- Special-interest groups that include travel medicine nurses and travel medicine pharmacists
- A biennial travel medicine meeting and annual regional submeetings
- A directory of domestic and international travel clinics affiliated with ISTM members
- An annual examination, leading to a Certificate of Knowledge in Travel Medicine, available to physicians, nurses, pharmacists, and other professionals offering travel advice

The Certificate of Knowledge in Travel Medicine has been administered by ISTM since 2003. The Body of Knowledge, which covers the scope of the specialty of travel medicine, forms the basis for examination questions. It was last updated in 2006 and is published on the ISTM website. Content areas in the Body of Knowledge include the following:

- Epidemiology related to travel medicine
- Immunology and vaccinology (including travel-related vaccines)
- Pre-travel consultation and management
  - > Patient evaluation
  - > Travelers with special needs
  - > Special itineraries
  - > Prevention and self-treatment
  - > Precautions
- Diseases contracted during travel
  - > Vectorborne diseases
  - > Diseases transmitted from person to person
  - > Foodborne and waterborne diseases
  - > Diseases related to bites and stings
  - > Diseases due to environmental hazards
- Other conditions associated with travel
  - > Conditions occurring during or after travel
  - > Conditions due to environmental factors
  - > Threats to personal safety and security
  - > Psychocultural issues
- Post-travel management
- General travel medicine issues
  - > Medical care abroad
  - > Travel clinic management
  - > Travel medicine information resources

Since it was introduced, the Certificate of Knowledge in Travel Medicine examination has been taken by more than 1,700 practitioners in 55 countries. Those who are successful in the examination are awarded a Certificate in Travel Health. The society hosts periodic examination preparation meetings. Practitioners offering travel medicine services or interested in the subject should strongly consider membership in ISTM. ISTM practitioners are listed on the organization's website, and those who have the Certificate of Knowledge in Travel Medicine are designated as such.

AMERICAN SOCIETY OF TROPICAL MEDICINE AND HYGIENE (ASTMH)

Formed in 1951 through the merger of predecessor organizations dating back to 1903, ASTMH (www.astmh.org) has a subsection that deals exclusively with tropical and travel medicine, known as the American Committee on Clinical Tropical Medicine and Travelers' Health.

ASTMH activities include the following:

- *The American Journal of Tropical Medicine and Hygiene*
- An annual meeting
- An electronic distribution list
- A tropical medicine clinic directory
- A biennial examination leading to a Certificate of Knowledge in Clinical Tropical Medicine and Travelers' Health, available to those who have passed an ASTMH-approved tropical medicine course or have sufficient tropical medicine experience

The content areas of the ASTMH Certificate of Knowledge in Clinical Tropic Medicine and Travelers' Health are as follows:

- Basic science and fundamentals
- Infectious and tropical diseases (including parasites, bacteria, fungi, and viruses)
- Other diseases and conditions
- Diagnostic and therapeutic approach to clinical syndromes
- Travelers' health
- Public health in the tropics
- Epidemiology and control of disease
- Laboratory diagnosis

More than 600 people who have passed the ASTMH examination are listed on the

ASTMH website. The society offers a periodic intensive update course in clinical tropical medicine and travelers' health, which is in part designed to prepare those planning to take the Certificate of Knowledge examination.

WILDERNESS MEDICAL SOCIETY

Organized in 1983, this society (www.wms.org) focuses on adventure travel, including wilderness travel and diving medicine. Its activities include the following:

- The journal *Wilderness and Environmental Medicine*
- Practice guidelines for emergency care in wilderness settings
- An annual meeting and subspecialty meetings
- Courses leading to certification in advanced wilderness life support
- A wilderness medical curriculum that, when successfully completed, qualifies members for fellowship in the Academy of Wilderness Medicine

INFECTIOUS DISEASES SOCIETY OF AMERICA (IDSA)

IDSA (www.idsociety.org) is the largest organization representing infectious diseases clinicians in the United States. Although IDSA does not deal exclusively with travel medicine, it maintains a strong interest in this topic. In 2006, IDSA published extensive evidence-based guidelines on the practice of travel medicine in the United States (Box A-1). It also publishes travel-related research in its

2 journals: *The Journal of Infectious Diseases* and *Clinical Infectious Diseases*.

INTERNATIONAL SOCIETY FOR INFECTIOUS DISEASES (ISID)

ISID (www.isid.org) was formed in 1986 and has approximately 20,000 members in 155 countries around the world. Like IDSA, ISID does not specifically focus on travel medicine. However, its international reach, particularly in low-resource countries, makes travel medicine an important topic in ISID and a valuable source of information for infectious diseases clinicians in many overseas travel destinations. Activities relevant to travel medicine that are supported by ISID include the following:

- *International Journal of Infectious Diseases*
- The biennial meeting International Congress on Infectious Diseases
- The Program for Monitoring Emerging Diseases (Pro-MED), an open-source electronic reporting system for reports of emerging infectious diseases and toxins, including outbreaks (www.promedmail.org)

AEROSPACE MEDICAL ASSOCIATION

This organization (www.asma.org) represents professionals in the fields of aviation, space, and environmental medicine who deal with air and space travelers. Its activities include the following:

- The journal *Aviation, Space, and Environmental Medicine*
- An annual meeting
- Continuing medical education in topics related to aerospace medicine

---

BOX A-1. ESSENTIAL ELEMENTS OF A QUALITY PRE-TRAVEL EVALUATION

The following elements, adapted from Spira and IDSA guidelines, provide an overview of a quality pre-travel evaluation:

- Evaluation of a traveler's health, including underlying health conditions and immunization history
- Careful analysis of the itinerary, including duration, season, activities, and style of travel
- Evaluation for vaccinations and other preventive measures
- Education for disease prevention and health maintenance, including access to medical care overseas

FINDING CARE WHILE TRAVELING OUTSIDE THE UNITED STATES

Both the ISTM and ASTMH websites contain the names of non-US-based clinics and health care providers affiliated with members of these organizations. Travelers are advised to review these lists before departure to identify health care resources at their travel destination. A number of countries or national travel medicine societies have websites related to travel medicine that also provide access to clinicians, including the following:

- Canada: Health Canada (www.hc-sc.gc.ca/hl-vs/travel-voyage/index_e.html)

- Great Britain: National Travel Health Network and Centre (www.nathnac.org) and British Travel Health Association (www.btha.org)
- South Africa: South African Society of Travel Medicine (www.sastm.org.za)
- Australia: Travel Medicine Alliance (www.travelmedicine.com.au)
- China: International Travel Healthcare Association (http://en.itha.org.cn)

Emergency travel-related medical care and medical evacuation may be accessed through a number of private companies. One example is International SOS, which operates throughout the world. Provider locations and details may be found at www.internationalsos.com.

BIBLIOGRAPHY

1. Hill DR, Ericsson CD, Pearson RD, Keystone JS, Freedman DO, Kozarsky PE, et al. The practice of travel medicine: guidelines by the Infectious Diseases Society of America. Clin Infect Dis. 2006 Dec 15;43(12):1499–539.

2. Kozarsky P. The body of knowledge for the practice of travel medicine—2006. J Travel Med. 2006 Sep–Oct;13(5):251–4.

3. Spira A. Setting the standard. J Travel Med. 2003 Jan–Feb;10(1):1–3.

APPENDIX B: ESSENTIAL ELECTRONIC RESOURCES FOR THE TRAVEL MEDICINE PRACTITIONER

David O. Freedman, Katherine J. Johnson

SELECTED ELECTRONIC RESOURCES IN TRAVEL MEDICINE

A variety of electronic resources is available for practitioners who provide pre- and post-travel medical care for international travelers (Table B-1). Checking more than 1 authoritative website on a specific issue is always recommended. Authoritative recommendations may contain some element of opinion, and some sites are updated more frequently than others. Fortunately, most sites now put an indicator at the bottom of each page stating when the last update was done or electronically notify interested users when changes are made.

ELECTRONIC NOTIFICATION AND DISCUSSION FORUMS

Electronic distribution lists (such as Listserv) use e-mail with or without a browser-based interface. Some lists are set up to provide information only. Others promote active discussion among members, whereby anyone who has joined a particular group can e-mail a posting to a central server, which is then disseminated to all members who have subscribed to the same list. On a moderated list, each posting is reviewed and accepted by a moderator or editor, while unmoderated lists disseminate each posting instantly to all other subscribers. TravelMed is an example of an unmoderated list, which focuses on issues related to the practice of travel medicine (see www.istm.org/WebForms/Members/MemberActivities/listserve.aspx for further information). CDC's website provides an information-only e-mail notification system called GovDelivery on a variety of health topics, including updates to the CDC Travelers' Health website. For more information or to subscribe, see www.cdc.gov/emailupdates/index.html.

Another common form of electronic notification is RSS (Really Simple Syndication). Many websites provide RSS feeds that instantly inform users when updates are made. To receive feeds, users must have an RSS reader on their computer or mobile device. Readers are commonly available as embedded features of most web browsers and e-mail applications or can be downloaded from commercial organizations. Users can customize notification settings to send multiple feeds directly to their e-mail account, or they can view feeds through their web browser, desktop, or mobile device.

Many of the resources below provide RSS feeds. CDC Travelers' Health generates feeds on 2 topics: travel notices and updates to the Yellow Book. For more information, see wwwnc.cdc.gov/travel/contentRss.aspx. Table B-2 highlights a subset of primary resources that provide RSS feeds that may be useful to travel medicine practitioners. Check the resources in Table B-1 for more information or updates through e-mail lists and other social media.

Note: *Tables B-1 and B-2 provide a representative but by no means exclusive sampling of resources that may be useful to the travel medicine practitioner. Brief descriptions of selected websites have been included to highlight resources that may be of particular interest. Please be advised that website URLs and content may change at any time.*

Table B-1. Selected websites for the travel medicine practitioner

Authoritative Travel Medicine Recommendations

CDC Travelers' Health homepage *Includes current travel health notices, disease- and destination-specific health recommendations, and guidance on a variety of topics in travel medicine*	www.cdc.gov/travel
CDC Travelers' Health Yellow Book homepage *Includes a searchable version of CDC Health Information for International Travel 2012 ("The Yellow Book") and a list of any updates occurring between print editions*	www.cdc.gov/yellowbook
US Department of State Bureau of Consular Services	www.travel.state.gov
US Department of State country-specific information, travel warnings, and travel alerts	http://travel.state.gov/travel/cis_pa_tw/cis/cis_4965.html
WHO international travel and health homepage *Includes the current edition of the International Travel and Health ("Green Book") publication, disease updates for travelers, International Health Regulations documents, and other disease-specific information*	www.who.int/ith/en
The Practice of Travel Medicine: Guidelines by the Infectious Diseases Society of America	www.journals.uchicago.edu/doi/pdf/10.1086/508782
US Department of Transportation aircraft disinsection requirements	http://ostpxweb.dot.gov/policy/safetyenergyenv/disinsection.htm

Emerging Diseases and Outbreaks

WHO global alert and response homepage *Includes current Disease Outbreak News and outbreaks sorted by country, disease, and year*	www.who.int/csr/en
PAHO epidemiologic alerts *Complements WHO's Disease Outbreak News (above) with information specific to the Americas*	http://new.paho.org/hq/index.php?option=com_content&task=view&id=1239&Itemid=1091
CDC Health Alert Network message archive	www2a.cdc.gov/HAN/ArchiveSys
GeoSentinel Surveillance Network of the International Society of Travel Medicine and CDC	www.geosentinel.org

continued

TABLE B-1. SELECTED WEBSITES FOR THE TRAVEL MEDICINE PRACTITIONER (continued)

ProMED-mail: program for monitoring emerging diseases *Includes moderated reporting of global infectious diseases and acute exposure to toxins*	www.promedmail.org
HealthMap: Global Disease Alert Map	www.healthmap.org/en
Global Health Facts (Kaiser Family Foundation)	www.globalhealthfacts.org
Surveillance and Epidemiologic Bulletins	
CDC MMWR Weekly, Recommendations and Reports, and Surveillance Summaries	www.cdc.gov/mmwr
WHO Weekly Epidemiological Record	www.who.int/wer/
PAHO list of links to National Bulletins in the Americas	www.paho.org/English/DD/AIS/vigilancia-en.htm
PAHO list of Ministries of Health in the Americas	www.paho.org/English/PAHO/MOHs.htm
WHO list of links to national travel and health websites	www.who.int/ith/links/national_links/en/index.html
Zoonotic disease surveillance: World Organization for Animal Health	www.oie.int
Eurosurveillance	www.eurosurveillance.org
Caribbean Epidemiology Centre	www.carec.org
ReliefWeb: administered by the UN Office for the Coordination of Humanitarian Affairs *Includes information on humanitarian emergencies and natural disasters from a variety of UN agencies and other sources*	www.reliefweb.int
WHO Crises and Emergencies: health-related situational updates	www.who.int/hac/crises/en
EpiNorth Europe	www.epinorth.org
EpiSouth Europe	www.episouth.org

continued

TABLE B-1. SELECTED WEBSITES FOR THE TRAVEL MEDICINE PRACTITIONER (continued)

Vaccine Resources

US Advisory Committee on Immunization Practices: recommendations on individual vaccines	www.cdc.gov/vaccines/pubs/ACIP-list.htm
CDC vaccine information statements for patients: download site	www.cdc.gov/vaccines/pubs/vis/default.htm
CDC information on vaccination shortages	www.cdc.gov/vaccines/vac-gen/shortages/default.htm
American Academy of Pediatrics table on status of licensure and recommendations for new vaccines	http://aapredbook.aappublications.org/news/vaccstatus.shtml
CDC Pink Book: Epidemiology and Prevention of Vaccine-Preventable Diseases *Includes an online version of the current edition, updates to the print edition, slide sets, and selected chapters from earlier editions*	www.cdc.gov/vaccines/pubs/pinkbook/default.htm
Vaccines and biologics used in US and foreign markets	www.immunize.org/catg.d/p5120.pdf
Translation of international vaccine-related terms into English	www.immunize.org/catg.d/p5121.pdf
Vaccine-preventable disease terms in multiple languages	www.immunize.org/catg.d/p5122.pdf
Vaccine information from the Immunization Action Coalition	www.vaccineinformation.org
WHO immunization, vaccines, and biologics *Includes links to national, regional, and international resources providing immunization information*	www.who.int/immunization/en
WHO country-specific routine immunization schedules	http://apps.who.int/immunization_monitoring/en/globalsummary/ScheduleSelect.cfm
Package inserts and manufacturers for some US-licensed vaccines and immunoglobulins	www.vaccinesafety.edu/package_inserts.htm
PATH vaccine resource library	www.path.org/vaccineresources

Consumer-Oriented Travel Health Information and Products

High Altitude Medicine Guide	www.high-altitude-medicine.com
Travel Health Online	www.tripprep.com

continued

TABLE B-1. SELECTED WEBSITES FOR THE TRAVEL MEDICINE PRACTITIONER (continued)

MDTravelHealth.com	www.mdtravelhealth.com
Chinook Medical Gear, Inc.	www.chinookmed.com
Magellan's Travel Supplies	www.magellans.com
Travel Medicine, Inc.	www.travmed.com
Overseas Medical and Safety Assistance	
US Department of State medical information for Americans abroad	http://travel.state.gov/travel/tips/brochures/brochures_1215.html
International Association for Medical Assistance to Travelers	www.iamat.org
International SOS: medical and security solutions, products, and assistance	www.internationalsos.com
MEDEX: worldwide travel assistance and international medical insurance	www.medexassist.com
Maps and Country Information	
US Overseas Security Advisory Council *Includes current US Department of State travel alerts, travel warnings, embassy Warden Messages, and safety and security resources*	www.osac.gov
US Central Intelligence Agency: The World Factbook	https://www.cia.gov/library/publications/the-world-factbook
US Department of State Background Notes	www.state.gov/r/pa/ei/bgn
US Federal Aviation Administration data on air safety standards in foreign countries	www.faa.gov/about/initiatives/iasa
European Commission Air Safety portal	http://ec.europa.eu/transport/air/index_en.htm
Falling Rain global gazetteer and place name altitude finder	www.fallingrain.com/world
Association for Safe International Road Travel	http://asirt.org
UN maps	www.un.org/Depts/Cartographic/english/htmain.htm
Perry-Castañeda Library map collection	www.lib.utexas.edu/Libs/PCL/Map_collection/map_sites/map_sites.html

continued

TABLE B-1. SELECTED WEBSITES FOR THE TRAVEL MEDICINE PRACTITIONER (continued)

Nations Online: destination guide to countries and nations	www.nationsonline.org
GeoNames geographic database	www.geonames.org
Lonely Planet travel information	www.lonelyplanet.com
Disability Information	
MossRehab ResourceNet: accessible travel	www.mossresourcenet.org/travel.htm
US Department of Transportation Aviation Consumer Protection and Enforcement	http://airconsumer.ost.dot.gov/publications/disabled.htm
Society for Accessible Travel and Hospitality	www.sath.org
Mobility International USA	www.miusa.org
Professional Medical Societies with a Focus on Travelers' Health	
International Society of Travel Medicine	www.istm.org
American Society of Tropical Medicine and Hygiene	www.astmh.org
Infectious Diseases Society of America	www.idsociety.org
Pediatric Infectious Diseases Society	www.pids.org
Divers Alert Network	www.diversalertnetwork.org
Wilderness Medical Society	www.wms.org
Undersea and Hyperbaric Medical Society	www.uhms.org
American Travel Health Nurses Association	www.athna.org
Global Health Council	www.globalhealth.org
Christian Medical and Dental Associations	www.cmda.org
Disease Information	
CDC diseases and conditions: A–Z list	www.cdc.gov/DiseasesConditions
WHO health topics: A–Z list	www.who.int/topics/en
PAHO health topics: A–Z list	http://new.paho.org/hq/index.php?option=com_joomlabook&Itemid=260
Oxford Malaria Atlas Project	www.map.ox.ac.uk

continued

CDC malaria map application	www.cdc.gov/malaria/map/index.html
CDC influenza homepage *Includes information about seasonal influenza, avian influenza, and others*	www.cdc.gov/flu
US Government Flu Portal	www.flu.gov
US Tropical Medicine Central Resource	http://tmcr.usuhs.mil/toc.htm#
UN special program on the diseases of poverty	www.who.int/tdr
WHO rabies bulletin: Europe	www.who-rabies-bulletin.org
WHO water supply and sanitation assessment	www.who.int/water_sanitation_health/monitoring/globalassess/en
WHO Global Schistosomiasis Atlas	www.who.int/schistosomiasis/epidemiology/global_atlas/en/index.html
Global Polio Eradication Initiative	www.polioeradication.org
General Travel Aids	
Embassies in the United States	www.state.gov/s/cpr/rls
Embassies in the United States web links	www.embassy.org/embassies/index.html
Times around the World	www.timeanddate.com/worldclock
Tourism Offices Worldwide Directory	www.towd.com
Visa/Plus ATM locator	http://visa.via.infonow.net/locator/global/jsp/SearchPage.jsp
MasterCard/Cirrus ATM locator	www.mastercard.com/cardholderservices/atm
US Organizations Offering Training in Travel Medicine	
International Society of Travel Medicine	www.istm.org
American Society of Tropical Medicine and Hygiene	www.astmh.org
Gorgas Memorial Institute	www.gorgas.org
Tulane Department of Tropical Medicine	www.sph.tulane.edu/tropmed
University of Washington School of Medicine	http://depts.washington.edu/cme/home
University of Minnesota Department of Medicine	www.globalhealth.umn.edu

Abbreviations: ATM, automated teller machine; MMWR, Morbidity and Mortality Weekly Report; PAHO, Pan American Health Organization; UN, United Nations; WHO, World Health Organization.

Table B-2. Selected travel medicine resources providing RSS feeds

CDC Travelers' Health *Feeds include travel notices, updates to the Yellow Book*	wwwnc.cdc.gov/travel/content/rss.aspx
CDC (agencywide) *Feeds on a variety of health topics*	www2c.cdc.gov/podcasts/rss.asp
US Department of State *Feeds include travel warnings, travel alerts, country-specific information, country background notes*	www.state.gov/misc/echannels/66791.htm
World Health Organization *Feeds include emergencies and disasters news, disease outbreaks, avian influenza*	www.who.int/about/licensing/rss/en
Pan American Health Organization	http://new.paho.org/hq/index.php?option=com_rss&feed=RSS2.0&no_html=1
US Government Flu Portal	www.flu.gov/rss/pandemicflu/news.xml
CDC MMWR Weekly, Recommendations and Reports, and Surveillance Summaries	www.cdc.gov/mmwr/rss/mmwr.xml
Zoonotic disease surveillance: World Organization for Animal Health	www.oie.int/en/animal-health-in-the-world/the-world-animal-health-information-system/info-list-rss/
ProMED-mail: program for monitoring emerging diseases	ww2.isid.org/rss/getrss.php
Global Health Reporting (Kaiser Family Foundation)	http://globalhealth.kff.org/Feeds.aspx
Eurosurveillance	www.eurosurveillance.org/Public/RSSFeed/RSSFeed.aspx
US Central Intelligence Agency: The World Factbook	http://www.cia.gov/news-information/your-news/index.html
ReliefWeb: administered by the United Nations Office for the Coordination of Humanitarian Affairs	www.reliefweb.int/rw/hlp.nsf/db900bykey/subscribe?OpenDocument&clickid=homepage
Divers Alert Network	www.diversalertnetwork.org/rss/index.asp
International Association for Medical Assistance to Travelers	www.iamat.org/blog/rss.cfm

Abbreviations: MMWR, Morbidity and Mortality Weekly Report.

BIBLIOGRAPHY

1. Freedman DO. Sources of travel medicine information. In: Keystone JS, Kozarsky PE, Freedman DO, Nothdurft HD, Connor BA, editors. Travel Medicine. 2nd ed. Philadelphia: Mosby; 2008. p. 29–34.

2. Keystone JS, Kozarsky PE, Freedman DO. Internet and computer-based resources for travel medicine practitioners. Clin Infect Dis. 2001 Mar 1;32(5):757–65.

APPENDIX C: TRAVEL VACCINE SUMMARY TABLE

David R. Shlim

Table C-1 is a quick reference for administering or prescribing travel-related vaccines. Before administering any vaccine, please review detailed instructions, precautions, and side effects under the specific vaccines discussed in this book or in the manufacturer's package insert. For other immunizations, refer to the corresponding disease section in Chapter 3.

Table C-1. Travel vaccine summary

VACCINE	BRAND NAME	DOSE	ROUTE	SCHEDULE	BOOSTER	AGE
Hepatitis A (adults)	Havrix	1.0 mL (1,440 ELISA units)	IM	0 and 6–12 months	None	≥19 years
	Vaqta	1.0 mL (50 units)	IM	0 and 6–18 months	None	≥19 years
Hepatitis A (pediatric)	Havrix	0.5 mL (720 ELISA units)	IM	0 and 6–12 months	None	1–18 years
	Vaqta	0.5 mL (25 units)	IM	0 and 6–18 months	None	1–18 years
Combined hepatitis A and hepatitis B	Twinrix	1.0 mL (20 µg of hepatitis B antigen and 720 ELISA units of hepatitis A antigen)	IM	0, 1 month, and 6 months; accelerated schedule: days 0, 7, and 21, with a fourth dose at 12 months	None	≥18 years
Japanese encephalitis	Ixiaro	0.5 mL	IM	0 and 28 days	To be determined	≥17 years
	JE-Vax[1]	0.5 mL for ages 1–2 years; 1.0 mL for ages ≥3 years	SQ	Days 0, 7, and 30	3 years[2]	≥1 year; limited by supply to children aged 1–16 years
Meningococcal conjugate (MenACWY)	Menactra (MenACWY_D)	0.5 mL	IM	1 dose	See Chapter 3, Meningococcal Disease	2–55 years
	Menveo (MenACWY_CRM)	0.5 mL	IM	1 dose	Not determined	11–55 years
Meningococcal polysaccharide (MPSV4)	Menomune	0.5 mL	SQ	1 dose	See Chapter 3, Meningococcal Disease	≥2 years

continued

TABLE C-1. TRAVEL VACCINE SUMMARY (continued)

VACCINE	BRAND NAME	DOSE	ROUTE	SCHEDULE	BOOSTER	AGE
Inactivated polio (adult)	Ipol	0.5 mL	SQ or IM	One dose at >18 years, if patient has already had an acceptable polio vaccine series	None	>18 years[3]
Rabies	Imovax	1.0 mL	IM	Preexposure series: days 0, 7, and 21 or 28	See Chapter 3, Rabies	No age restrictions
	RabAvert	1.0 mL	IM	Preexposure series: days 0, 7, and 21 or 28	See Chapter 3, Rabies	No age restrictions
Typhoid capsular polysaccharide	Typhim Vi	0.5 mL	IM	1 dose	Every 2 years	>2 years
Typhoid oral, live, attenuated	Vivotif	1 pill	Oral	1 pill every other day for 4 doses	Every 5 years	>6 years
Yellow fever	YF-Vax	0.5 mL	SQ	1 dose	Every 10 years	>9 months, same dose for children and adults[4]

Abbreviations: ELISA, enzyme-linked immunosorbent assay; IM, intramuscular; SQ, subcutaneous.

[1] This vaccine is no longer manufactured, and supplies are limited to stockpiled vaccine. Ixiaro may be approved for use in children when studies are completed. JE-Vax will remain the vaccine of choice for children <17 years until supplies are exhausted or Ixiaro is approved for children.

[2] Booster recommendations beyond the first booster have not been established. A booster dose may be given 2 years after the primary series; however, most authorities recommend every 3 years if the traveler remains at risk.

[3] For catch-up immunization in pediatric population, see Table 7-4.

[4] Special considerations apply in deciding whether to administer yellow fever vaccine. Please review Chapter 3, Yellow Fever before administration. Yellow fever vaccine is never given to infants <6 months and is given only under special circumstances for ages 6–8 months.

APPENDIX D: THE HEALTHMAP SYSTEM

Amy L. Sonricker, Clark C. Freifeld, John S. Brownstein

SYSTEM OVERVIEW

In the past 15 years, internet technology has become an integral part of public health surveillance. Information about infectious disease outbreaks is disseminated not only through online communications by government agencies but also through informal channels, ranging from press reports to blogs to chat rooms. Collectively, these sources provide a view of global health that is fundamentally different from that yielded by traditional public health infrastructure. Web-based sources provide valuable epidemic intelligence by disseminating current, highly localized information about outbreaks, especially in areas that have limited public health capacity.

HealthMap (www.healthmap.org) was developed with the aim of creating an integrated global view of emerging infectious diseases, based not solely on traditional public health datasets but rather on a broad range of available information sources, including these informal Internet channels. HealthMap is a publicly available online resource that collects, filters, and visualizes disease outbreak reports in real time, by means of a series of automated text-processing algorithms. Sources include online news through aggregators such as Google News, expert-curated discussion such as ProMED-mail, and validated official reports from organizations such as the World Health Organization (WHO). Disease outbreak reports are collected in 7 languages (English, French, Russian, Spanish, Arabic, Chinese, and Portuguese), classified by disease and location, and then mapped to a user-friendly, interactive display (see Figure D-1).

The system also allows disease experts and public health professionals to submit events not collected by the automated system, through both the web interface and by mobile applications (www.healthmap.org/outbreaksnearme). The "Outbreaks Near Me" mobile application uses GPS technology to show health alerts and ongoing outbreak news in the vicinity of the user. The application also allows users to search for outbreaks in specific locations worldwide.

Currently, HealthMap serves as a direct information source for over a million visitors a year and serves as a resource for libraries, physicians, international travelers, local health departments, governments, and multinational agencies (such as WHO), which use the HealthMap data stream for day-to-day surveillance activities. CDC has a relationship with HealthMap that includes a specific layer of the map used to geolocate travel-related illness detected by the GeoSentinel global surveillance system. HealthMap extracts data and provides a user interface that is particularly focused on providing users with news of immediate interest, while reducing information overload.

HEALTHMAP DATA VISUALIZATION AND DISSEMINATION

The freely available HealthMap site presents users with a customizable map view of worldwide infectious disease alerts. An advanced search area allows users to control the map view, including the ability to filter by source, date, disease, and region. "Full screen" mode expands the map to cover the full browser window, allowing richer visual display and navigation.

Automated e-mail alerts of infectious disease reports are also available from HealthMap. As with the website, users may customize these e-mails to receive only information corresponding to specific parameters.

Automated surveillance of Internet information sources provides a method for creating a timely, sensitive, and comprehensive view of worldwide emerging infectious diseases. Mining the web is a valuable new approach that can play a useful role in the efforts of public health practitioners and clinicians. Ultimately, HealthMap's integration of real-time, web-based infectious disease surveillance works to augment epidemic intelligence with information from outside the traditional public health infrastructure to enhance situational awareness of disease threats.

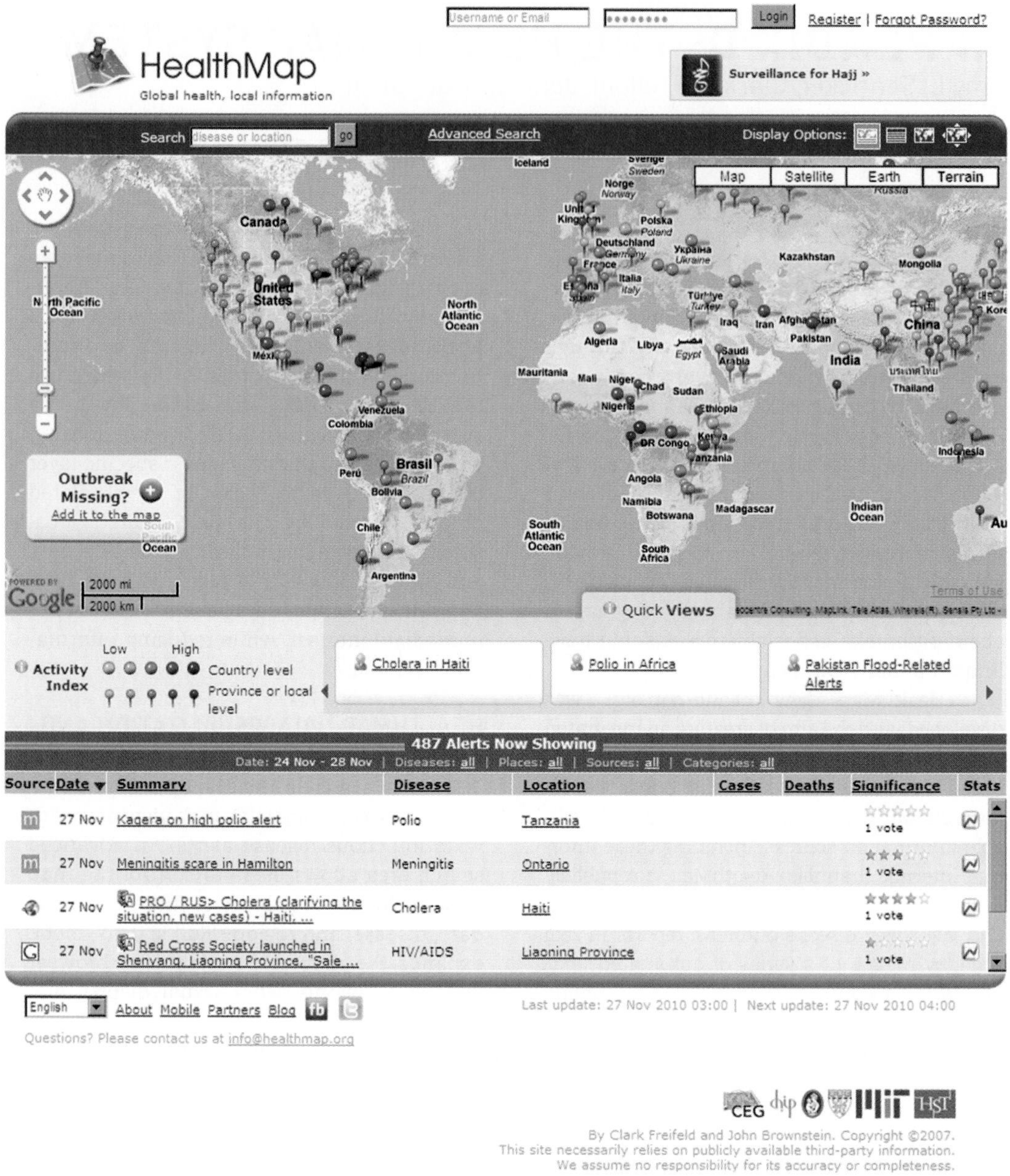

HealthMap
Global health, local information

Username or Email | •••••••• | Login Register | Forgot Password?

Surveillance for Hajj »

Search [disease or location] [go]   Advanced Search   Display Options:

| Map | Satellite | Earth | Terrain |

Outbreak Missing?
Add it to the map

POWERED BY Google   2000 mi / 2000 km

Terms of Use

Quick Views

Activity Index   Low   High   Country level   Province or local level

Cholera in Haiti | Polio in Africa | Pakistan Flood-Related Alerts

487 Alerts Now Showing
Date: 24 Nov - 28 Nov | Diseases: all | Places: all | Sources: all | Categories: all

Source	Date ▼	Summary	Disease	Location	Cases	Deaths	Significance	Stats
m	27 Nov	Kagera on high polio alert	Polio	Tanzania			☆☆☆☆☆ 1 vote	
m	27 Nov	Meningitis scare in Hamilton	Meningitis	Ontario			★★★☆☆ 1 vote	
🌐	27 Nov	PRO / RUS> Cholera (clarifying the situation, new cases) - Haiti, ...	Cholera	Haiti			★★★★☆ 1 vote	
G	27 Nov	Red Cross Society launched in Shenyang, Liaoning Province, "Sale ...	HIV/AIDS	Liaoning Province			★☆☆☆☆ 1 vote	

[English ▼] About Mobile Partners Blog fb

Last update: 27 Nov 2010 03:00 | Next update: 27 Nov 2010 04:00

Questions? Please contact us at info@healthmap.org

CEG dip MIT HST

By Clark Freifeld and John Brownstein. Copyright ©2007.
This site necessarily relies on publicly available third-party information.
We assume no responsibility for its accuracy or completeness.

FIGURE D-1. SCREENSHOT OF HEALTHMAP

BIBLIOGRAPHY

1. Brownstein JS, Freifeld CC, Madoff LC. Digital disease detection—harnessing the web for public health surveillance. N Engl J Med. 2009 May 21;360(21):2153–5, 7.

2. Brownstein JS, Freifeld CC, Reis BY, Mandl KD. Surveillance sans frontieres: internet-based emerging infectious disease intelligence and the HealthMap project. PLoS Med. 2008 Jul 8;5(7):e151.

3. Freifeld CC, Mandl KD, Reis BY, Brownstein JS. HealthMap: global infectious disease monitoring through automated classification and visualization of Internet media reports. J Am Med Inform Assoc. 2008 Mar–Apr;15(2):150–7.

Index

Note: Page numbers followed by the letter b refer to boxes; those followed by the letter f refer to figures; those followed by the letter m refer to maps; and those followed by the letter t refer to tables.

Photography Credits

FRONT COVER IMAGES
Camels: Abraham Nowitz/National Geographic Stock
Zebras: David J. Maddy/Personal Collection
Tree: David J. Maddy/Personal Collection
Great Wall: Shutterstock

BACK COVER IMAGES
China temple: stock
Night scene: Kelly Holton/Personal Collection
Market: David Snyder/CDC Foundation
Beach: David Snyder/CDC Foundation

BANNER IMAGES FOR SELECT DESTINATIONS
from left to right

The Caribbean (p. 399): Frhojdysz/Dreamstime, David Grayer/Personal Collection, Dream69/Dreamstime

China (p. 404): Gary W. Brunette/Personal Collection, Ronnie Henry/Personal Collection, Jarnogz/Dreamstime

Cuzco–Machu Picchu, Peru (p. 408): David Snyder/David Snyder Photography, Dan Breckwoldt/Dreamstime, David Snyder/David Snyder Photography

Egypt and Nile River Cruises (p. 412): Andrew Kaplan/Personal Collection, Andre Klaassen/Dreamstime, Francisco Caravana/Dreamstime

Guatemala and Belize (p. 415): all photos, Stephen N. Molnar/Personal Collection

Hajj Pilgrimage, Saudi Arabia (p. 419): Aidar Ayazbayev/Dreamstime, Ziad A Memish/Personal Collection, Zambezishark/Dreamstime

Iguassu Falls, Brazil/Argentina (p. 422): David Davis/Dreamstime, Rodrigo Arena/Dreamstime, Casadphoto/Dreamstime

India (p. 425): David Snyder/CDC Foundation, Peter Hazlett/Dreamstime, David Snyder/CDC Foundation

Kilimanjaro, Tanzania (p. 430): David J. Maddy/Personal Collection, David J. Maddy/Personal Collection, Kevin C. Kain/Personal Collection

Mexico (p. 433): David J. Maddy/Personal Collection, Enrique Gomez/Dreamstime, Dongfan Wang/Dreamstime

Nepal (p. 436): David R. Shlim/Personal Collection, David R. Shlim/Personal Collection, Dénes Egervari/Personal Collection

Safaris in East and Southern Africa (p. 440): David J. Maddy/Personal Collection, Troy R. Inman/Personal Collection, David J. Maddy/Personal Collection

South Africa (p. 443): Richard Mackinnon-Little/Personal Collection, Richard Mackinnon-Little/Personal Collection, Owen B. Lever/Dreamstime